Rehabilitation for Nerve Transfers of the Upper Extremity

Lorna C. Kahn • Macyn M. Stonner
Christopher J. Dy
Editors

Rehabilitation for Nerve Transfers of the Upper Extremity

A Clinical Manual

Springer

Editors
Lorna C. Kahn
Milliken Hand Rehabilitation Center
WashU Medicine
St. Louis, MO, USA

Macyn M. Stonner
Milliken Hand Rehabilitation Center
WashU Medicine
St. Louis, MO, USA

Christopher J. Dy
Department of Orthopedic Surgery, Division of Hand and Microsurgery
WashU Medicine
St. Louis, MO, USA

ISBN 978-3-031-92007-3 ISBN 978-3-031-92008-0 (eBook)
https://doi.org/10.1007/978-3-031-92008-0

This Springer imprint is published by the registered company Springer Nature Switzerland AG
The registered company address is: Gewerbestrasse 11, 6330 Cham, Switzerland

For almost 20 years, I have enjoyed the privilege of working with the brilliant nerve surgeon, Dr. Susan Mackinnon. Without her mentorship, empowerment, and appreciation of hand therapy, this book would not have been possible. I gratefully dedicate this book to her.

Lorna C. Kahn

For Ellen King—a beloved therapist, mentor, and friend. She was the most compassionate clinician I have ever known, and she is missed on this earth every day. I dedicate this book to her with love.

Macyn M. Stonner

Contents

Contributors

Mike Cricchio University of Florida Hand and Upper Extremity, Gainesville, FL, USA

Jennifer Dodson OrthoCarolina, Charlotte, NC, USA

Christopher J. Dy Department of Orthopedic Surgery, Division of Hand and Microsurgery, WashU Medicine, St. Louis, MO, USA

Jennifer Erickson Harborview Medical Center, Seattle, WA, USA

Jennifer Q. Farrar Vanderbilt Health Belle Meade Clinic, Vanderbilt University Medical Center, Nashville, TN, USA

Lourdes Filippi Johns Hopkins Hospital, Baltimore, MD, USA

Jamie Findeiss Athletico Physical Therapy, St. Louis, MO, USA

Lorna C. Kahn Milliken Hand Rehabilitation Center, WashU Medicine, St. Louis, MO, USA

Alexandra MacKenzie Hand and Upper Extremity Therapy Center, Hospital for Special Surgery, New York, NY, USA

Zachary D. Randall Department of Orthopedic Surgery, WashU Medicine, St. Louis, MO, USA

Eshan Sane Department of Orthopedic Surgery, WashU Medicine, St. Louis, MO, USA

Macyn M. Stonner Milliken Hand Rehabilitation Center, WashU Medicine, St. Louis, MO, USA

Elizabeth Westland Athletico Physical Therapy/ Hand Therapy, Saint Louis, MO, USA

Amy M. Young Northwestern Medicine Center for Surgery of the Hand, Chicago, IL, USA

Principles of Rehabilitation after Nerve Transfers

Introduction to Nerve Transfers

Zachary D. Randall, Eshan Sane, and Christopher J. Dy

A nerve transfer is a surgical technique that reroutes a nerve from one muscle or muscle group to another to restore important lost function [1]. In this procedure, healthy nerves are redirected to a damaged nerve to reinnervate a targeted muscle or sensory area. This approach relies on the principle that the donor nerve's original function is either redundantly innervated or less essential to daily function than the injured nerve's function being reconstructed. Nerve transfers are often indicated when crucial functional muscles, such as the elbow flexors in the upper extremity after a brachial plexus injury, are not expected to spontaneously recover. Performing a nerve transfer involves selecting a redundant or expendable donor nerve, transecting it, redirecting it to the damaged nerve's terminal branches, and performing a microsurgical nerve coaptation [2]. While there may be some decrease in donor muscle strength, the recipient muscle gradually reinnervates, regaining some of its previous function. Following the nerve transfer, reinnervation of the target muscle typically begins 3–9 months post-surgery, with gradual improvements in function as reinnervation of the muscle units increases [3]. Full recovery can take up to 2–3 years, depending on the distance the nerve fibers need to grow, the patient's regeneration potential, and the condition of the donor nerves. Rehabilitation plays a crucial role in optimizing the outcomes, as targeted exercises help with cortical plasticity, retraining the muscle, and maximizing functional recovery [4]. Although nerve transfers may not completely restore pre-injury strength, they often enable significant improvements in mobility and quality of life for patients who would otherwise face long-term deficits.

Z. D. Randall · E. Sane
Department of Orthopedic Surgery, WashU Medicine, St. Louis, MO, USA

C. J. Dy (✉)
Department of Orthopedic Surgery, Division of Hand and Microsurgery, WashU Medicine, St. Louis, MO, USA
e-mail: dyc@wustl.edu

History of Nerve Transfers

The history of nerve transfer is rich with innovations and milestones that have significantly improved outcomes for patients with severe nerve injuries. This section delves into the key historical developments in nerve transfers and highlights the contributions of pioneering surgeons and the evolution of techniques that laid the groundwork for modern nerve reconstruction.

Early Pioneers and Initial Discoveries

The first reported nerve transfer was performed by Ballance in 1903, who described the transfer of the spinal accessory nerve to the facial nerve to restore facial movement [5]. This initial groundbreaking work demonstrated the potential of nerve transfers to restore function in denervated muscles. In 1913, Tuttle became the first to apply nerve transfer techniques to repair brachial plexus injuries [6]. He utilized the healthy fourth cervical nerve transferred end-to-end just distal to a damaged upper trunk and reported encouraging results.

The 1920s through mid-twentieth century saw further advancements in nerve transfer applications with Vulpius and Stoffel, in 1920, describing the use of the medial pectoral nerve as a donor nerve for transfers to the musculocutaneous nerve [7], and Harris, in 1921, who reported the first transfer of the radial nerve to the median nerve [8]. In 1948, Lurje reported an approach to transfers of the pectoral and thoracodorsal nerves to the musculocutaneous nerve [9].

Advances in the Late Twentieth Century

The late twentieth century saw a surge in the development and refinement of nerve transfer techniques. These paralleled advancements in surgical technologies such as the incorporation of intraoperative microscopes allowed for ster-

L. C. Kahn et al. (eds.), *Rehabilitation for Nerve Transfers of the Upper Extremity*,
https://doi.org/10.1007/978-3-031-92008-0_1

ile magnification and visualization of tissues. This, along with specifically designed fine forceps, clamps, scissors, sutures, and fixtures, enabled the growth of microsurgery as a field. With these new developments, in 1980, Samardzic et al. performed the first double-nerve transfer, using the pectoral nerve as a donor to the axillary and the thoracodorsal transferred to the musculocutaneous nerve [10]. This innovative approach demonstrated for the first time the potential of combining multiple nerve transfers to achieve better functional outcomes. Bedeschi et al., in 1984, introduced sensory nerve transfers in hand surgery, further expanding the scope of nerve transfer surgery beyond the previously reported motor function applications [11].

In 2002, Mackinnon reported on the pronator quadratus to ulnar nerve motor fascicle transfer for proximal ulnar nerve lesions [12]. This technique provided a new option for patients with severe ulnar nerve injuries. In 1993, Brandt and Mackinnon reported their experience with the pectoral to musculocutaneous transfer, further refining the application of pectoral nerve transfers in brachial plexus injuries [13]. Their work demonstrated the importance of detailed anatomical knowledge and precise surgical technique in achieving successful outcomes.

The twentieth century also saw increasing implementation of electrodiagnostics as a technique to test nerve characteristics and provide valuable insight into preoperative planning for nerve transfers. Electrodiagnostics (EDX) consists of two main tests: nerve conduction studies (NCSs) and electromyography (EMG). Nerve conduction studies use surface electrodes to stimulate underlying nerves and measure electrical response rate and speed of conduction. EMG uses intramuscular needles to record electrical impulses corresponding to muscular contraction after stimulation. After three or more months following acute nerve injury, EMGs show fibrillations and positive sharp waves (PSWs) that allow for identification of deinnervated muscles, while the presence of motor unit action potentials (MUAPs) identifies if a muscle is beginning to spontaneously recover or would benefit from nerve surgery to enable salvage of the muscle before terminal muscle atrophy occurs at around 18 months post-injury. In acute nerve transections, the distal portion of the nerve is separated from its cell body, and Wallerian degeneration will occur within days [14]. The neuromuscular junctions will degrade before the axons, thereby affecting nerve transmission. For this reason, EDX can identify complete nerve transection much earlier. In chronic nerve injury such as chronic cubital tunnel syndrome, there can be damage to the axons of the nerve, and EMGs highlight the presence of fibrillations, PSWs, and chronic reinnervation changes in the MUAPs. Despite the chronicity of such conditions, these patients may also benefit from nerve transfer [15]. Donor nerves can also be identified and confirmed with electrodiagnostic testing. NCS will ensure that the motor nerves are healthy and have no latency in nerve conduction, and EMG will confirm that they are innervated or, as with some salvage procedures, that they are reinnervating. In cases where donor nerves are limited, a less-than-ideal but potentially reinnervating motor nerve may be used for a transfer.

The Oberlin Transfer

One of the most significant advancements in the early 1990s was the introduction of the transfer described by Oberlin et al. in 1994 [16]. This technique involves the transfer of fascicles of the ulnar nerve to the biceps muscle nerve to restore elbow flexion. The Oberlin transfer quickly became a cornerstone of nerve transfer surgery due to its high success rate, reproducibility, and relatively straightforward application.

Twenty-First-Century Progress

The period leading up to the early twenty-first century saw a rapid increase in the adoption and refinement of nerve transfer techniques. Surgeons around the world reported various nerve transfers, each contributing to the growing body of knowledge and experience in this field. These advancements allowed for greater flexibility in surgical planning, as surgeons could tailor their approach to the specific needs of each patient. From the early work of Ballance and Tuttle to the modern techniques developed by Mackinnon and Oberlin, each advancement had built upon the previous ones, creating a robust foundation for contemporary nerve reconstruction surgery.

With the turn of the century came new nerve transfer procedures that enhanced specific movement abilities while maintaining the integrity of motion at donor sites. Among these included the popularized procedure by Leechavengvongs et al. in 2003 [17], to restore deltoid function following brachial plexus injury. This procedure achieved shoulder abduction restoration with a posterior approach of transferring triceps nerve fascicles from the radial nerve to the anterior axillary nerve. Importantly, there was no significant weakness in triceps extension after this surgery. This procedure is commonly combined with the single fascicular Oberlin transfer or the double-fascicular transfer (DFT) described by Mackinnon, and the spinal accessory to suprascapular nerve transfer, forming the "triple transfer" commonly used for upper trunk brachial plexus injuries.

The following decade marked significant contributions to using nerve transfers in treating injuries and nerve impairments, which were previously addressed by nerve grafts. These included the median to radial nerve transfers developed by Mackinnon from 2007 to 2010, which created "a more reliable intervention alternative than grafting when addressing proximal nerve injuries, injuries involving a long segment of the nerve, or complicated injuries involving an indiscrete or multilevel insult" [18]. Mackinnon replicated her success of the median to radial nerve transfer, with a median-to-ulnar nerve transfer for patients with proximal ulnar nerve injuries [19].

Bertelli introduced nerve transfers distal to the wrist to improve intrinsic thumb and finger motion. These include the abductor digiti minimi (ADM) to thenar motor nerve transfer in high median nerve injuries. With this nerve transfer, individuals may recover multidirectional thumb use, a novel option and a vast functional improvement from the unidirectional opponensplasty tendon transfer. This and the opponens pollicis-to-terminal ulnar motor nerve transfer (to improve lateral pinch) have minimal to no donor loss, and due to the proximity of donor and recipient muscles, the time to reinnervation is much faster than more proximal transfers. [20–22]

The advancement of these end-to-end nerve transfers also spurred investigation into end-to-side reversible or "supercharged" nerve transfers, which entail "diverting the end of an expendable, functioning donor nerve into the side of an injured recipient nerve that remains in continuity" [23]. These are utilized in the case of incomplete and mixed nerve injuries, where "axonal regeneration does occur but only partial motor recovery is expected" [23]. In 2015, Mackinnon et al. clarified the indications for these supercharged end-to-side nerve transfers in the context of anterior interosseous-to-ulnar motor nerve transfers [23]. Yet, the uncertainty described in quantifying the proportion of recovery attributable to this nerve transfer versus the normal healing process presents a challenge to be addressed by the field going forward.

Modern Applications of Nerve Transfers (2016–2024)

The development of the above-described techniques and a maturation of the field as a whole have led to an increase in the frequency of nerve transfers relative to other types of nerve reconstruction. Specifically, the implementation of nerve transfers as a reliable surgical option in brachial plexus injury has preempted a rise in their use throughout peripheral nerve surgery and microsurgery [24]. Compared with tendon transfers, nerve transfers preserve native muscle biomechanics and can decrease the time to muscle and sensory reinnervation. When a nerve is injured to an extent that primary nerve repair is not an option, nerve transfers provide a suitable option. For these reasons, they offer an appealing alternative or addition to existing reconstructive options [24].

Adoption of nerve transfers has extended from nerve transfers in the upper extremity, where they were first explored, now to the lower extremity as well. Indications for nerve transfers in the lower extremity are still evolving, but transfers have been utilized for non-recovering peroneal, obturator, femoral, or tibial nerve palsies as well as plantar neuropathies [25]. Moreover, the preliminary results show that nerve transfers may be more reliable than nerve repair utilizing graft reconstruction in lower extremity cases. This is likely related to a single coaptation site having less axonal loss across coaptation sites; however, more research is required to clarify [26].

Emerging Trends and Future Directions in Nerve Transfer (2025–)

Going forward, several new trends have emerged regarding functional and injury-specific advances in both nerve transfer surgical techniques and postoperative rehabilitation. The new frontier, beyond improving operative techniques in isolation or examining new transfer options, is to help patients tailor their rehabilitation protocol to their individual injury mechanisms and surgical approach. Examples of these new protocols include protecting the length of the recovering muscle during early rehabilitation and promoting donor activation by "flooding" the donor nerves with high-volume, low-intensity exercises in the early phases of the postoperative period [27]. Furthermore, the donor-recipient muscle relationship is continuously being studied, with therapies now focusing on combining donor and recipient muscle exercises together given that coactivation of the donor increases the strength of the recipient for several years post-transfer [28].

Regarding surgical improvements, further standardization of nerve transfer procedures is required to quantify their benefit over nerve grafting [29]. Recovery of shoulder function is a vast area of future study and improvement, relative to recovery of elbow flexion in which nerve transfers are starting to become the standard protocol. Comparative studies will also be key in determining the effectiveness of nerve transfers when compared to other treatment options [29]. However, in order for effective comparative analysis, researchers will need to agree upon standardized outcome measurements and timelines. Still, nerve transfers have yielded promising results in all of these cases.

The field of nerve transfers and combined nerve surgeries is rapidly advancing, both independently and relative to other nerve reconstruction techniques. Surgeons now have access to new methods like supercharged end-to-side nerve transfers and alternative approaches for obtaining donor nerves, enabling them to tailor their techniques to individual patients. As this field expands, further exploration is necessary to understand the unique isolated benefits of each surgical approach while giving more consideration to rehabilitation protocols. Although there is still significant work to be done to achieve this goal, the ultimate aim is to clarify these techniques and effectively treat specific functional deficits through optimal operative and postoperative plans.

References

1. Moore AM, Novak CB. Advances in nerve transfer surgery. J Hand Therapy. 2014;27(2):96–105.
2. Mackinnon SE. Nerve surgery. Thieme; 2015.
3. Mackinnon SE, Colbert SH. Nerve transfers in the hand and upper extremity surgery. Tech Hand Up Extrem Surg. 2008;12(1):20–33.
4. Larocerie-Salgado J, Chinchalkar S, Ross DC, Gillis J, Doherty CD, Miller TA. Rehabilitation following nerve transfer surgery. Tech Hand Up Extrem Surg. 2022;26(2):71–7.
5. Ballance CA, Ballance HA, Stewart P. Remarks on the operative treatment of chronic facial palsy of peripheral origin. Br Med J. 1903;1(2209):1009–13. https://doi.org/10.1136/bmj.1.2209.1009.
6. Tuttle HK. Exposure of the brachial plexus with nerve-transplantation. J Am Med Assoc. 1913;61(1):15–7. https://doi.org/10.1001/jama.1913.04350010017006.
7. Vulpius O, Stoffel A. Orthopädische Operationslehre. Ferdinand Enke; 1920.
8. Harris RI. The treatment of irreparable nerve injuries. Can Med Assoc J. 1921;11(11):833–41.
9. Lurje AS, On the Use of N. Musculocutaneous for neurotization of N. radialis in cases of very large defects of the latter. Ann Surg. 1948;128(1):110–5.
10. Samardzic MM, Grujicic DM, Rasulic LG, Milicic BR. The use of thoracodorsal nerve transfer in restoration of irreparable C5 and C6 spinal nerve lesions. Br J Plast Surg. 2005;58(4):541–6. https://doi.org/10.1016/j.bjps.2003.12.027.
11. Bedeschi P, Celli L, Balli A. Transfer of sensory nerves in hand surgery. J Hand Surg Br. 1984;9(1):46–9. https://doi.org/10.1016/0266-7681(84)90013-5.
12. Novak CB, Mackinnon SE. Distal anterior interosseous nerve transfer to the deep motor branch of the ulnar nerve for reconstruction of high ulnar nerve injuries. J Reconstr Microsurg. 2002;18(6):459–64. https://doi.org/10.1055/s-2002-33326.
13. Brandt KE, Mackinnon SE. A technique for maximizing biceps recovery in brachial plexus reconstruction. J Hand Surg Am. 1993;18(4):726–33. https://doi.org/10.1016/0363-5023(93)90328-z.
14. Ferrante MA. The assessment and management of peripheral nerve trauma. Curr Treatment Opt Neurol. 2018;20:1–18.
15. Power HA, Sharma K, El-Haj M, Moore AM, Patterson MM, Mackinnon SE. Compound muscle action potential amplitude predicts the severity of cubital tunnel syndrome. JBJS. 2019;101(8):730–8.
16. Oberlin C, Béal D, Leechavengvongs S, Salon A, Dauge MC, Sarcy JJ. Nerve transfer to biceps muscle using a part of ulnar nerve for C5–C6 avulsion of the brachial plexus: anatomical study and report of four cases. J Hand Surg Am. 1994;19(2):232–7. https://doi.org/10.1016/0363-5023(94)90011-6.
17. Leechavengvongs S, Witoonchart K, Uerpairojkit C, Thuvasethakul P. Nerve transfer to deltoid muscle using the nerve to the long head of the triceps, part II: a report of 7 cases. J Hand Surg Am. 2003;28(4):633–8. https://doi.org/10.1016/s0363-5023(03)00199-0.
18. Brown JM, Tung TH, Mackinnon SE. Median to radial nerve transfer to restore wrist and finger extension: technical nuances. Neurosurgery. 2010;66(Suppl. 3):75–83.; discussion 83. https://doi.org/10.1227/01.NEU.0000354364.13224.C8.
19. Brown JM, Yee A, Mackinnon SE. Distal median to ulnar nerve transfers to restore ulnar motor and sensory function within the hand: technical nuances. Neurosurgery. 2009;65(5):966–77.; discussion 977–8. https://doi.org/10.1227/01.NEU.0000358951.64043.73.
20. Bertelli JA, Tuffaha S, Sporer M, et al. Distal nerve transfers for peripheral nerve injuries: indications and outcomes. J Hand Surg (European Volume). 2024;49(6):721–33.
21. Bertelli JA, Soldado F, Rodrígues-Baeza A, Ghizoni MF. Transferring the motor branch of the opponens pollicis to the terminal division of the deep branch of the ulnar nerve for pinch reconstruction. J Hand Surg. 2019;44(1):9–17.
22. Bertelli JA, Soldado F, Rodrígues-Baeza A, Ghizoni MF. Transfer of the motor branch of the abductor digiti quinti for thenar muscle reinnervation in high median nerve injuries. J Hand Surg. 2018;43(1):8–15.
23. Davidge KM, Yee A, Moore AM, Mackinnon SE. The supercharge end-to-side anterior interosseous-to-ulnar motor nerve transfer for restoring intrinsic function: clinical experience. Plast Reconstr Surg. 2015;136(3):344e–52e. https://doi.org/10.1097/PRS.0000000000001514.
24. Morris M, Brogan DM, Boyer MI, Dy CJ. Trends in nerve transfer procedures among board-eligible orthopedic hand surgeons. J Hand Surg Glob Online. 2021;3(1):24–9. https://doi.org/10.1016/j.jhsg.2020.10.003.
25. Duraku LS, Buijnsters ZA, Power DM, George S, Walbeehm ET, de Jong T. Motor and sensory nerve transfers in the lower extremity: systematic review of current reconstructive possibilities. J Plast Reconstr Aesthet Surg. 2023;84:323–33. https://doi.org/10.1016/j.bjps.2023.06.011.
26. Campbell AA, Eckhauser FE, Belzberg A, Campbell JN. Obturator nerve transfer as an option for femoral nerve repair: case report. Neurosurgery. 2010;66(Suppl. 6):375.; discussion 375. https://doi.org/10.1227/01.NEU.0000369649.31232.B0.
27. Kahn LC, Stonner MM, Dy CJ. Key considerations for nerve transfer rehabilitation after surgical reconstruction for brachial plexus and peripheral nerve injuries. J Hand Surg Am. 2024;49(2):160–8. https://doi.org/10.1016/j.jhsa.2023.09.016.
28. Brogan DM, Osei DA, Colorado BS, Sneag DB, Van Voorhis A, Dy CJ. Team approach: management of brachial plexus injuries. JBJS Rev. 2022;10(4):e21.00222. https://doi.org/10.2106/JBJS.RVW.21.00222.
29. Domeshek LF, Novak CB, Patterson JMM, et al. Nerve transfers—a paradigm shift in the reconstructive ladder. Plast Reconstr Surg Glob Open. 2019;7(6):e2290. https://doi.org/10.1097/GOX.0000000000002290.

Rehabilitation Following Nerve Transfers in the Brachial Plexus Population

Lorna C. Kahn

Introduction

Functional recovery is not guaranteed following nerve transfers, and it is the role of the rehabilitation team to guide the patient through the motor reeducation process to maximize recovery of limb function [1–3]. Historically, therapy has not been recognized as an important part of nerve transfer reconstruction. Even today, many physicians do not utilize physical or occupational therapy services to improve functional outcomes following nerve transfers. This may be due to the lack of recognition of therapists' role in postoperative management. It may also be due to a limited number of therapists who have familiarity with the surgery and know how to effectively manage a comprehensive postoperative program. Additionally, there is a paucity of literature to support rehabilitation following nerve transfers. In a 2015 literature review of nerve transfers to restore elbow flexion by Beers et al., 12 peer-reviewed articles were found. Of these, four did not mention therapy services provided, four mentioned general therapy with no specific approach geared to nerve transfers, and the remaining four mentioned a specific approach to rehabilitation following nerve transfer. Of this limited sample, the four that mentioned a specific approach to rehabilitation reported superior outcomes [4]. Like anything new, it will take time for new information to disseminate to the therapy world and become a routine part of physical and occupational therapy education curricula.

Initially, nerve transfer rehabilitation was considered very similar to tendon transfer rehabilitation. They both involve a "donor" and "recipient," and at some point, co-contraction of the two is encouraged. Beyond this, the two are very different reconstruction strategies. Tendon transfer recovery is typically completed around 3 months following the surgery [5, 6]. At 3 months, some nerve transfers are beginning to show early signs of muscle reinnervation, while others will not start for another 3–4 months. This protracted length of time for functional recovery is a hallmark of nerve transfers. Once the coaptation of the two nerves is performed, the timeline for motor recovery begins. The estimated length of time to recovery is based on the approximate distance the axons must grow to reach the motor end plates of the recipient muscle(s). Patient age, diabetes, and quality of the donor nerve(s) also impact the recovery of the regenerating nerve [7]. Once it reaches the likely atrophied and often long denervated muscle(s), it will need time to reinnervate enough muscle fibers before visual or palpable confirmation of recovery is noted with the first twitch of movement.

Given that the therapist will likely have longer and more frequent sessions with the patient compared to the surgeon, it is the responsibility of the therapist to have a clear understanding of the surgery so that accurate patient education is conveyed, and correct details are used to develop a comprehensive motor reeducation program. Obtaining a copy of the operative note is ideal if verbal communication with the physician is not available.

The Surgery

In a perfect scenario, the following information is available to guide the therapist.

1. **In what timeframe was this nerve transfer performed?**

   The timing of the nerve transfer relative to the onset of motor loss (trauma or other) will greatly affect one's expectations of recipient muscle outcomes. As noted in the pioneer clinical text *Nerve Surgery* by Dr. Susan

Supplementary Information The online version contains supplementary material available at https://doi.org/10.1007/978-3-031-92008-0_2.

L. C. Kahn (✉)
Milliken Hand Rehabilitation Center, WashU Medicine, St. Louis, MO, USA
e-mail: Kahn.lorna.c@wustl.edu

L. C. Kahn et al. (eds.), *Rehabilitation for Nerve Transfers of the Upper Extremity*,
https://doi.org/10.1007/978-3-031-92008-0_2

Mackinnon, "recovery of motor function depends on a critical number of motor axons reaching the target muscle and reinnervating muscle fibers within a critical time period" [8]. In other words, *time is muscle*.

The longer the muscle remains denervated, the more degradation and atrophy will occur. After about 12 months from the onset of denervation, there is a greater likelihood that fatty infiltrate will set in and the muscle will not reinnervate [9]. Thus, distance (from the nerve transfer coaptation to the recipient muscle motor end plates) and time are the key influencing factors to nerve transfer outcomes. The sooner the nerve transfer is performed, the greater the likelihood of motor recovery. A nerve transfer performed more than 10 months post-injury will have a lower expectation for functional motor recovery than one performed before 6 months [10].

2. **What specific branches of the donor nerve were used**?

   For example, were median nerve fascicles to flexor carpi radialis (FCR) used or was this not delineated and a mix of median motor nerve fascicles were used as donors? Identifying the exact donor branches will make the donor activation exercises more specific and accurate. In some cases, all fascicles of a motor nerve are taken. Knowing this will prepare one to explain the potential loss of power or altered kinematics of the joint following the transfer if there was no redundant muscle for the donor. This is generally rare and more often occurs in severe plexopathies where donor options are greatly limited.

3. **Were the donors normal?**

   There are often situations such as a complex brachial plexopathy, in which the only available donor is damaged but appears to be recovering, and the nerve transfer may be qualified as a salvage procedure. It is performed with the hope that damaged donor nerve will recover into the recipient muscle to provide movement and function that is deemed more important than the donor muscle. For example, following an incomplete plexus injury where there is no arm function except some median motor fibers, these may be transferred into the musculocutaneous nerve in an effort to restore elbow flexion and the ability to bring the hand to the face. Expectations of recipient (biceps) strength outcomes would be guarded in this situation. In the opposite scenario, outcome expectations would be much higher for a young patient with a healthy, neurologically intact, and well-developed donor muscle. Knowledge of the donor viability will help guide the rehabilitation program and the functional expectations for the patient.

   Occasionally, an operative report will mention a good "size match" between donor and recipient nerves. This refers to the approximate number of axons present. An ideal nerve transfer involves similar axonal counts in both the donor and recipient motor nerves. Conversely, when the donor is weak and/or has a limited number of axons (making a less ideal axon match), expectations for functional outcome will be diminished. Schreiber et al. describe inferior outcomes in elbow flexor strength following nerve transfers where the donor-to-recipient fiber count ratio was $<0.7:1$ [11].

4. **Was this an end-to-end or end-to-side transfer?**

   An end-to-end (ETE) nerve transfer means the donor and recipient fascicles are transected and sewn together. A reverse or supercharge end-to-side (R/SETS) procedure involves the creation of an epineural window in the recipient nerve, transection, and transfer of the donor nerve to this "window" in the recipient nerve [12] (Image 1). Mackinnon et al. demonstrated the success of this model in a rodent study finding equivalence relative to the total number of regenerating donor axons when compared to the ETE model [8]. The importance of this knowledge to the rehabilitation team relates to timelines and expectations. The fact that the recipient nerve remains intact leaves the potential for the native nerve to recover into the recipient muscle. For example, following a SETS of the pronator quadratus (PQ) branch of the anterior interosseous nerve (AIN) to the ulnar motor nerve in the distal forearm, a minimum of 6 months would be expected for early motor recovery [13]. If motor recovery is seen significantly earlier, it is more likely that the recovery is related either to the concomitant decompression of the recipient ulnar nerve at the wrist or to native ulnar nerve recovery.

5. **Was a nerve graft included in the surgery?**

   If there is not enough nerve length of the donor and recipient nerves to create a tension-free coaptation, a nerve graft is used to fill this gap. Having knowledge of the graft and its length will help more accurately gauge the length of the transfer. Remember that nerve length or distance correlates with time to recovery. If a 6 cm graft is used, that would potentially add 3 months to the estimated recovery time. This may explain why the use of nerve grafts with nerve transfers has been associated with poorer outcomes [14].

6. **Does the patient have cervical spine issues that led to motor loss?**

   An individual with significant degenerative joint disease involving the cervical spine who undergoes an upper-extremity nerve transfer has a risk of donor degradation (if the donor involves an upper-extremity peripheral nerve) over time. Outcome expectations should be more guarded in these situations.

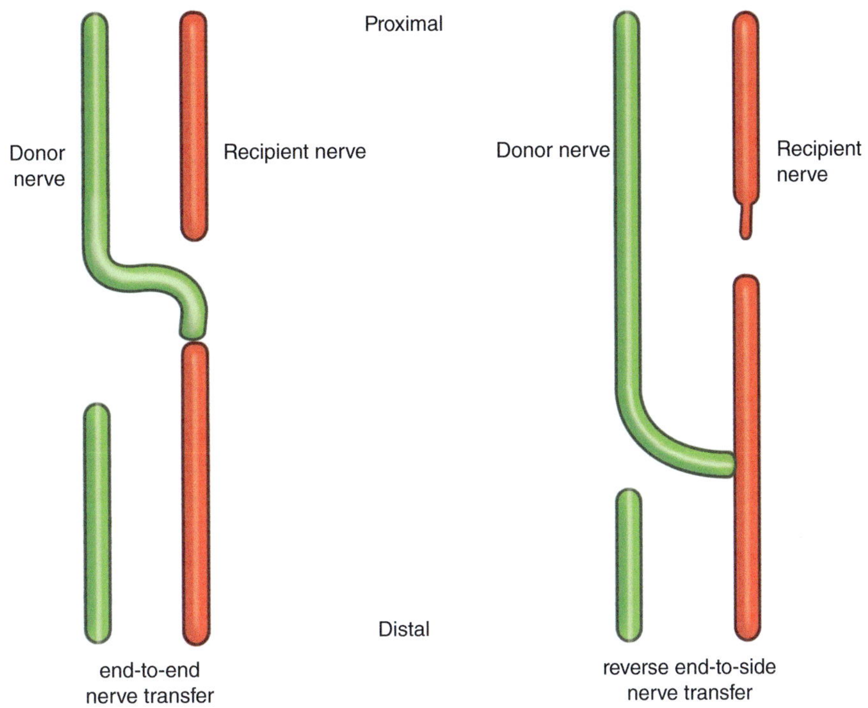

Image 1 The end to end (ETE) nerve transfer involves neurotomy of the donor and recipient nerves and coaptation of the proximal donor to the distal recipient nerve. The reverse end to side (RETS) nerve transfer involves neurotomy of the donor nerve and coaptation of the proximal end to the side of the recipient nerve

The Patient

Nerve transfers are complex, and developing a thorough understanding of the procedure can be challenging for even the well-educated patient. To be successful with motor reeducation, it is important for the clinician to understand how patients learn. Some of the physical traumas that lead to nerve transfers often involve traumatic brain injury (TBI), potentially putting the individual at a tremendous disadvantage to learn complex concepts. Patients may have memory and attention deficits, including early dementia, which can limit one's ability to learn. An awareness of a patient's general cognitive function will help guide the therapist in creating a program that is tailored to his or her needs. Patients with limited cognition will benefit from more simplified verbal instructions, clearly written handouts, frequent therapy visits, and potentially more assistance from a family member [15].

Socioeconomic status should also be considered as this often leads to barriers to therapy including social and financial support. The literature states that high socioeconomic deprivation is associated with limited access to and participation in therapy, thus leading to poor outcomes [16]. Pain is another factor that the rehabilitation team should assess. Pain frequently coexists with a peripheral nerve injury and can be severe [17–19]. It has been shown to negatively affect functional outcomes as well as health-related quality of life [17]. A multimodal pain evaluation should be completed at the onset of care so that pain can be appreciated and better managed, allowing the patient to succeed with the motor reeducation program.

Timelines

Setting expectations is a difficult yet important part of the rehabilitation program. At the onset of care, the individual should understand that the intent of surgery is to restore some motor function, but this does not mean that it will restore pre-injury function. By setting realistic expectations, it will be easier to work with the individual and enable them to celebrate the small achievements made throughout the two (or more) year process. By informing patients of the timelines relating to nerve, muscle, and rehabilitation, their understanding and acceptance of the process may be enhanced, and more realistic expectations may be possible.

Axonal injuries (Seddon's axonotmesis; Sunderland 2 + 3) and repaired nerves (following neurotmesis/Sunderland 4 + 5) have been described as recovering at a rate of an inch (or 2.5 cm) per month [20]. Considering that many factors influence recovery, one can cautiously estimate the time to muscle response following coaptation of the donor to recipient nerve. For instance, following a nerve transfer from the AIN branch to the PQ to the deep motor ulnar nerve, one can estimate the number of months to response in the first dorsal interossei muscle by measuring the distance from the proximal third of the forearm incision to the distal palmar crease (DPC) and then across the DPC to the second ray (region of the first dorsal interosseous and adductor pollicis). This transfer has been described as correlating with an average of 7–9 months to see movement [13].

The muscle recovery timeline is best described in terms of manual muscle testing grades or Medical Research Council (MRC) grading. By showing the patient what "normal" or 5/5 MRC strength is on the uninvolved side, one can begin a conversation that illustrates each level from zero to five, with zero being the recipient muscle(s). Manual muscle testing (MMT) is an assessment generally used by therapists to quantify muscle strength from zero to five. MMT scoring includes pluses (+) and minuses (−), which allows for greater responsiveness to change [21].

Education through metaphors may augment patient understanding of complex concepts. Using the metaphor of a dimmer switch on a light may illustrate the gradual nature of motor and functional recovery over time. A graph of this relationship can easily be demonstrated by plotting MMT muscle grades on the *x*-axis (with spacing that represents time in months) and force development on the *y*-axis. In this way, one can visualize the gradual recovery of strength over time. This graph can be used to discuss estimated outcomes by 6, 12, and 24 months. For those who have had a salvage procedure or less than ideal nerve transfer, it may be beneficial to eliminate the 5/5 score to help solidify a realistic expectation and help patients recognize other factors that may affect their outcomes (see Appendix 1).

The timeline for rehabilitation is divided into three phases which guide the progression of care that corresponds with the recovery level [2]. Phase 1 begins with a pre-op evaluation (when possible) and lasts until the first twitch of muscle recovery motion is noted in the recipient muscle (1/5 MMT grade). Phase 2 starts when a twitch of muscle contraction produces early movement in gravity lessened planes (2-/5 MMT grade) and continues through recovery of full joint movement through available passive range against gravity (3/5 MMT grade). Phase 3 begins once there is full movement against gravity, and the recipient muscle can withstand slight pressure. Strengthening the recipient muscle with resistance is the hallmark of this phase. It is important to recognize that not all patients progress to phase 3.

Patient Education: Applying the Concepts of Cortical Plasticity

The discussion of recovery and expectations is a crucial component of rehabilitation. It is often difficult to translate this complex information to an average adult in a way that can be easily understood and retained. General models of motor learning should be considered when approaching this conversation and developing the treatment plan. These include the following:

1. A three-stage model that recognizes novice, advanced, and expert levels of familiarity and knowledge of the topic. Based on the individual's understanding of the current level of recovery, one would appropriately select and revise the training approach [22].
2. The Fitts and Posner model is based on the available level of attention (cognitive, associative, and autonomous). The better attention patients have, the better suited they are for cognitive learning where they understand the nature of the task. The associative level involves selecting the best strategy suited for the individual patient. The autonomous level is suited for those individuals with the poorest attention [23]. They may do best with a strategy that involves an automatic response or skill, for example, creating a new movement habit that incorporates both donor and recipient muscles (Image 2).
3. Practice and feedback should be structured to optimize learning. Learning does not occur in the absence of practice.
4. Feedback from the therapist should be distinguished as different from encouragement.

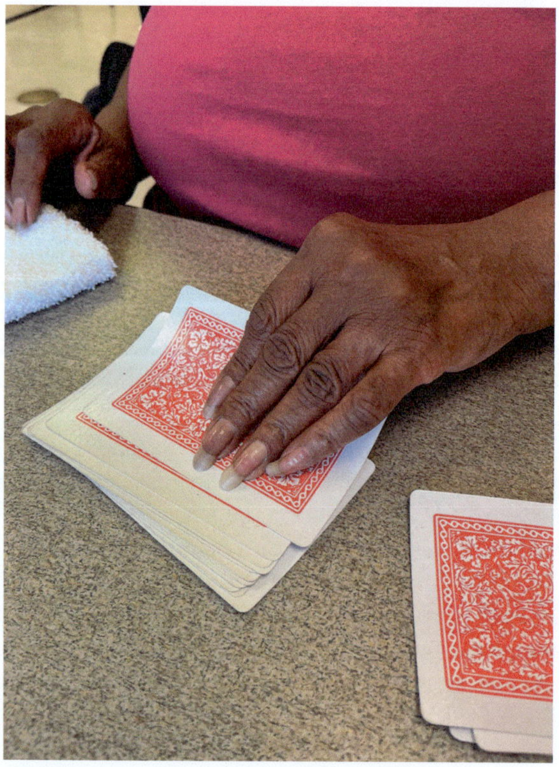

Image 2 An automatic response in the form of a skill involving both donor and recipient muscles is demonstrated here as the individual performs card counting (forearm pronation with intrinsic plus positioning) following an AIN/PQ to ulnar nerve transfer

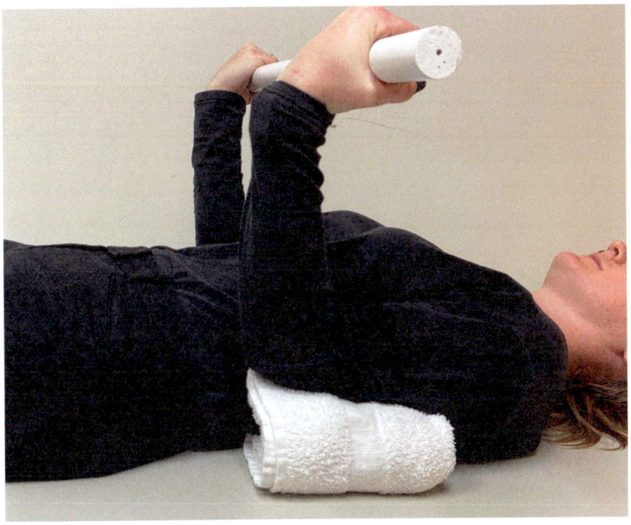

Image 3 A dowel is used to aid with bilateral exercises for elbow flexion following median and ulnar to musculocutaneous nerve transfers

5. Feedback strategies include intrinsic and extrinsic feedback. Intrinsic or internal feedback may be visual, somatosensory, or auditory. Extrinsic feedback includes verbal, visual, and auditory feedback. Extrinsic feedback is more effective when provided after a task and should be limited.
6. Bilateral activity engages higher-level cortical thinking than unilateral activities. For example, using a dowel when repetitively flexing the elbows while activating the finger and wrist flexors (as with the double fascicular transfer for musculocutaneous function) will aid with the cortical plasticity that is promoted to recover independent elbow flexion [24, 25] (Image 3).

The focus of patient education is typically on the loss of movement, but as we consider the appropriate learning model, one must first recognize the additional changes that occur on a cortical level. The motor cortex, situated in the frontal lobe of the brain, directs signals to the motor neurons via the spinal cord [26]. The homunculus has been long accepted as the metaphorical "little man" representation of the cortical map of motor function since the groundbreaking research of Wilder Penfield in the 1930s. This linear model with exaggerated representations of the hands, feet, and mouth mirrors the amount of "neural real estate" in the motor cortex [27]. Modern advances in functional magnetic resonance imaging (fMRI) have suggested an updated version of the homunculus that recognizes interconnectivity between the big three areas. These interconnected areas are responsible for various tasks, planning, and thoughts of movement, supporting the concept of mind-body connection [28].

Interconnectivity also supports the concepts of cortical plasticity. Anastakis and colleagues stress the importance of understanding and incorporating concepts of cortical plasticity training with motor reeducation. Their 2008 article eloquently states that "rehabilitation uses repeated practice or experience and patient engagement to drive adaptive plasticity in neural circuits to support recovery of normal function. Practice results in neural activity while motivation yields neuromodulatory release, and these components act synergistically to drive neural plasticity in active circuits. In many cases, rehabilitation engages these components and is sufficient to improve recovery." [29]

The following treatment strategies incorporate an understanding of these cortical changes which occur following peripheral nerve injury and nerve transfer reconstruction [29]:

1. Preoperative training and practice of the movements required to activate a future nerve transfer
2. Reinforcement of the importance of practice and repetition
3. Early activation of the motor movement with resistance and/or gravity removed
4. Focused practice and repetition with a therapist during early stages of motor learning
5. Strengthening and endurance exercises for up to and possibly beyond 2 years following motor reinnervation

Muscle Length and Recovery of Function

The relationship between the length of a muscle and the amount of force it can produce was first described by Magnus Blix in the 1800s. The Blix curve, also referred to as the length-tension curve, illustrates the relationship between the tension a muscle can develop and the length of the muscle [30, 31] (Image 4). We now know that this relates to the amount of overlap between the muscle components: myosin and actin. A "sweet spot" exists where the degree of overlapping actin and myosin components correlates with the greatest percent of force the muscle can generate. When the muscle is too short or too long, there is diminished ability to generate adequate force [32, 33]. Surgeons performing tendon transfers consider this relationship when setting the ten-

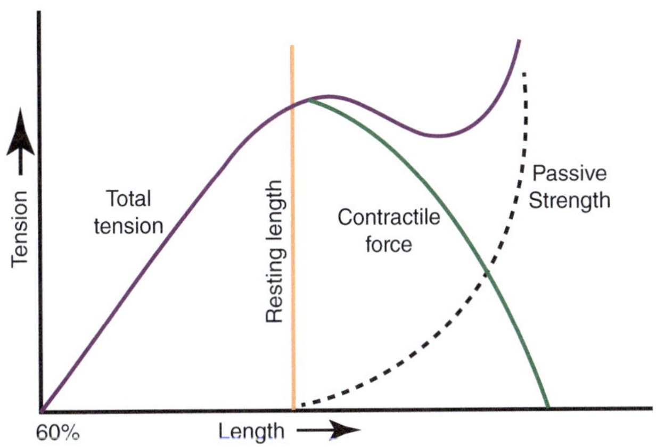

Image 4 The BLIX or length-tension curve

sion of the donor muscle by the length of its position in the transfer [12, 34]. Recipient muscles are not surgically altered during nerve transfers, and the surgical coaptation site does not require protection for more than 2–3 weeks. Yet, consideration should be given to the effects of gravity, strong antagonist muscle forces, and length of the recipient muscle when determining optimal positioning both before and after surgery. Optimal recipient muscle length should be maintained *until reinnervation occurs* and adequate strength is recovered in order to create balance at the joint [32, 33, 35]. This is especially important when the nerve injury is isolated, meaning that the antagonist muscle is likely intact. In this situation, the strong antagonist becomes dominant and unopposed, which will pull the denervated muscle to a stretched position. This is obvious in isolated musculocutaneous nerve palsies where elbow hyperextension posturing often occurs.

Another example is an upper trunk injury of the brachial plexus involving musculocutaneous nerve palsy. Without active elbow flexor function, the triceps becomes dominant for any attempt at elbow movement, pulling the elbow into full extension (Image 5). Over time, the lack of antagonistic flexion may lead to triceps shortening (limiting passive end-range elbow flexion) as well as overlengthening of the biceps and brachialis muscles. When unopposed, this will interfere with the patient's ability to isolate the recovering recipient muscle(s) following a single- or double-fascicular nerve transfer as he or she tries to regain elbow flexion [35]. An appropriate intervention in this scenario would be patient education in the importance of avoiding overlengthening of the denervated muscle and advocating the use of a device to protect it. A sling is useful as well as a hip-based support used by caretakers of infants or toddlers who need extra support to hold the child's weight (Image 6). Alternatively, the muscle(s) can become too short, as seen with mid/lower brachial plexus injuries. The loss of extrinsic flexor muscle function may lead to flexor muscle shortening and joint contractures. Following a nerve transfer to provide hand closing, the extrinsic flexors' ability to provide finger flexion will be limited if unopposed and starting from the muscles' shortened positions. In this scenario, forearm or hand-based orthoses are useful to prevent and/or restore joint and muscle length (Image 7).

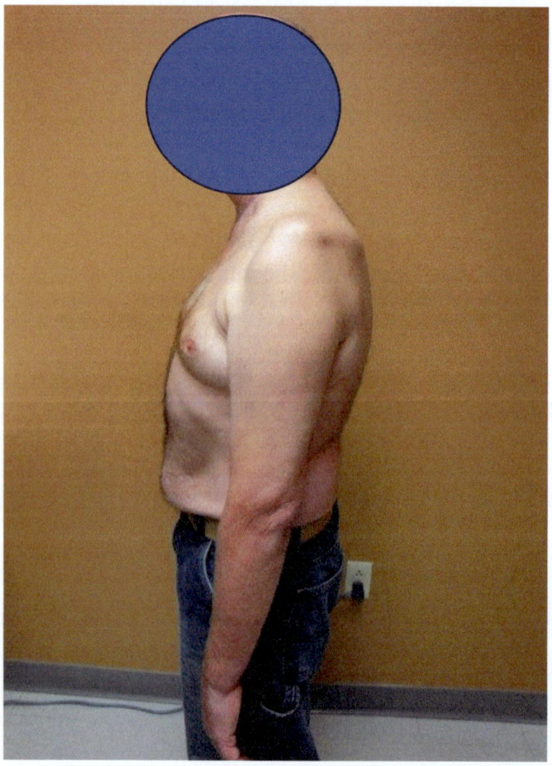

Image 5 With an upper trunk plexus injury, the triceps is often unopposed leading to elbow hyperextension or triceps dominance that can interfere with elbow flexor recovery

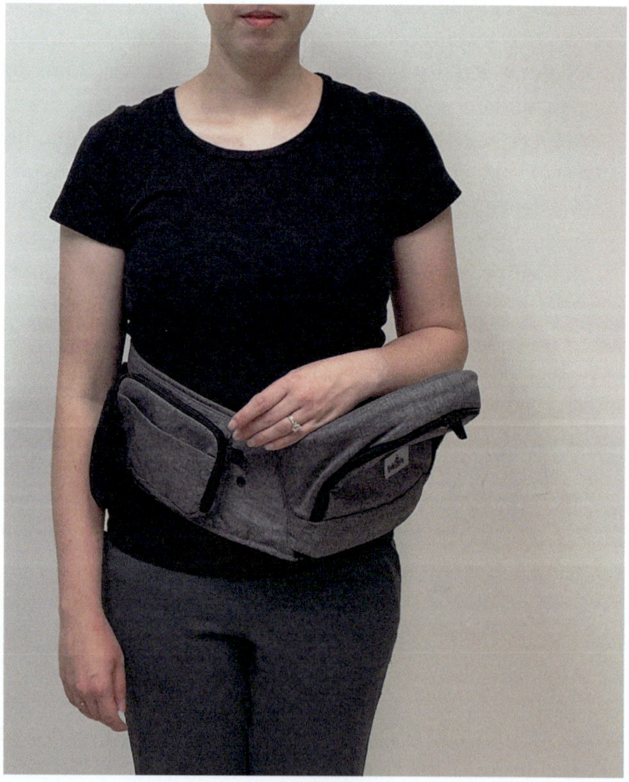

Image 6 A hip support such as those that are designed for young infants is useful in supporting the weight of an arm lacking shoulder and or elbow motor function. This may be used both to support the elbow flexor length and the reduce glenohumeral subluxation

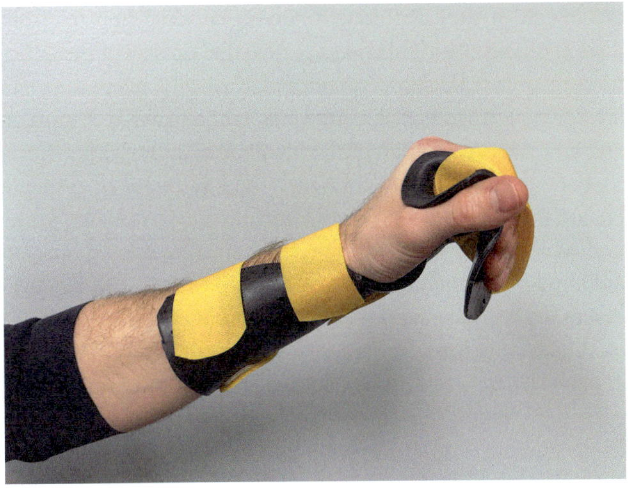

Image 7 An orthosis such as this resting hand orthosis is recommended to support the length of the recipient flexors when limited active intrinsic and extrinsic function may lead to hand posturing that encourages excess shortening of the flexor muscles

Donor Activation (DAFRA)

Donor activation is the central construct for motor reeducation following nerve transfers. By acknowledging the altered neural pathways produced by transferring a motor nerve from a donor muscle(s) to a recipient motor nerve, a patient can begin the process of regaining function in the denervated recipient muscle. DAFRA refers to "**donor activation focused rehabilitation approach**" to nerve transfers. This approach focuses on strengthening these new neural pathways with simplified patient education and exercises to promote learning a new motor pattern with the goal of improved functional outcomes [36]. Donor activation may be introduced with a variety of metaphors to help clarify these concepts. A "gas pedal" is likened to donor activation because the greater the activation or contraction of the donor muscle, the more the response that is ultimately seen in the recipient muscle. "Step on the gas" is a simple phrase that encourages recipient muscle response by contracting the donor muscle (see Appendix 2). Although not yet scientifically proven with electromyography studies, there is anecdotal evidence that promoting donor activation early in the recovery phase will enhance reinnervation and recovery in the recipient muscle(s).

The DAFRA program was adapted from the tendon transfer rehabilitation model and the work of Anastakis and colleagues. Co-contraction of the donor and recipient muscles in a repetitive way promotes cortical plasticity that supports functional recovery [21]. Patients with *tendon* transfers can perform this early on because the innervated muscles are transferred and surgically "tied" to denervated tendon/muscle units. Within weeks, as the healing tendon coaptation is complete, patients can actively move in the newly created movement pattern, which benefits the learning process. Following a *nerve* transfer, nerve growth into the denervated muscle takes many months before actual movement occurs. Despite this prolonged recovery, it is believed that early "pairing" or "patterning" of the new combination of donor contraction with passive or assisted movement of the recipient muscle (long before the reinnervated active movement occurs) will benefit the process of cortical plasticity and motor recovery.

The motor reeducation program is divided into three phases. Phase 1 begins preoperatively with a comprehensive assessment of motor and sensory deficits, functional limitations, and social support. In the ideal setting, the therapist will collaborate with the surgeon team prior to surgery. The contribution of the therapists' clinical assessments and understanding of the patient's abilities, functional goals, and needs will enhance discussion of surgical options. Additionally, the therapists' expertise on synergistic movement patterns that will enable easier rehabilitation is helpful for the surgeon and ultimately benefits the patient.

Phase 1

Preoperative Management

Preoperative treatment should address any passive range-of-motion (PROM) deficits brought about by joint contractures or antagonistic muscle shortening. Fitting or fabrication of braces or orthoses to aid with pain, function, and muscle imbalance is best initiated before significant joint changes occur or strong muscle substitution patterns emerge [37]. For example, someone with an isolated low median nerve injury will, over time, develop a thumb web space contracture from a lack of palmar abduction and unopposed adduction. A C-bar orthosis, also called a web spacer, may correct an adduction contracture, and a hand-based thumb opposition orthosis will help maintain thumb adductor length and functional thumb opposition to other digits [38] (Image 8).

Once nerve transfer surgical planning is complete, preoperative visits will include education regarding donor and recipient muscles and their functional importance. The exercise algorithm of a) donor activation and b) active donor with passive recipient patterning is introduced. Initial donor activation exercises should be simple movements that can be performed easily (without equipment, i.e., bands, weights) to improve patient compliance. Recovery timelines are introduced, and realistic expectations of the surgery(ies) are discussed.

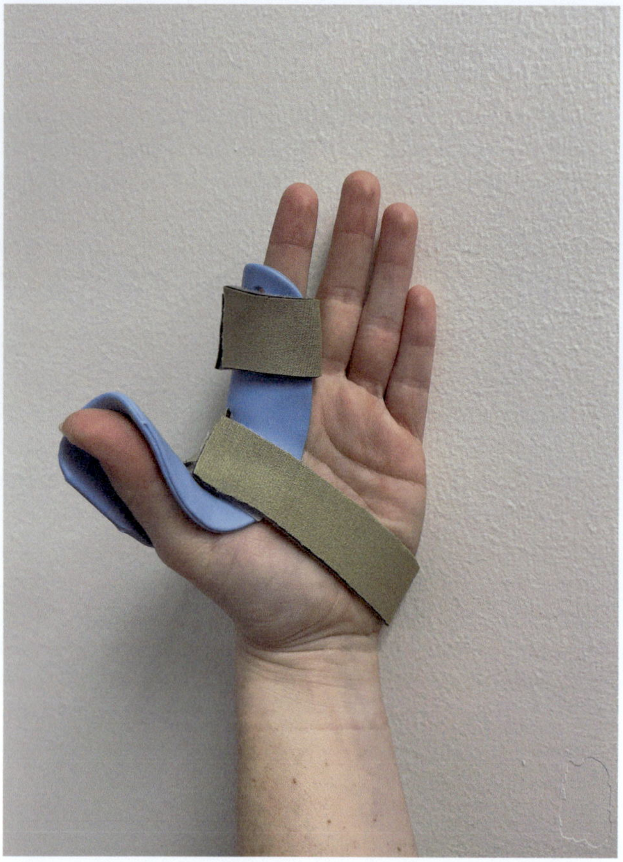

Image 8 A C-bar orthosis is used to prevent or improve thumb adduction contractures

Postoperative Management

Postoperative therapy should commence within 2–4 weeks of surgery. The operative report is reviewed, and donor and recipient targets are confirmed with the surgeon to ensure accuracy of the motor reeducation program. Therapists should be aware of any muscle or tendon alterations that may have been necessary to access the nerves. The subsequent repair of these tendons requires a delay of typically 4 weeks before ROM of the affected joint is addressed [39].

If the patient was not seen preoperatively, the same assessments mentioned above are performed after surgery. Basic scar and edema management is addressed, if needed. For proximal transfers involving the elbow and shoulder, strong precautions are outlined to limit use and excessive movement of the involved joint(s). This may include use of a sling or shoulder immobilizer, which is guided by individual surgeon preference. Sling use should include instruction to perform gentle elbow ROM throughout the day to avoid ulnar nerve irritation at the cubital tunnel. Avoiding excessive limb use and motion will reduce the likelihood of seroma formation and wound complications. For distal procedures of the wrist and hand, 2–3 weeks of immobilization with an orthosis is advised, per general guidelines following any nerve repair to reduce edema and protect the repair/coaptation [15]. The literature varies on the length of time required following a nerve transfer from days to weeks [40]. This may relate to the quality of the structures involved and surgeon preference. Ideally, nerve transfers are performed with tension-free coaptation to avoid disruption and allow earlier motion of the involved anatomy [8].

Patient education begins early and is repeated often to ensure that patients understand how the nerve transfer works and what they can do to improve their outcomes. Pertinent anatomy is identified, and a synopsis of the operative note is discussed with the patient. Use of illustrations, metaphors, or analogies may improve patient's understanding of these concepts. Written instructions capturing all this information will help individuals digest and decipher instructions at home (Appendices 3 and 4; Supplementary Video 1).

A primary goal of the first (or second) therapy visit should be to describe what "drives" the recovery of the denervated muscle. Identifying the exact donor muscle is not as important as describing what the donor muscle action does and demonstrating it. Donor activation is demonstrated as a simple movement that can be performed in any environment and without equipment. For example, when the triceps is the donor, patients may press on their thigh while sliding it forward towards the knee. This actively straightens the elbow by eliciting a triceps contraction and can be performed anywhere. Donor activation is the foundation of motor reeducation, and compliance may improve with clear and feasible exercise instruction [2]. Donor activation is performed for all transfers, including those in which the donor nerve has technically been completely transected for the transfer. In most cases, the donor muscle function is redundant, and once sacrificed, the residual redundant muscle will move the joint in a similar way and drive the brain to send messages in this pathway. For example, the AIN-to-ulnar nerve transfer typically involves sacrificing the entire PQ branch of the AIN. "Donor activation" remains possible as the individual will continue to be able to pronate the forearm using the pronator teres muscle. Expectations for frequency of donor activation movements are set high, at a rate of 10 per hour, with the hope that this is performed at least several times throughout the day [36].

The second exercise introduced early in phase 1 is one that drives cortical plasticity by patterning the combined movements of the donor and recipient structures. Given the lack of function in the recipient muscle throughout this phase, movement of the recipient muscle action is performed passively while the donor muscle contraction is performed actively (or with resistance) [41]. Some nerve transfer patterning exercises are simple, while others require creativity to make this combined motion easy for the patient to perform at home. The double-fascicular nerve transfer for elbow flexion, "DFT," lends itself to relatively easy donor-recipient pairing. The patient is instructed to make a fist (flexor digitorum superficialis, FDS) and flex the wrist (flexor carpi ulnaris, FCU), as if scooping ice cream while passively flexing the elbow with the uninvolved hand. Conversely, pairing the spinal accessory to suprascapular nerve transfer may involve using a long dowel held in both hands with the elbow supported to push the

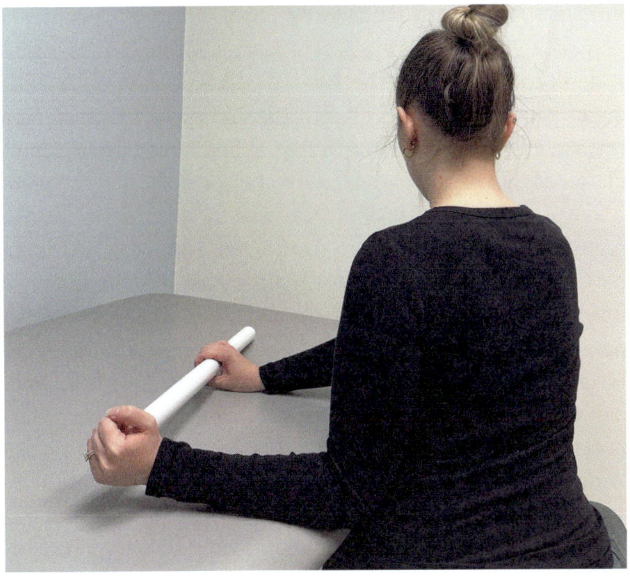

Image 9 Following a SAN-SS nerve transfer co-contraction of active trapezius donor with passive recipient infra and supraspinatus muscle is encouraged early on. Here a dowel is used to assist with passive externals rotation while the scapula retracts

involved arm into external rotation while having the patient to retract the scapula in supine [15] (Image 9).

It is assumed that for each nerve transfer described in the subsequent chapters, the assessment for additional therapeutic interventions will be performed based on individual patient needs. Loss of muscle function in one or more muscles results in disuse, weakness, joint changes, and functional change or loss [42]. Addressing functional independence with orthoses and/or adaptive equipment is also important to the treatment plan. Weakness of uninvolved muscles should also be addressed with a comprehensive exercise plan.

A comprehensive plan of care following any nerve transfer will ideally include the following:

- Perform baseline and follow-up motor evaluation.
- Address pain management.
- Provide patient education.
- Maintain function while minimizing substitution patterns.
- Prevent joint contractures.
- Manage edema.
- Optimize strength of uninvolved and donor muscles.
- Limit subluxation of the humeral head, when applicable.
- Train with specific exercises to enhance new motor patterns.

Therapy Frequency

A visit frequency of one time per week is typical for the first 4–8 weeks of phase 1. It is based on the patients' needs and the complexity of their condition. Once initial goals are met, and accurate performance and understanding of the home exercise program (HEP) are achieved, monthly therapy visits are adequate. Given the protracted length of recovery and the often-finite insurance coverage for many patients, conservative use of therapy visits is encouraged. Monthly visits are recommended until muscle twitch recovery is identified.

Assessment of Recovery

Assessment of motor return is performed during monthly therapy visits and helps to define recipient muscle status. The first sign of recovery is often described, unknowingly, by the patient as new onset of pain or tenderness in the denervated muscle and may be accompanied by new reports of "electric shocks" in the recipient muscle. Lee described this *tender muscle sign* as a predictor of muscle reinnervation that occurs before any muscle twitch is palpated or visualized [43]. This tenderness should be conveyed as a promising event of the patient's recovery as it predicts muscle contraction in the previously denervated muscle. This interpretation is motivating to patients by giving them hope and may renew their compliance with home exercises for their long motor recovery journey. The *tender test* is performed by gently pinching the recipient muscle belly and asking if this elicits pain or tenderness relative to the same pinch applied to uninvolved side or other neurologically intact muscles [43].

At some point following the tenderness sign, early movement will emerge in the recipient muscle in the form of a twitch, referred to in the MRC/MMT grading system as a 1/5 strength. This time period is often described between 8 and 12 weeks following the onset of muscle tenderness [13]. To test for a twitch in a recovering muscle in phase 1, the patient should be positioned so both examiner hands are readily available and not needed to support a limb. The therapist or surgeon resists the donor muscle action by applying force in the opposite direction of the donor action while palpating the recipient muscle. For some muscles, like the biceps, it may be easier to detect a muscle contraction in the region of the distal tendon than in the muscle belly. At the distal tendon, it can be more easily differentiated from a brachialis muscle contraction, which is palpated at either side of the biceps tendon (Image 10).

Knowledge of a muscle's innervation pattern is also helpful. In general, the more proximal fibers will recover sooner than the distal fibers. For example, the course of the axillary nerve runs from the posterior deltoid muscle to the middle deltoid and eventually to the anterior deltoid fibers. Therefore, following the triceps-to-axillary nerve transfer, one would expect posterior deltoid muscle fibers to recover before the others and palpation would begin there. An estimated timeframe to perceive a positive tender sign and the first muscle twitch following common nerve transfers is outlined in a paper by Hill and colleagues, which serves as a good resource for estimating a patient's recovery [13].

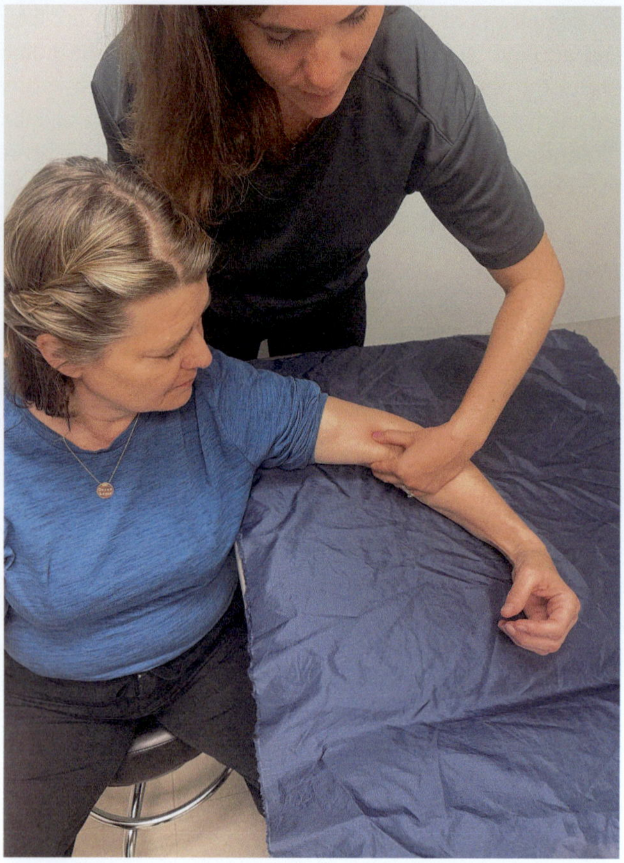

Image 10 Assessment for recovery of biceps function is demonstrated with palpation at the distal tendon in the antecubital fossa

Factors Affecting Recovery Time

A nerve transfer may be performed with an end-to-end (ETE) or an end-to-side (ETS) neurorrhaphy, more specifically a reverse end-to-side neurorrhaphy. When a reverse or supercharge end-to-side procedure is performed, the recipient nerve remains intact, leaving potential for this native nerve to recover independently from the transfer [44, 45]. This is, in part, because these procedures typically involve decompressing the native nerve. There are situations where the motor nerve injury is mixed (referred to by some as a Sunderland level 6) such that some fascicles of the nerve may have axonal injury (Sunderland levels 2–4) and others may be neuropraxic (Sunderland level 1) [46, 47]. Mackinnon describes a "Sunderland 0" as well [48]. This refers to a scenario in which loss of nerve function is due to compression-related blood flow to the nerve. If limited blood flow was contributing to motor loss preoperatively, after the decompression that typically accompanies the ETS nerve transfer, an individual may demonstrate some recovery as early as days to weeks following surgery [49, 50]. If some of the motor fibers were a level 1 injury with a local conduction block, following the decompression, myelin recovery would occur within weeks to months with potential early motor recovery at that time. These recoveries are *independent of the nerve transfer* and therefore will demonstrate motor function earlier than expected and without the need for concomitant donor activation (Table 1, rehab).

Table 1 Degree of nerve injury and anticipated recovery [46]

Degree of nerve injury	Definition of nerve injury	Prognosis	Tinel sign	Potential surgical interventions
First (Neurapraxia)	Segmental demyelination Axonal continuity maintained; endoneurium, perineurium and epineurium, intact	Favorable	None	None, distal decompression
Second (Axonotmesis)	Discontinuity of axon and myelin; endoneurium, perineurium, and epineurium intact	Favorable	Present, progressive	None, distal decompression, supercharge procedure
Third	Discontinuity of axon, myelin and endoneurium; perineurium and epineurium intact	Favorable	Present, progressive	None, distal decompression, supercharge procedure
Fourth	Only the epineurium remains intact	Unfavorable	Present; no progression	Nerve repair, graft, transfer
Fifth (Neurotmesis)	Complete nerve transection	Unfavorable	Present; no progression	Nerve repair, graft, transfer
Sixth	Mixed injury pattern	Variable	Variable	All options may be appropriate

Phase 2

Progression of the motor reeducation program to phase 2 is marked by a trace muscle contraction that is referred to as 1 to 2−/5 MMT grade [51]. This is a sign of early recovery and suggests that the recipient muscle is starting to reinnervate. Phase 2 will continue until the recipient muscle is able to move against gravity through the entire available range of motion (Table 2, rehab).

The exercise progression in this phase is designed to *gradually* increase demand as function recovers [36]. Outlined here are recommendations for this progression, but these should not be considered as comprehensive or strict guidelines.

- Donor activation exercises should continue throughout the day to promote nerve growth and reinnervation via the new neural pathways. Co-contraction of donor-recipient muscles is performed in gravity-lessened (or gravity-assisted) planes of motion to allow for active-assisted motion to occur in the weak muscle(s). For example, elbow flexion following the DFT may now progress to sitting with the arm supported at shoulder height on a table. An arm skate or slick nylon cloth under the arm is recommended to reduce the frictional forces incurred by sliding the limb. The goal is to make the task as easy as possible for the recipient muscle to move independently, if only in a short range. It is important to convey this concept to the patient, so they understand the expectations at this point in their motor recovery and are not tempted to demand too much. Exercises that demonstrate independent movement are very encouraging for patients and may motivate them to improve compliance with their home exercise program.
- As strength in the recipient advances to 2 and 2+ out of 5 MMT grade, exercises may be advanced to include "place and hold" exercises. Gravity-lessened planes may still be used. The therapist (or the patient's contralateral hand) will place the muscle in its shortened position at end range, and the patient contracts the donor muscle while attempting to actively maintain the position once the support is removed. Using the example of the DFT again, one would position the arm at shoulder height resting on a table. While activating the donors (finger and wrist flexion), the elbow is passively flexed through maximal ROM, and the patient attempts to maintain the position while maintaining donor activation as the support is removed (Image 11).
- "Place and hold" exercises will advance to the antigravity position once the recipient muscle achieves 3−/5 strength grade. Patients should continue to practice gravity-lessened or -assisted motion with donor activation as this will enable them to exercise with greater duration with less fatigue. Once the individual can flex the joint through full ROM in an antigravity position, the rehabilitation program advances to phase 3.

Advance According to Strength Level

The three phases of rehabilitation are not intended to be strict cutoffs but are rather a guide for the therapist in advancing the motor reeducation program. The goal of the phases is to outline exercises that are appropriate for the current strength level of the recipient muscle. For this reason, continued monthly assessment of the recipient strength is recommended. There is no response in the recipient muscle for the majority of phase 1, which is why the focus is on donor activation, followed by passive pairing of recipient movement with co-contraction of the donor muscle(s). As patients advance through phase 2, the exercises are modified to accommodate the strength and available endurance of the recipient muscle(s). Starting with active-assisted motion, patients can advance to "place and hold" exercises [2, 15]. By the end of phase 2, antigravity exercises are initiated with end-range or early-range assistance. Ultimately, if patients achieve full antigravity motion, phase 3 resistive exercises may be introduced. Therapists should keep in mind that this scale is altered for fingers and thumb muscles. Given the relative size of small body parts, gravity's effect is negligible. A 3/5 MMT score in the hand refers to full active ROM no matter the position relative to gravity, and partial ROM is considered 2/5 MMT grade [51].

Historically, the literature has supported the use of exercise for recovery of muscle strength [52, 53]. There is little controversy when discussing neurologically intact muscle. Exercise has been shown to improve muscle strength in intact or even moderately denervated muscle [54]. There is conflicting evidence in the literature, however, when discussing the effects of exercise on denervated muscle or peripheral motor nerve regeneration [52, 54–57]. The timing, type, and intensity of exercise are key factors in the variability of evidence. Some theorize that simple passive ROM exercises may preserve motor end-plate structures in denervated muscle by increasing trophic factor release on regenerating axons and modulating central neuronal plasticity [52]. Hence, we advocate for passive recipient exercises throughout phase 1.

Once there is evidence of motor recovery after a nerve transfer, the temptation during phase 2 may be to use whatever muscle function is available to improve its strength. However, if the exercise program is advanced too quickly and/or the demand is too great, recovery of the reinnervating muscle can be hampered. Work by Tam and colleagues

Table 2 Manual muscle testing (MMT) grading system

Numerical grade	Grade	Muscle description that aligns with the grade	Comments
0	Zero	No evidence of contraction	
+T	Tender sign	No contraction but the muscle is unusually tender to pinching	Not a MMT grade but useful for predicting recovery
1	Trace	Small muscle contraction palpable but no movement	
1+	Trace plus	Contraction noted with the initiation of movement	Not officially part of the established grading system[a]
2-	Poor minus	Movement through partial available range in a *gravity lessened* plane	Measure arc of available motion to monitor change
2	Poor	Movement of the joint through the complete available range when in a *gravity lessened* plane	Measure arc of available motion to monitor change
2+	Poor plus	Movement of the joint through the complete available range when in a *gravity lessened* plane AND through a partial range in an *antigravity* plane	Measure arc of available motion to monitor change
3-	Fair minus	Movement of the joint through most of the range against gravity	The position is not sustained and gradually loses its ability to stay in the test position
3	Fair	Movement of the joint through the full available antigravity range but not tolerate any pressure	Able to maintain the test position
3+	Fair plus	Movement of the joint through the full available antigravity range and tolerates minimal pressure in the test position	
4-	Good minus	Movement of the joint through the full available antigravity range and tolerates minimal-moderate pressure in the test position	
4	Good	Movement of the joint through the full available antigravity range and tolerates moderate pressure in the test position	
4+	Good Plus	Movement of the joint through the full available antigravity range and tolerates moderate to very firm pressure in the test position	
5	Normal	Movement of the joint through the full available antigravity range and tolerates very firm pressure in the test position	This is not intended to mean the maximum force that the examiner can apply but rather a reasonable amount for normal functional use

[a]This grade is not officially part of the established MMT grading system but is useful when monitoring for early recovery of muscle function following a nerve transfer. The authors use this to delineate a subtle muscle contraction from a distinct contraction with minimal degrees of movement in the associated joint

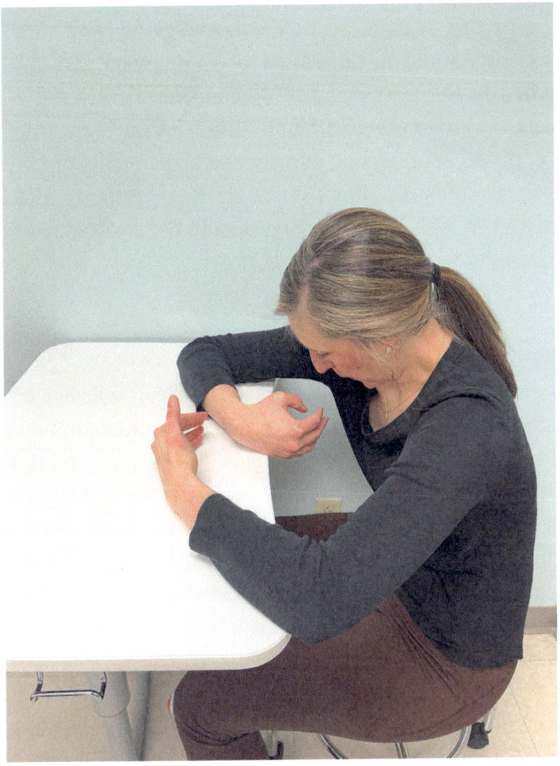

Image 11 End range elbow flexion "place and hold" exercise is demonstrated in a gravity lessened plane following nerve transfers to recover biceps and brachialis function

looked at the effect of exercise on the ability of the recovering motor neurons to sprout and for motor units to enlarge [54, 57]. They acknowledge the earlier work of others who demonstrate that exercise enhances muscle recovery in neurologically intact or even in moderately denervated muscles. However, when the denervation is severe, the effect of increased neuromuscular activity was a reduction in axonal spouting and therefore a reduction of motor recovery [54, 57]. For this reason, advancement of exercise in phases 2 and 3 should be done carefully and with awareness of the individual's MMT grade and endurance [2, 15].

Phase 3

Phase 3 begins when the reinnervated muscle can contract through the associated joint's full PROM against gravity. This does not include the intrinsic muscles of the hand. Gravity is not a factor in achieving 3/5 strength in muscles of the hand where full motion in any plane is considered 3/5 [51]. There is great variability in outcomes for many nerve transfers, and some transfers will never achieve full active movement through a full range. For those that do, the introduction of resistance exercise is the hallmark of this phase.

Full active movement against gravity is the first exercise in this phase. Once the individual can fully contract through the available range, light resistance is added to the exercise program. For individuals with 3+/5 strength where they can sustain a muscle contraction against minimal force, therapists should introduce the smallest amount of resistance that they can maintain. In the early months of phase 3, donor activation will continue, as it aids with building muscle strength needed for function.

Once significant control of the recipient muscle is attained, isolation or "donor deactivation" exercises are introduced [1, 15]. Active and resisted exercises are demonstrated in a variety of ways to strengthen the new neural pathway without co-contraction of the donor muscle. These include bilateral activities, exercises that demand contralateral limb participation, mirrored actions, and task-oriented actions that have been shown to enhance cortical plasticity [58] (Image 12). As strength against gravity is re-established, exercise continues to advance but at a slower pace that one would set for an uninjured muscle with non-neuropathic weakness. Recovery of strength after nerve transfer may continue for several years [59].

Endurance

To develop a functional contraction, a muscle needs only 20–30% of its total motor axons to be innervated [57]. However, reinnervation that attains muscle contraction through full range, even with resistance, does not equate to endurance. The limited number of motor fibers available for some nerve transfers may explain why endurance in the recipient muscle following a nerve transfer is notoriously poor for a long time. Fiber count may also explain why many recipient muscles do not regain full strength. It has been demonstrated in the literature that a reduction in the number of axons reinnervating a denervated muscle is associated with a reduction in the muscle's ability to generate force [60].

The takeaway here is to advance the motor reeducation program according to the individual transfer and the results of recipient muscle assessment for each patient. Every patient will be different. The second point is to respect fatigue. Throughout phase 1, phase 2, and early in phase 3, the intensity of exercise should be maintained at a low level with high frequency (fewer repetitions, more often through-

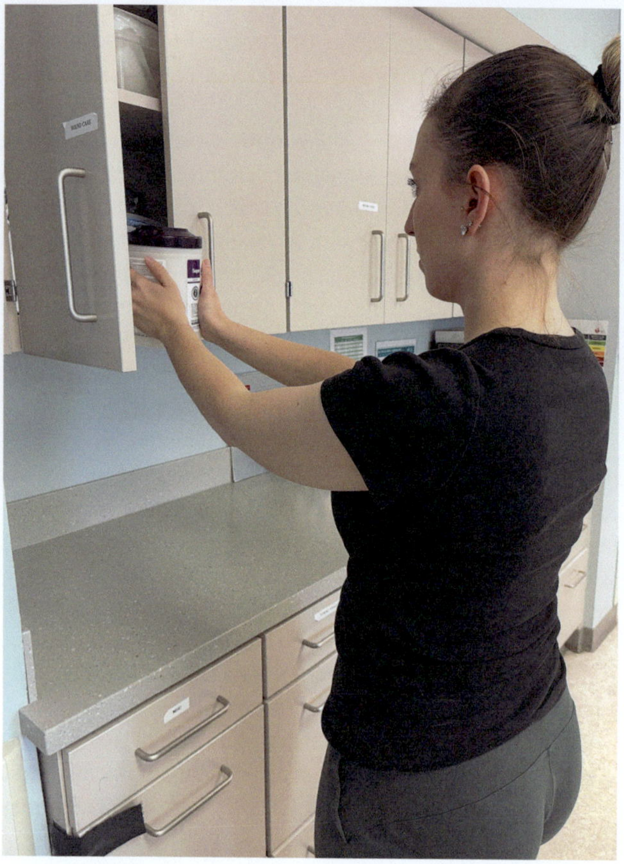

Image 12 This bilateral and task-oriented activity encourages cortical plasticity and is used for donor deactivation to strengthen the new neural pathway without co-contraction of the donor muscle

out the day) to allow the muscle to recover, thus avoiding fatigue. Studies with rodents using low-intensity treadmill training have demonstrated increased length of regenerated axons following nerve repair [53, 61]. Endurance tends to progress slowly in reinnervating muscles. After several repetitions of newly reacquired volitional movement, a patient may not be able to replicate the movement for several minutes. For this reason, spacing out exercises over time and respecting fatigue may augment motor recovery and strength. And finally, there are situations where completely resting the muscle may be your treatment "prescription" or home program. If you believe their current exercise level is too intense and they are struggling to progress, instructing them to reduce exercise and or activity, resting the muscle for a few weeks, may lead to strength gains.

How to Use This Book

This book is meant to be a resource for therapists who treat individuals following nerve transfer procedures and the surgeons who performed these surgeries. It should be considered a guide to the concepts of motor reeducation and rehabilitation. The information described in each of the individual transfer chapters is not intended to be comprehensive but rather a starting point from which you can adapt to a patient's individual needs and interests. Do not consider this as a rigid protocol but rather a format that enables one to start treatment and advance exercises based on the individual's goals and needs.

You will find that some nerve transfers are more synchronous and intuitive as with the ECRB to AIN, whereas others may involve antagonistic donor and recipient muscles, such as thoracodorsal to long thoracic nerve transfer. The information here should enable you to use your own creativity to develop exercise programs that best suit the individual.

The individual transfer chapters are designed to guide a therapist through the basics of a rehabilitation program. Addendums include handouts that may be used to start a home exercise program for the patient. Keep in mind that individual needs may vary based on aspects of their injury that are not assumed for the material covered in the chapter. Some exercises may be unreasonable for individuals with concomitant injuries including complete plexus injuries.

Appendix 1

See Image 13.

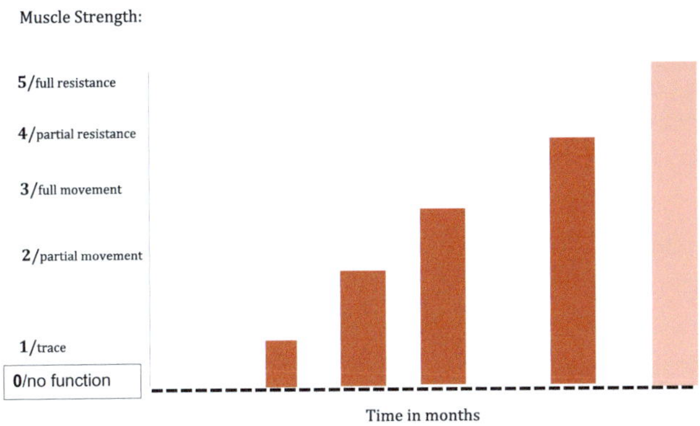

Image 13 Muscle strength recovery in terms of muscle grades over time on the X axis is plotted against theoretical force that muscle exerts during nerve transfer recovery on the Y axis to help explain the recovery expectations

Appendix 2

See Image 14.

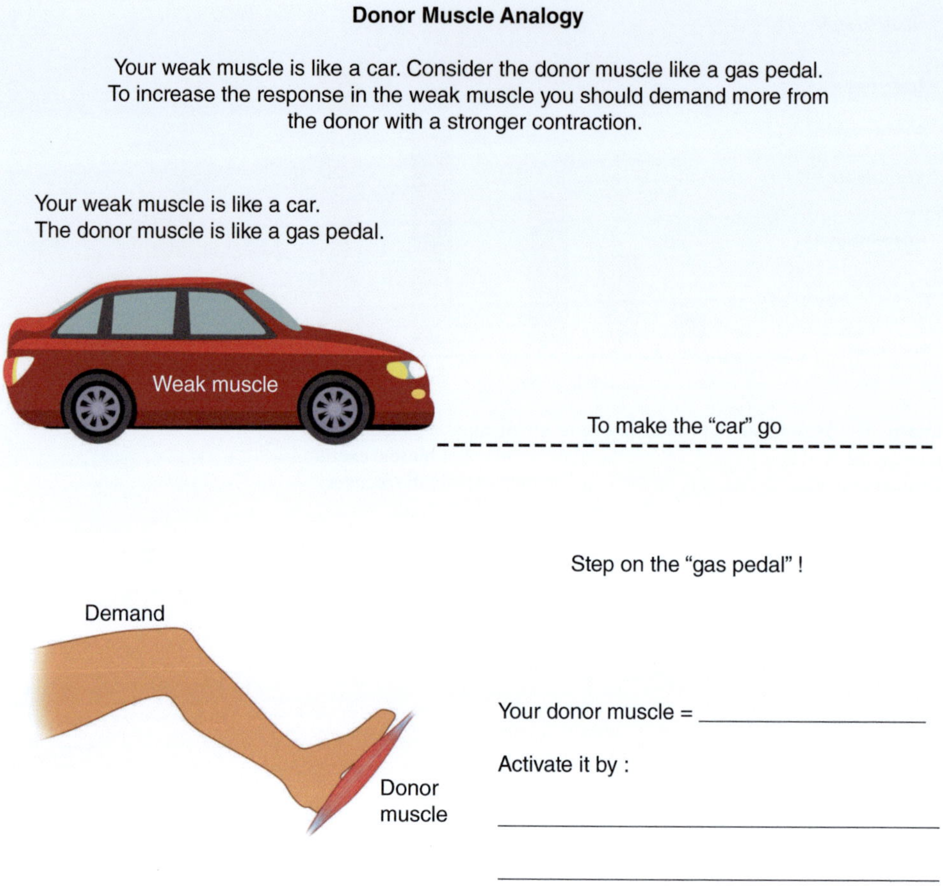

Image 14 A sample patient handout to aid in explaining the recovery process

Appendix 3

See Image 15.

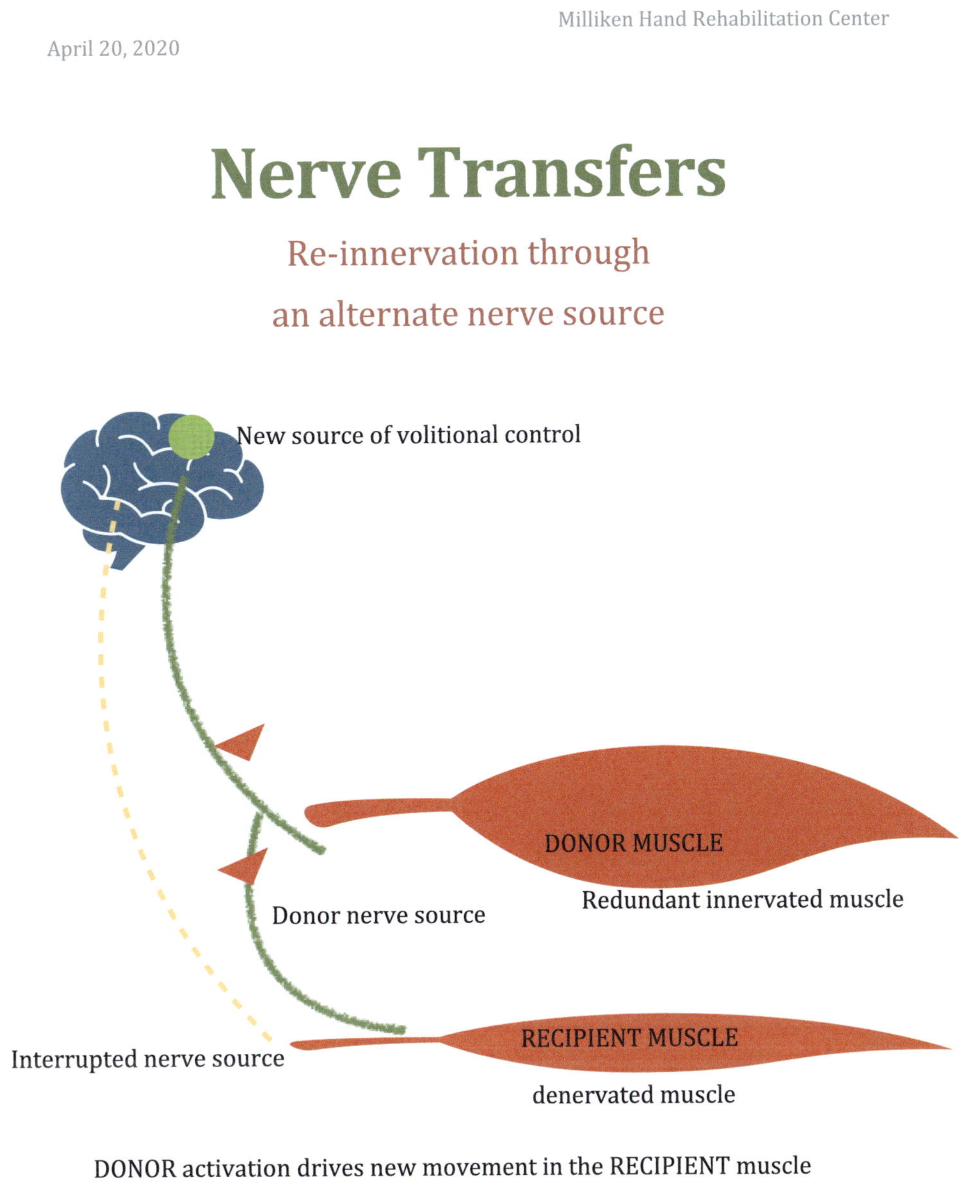

Image 15 A visual aid that may be helpful when explaining the altered neural pathway following a nerve transfer to a patient

Appendix 4

See Image 16.

Image 16 This sample patient handout identifies donor and recipient muscles and their functions and may be used for early instruction

Nerve Transfer Instructions

Date of Surgery:

General Advice:

1. Practice donor activation often.
2. Practice combined motions frequently for short periods/low reps.
3. Respect fatigue; stop and try again later.
4. More is more when it comes to donor ms contractions.
5. Be patient! This will take a long time.

Transfer

________________ nerve (________________ muscle) **TO**
________________ nerve (________________ muscle)

"Donor" = ________________ muscle

action = ________________

"Recipient" = ________________ m

action = ________________

Exercise #1

ACTIVATE THE DONOR:

10x/hour

Exercise #2:

COMBINE DONOR + RECIPIENT ACTION:

Several times/day

References

1. Larocerie-Salgado J, Chinchalkar S, Ross DC, Gillis J, Doherty CD, Miller TA. Rehabilitation following nerve transfer surgery. Tech Hand Up Extrem Surg. 2022;26(2):71–7.
2. Kahn L, Moore A. Donor activation focused rehabilitation approach: maximizing outcomes after nerve transfers. Hand Clin. 2016;32(2):263–77.
3. Hill JL, Turner LC, Jones RD, et al. The stages of rehabilitation following motor nerve transfer surgery. J Musculoskelet Surg Res. 2019;3(60)
4. Beers A, Ivens R, Kahn L, Mackinnon S. Functional outcomes following nerve transfer surgery for a C5–C7 brachial plexus palsy are improved with DAFRA rehabilitation technique. Paradise Island, Bahamas: Washington University School of Medicine; 2015.
5. Sultana SS, MacDermid JC, Grewal R, Rath S. The effectiveness of early mobilization after tendon transfers in the hand: a systematic review. J Hand Therapy. 2013;26(1):1–21.
6. Compton J, Owens J, Day M, Caldwell L. Systematic review of tendon transfer versus nerve transfer for the restoration of wrist extension in isolated traumatic radial nerve palsy. JAAOS Glob Res Rev. 2018;2(4):e001.
7. Ruijs ACJ, Jaquet JB, Kalmijn S, Giele H, Hovius SER. Median and ulnar nerve injuries: a meta-analysis of predictors of motor and sensory recovery after modern microsurgical nerve repair. Plastic Reconstruct Surg. 2005;116(2):484–94.
8. Mackinnon S. Nerve surgery. Theime; 2015.
9. Chaudhry V, Cornblath DR. Wallerian degeneration in human nerves: serial electrophysiological studies. Muscle Nerve. 1992;15(6):687–93.
10. Mackinnon SE, Yee A. Nerve surgery. New York: Thieme; 2015.
11. Schreiber JJ, Byun DJ, Khair MM, Rosenblatt L, Lee SK, Wolfe SW. Optimal axon counts for brachial plexus nerve transfers to restore elbow flexion. Plastic Reconstruct Surg. 2015;135(1):135e–41e.
12. Fujiwara T, Matsuda K, Kubo T, et al. Axonal supercharging technique using reverse end-to-side neurorrhaphy in peripheral nerve repair: an experimental study in the rat model. J Neurosurg. 2007;107(4):821–9.
13. Hill JL, Turner LC, Jones RD, Jimulia DT, Miller C, Power DM. The stages of rehabilitation following motor nerve transfer surgery. J Musculoskelet Surg Res. 2019;3:60.
14. Bertelli JA, Ghizoni MF. Reconstruction of C5 and C6 brachial plexus avulsion injury by multiple nerve transfers: spinal accessory to suprascapular, ulnar fascicles to biceps branch, and triceps long or lateral head branch to axillary nerve. J Hand Surg. 2004;29(1):131–9.
15. Kahn LC, Stonner MM, Dy CJ. Key concepts for nerve transfer rehabilitation after surgical reconstruction for brachial plexus and peripheral nerve injuries. J Hand Surg. 2023;
16. Stonner MM, Keane G, Berlet L, Goldfarb CA, Pet MA. The impact of social deprivation and hand therapy attendance on range of motion after flexor tendon repair. J Hand Surg Am. 2022;47(7):655–61. https://doi.org/10.1016/j.jhsa.2022.03.018.
17. Novak CB, Anastakis DJ, Beaton DE, Mackinnon SE, Katz J. Biomedical and psychosocial factors associated with disability after peripheral nerve injury. J Bone Joint Surg Am. 2011;93(10):929–36. https://doi.org/10.2106/jbjs.J.00110.
18. Novak CB, Katz J. Neuropathic pain in patients with upper-extremity nerve injury. Physiother Can Summer. 2010;62(3):190–201. https://doi.org/10.3138/physio.62.3.190.
19. Jensen MP, Chodroff MJ, Dworkin RH. The impact of neuropathic pain on health-related quality of life: review and implications. Neurology. 2007;68(15):1178–82. https://doi.org/10.1212/01.wnl.0000259085.61898.9e.
20. Seddon H, Medawar P, Smith H. Rate of regeneration of peripheral nerves in man. J Physiol. 1943;102(2):191.
21. Paternostro-Sluga T, Grim-Stieger M, Posch M, et al. Reliability and validity of the Medical Research Council (MRC) scale and a modified scale for testing muscle strength in patients with radial palsy. J Rehab Med. 2008;40(8):665–71.
22. Salehi SK, Tahmasebi F, Talebrokni FS. A different look at featured motor learning models: comparison exam of Gallahue's, Fitts and Posner's and Ann Gentile's motor learning models. Movement Sport Sci. 2021;2:53–63.
23. Fitts PM, Posner MI. Human performance; 1967;
24. Lundborg G. Nerve injury and repair; 1988;
25. Taylor JA, Ivry RB. The role of strategies in motor learning. Ann N Y Acad Sci. 2012;1251(1):1–12.
26. Yip DW, Lui F. Physiology, motor cortical. In: StatPearls. StatPearls Publishing Copyright © 2024, StatPearls Publishing LLC; 2024.
27. Penfield W, Boldrey E. Somatic motor and sensory representation in the cerebral cortex of man as studied by electrical stimulation. Brain. 1937;60(4):389–443.
28. Gordon EM, Chauvin RJ, Van AN, et al. A somato-cognitive action network alternates with effector regions in motor cortex. Nature. 2023;617(7960):351–9. https://doi.org/10.1038/s41586-023-05964-2.
29. Anastakis DJ, Malessy MJ, Chen R, Davis KD, Mikulis D. Cortical plasticity following nerve transfer in the upper extremity. Hand Clin. 2008;24(4):425–44.
30. Gardenier J, Garg R, Mudgal C. Upper extremity tendon transfers: a brief review of history, common applications, and technical tips. Indian J Plastic Surg. 2020;53(2):177–90. https://doi.org/10.1055/s-0040-1716456.
31. Gordon AM, Huxley AF, Julian FJ. The variation in isometric tension with sarcomere length in vertebrate muscle fibres. J Physiol. 1966;184(1):170–92. https://doi.org/10.1113/jphysiol.1966.sp007909.
32. Gossman MR, Sahrmann SA, Rose SJ. Review of length-associated changes in muscle: experimental evidence and clinical implications. Phys Therapy. 1982;62(12):1799–808.
33. Goldspink G, Tabary C, Tabary JC, Tardieu C, Tardieu G. Effect of denervation on the adaptation of sarcomere number and muscle extensibility to the functional length of the muscle. J Physiol. 1974;236(3):733–42.
34. Livermore A, Tueting JL. Biomechanics of Tendon Transfers. Hand Clinics. 2016;32(3):291–302. https://doi.org/10.1016/j.hcl.2016.03.011.
35. Lieber RL. Skeletal muscle structure, function, and plasticity. Lippincott Williams & Wilkins; 2002.
36. Kahn LC, Moore AM. Donor activation focused rehabilitation approach: maximizing outcomes after nerve transfers. Hand Clin. 2016;32(2):263–77. https://doi.org/10.1016/j.hcl.2015.12.014.
37. Colditz JC. Splinting the hand with a peripheral nerve injury. In: Hunter J, Mackin E, Callahan A, editors. Rehabilitation of the hand and upper extremity. Mosby; 2002. p. 622–34.
38. Lohman H, Coppard BM, Raber M. Orthotic intervention for nerve injuries. In: Introduction to orthotics-E-Book: a clinical reasoning and problem-solving approach; 2014. p. 293.
39. Manske RC, Prohaska D. Pectoralis major tendon repair post-surgical rehabilitation. North Am J Sports Phys Therapy. 2007;2(1):22.
40. Novak CB, von der Heyde RL. Evidence and techniques in rehabilitation following nerve injuries. Hand Clin. 2013;29(3):383–92.
41. Power HA, Kahn LC, Patterson MM, Yee A, Moore AM, Mackinnon SE. Refining indications for the supercharge end-to-side anterior interosseous to ulnar motor nerve transfer in cubital tunnel syndrome. Plastic Reconstruct Surg. 2020;145(1):106e–16e.
42. Akeson W, Amiel D, Abel M, Garfin S, Woo SL. Effects of immobilization on joints. Clin Orthop Relat Res. 1987;219:28–37.

43. Lee EY, Karjalainen TV, Sebastin SJ, Lim AY. The value of the tender muscle sign in detecting motor recovery after peripheral nerve reconstruction. J Hand Surg. 2015;40(3):433–7.
44. Doherty CD, Miller TA, Larocerie-Salgado J, Byers BA, Ross DC. Reverse end-to-side anterior interosseous nerve–to–ulnar motor transfer for severe ulnar neuropathy. Plastic Reconstruct Surg. 2020;146(3):306e–13e.
45. Kale SS, Glaus SW, Yee A, et al. Reverse end-to-side nerve transfer: from animal model to clinical use. J Hand Surg. 2011;36(10):1631–9. e2
46. Moore AM, Wagner IJ, Fox IK. Principles of nerve repair in complex wounds of the upper extremity. Thieme Medical Publishers; 2015. p. 040–7.
47. Chhabra A, Ahlawat S, Belzberg A, Andreseik G. Peripheral nerve injury grading simplified on MR neurography: As referenced to Seddon and Sunderland classifications. Indian J Radiolo Imaging. 2014;24(03):217–24.
48. Peters BR, Pripotnev S, Chi D, Mackinnon SE. Complete foot drop with normal electrodiagnostic studies: Sunderland "zero" ischemic conduction block of the common peroneal nerve. Ann Plastic Surg. 2022;88(4):425–8.
49. Jung J, Hahn P, Choi B, Mozaffar T, Gupta R. Early surgical decompression restores neurovascular blood flow and ischemic parameters in an in vivo animal model of nerve compression injury. JBJS. 2014;96(11):897–906.
50. Mackinnon SE. Pathophysiology of nerve compression. Hand Clin. 2002;18(2):231–41.
51. Kendall HO, Kendall FP, Wadsworth GE. Muscles, testing and function. American Journal of Physical Medicine & Rehabilitation. 1973;52(1):43.
52. Udina E, Cobianchi S, Allodi I, Navarro X. Effects of activity-dependent strategies on regeneration and plasticity after peripheral nerve injuries. Ann Anat Anatomischer Anzeiger. 2011;193(4):347–53.
53. Udina E, Puigdemasa A, Navarro X. Passive and active exercise improve regeneration and muscle reinnervation after peripheral nerve injury in the rat. Muscle Nerve. 2011;43(4):500–9.
54. Tam SL, Gordon T. Neuromuscular activity impairs axonal sprouting in partially denervated muscles by inhibiting bridge formation of perisynaptic Schwann cells. J Neurobiol. 2003;57(2):221–34.
55. English AW, Wilhelm JC, Sabatier MJ. Enhancing recovery from peripheral nerve injury using treadmill training. Ann Anat Anatomischer Anzeiger. 2011;193(4):354–61.
56. van Meeteren NL, Brakkee JH, Hamers FP, Helders PJ, Gispen WH. Exercise training improves functional recovery and motor nerve conduction velocity after sciatic nerve crush lesion in the rat. Arch Phys Med Rehab. 1997;78(1):70–7.
57. Tam SL, Archibald V, Jassar B, Tyreman N, Gordon T. Increased neuromuscular activity reduces sprouting in partially denervated muscles. J Neurosci. 2001;21(2):654–67.
58. Nudo RJ, Plautz EJ, Frost SB. Role of adaptive plasticity in recovery of function after damage to motor cortex. Muscle Nerve. 2001;24(8):1000–19.
59. Merrell GA, Barrie KA, Katz DL, Wolfe SW. Results of nerve transfer techniques for restoration of shoulder and elbow function in the context of a meta-analysis of the English literature. J Hand Surg. 2001;26(2):303–14.
60. Cederna PS, Youssef MKH, Asato H, Urbanchek MG, Kuzon WM Jr. Skeletal muscle reinnervation by reduced axonal numbers results in whole muscle force deficits. Plastic Reconstruct Surg. 2000;105(6):2003–9.
61. Tam SL, Archibald V, Tyreman N, Gordon T. Tetrodotoxin prevents motor unit enlargement after partial denervation in rat hindlimb muscles. J Physiol. 2002;543(2):655–63.

The Role of Cortical Reorganization in Nerve Transfers

Amy M. Young, Jennifer Erickson, and Jennifer Dodson

Introduction

Cortical plasticity refers to the brain's inherent ability to modify its functional and structural neural organization based on internal and external influences such as sensorimotor learning, age, injury, and recovery. Cortical reorganization can be considered both a process and an outcome of rehabilitation following nerve transfer. Remapping at the cortical level is required for the donor nerve to obtain motor control over recipient musculature [1]. Understanding the role of cortical reorganization is therefore essential during the rehabilitation process following nerve transfer surgery. This chapter highlights factors that influence cortical plasticity and therapy interventions to consider when treating this population to optimize function.

Sensorimotor Learning

When first learning a new motor skill, cortical areas representing the involved muscles expand [2]. The extent of neuroplastic changes with sensorimotor learning correlates with function. Both short- and long-duration practices of a specific motor skill elicit cortical reorganization in healthy individuals. Evidence suggests that cortical maps representing the abductor pollicis brevis (APB) muscle enlarge following 10 min of texting practice [2]. After 4 weeks of practicing a dynamic balance task, Lehmann observed that cortical changes in the premotor and primary sensorimotor cortices correlated with improved learning, motor planning, and motor control [3].

Aging

The brain retains the potential for cortical reorganization over the span of one's lifetime. However, the capacity for neural plasticity diminishes with age [1]. Age has been found to be a powerful predictor of outcomes following nerve transfer surgery [4]. Following median or ulnar nerve to musculocutaneous nerve transfer, the extent of independent elbow flexion control achieved has been found to be excellent in patients up to 16 years of age. In patients older than 17, the degree of independent recipient function is significantly less, which may indicate fewer neuroplastic changes with age [1]. In this study, plasticity was measured using a Plasticity Grading Scale, which was developed to determine the amount of independent recipient muscle control achieved following nerve transfer surgery [5].

The association between bicep strength and age is similarly noted following intercostal nerve-to-musculocutaneous nerve transfers. Elbow flexion Medical Research Council (MRC) grade 3 or more is achieved by a greater percentage of patients under age 30 compared to older patients [6]. Following triceps-to-axillary nerve transfer, a significant negative correlation between age and deltoid strength was similarly noted by Spinner and colleagues at the Mayo Clinic. A greater percentage of patients under 40 years of age achieved deltoid strength of MRC grade 3 or better compared to older patients [7]. Similarly, Sallam and colleagues demonstrated that functional outcome following nerve transfer surgery rapidly declines after the age of 35 [8]. These data suggest that therapeutic interventions to enhance cortical plasticity may be of particular importance for older patients to obtain optimal strength and independent control of the recipient muscle(s) [1]. However, the age that defines "older" has not yet been clearly identified as it relates to the

A. M. Young (✉)
Northwestern Medicine Center for Surgery of the Hand, Chicago, IL, USA

J. Erickson
Harborview Medical Center, Seattle, WA, USA

J. Dodson
OrthoCarolina, Charlotte, NC, USA

L. C. Kahn et al. (eds.), *Rehabilitation for Nerve Transfers of the Upper Extremity*,
https://doi.org/10.1007/978-3-031-92008-0_3

potential for cortical plasticity following nerve transfer surgery [1]. Moreover, it is important to note that there are other neurophysiological factors that may explain the negative correlation between age and functional outcome following nerve transfer.

Cortical Plasticity Following Peripheral Nerve Injury

There are several animal studies correlating the functional reorganization in the sensory and motor cortices after injuries such as amputations, brachial plexus injuries, and nerve compression. As early as 1983, there has been evidence that reorganization in the somatosensory cortex begins immediately following peripheral nerve injury [9, 10]. Peripheral nerve injuries have a larger zone of injury than the localized site of physical trauma. Severe brachial plexus and peripheral nerve injuries can result in the complete loss of afferent and efferent flow of information within the central nervous system (CNS). Injury to a peripheral nerve prompts a synchronous cascade of functional changes along the entire pathway from peripheral nerve to cerebral cortex. Structural alterations begin with the degeneration of central axons and termination of peripheral sensory neurons and may continue along nerve synapses inducing structural atrophy and degeneration at spinal, brain stem, thalamic, and cortical levels [11]. This reorganization of neural circuits leads to changes in sensory perception, motor function, and pain processing.

As the somatosensory cortex undergoes reorganization, the cortical areas corresponding to the affected body part may shrink while the neighboring areas, representing intact body parts, may expand [9]. Ultimately, these changes in the motor cortex affect movement planning and execution, especially if the injury impacts motor nerves. The literature supports this concept—that human grey and white matters demonstrate structural changes that relate to these alterations in function [12]. Changes in the connectivity between the brain and regions of perception may also show increased activation, ultimately contributing to maladaptive responses and the experience of neuropathic pain. Increased activation in the amygdala and prefrontal cortex leads to cortical changes in regions involved in emotional processing, resulting in altered perception, abnormal responses to sensory stimuli, and emotional responses to pain [13, 14].

Overall, cortical changes reflect the brain's adaptive response to peripheral nerve injury. This may lead to compensation for lost functions involving sensory processing, motor control, and pain modulation. These occurrences may contribute to altered perception and response to sensory stimuli [13].

Cortical Plasticity Following Peripheral Nerve Repair

Axons begin to regenerate following peripheral nerve repair. However, instead of reinnervating their original targets, axons may become mismatched from their initially intended anatomic and physiologic targets. These altered neural connections lead to novel cortical mapping that represents the injured body part. After nerve repair, end organs such as muscle and skin that were previously unable to communicate with the central nervous system (CNS) may once again contribute to motor control and perception [4]. Thus, a neural catch-22 is created between cortical structure and function [12]. Distorted sensorimotor information enters the CNS, and distorted efferent signals leave the CNS, contributing to continued motor and sensory deficits. Therapeutic interventions such as sensorimotor relearning techniques or modulation of sensorimotor information may be beneficial to gain and organize cortical representation of the injured body part to optimize function [15]. Examples of therapy interventions may include sensory reeducation, bilateral training, graded motor imagery, biofeedback, and sensory substitution strategies [16].

Cortical Plasticity Following Nerve Transfer

A study of the intercostal or phrenic nerve-to-musculocutaneous (MCN) transfer to restore elbow flexion may inform our understanding of the cortical reorganization that occurs. After connecting the ICN to the injured neural pathway from the cortex to cervical motor neuron pool by C6 to the MCN, contraction of the biceps is activated by sustained inspiration and expiration [17]. This occurs due to the ICN's primary motor cortex's midline location. Months later, patients learn to activate the biceps with normal respiration due to the cortical activation occurring laterally in the biceps' original primary motor cortex area. A shift occurs from the medial to lateral because of changes in the cortex that are directed by neuroplasticity. Phrenic nerve-to-MCN transfers have demonstrated a higher rate of patients achieving an MRC grade of 3 for elbow flexion, but respiratory concerns have limited its acceptance [18, 19]. Although good biceps strength may be achieved following hypoglossal nerve-to-MCN transfer [20], Socolovsky elucidates the poor functional outcomes for this nerve transfer. As the tongue relaxes, the biceps will also relax. Chewing or talking will activate the donor hypoglossal nerve as the tongue is pushed against the roof of the mouth, which would cause involuntary elbow flexion [21]. This transfer therefore demonstrates less successful skill acquisition (compared with other musculocutaneous nerve transfers) due to lack of cortical connection between elbow flexion and the tongue. These data suggest that choosing transfers that have a preexisting connection between the cortex of the donor and recipient is essential to successful outcomes [21].

It is important to note that there are several factors that impact outcomes following surgical interventions for nerve reinnervation: [22]

- There is a positive correlation to close proximity of donor and recipient muscle cortical representations on the motor cortex.
- The presence or absence of minimally active interneural connections should be considered.
- Recovery of gross motor function is more reliable than fine motor function, including finger dexterity and in-hand manipulation tasks.
- Patients who engage in rehabilitation demonstrate superior long-term function compared to those who do not.
- Patient age, delay from injury to surgery, and extent of nerve injury are among the strongest predictors of nerve transfer success [6, 23].
- Concomitant brain injury may contribute to poorer functional results [14].

Therapy Interventions to Enhance Cortical Representation of Recipient Muscle(s)

Graded Motor Imagery

Graded motor imagery (GMI) is a behavioral therapy technique that helps patients retrain the brain and normalize central processing. GMI was originally developed for patients with chronic pain or phantom limb pain following amputation. The purpose of GMI is to help patients gradually and systematically move an injured body part without triggering a painful response. Evidence now supports the role of GMI for patients following nerve transfer surgery to optimize motor reeducation and strengthen the new neural pathway from the central to peripheral nerve system [24, 25]. The three components of GMI include laterality training, motor imagery, and mirror visual feedback.

The principles of GMI coincide with those of the DAFRA model (donor activation focused rehabilitation approach), a treatment approach that emphasizes frequent, volitional activation of the donor muscle(s) to augment motor control in the target muscle(s) [26, 27]. GMI strategies may be used to promote activation and remapping of sensorimotor cortical areas representing target muscle(s) to enhance motor learning [22, 28, 29]. These techniques may begin in the early phase of therapy as volitional movement in the target muscle is not required for successful implementation.

- **GMI Part 1: Laterality Training**
  Laterality training involves discriminating between right and left sides of the body, which activates premotor areas of the brain, similar to actual movement [30]. Actual movement activates the primary motor and somatosensory cortices, whereas laterality training does not [30, 31]. Activation of the premotor areas of the brain that are otherwise inactive due to muscle denervation may lead to growth of cortical representation for the target muscle(s) [32, 33].
  During laterality training, images of hands or arms using cards or smart phone-based applications are presented to the patient from various views (dorsal, superior, lateral, anterior, etc.) and various positions (flexion, extension, supination, abduction, etc. and combinations of these). The patient is instructed to identify the image as a right versus left extremity as quickly and accurately as possible. It is important to prioritize accuracy over speed. Norm for discrimination between right- and left-hand cards is >80% accuracy at a rate of <2 ± 0.5 s [34].
  Pictures presented at 0 degrees of rotation in relation to the patient's viewpoint are most accessible and align the hand in the patient's visual field as one would view their own hand: wrist proximal, and fingers distal. If this activity does not induce any pain in the hand or arm, the challenge may be increased by rotating the image clockwise from 0° to 90°, 180°, or 270° [34]. Laterality training may be further advanced by increasing the number of images presented, including images of more dynamic hand postures, and adding images of the lower extremity [31, 35]. It is important to note that GMI activities should not be advanced if the patient experiences pain with the preceding task. Once patients are proficient with laterality training for 2 weeks without neuropathic symptoms, they may progress to GMI part 2 or motor imagery.
- **GMI Part 2: Motor Imagery**
  Motor imagery is the mental simulation of movement without production of actual movement. The primary motor cortex, premotor cortex, and supplementary motor areas of the brain are similarly active with both volitional and imagined movements [36]. Visual imagery, or how a movement looks, may be performed from the first- or third-person perspective. First-person perspective is the view from within one's own body looking out. The third-person point of view is picturing oneself or someone else completing a movement or task as an outside observer. Kinesthetic imagery, or how the movement feels, focuses on the proprioceptive qualities of movement such as direction, force, effort, and speed [36].

  A quiet space to perform motor imagery may be useful as it requires focus and sustained attention. The patient may perform visual imagery, kinesthetic imagery, or both.

The patient chooses what type of imagery is most appropriate for their learning. If the patient identifies lower-body dressing as a painful or difficult task, he or she may first imagine the task being performed by someone else who does not have a nerve injury. With repetition and practice, the patient may progress to self-visualizing this activity, perhaps imagining a specific article of clothing he or she owns. Furthermore, if actual lower-body dressing induces pain at baseline, the patient may first imagine putting on comfortable clothes such as loose sweatpants and slippers. He or she may progress to visualizing putting on dress pants and formal shoes.

Upper extremity function may be enhanced when motor imagery is performed in combination with physical practice [31]. For example, following nerve transfer, a patient may perform donor muscle activation combined with *imagined* recipient muscle activation. This technique can be incorporated into functional activities that are familiar and meaningful to the patient. For example, a patient's goal may be to return to basketball following AIN-to-ulnar nerve transfer. The patient may hold a basketball and actively pronate the forearm (donor activation for PQ) while imagining maximal finger abduction (imagery of recipient activation for dorsal interossei).

- **GMI Part 3: Mirror Visual Feedback**

Mirror visual feedback involves occluding the affected limb from view behind a mirror in the sagittal plane and gazing at the reflection of movement produced by the unaffected limb in the mirror. Mirror visual feedback can be considered a sensory substitution strategy [16]. Visual information is prioritized over proprioceptive input at the cortical level [31]. Movement in the mirror's reflection activates brain areas similar to actual movement, substituting quality visual sensory information for impaired movement and proprioception of the recipient muscle(s). The mirror creates the visual illusion of volitional movement of the denervated upper extremity to activate the primary motor cortex of the recipient muscle(s) [28, 29].

Mirror visual feedback in phase 1 of rehabilitation [26] may include bilateral donor muscle activation (Image 1), recipient muscle activation on the *uninjured* side (Images 2, 3, and 4), and task-based activities requiring recipient muscle activation on the *uninjured* side. In phase 2 of therapy, combined donor movement with bilateral recipient muscle activation may be performed (Images 5, 6, and 7). At the end of phase 2 and beginning of phase 3, the patient may complete task-based activities requiring bilateral recipient muscle activation (Image 8). The progression of these mirror exercises is based on the muscle strength of the recipient muscle and the skill acquisition of the patient, which are derived from the DAFRA rehabilitation approach [26]. This model suggests that patients must demonstrate evidence of motor return in the recipient muscle in order to perform bilateral movements during mirror therapy.

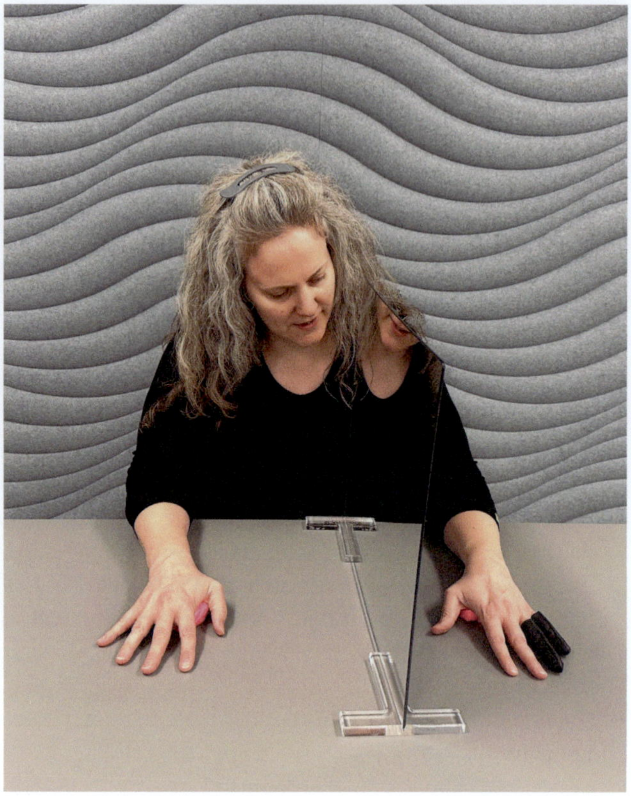

Image 1 MVF is depicted for Phase I following AIN to ulnar motor nerve transfer. The left hand, which is the affected upper extremity, is hidden from view behind the mirror. The patient gazes at the reflection of the unaffected upper extremity in the mirror during [1] bilateral isometric forearm pronation into putty with finger tube orthoses donned at affected ring and small fingers. The radial aspect of right and left palms rest on therapy putty

Evidence by Chen et al. reveals that following median and/or ulnar nerve injury, participation in mirror visual feedback results in greater improvement in grip strength, finger dexterity, and manual dexterity compared to classic sensory relearning [29]. Abolfazli and colleagues looked at outcomes of mirror visual feedback following general reconstructive hand surgery, which included cases of peripheral nerve injures. They found that when mirror therapy was combined with standard rehabilitation, patients experience significantly greater improvement in pain, perceived disability, range of motion, and dexterity compared to the control group [37]. In a study by Hsu, mirror visual feedback incorporating touch-observation and task-based activities significantly improved sensorimotor control and hand dexterity in patients with peripheral nerve injuries [38]. Mirror therapy has historically been used in the phantom limb population, reducing pain signals associated with amputation. However, more recent literature clearly highlights the impact of mirror feedback

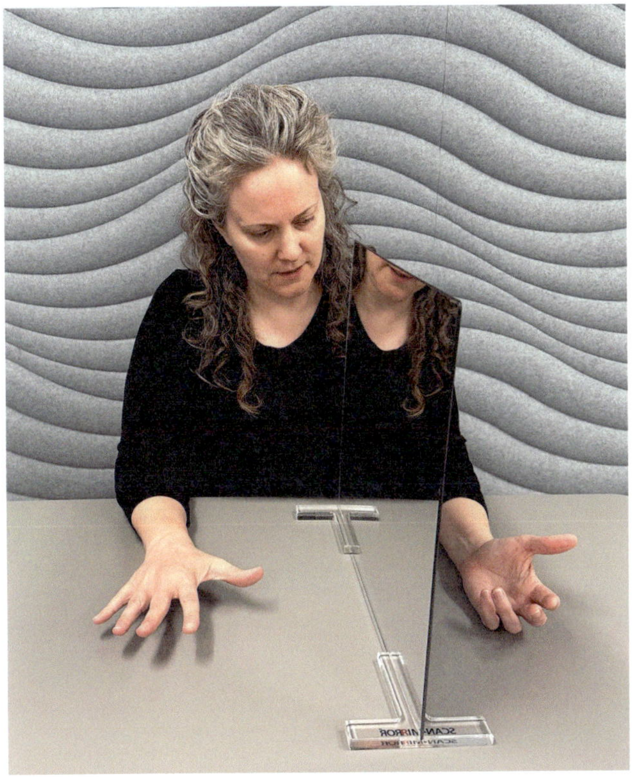

Image 2 MVF is depicted for Phase I following AIN to ulnar motor nerve transfer. The patient gazes at the reflection of the unaffected upper extremity in the mirror, completing *unilateral* donor activation (forearm pronation) with simultaneous active recipient movement: **finger abduction for dorsal interossei.** The affected upper extremity remains at rest, hidden behind the mirror

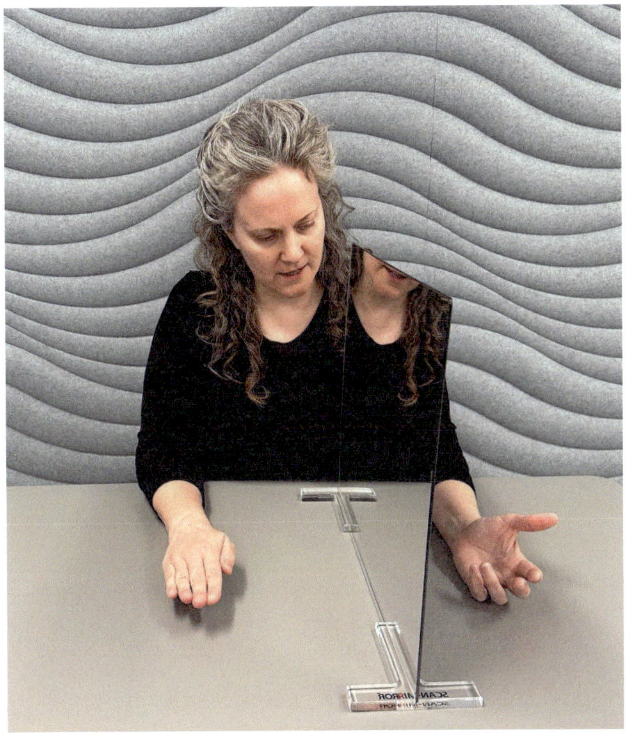

Image 3 MVF is depicted for Phase I following AIN to ulnar motor nerve transfer. The patient gazes at the reflection of the unaffected upper extremity in the mirror, completing *unilateral* donor activation (forearm pronation) with simultaneous active recipient movement: **finger adduction for palmar interossei.** The affected upper extremity remains at rest, hidden behind the mirror

on other more functional-related goals in the context of peripheral nerve injury, including dexterity, strength, range of motion, and disability.

Sensory Reeducation

This clinical manual provides rehabilitation guidelines specifically for motor nerve transfers, yet many surgeons perform sensory nerve transfers in addition to motor transfers. In the case of median nerve injury, for example, patients lose not only movement of the thumb, index, and middle fingers, but also sensation in two-thirds of the hand. Sensory nerve transfers take a healthy sensory nerve to a "less critical" area and reroute it to an injured nerve of a "more critical" area, providing tactile sensation and proprioception to a denervated area of skin [39]. For example, following ulnar nerve injury, the median nerve sensory fascicles of the third web space can be transferred to the ulnar territory of the hand, which can be argued as a more functional and crucial area of sensory input. Sensory nerve transfers have not been accepted by all. A recent systematic review revealed that they may lead to donor-site neuroma, long-standing neuropathic pain, ongoing paresthesia, and dysfunction [39]. In these cases, the concept of sensory reeducation is introduced.

Sensory reeducation, or sensory retraining, is a method used to improve sensory perception after nerve injury. It involves exercises and activities to stimulate the senses, such as touch, by helping the brain relearn and interpret signals directly [40]. Early sensory relearning programs are encouraged for the purpose of supplying the sensory cortex with relevant information to maintain the cortical map of the affected extremity [41]. It is important to recognize the possibility of limited or absent protective sensibility after a complete nerve injury. Therapists should educate patients on the risk of burns and frostbite and emphasize the importance of carefully watching the hand during use to prevent further injury.

Soon after peripheral nerve injury, a greater stimulus intensity may be necessary for the patient make a distinction between constant versus moving touch. However, during sensory reeducation exercises, the intensity provided should never evoke pain. Hypersensitivity to normal touch is common during this period. Desensitization is a method to gradually increase tolerance to tactile stimuli in patients experiencing allodynia and/or hyperalgesia [42]. Techniques may include texture discrimination, light touch discrimina-

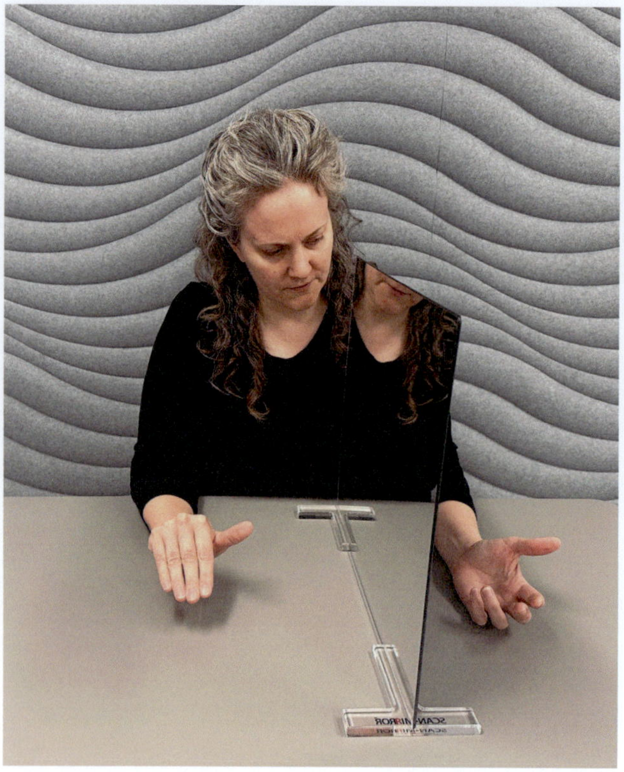

Image 4 MVF is depicted for Phase I following AIN to ulnar motor nerve transfer. The patient gazes at the reflection of the unaffected upper extremity in the mirror, completing *unilateral* donor activation (forearm pronation) with simultaneous active recipient movement: **intrinsic plus position for lumbricals**. The affected upper extremity remains at rest, hidden behind the mirror

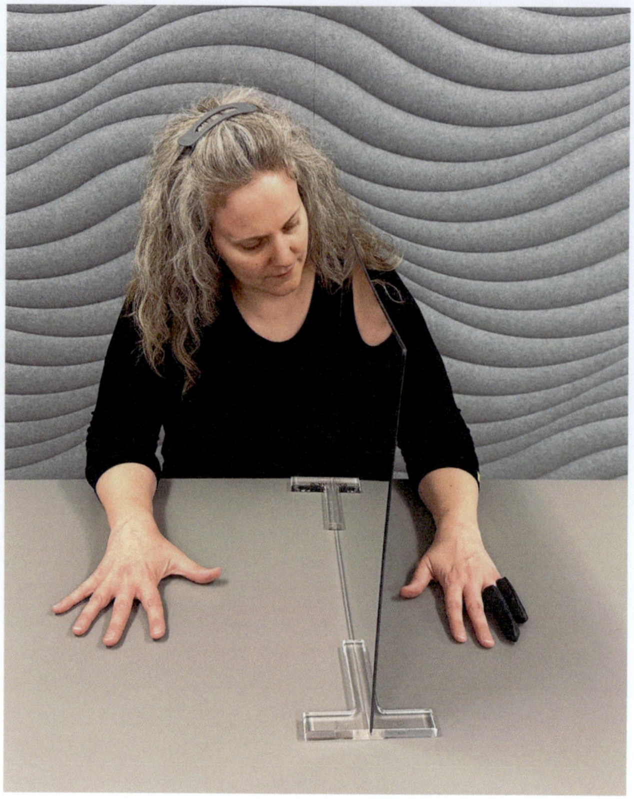

Image 5 MVF is depicted for Phase 2 following AIN to ulnar motor nerve transfer. The patient completes *bilateral* donor activation (forearm pronation) with simultaneous active recipient movement: **finger abduction for dorsal interossei.** Ring and small finger tube orthoses are worn to assist in maintaining IP extension

tion, massage with various textures, deep touch, and vibration. Evidence shows that following peripheral nerve repair, patients undergoing a formal program of sensory reeducation achieve better functional sensibility, in less time, than those without retraining [43]. Furthermore, Goransson and Cederlund found that after a 6-week formal desensitization program, patients experienced significantly decreased pain, decreased size of the sensitive area, and improved performance of daily activities [44]. However, this study was not specific to patients with upper extremity nerve transfer. Additional higher-level studies are needed to provide desensitization guidelines and functional outcomes for patients undergoing nerve transfer surgery.

Bilateral Movements

Incorporating bilateral movements into therapy after nerve transfer surgery may have several benefits, including improving adaptive neural plasticity, range of motion, coordination, symmetry, and neural coupling [45]. Bilateral touch activates both ipsilateral and contralateral cerebral hemispheres, supporting the concept that using the uninjured hand may provide accurate tactile information to the cerebral cortex, facilitating sensorimotor relearning [45]. During bilateral hand movements, an automatic reflex of activity takes place at both the ipsilateral and contralateral sites of stimulation [46]. Additionally, bilateral arm movements have been shown to induce large-scale neuronal activation [47]. Therapy exercises requiring bilateral arm movements are therefore fundamental to enhancing sensorimotor relearning and may be used in all phases of rehabilitation to augment skill acquisition over time.

Biofeedback

Use of biofeedback after nerve transfer surgery is cited in various rehabilitation guidelines to enhance motor relearning and promote cortical reorganization [24, 26, 28, 48]. Although the use of surface electromyographic (sEMG) biofeedback is included in rehabilitation guidelines, there are currently no high-level studies that demonstrate its effectiveness. Optimal frequency, duration of use, and timing of initiation are not well understood. Recommendations for use following nerve transfer surgery are similarly limited [28, 49].

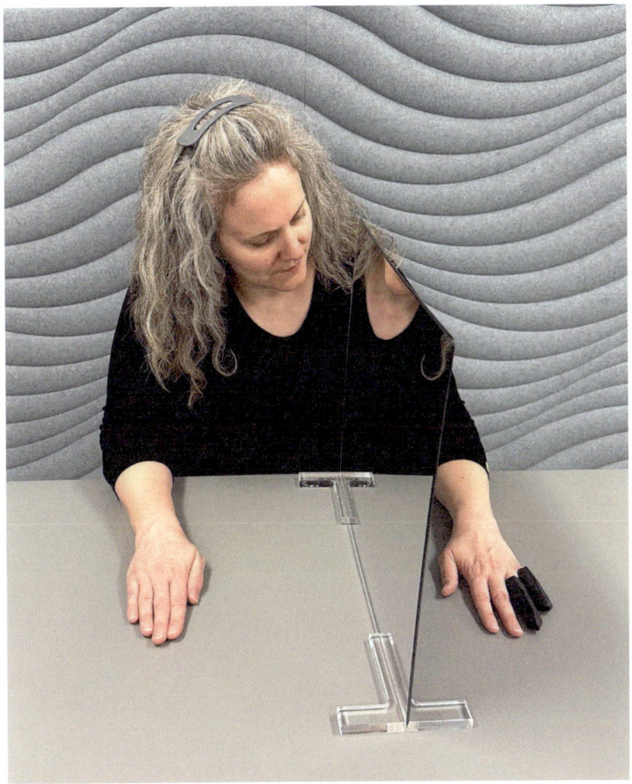

Image 6 MVF is depicted for Phase 2 following AIN to ulnar motor nerve transfer. The patient completes *bilateral* donor activation (forearm pronation) with simultaneous active recipient movement: **finger adduction for palmar interossei**. Ring and small finger tube orthoses are worn to assist in maintaining IP extension

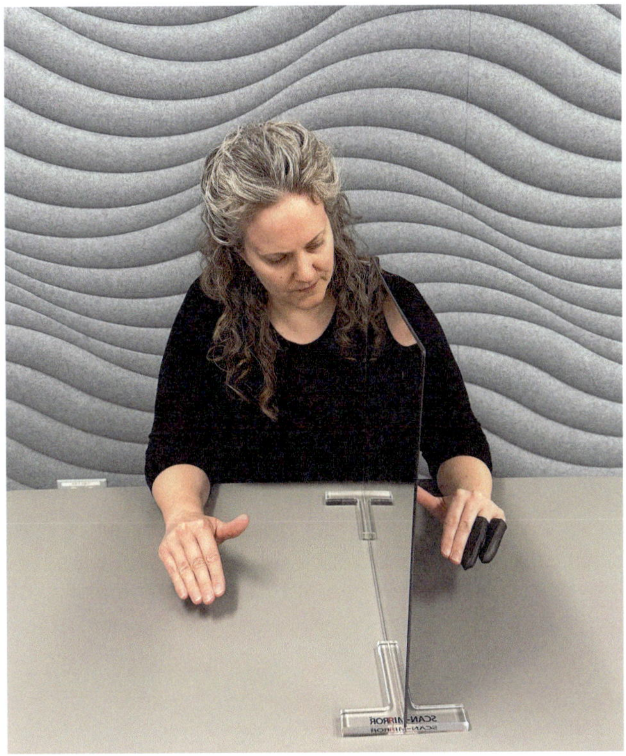

Image 7 MVF is depicted for Phase 2 following AIN to ulnar motor nerve transfer. The patient completes *bilateral* donor activation (forearm pronation) with simultaneous active recipient movement: **intrinsic plus position for lumbricals**. Ring and small finger tube orthoses are worn to assist in maintaining IP extension

Donor activation is an essential component of the early phases of therapy. Successful rehabilitation following nerve transfer surgery depends on obtaining selective reinnervation or the ability of the recipient muscle to obtain motor control without activation of the donor muscle [50]. Surface EMG biofeedback may be utilized in both scenarios (Image 9). Sturma et al. provide a surface EMG-guided rehabilitation process to assist with cortical remapping and offer valuable feedback to the patient when performing sensorimotor reeducation [28]. The approach Sturma describes correlates with the three phases of the DAFRA model [26] that are presented below:

Phase 1:

Characterized by the following:

- The recipient muscle is silent.
- There is axonal regeneration into the recipient muscle(s).
- Therapy emphasizes patient education due to lack of movement in the recipient muscle(s).
- There is early cortical activation of the formerly denervated area with mirror therapy, motor imagery, and observation of movements.

Phase 2:

Characterized by the following:

- There is axonal regeneration into the recipient muscle(s).
- First volitional contractions are noted.
- Guided sEMG training is facilitated to the donor to enhance cortical activity.
- sEMG facilitates awareness of the recipient.

Phase 3:

Characterized by the following:

- Treatment emphasizes the relearning of original movement patterns.
- sEMG is used to separate the donor from recipient (selective activation).
- Refinement of motor skills indicates the end of rehabilitation.

Three key points for therapists are illustrated below; sEMG biofeedback should be used:

- On the donor muscle to enhance cortical activity
- On the recipient muscle once trace contraction is noted

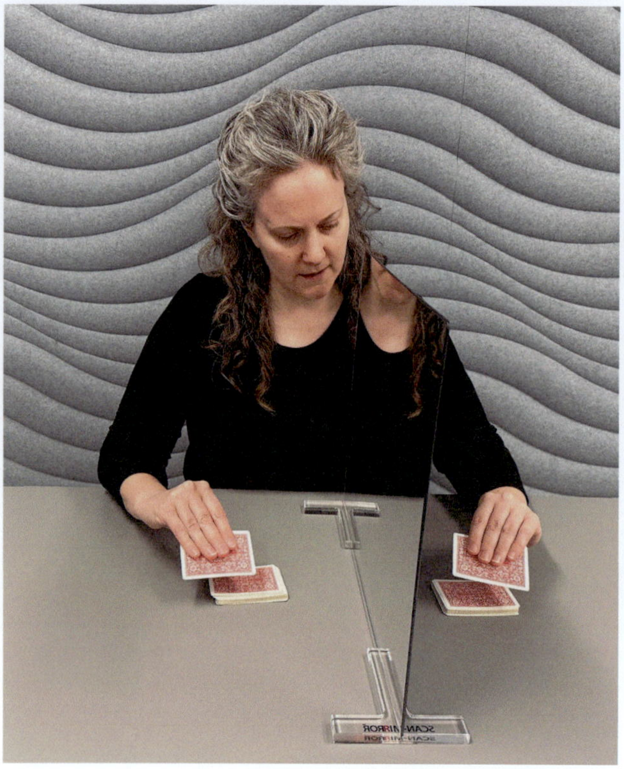

Image 8 MVF is depicted for Phase 3 following AIN to ulnar motor nerve transfer. The patient completes a *bilateral* task requiring donor activation (forearm pronation) with simultaneous recipient activation: intrinsic plus position using a deck of cards. The patient no longer requires ring and small finger tube orthoses to maintain IP extension

- To increase patients' ability to separate the donor from recipient (selective activation) after mastery of recipient activation is achieved

Therapists may not have access to an sEMG biofeedback unit in their clinic and therefore will use other methods of cortical reorganization, including all or partial stages of graded motor imagery, tactile/verbal/visual feedback, etc. Higher-level studies are needed to demonstrate the benefit of sEMG to allow therapists to advocate for purchase of a biofeedback unit in their clinic. As the healthcare landscape continues to evolve and reimbursements decline, therapists and surgeons struggle with the fact that the rehabilitation process is protracted for this population. As surgical advances are being made, rehabilitation approaches must also demonstrate efficiency and effectiveness to decrease healthcare costs in a population that will require prolonged medical management. In the absence of high-level studies, clinicians must rely on available evidence and expert opinion, which supports the use of sEMG in the brachial plexus population for successful rehabilitation.

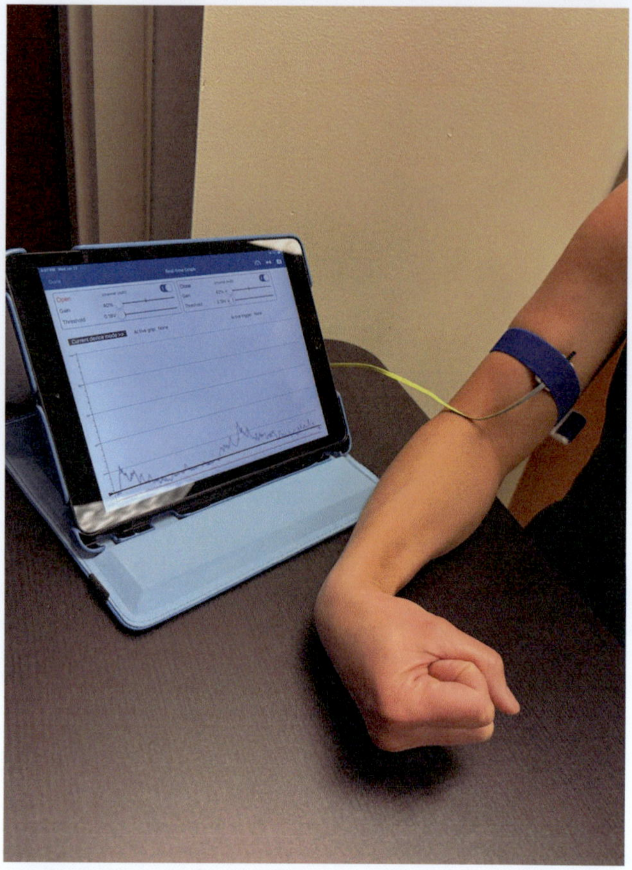

Image 9 Surface EMG biofeedback is performed to enhance motor re-education and promote cortical reorganization following nerve transfers

Neuromuscular Electrical Stimulation (NMES)

The use of neuromuscular electrical stimulation (NMES) has been shown to enhance muscle activation in neurologically intact muscles; however, its role after a peripheral nerve injury is contradictory. According to a recent literature review, the use of NMES as an adjunctive treatment for patients with peripheral nerve injuries, specifically after nerve transfers, has not been solidly established [51, 52]. Activation of paretic muscle groups affected by nerve injury with electric stimulation has been attempted for many years; however, there is conflicting research with a lack of pragmatic clinical protocols to support its use.

It is important to distinguish this research from that involving "nerve stimulation." There has been considerable support in the recent literature for *intraoperative* nerve stimulation. Electric stimulation of the peripheral nerve immediately following repair has been shown to accelerate nerve recovery and improve patient outcomes [53]. This is performed by the nerve surgeon while the patient is still recovering in the postanesthesia care unit (PACU). Note that nerve stimulation greatly differs from muscle stimulation.

Stimulation of denervated *muscle* requires direct current (DC) stimulators at parameters that may cause discomfort and, in some cases, burns on the skin [54]. (These often require the pulse duration to be 100–1000 times more than that which is used in innervated muscle for strengthening.) Some studies demonstrate the enhancement of nerve regeneration with electrical stimulation, yet others suggest that high frequency or increased use will lead to muscle fatigue and weaken the effect of nerve recovery, potentially exacerbating nerve damage [55, 56]. There is promising research to support the use of electric stimulation of paralyzed muscle in the peripheral nerve population, yet more research is needed before the findings in the animal models translate to human population in a manner that is safe and effective. It is important to note that NMES is usable in some instances in the spinal cord population where the volitional motor loss relates to an upper motor neuron (UMN) injury—proximal to the motor cell body (in the spinal cord). This preserves the ability to respond to alternating current (AC) stimulators that are typically seen in rehabilitation departments. In lower motor neuron or peripheral nerve injuries, however, the axon is injured, separating it from the cell body, triggering Wallerian degeneration and a cascade of chemical changes which limit the muscles' ability to respond to the standard NMES units (AC current stimulators) with a muscle contraction [57]. There are new muscle stimulation interventions on the horizon which show promise in augmenting exercise programs that promote recovery in denervated muscle. We look forward to future research to support this in the nerve transfer rehabilitation realm.

For the abovementioned reasons, it is not in the practice of the authors to use NMES during **early** phases of therapy following nerve transfer surgery. Without further evidence, standard NMES should not be utilized on denervated muscle that demonstrates no motor function. However, when muscle reinnervation is apparent, there may be some benefit for use of NMES to augment the motor reeducation program.

References

1. Socolovsky M, Lovaglio A, Bonilla G, Di Masi G, Barillaro K, Malessy M. Brain plasticity and age after restoring elbow flexion with distal nerve transfers in neonatal brachial plexus palsy and nonneonatal traumatic brachial plexus injury using the plasticity grading scale. J Neurosurg. 2023;139(6):1568–75.
2. Meek AW, Perez J, Poston B, Riley ZA. Cortical representation and excitability increases for a thenar muscle mediate improvement in short-term cellular phone text messaging ability. Brain Sci. 2021;11(3):406.
3. Lehmann N, Aye N, Kaufmann J, et al. Changes in cortical microstructure of the human brain resulting from long-term motor learning. J Neurosci. 2023;43(50):8637–48.
4. Socolovsky M, Malessy M. Brain changes after peripheral nerve repair: limitations of neuroplasticity. J Neurosurg Sci. 2021;65(4):421–30.
5. Socolovsky M, Barillaro K, Bonilla G, Di Masi G, Malessy M. Nerve transfers for brachial plexus injuries: grading of volitional control. J Neurosurg. 2022;138(5):1419–25.
6. Bhatia A, Kulkarni A, Zancolli P, et al. The effect of age and the delay before surgery on the outcomes of intercostal nerve transfers to the musculocutaneous nerve: a retrospective study of 232 cases of posttraumatic total and near-total brachial plexus injuries. Indian J Plast Surg. 2020;53(02):260–5.
7. Lee JY, Kircher MF, Spinner RJ, Bishop AT, Shin AY. Factors affecting outcome of triceps motor branch transfer for isolated axillary nerve injury. J Hand Surg Am. 2012;37(11):2350–6.
8. Sallam AA, El-Deeb MS, Imam MA. Useful functional outcome can be achieved after motor nerve transfers in management of the paralytic hand. An observational study. HSS J. 2016;12(1):2–7.
9. Wall JT, Kaas JH, Sur M, Nelson RJ, Felleman DJ, Merzenich MM. Functional reorganization in somatosensory cortical areas 3b and 1 of adult monkeys after median nerve repair: possible relationships to sensory recovery in humans. J Neurosci. 1986;6(1):218–33.
10. Merzenich MM, Kaas JH, Wall J, Nelson RJ, Sur M, Felleman D. Topographic reorganization of somatosensory cortical areas 3b and 1 in adult monkeys following restricted deafferentation. Neuroscience. 1983;8(1):33–55.
11. Wall JT, Xu J, Wang X. Human brain plasticity: an emerging view of the multiple substrates and mechanisms that cause cortical changes and related sensory dysfunctions after injuries of sensory inputs from the body. Brain Res Rev. 2002;39(2–3):181–215.
12. Taylor KS, Anastakis DJ, Davis KD. Cutting your nerve changes your brain. Brain. 2009;132(11):3122–33.
13. Davis KD, Taylor KS, Anastakis DJ. Nerve injury triggers changes in the brain. Neuroscientist. 2011;17(4):407–22.
14. Tajerian M, Alvarado S, Millecamps M, et al. Peripheral nerve injury is associated with chronic, reversible changes in global DNA methylation in the mouse prefrontal cortex. PLoS One. 2013;8(1):e55259.
15. Navarro X, Vivó M, Valero-Cabré A. Neural plasticity after peripheral nerve injury and regeneration. Prog Neurobiol. 2007;82(4):163–201.
16. Zink PJ, Philip BA. Cortical plasticity in rehabilitation for upper extremity peripheral nerve injury: a scoping review. Am J Occup Ther. 2020;74(1):7401205030p1–7401205030p15.
17. Malessy MJA, Van Dijk JG, Thomeer RTWM. Respiration-related activity in the biceps brachii muscle after intercostal-musculocutaneous nerve transfer. Clin Neurol Neurosurg. 1993;95:95–102.
18. Socolovsky M, Di Masi G, Bonilla G, Paez MD, Robla J, Cabrera CC. The phrenic nerve as a donor for brachial plexus injuries: is it safe and effective? Case series and literature analysis. Acta Neurochir. 2015;157:1077–86.
19. Liu Y, Lao J, Zhao X, Gao K. Comparative study of phrenic and intercostal nerve transfers for elbow flexion after global brachial plexus injury. Hand. 2016;11(Suppl. 1):21S–2S.
20. Malessy MJA, Hoffmann CFE, Thomeer R. Initial report on the limited value of hypoglossal nerve transfer to treat brachial plexus root avulsions. J Neurosurg. 1999;91(4):601–4.
21. Socolovsky M, Malessy M, Lopez D, Guedes F, Flores L. Current concepts in plasticity and nerve transfers: relationship between surgical techniques and outcomes. Neurosurg Focus. 2017;42(3):E13.
22. Rosén B, Vikström P, Turner S, et al. Enhanced early sensory outcome after nerve repair as a result of immediate post-operative re-learning: a randomized controlled trial. J Hand Surg Eur Vol. 2015;40(6):598–606.
23. Haldane C, Frost G, Ogalo E, Bristol S, Doherty C, Berger M. A systematic review and meta-analysis of patient-reported outcomes following nerve transfer surgery for brachial plexus injury. PM&R. 2022;14(11):1368–81.
24. Larocerie-Salgado J, Chinchalkar S, Ross DC, Gillis J, Doherty CD, Miller TA. Rehabilitation following nerve transfer surgery. Tech Hand Up Extrem Surg. 2022;26(2):71–7.
25. Eren T, Kuru CA, Harput G, Leblebicioglu G. Case-based report of graded motor imagery experience in traumatic brachial plexus injury: the art of moving without moving. J Hand Ther. 2024;37(1):161–9.
26. Kahn L, Moore A. Donor activation focused rehabilitation approach: maximizing outcomes after nerve transfers. Hand Clin. 2016;32(2):263–77.
27. Kahn LC, Evans AG, Hill EJ, Fox IK. Donor activation focused rehabilitation approach to hand closing nerve transfer surgery in individuals with cervical level spinal cord injury. Spinal Cord Ser Cases. 2022;8(1):1–9.
28. Sturma A, Hruby LA, Farina D, Aszmann OC. Structured motor rehabilitation after selective nerve transfers. J Vis Exp. 2019;150(e59840):1–11.
29. Chen YH, Siow TY, Wang JY, Lin SY, Chao YH. Greater cortical activation and motor recovery following mirror therapy immediately after peripheral nerve repair of the forearm. Neuroscience. 2022;481:123–33.
30. Parsons LM, Fox PT. The neural basis of implicit movements used in recognising hand shape. Cogn Neuropsychol. 1998;15:583–616.
31. Stralka S. Graded motor imagery. In: Skirven T, Osterman A, Fedorczyk J, Amadio P, Shin E, editors. Rehabilitation of the hand and upper extremity. Elsevier; 2021. p. 1410–4.
32. Lou L, Shou T, Li Z, Li W, Gu Y. Transhemispheric functional reorganization of the motor cortex induced by the peripheral contralateral nerve transfer to the injured arm. Neuroscience. 2006;138(4):1225–31.
33. Shen J. Plasticity of the central nervous system involving peripheral nerve transfer. Neural Plast. 2022;2022(1):5345269.
34. Moseley GL, Butler DS, Beames TB, Giles TJ. The graded motor imagery handbook. NOI Group Publications; 2012.
35. Priganc VW, Stralka SW. Graded motor imagery. J Hand Ther. 2011;24(2):164–9.
36. Walsh NE, Jones L, McCabe CS. The mechanisms and actions of motor imagery within the clinical setting. In: Textbook of neuromodulation: principles, methods and clinical applications. Springer; 2014. p. 151–8.
37. Abolfazli M, Lajevardi L, Mirzaei L, Abdorazaghi HA, Azad A, Taghizadeh G. The effect of early intervention of mirror visual feedback on pain, disability and motor function following hand reconstructive surgery: a randomized clinical trial. Clin Rehabil. 2019;33(3):494–503.
38. Hsu HY, Chen PT, Kuan TS, Yang HC, Shieh SJ, Kuo LC. A touch-observation and task-based mirror therapy protocol to improve sensorimotor control and functional capability of hands

for patients with peripheral nerve injury. Am J Occup Ther. 2019;73(2):7302205020p1–7302205020p10.
39. Duraku LS, Hundepool CA, Moore AM, et al. Sensory nerve transfers in the upper limb after peripheral nerve injury: a scoping review. J Hand Surg Eur Vol. 2024;49(8):946–55.
40. Dellon A. Re-education of sensation. In: Evaluation of sensibility and re-education of sensation in the hand. Baltimore, MD: Williams & Wilkins; 1988.
41. Rosén B, Lundborg G. Sensory re-education after nerve repair: aspects of timing. Handchir Mikrochir Plast Chir. 2004;37(01):8–12.
42. Rosén B, Björkman A, Lundborg G. Sensory relearning and the plastic brain. In: Skirven T, editor. Rehabilitation of the hand and upper extremity. 7th ed. Elsevier; 2020.
43. Daniele HR, Aguado L. Early compensatory sensory re-education. J Reconstr Microsurg. 2003;19(02):107–10.
44. Göransson I, Cederlund R. A study of the effect of desensitization on hyperaesthesia in the hand and upper extremity after injury or surgery. Hand Therapy. 2011;16(1):12–8.
45. Oliveri M, Rossini PM, Pasqualetti P, et al. Interhemispheric asymmetries in the perception of unimanual and bimanual cutaneous stimuli: a study using transcranial magnetic stimulation. Brain. 1999;122(9):1721–9.
46. Thomas FA, Dietz V, Schrafl-Altermatt M. Automatic gain control of neural coupling during cooperative hand movements. Sci Rep. 2018;8(1):5959.
47. Jang SH, Seo JP, Lee SH, Jin SH, Yeo SS. The cortical activation pattern during bilateral arm raising movements. Neural Regen Res. 2017;12(2):317–20.
48. Hill JL, Turner LC, Jones RD, et al. The stages of rehabilitation following motor nerve transfer surgery. J Musculoskelet Surg Res. 2019;3(60)
49. Deveza LA, Robbins SR, Duong V, et al. Efficacy of a combination of conservative therapies vs an education comparator on clinical outcomes in thumb base osteoarthritis: a randomized clinical trial. JAMA Intern Med. 2021;181(4):429–38. https://doi.org/10.1001/jamainternmed.2020.7101.
50. Novak CB, Von der Heyde RL. Evidence and techniques in rehabilitation following nerve injuries. Hand Clin. 2013;29(3):383–92.
51. Costello MC, Errante EL, Smartz T, Ray WZ, Levi AD, Burks SS. Clinical applications of electrical stimulation for peripheral nerve injury: a systematic review. Front Neurosci. 2023;17:1162851.
52. Piccinini G, Cuccagna C, Caliandro P, et al. Efficacy of electrical stimulation of denervated muscle: a multicenter, double-blind, randomized clinical trial. Muscle Nerve. 2020;61(6):773–8.
53. Juckett L, Saffari TM, Ormseth B, Senger JL, Moore AM. The effect of electrical stimulation on nerve regeneration following peripheral nerve injury. Biomolecules. 2022;12(12):1856.
54. Pieber K, Herceg M, Paternostro-Sluga T, Schuhfried O. Optimizing stimulation parameters in functional electrical stimulation of denervated muscles: a cross-sectional study. J Neuroeng Rehabil. 2015;12:1–7.
55. Haastert-Talini K, Schmitte R, Korte N, Klode D, Ratzka A, Grothe C. Electrical stimulation accelerates axonal and functional peripheral nerve regeneration across long gaps. J Neurotrauma. 2011;28(4):661–74.
56. Vanderthommen M, Duchateau J. Electrical stimulation as a modality to improve performance of the neuromuscular system. Exerc Sport Sci Rev. 2007;35(4):180–5.
57. Chandrasekaran S, Davis J, Bersch I, Goldberg G, Gorgey AS. Electrical stimulation and denervated muscles after spinal cord injury. Neural Regen Res. 2020;15(8):1397–407.

The Psychosocial Impact of Traumatic Brachial Plexus Injuries

Macyn M. Stonner

The implications of brachial plexus injuries (BPIs) extend far beyond the physical deficits of weakness, paresthesia, and pain. These injuries impact all aspects of patients' lives, including their work, financial security, sense of self-worth, confidence in their appearance, and psychosocial well-being. Even in the most optimal scenarios in which native reinnervation occurs without surgery or if timely nerve transfer is performed, upper-extremity function is never fully restored. Use of the injured arm will always be inferior to pre-injury function, and patients should expect multiple surgeries [1] and a 2–3-year recovery period. No matter how thoroughly this information is shared, patients are never fully prepared for the functional, economic, and psychological consequences that accompany a BPI.

Functional Impact

An epidemiological study in 2012 found that 98% of traumatic BPI cases affect males, and 90% result from motorcycle accidents [2, 3]. These injuries disproportionately affect those who are young, active, and in their prime wage-earning years. Patients with BPI maintain a high level of work disability even after years of surgery and dedicated rehabilitation. The surgery team from a high-volume brachial plexus center in Coimbatore, India, found that at 8.6 months from surgery, only 57% of patients were working. Of those who returned to work (83 out of 144 people), 59% returned to less physically demanding jobs [2]. However, patients who maintained some level of employment felt more satisfied and integrated with society [4]. Furthermore, this study also concluded that it took a mean of 6.8 months for patients to write with their affected extremity [2]. In a systematic review of the literature conducted as part of an economic analysis, Hong et al. demonstrated that 40% of BPI patients do not return to work, 27% return to work in a different job, and 33% return to work in the same job [5]. Surgeons and therapists should encourage BPI patients to maintain some level of community engagement during recovery [6]. This helps restore meaning and sense of self-worth. Furthermore, surgeons and therapists should consider the impact that the uncertainty of the ultimate functional outcome has on the patient's ability to adjust to life after BPI [7]. Patients who actively engage in their BPI care are less likely to express frustration about their experience and are more likely to accept the new functional status of their injured arm [7].

Economic Impact

Not only does the abrupt change in employment status contribute to financial stress, but the direct healthcare costs from the medical, surgical, and therapy providers do as well. One-third of BPI patients are at risk for catastrophic health expenditure after reconstructive surgery, demonstrating the substantial financial strain to the individual [8]. A 2021 study revealed that the median total cost of a single BPI case was $840,539 [9]. This includes both the direct healthcare cost and the indirect cost of lost wages. However, this study only captured privately insured patients, and evidence shows that a large portion of BPI patients have federally funded insurance. Bucknor and colleagues found that 25.9% of their cohort had Medicare or Medicaid, but when examining those treated through the emergency department, the percentage of government-funded patients was 39.2% [10]. Zeyl and colleagues found that 41.78% of their 23,755 BPI hospital admissions were either uninsured or had Medicaid or Medicare. They found that these patients also had significantly longer hospital length of stay (LOS) compared to privately insured patients, which clearly contributes to increased healthcare costs for an already under-resourced population. Furthermore, Zeyl revealed that postoperative rehabilitation

M. M. Stonner (✉)
Milliken Hand Rehabilitation Center, WashU Medicine, St. Louis, MO, USA
e-mail: macyn.stonner@wustl.edu

L. C. Kahn et al. (eds.), *Rehabilitation for Nerve Transfers of the Upper Extremity*,
https://doi.org/10.1007/978-3-031-92008-0_4

is the most expensive aspect of the direct costs following BPI surgery, and access to adequate therapy is imperative for optimal recovery. In the state of Missouri for example, outpatient occupational and physical therapy is not covered by Medicaid unless the patient is either pregnant or under the age of 21 [11]. Because a large portion of BPI patients have Medicaid, this poses a great barrier to accessibility to rehabilitation and increases the risk of poor functional outcomes [12]. Hand and nerve surgeons and therapists must advocate for improving coverage and reimbursement and should consider these barriers when treatment planning. Beyond the direct cost to the individual patient, there are indirect costs to society when patients are not physically or mentally able to return to employment. Hong et al. estimated that the mean total indirect cost for BPI was $1,113,962 per patient [5].

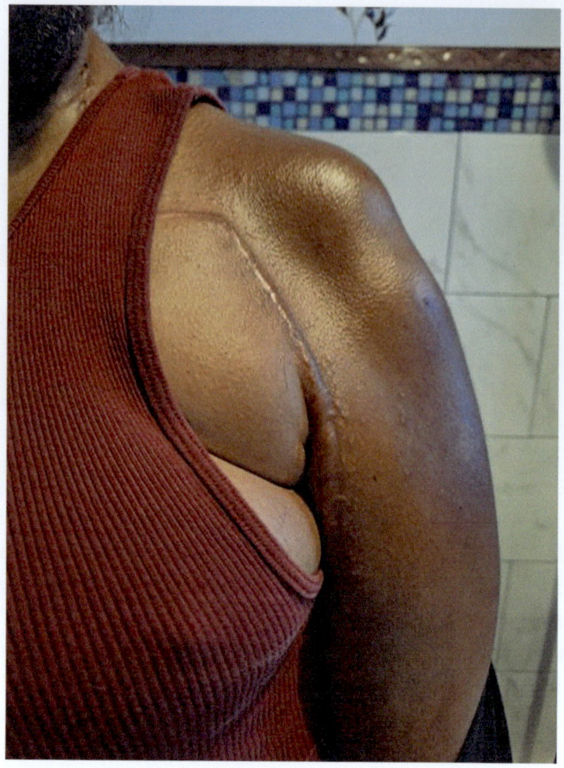

Image 1 Glenohumeral subluxation from a pan-plexus injury is shown anteriorly due to lack of deltoid and rotator cuff function to stabilize the shoulder

Psychological Impact

Patients with BPI are at increased risk of anxiety, depression, and strained relationships. Half of BPI patients develop either depression or anxiety after their injury, with one-quarter having symptoms of both depression and anxiety [13]. There are many contributing factors, including post-traumatic stress disorder (PTSD), neuropathic pain, and an abrupt change in functional and employment status [14]. As expected, there is an association between the magnitude of depressive symptoms and the severity of disability prior to BPI surgery [15]. Early identification of patients with depression provides an opportunity to treat these symptoms during the lengthy wait for reinnervation after BPI surgery.

More than 70% of patients with BPI develop chronic pain that is severe in nature [16, 17]. Neuropathic pain has a strong, well-documented relationship with depression and anxiety in the peripheral nerve injury population [18, 19]. Patients will often prioritize the management of their pain over the restoration of any motor or sensory function. They long for a moment without all-consuming pain over the ability to use the arm. Patients may describe the pain as an "intense itch" that is not alleviated by scratching or a hand that feels like it is on fire or "going to explode" from a burning pressure. These individuals have expressed a strong need for alternative options to the traditional pharmacologic treatments (such as gabapentinoids and opioids) to treat their neuropathic pain [20].

Shoulder subluxation is another potential source of pain that results from the heavy weight of the flail limb in the setting of inadequate muscular support. This may lead to traction on the injured plexus and/or excessive muscle substitution, resulting in severe neck and shoulder pain (Images 1 and 2). Some patients even request a forequarter amputation to eliminate upper extremity pain. Although this is relatively uncommon, amputation following pan-plexus injury has promising outcomes for a specific subset of

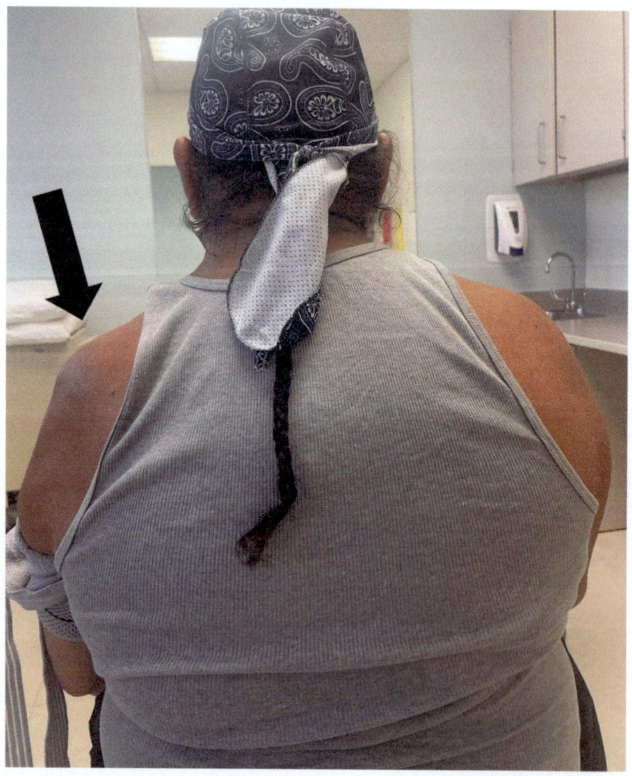

Image 2 Glenohumeral subluxation from a pan-plexus injury is shown posteriorly, highlighting the markedly depressed shoulder position compared to the contralateral side

patients [21]. Amputation may be an effective option for shoulder subluxation pain from excessive limb weight, but not for neuropathic pain given that the nerve injury (in the supraclavicular fossa) is proximal to the site of amputation.

A study by Landers found that 33% of their BPI cohort had suicidal ideation, and another study revealed that one patient who was a laborer with a pan-plexus injury did commit suicide [2, 22]. Traumatic plexus injuries create a clear psychological burden that warrants an interdisciplinary clinical team approach including social work, physiatry, pain management, pain psychology, and hand therapy (Image 4) [13, 14, 23].

Risk of Opioid Misuse

Because patients with BPI are often followed by multiple providers from multiple specialties, they have an increased likelihood of being prescribed opioids [24] even though opioids are considered a "third-line medication" for the management of neuropathic pain, after gabapentin and/or pregabalin followed by selective serotonin reuptake inhibitors (SSRIs). Patients with BPI are additionally at risk for misuse of opioids due to chronic pain, depression, anxiety, and socioeconomic challenges [13, 25]. A large US study of 1936 BPI patients showed that 27.7% of patients had prolonged opioid dependence (defined as continued opioid use between 90 and 180 days of BPI surgery) [26]. This is significantly higher than the 0.11% found in the study's control group. However, patients who were opioid naïve (did not receive opioid prescription within 1 year prior to surgery) demonstrated a postoperative opioid dependence percentage of 10.8%. Results demonstrate that BPI providers should recognize drug dependency risk factors in order to provide counseling, resiliency training, and mental health support as appropriate [27].

The Role of the Therapist

Hand therapists are in a unique position to address the psychological aspect of the brachial plexus journey. Therapists and patients benefit from more frequent and longer sessions than physicians. During 45–60 minute appointments, therapists may see patients preoperatively for a few weeks or months and then postoperatively for potentially 12–24 months. The professional relationship often develops into a friendship where patients feel vulnerable and share personal and sensitive information. Patients with nerve injuries view their hand therapists as a valuable resource for education and counseling about treatment options [28]. Although physical and occupational therapists are not licensed mental health professionals, they are equipped to provide coping techniques for the management of stress and pain. Additionally, therapists may guide patients in graded motor imagery (GMI), a three-stage treatment program that helps to improve cortical reorganization following peripheral nerve injury without inducing pain [29] (Image 3). This was originally created for patients with phantom limb pain but has evolved to also benefit patients with neuropathic pain and complex regional pain syndrome (CRPS). Recent evidence also highlights the unique potential role of the hand therapist in educating patients about safe disposal of excess opioid medication after upper-extremity surgery [30]. Lastly, therapists should address sleep positioning with their BPI patients as sleep quality is a significant predictor of disability and work performance among patients with brachial plexus injuries [6]. These patients struggle with sleep due to neuropathic pain, the heavy weight of the arm, and musculoskeletal shoulder pain from faulty positioning. A simple yet helpful sleep position is for patients to be supine with a pillow supporting the head and neck in a neutral position, a pillow supporting the upper arm in slight shoulder flexion with the elbow at or above the shoulder height, and a pillow on the abdomen to support the elbow, forearm, and hand (Image 4).

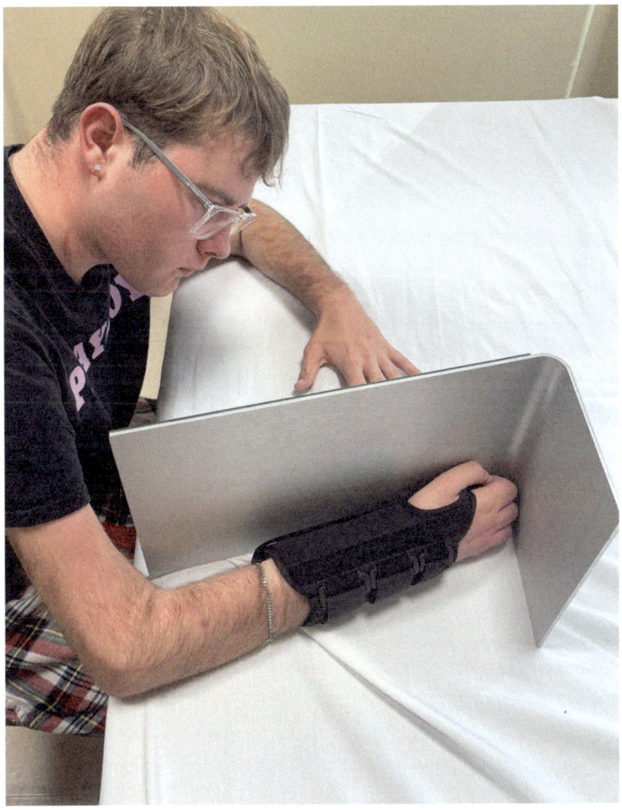

Image 3 Using a mirror, the patient looks at the reflection of his uninjured hand, while his injured hand is occluded behind the mirror. He performs bilateral hand movements in a pain-free range to improve cortical plasticity

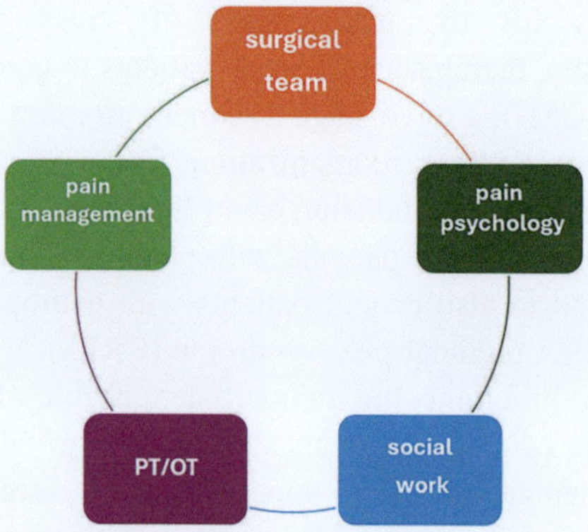

Image 4 An interdisciplinary team approach is recommended to address the multitude of psychosocial issues that may burden the individual with a brachial plexus injury

Clinical Implications

Brachial plexus injuries are clearly life-altering. It is important for providers to approach care with empathy. Physicians (and/or therapists) are often tasked with difficult patient conversations. These may include informing patients that their arm will never be the same, that their available surgical options are suboptimal, or that their EMG results suggest failure of the surgery. Difficult news should be delivered delicately and include the provider's acknowledgement of the devastating nature of their functional loss. Prior to surgery, some BPI patients have unrealistic expectations with regard to functional recovery and return to work [31]. Setting realistic expectations throughout the continuum of care is also helpful in minimizing disappointment. This begins after the initial injury and continues during surgical planning and throughout postoperative follow-up appointments. For example, patients should understand the timeline of nerve reinnervation and should expect a one to two+ year period of recovery. Coupling these realistic expectations with hope and optimism is also important. Patients with BPI benefit from ongoing care from multiple providers, including the surgery team, social work, therapy, pain psychology, and/or pain management. Having multiple providers with regular patient contact may help individuals feel heard while addressing an array of physical and psychosocial concerns. Additionally, this may make it more likely for providers to detect mental health concerns in a timely manner, communicate them, and refer patients appropriately to supportive services.

References

1. Jain DKA, Bhardwaj P, Venkataramani H, Sabapathy SR. An epidemiological study of traumatic brachial plexus injury patients treated at an Indian centre. Indian J Plast Surg. 2012;45(3):498–503.
2. Narakas AO, Hentz VR. Neurotization in brachial plexus injuries: indication and results. Clin Orthop Relat Res. 1988;237:43–56.
3. Songcharoen P. Brachial plexus injury in Thailand: a report of 520 cases. Microsurgery. 1995;16:35–9.
4. Terzis JK, Verkis MD, Soucacos PN. Outcomes of brachial plexus reconstruction in 204 patients with devastating paralysis. J Plastic Reconstruct Surg. 1999;104:1221–40.
5. Hong TS, Tian A, Sachar R, Ray WZ, Brogan DM, Dy CJ. Indirect cost of traumatic brachial plexus injuries in the United States. JBJS. 2019;101(16):e80.
6. Stonner MM, Mackinnon SE, Kaskutas V. Predictors of functional outcome after peripheral nerve injury and compression. J Hand Ther. 2020; https://doi.org/10.1016/j.jht.2020.03.008.
7. Dy CJ, Brogan DM, Rolf L, James AS. 'Being a patient the rest of my life'–the influence of patient participation during recovery after brachial plexus injury. J Hand Ther. 2023;36(1):60–5.
8. Kay HF, Buss JL, Keller MR, Olsen MA, Brogan DM, Dy CJ. Catastrophic health care expenditure following brachial plexus injury. J Hand Surg Am. 2023;48(4):354–60.
9. Dy CJ, Lingampalli N, Peacock K, Olsen MA, Ray WZ, Brogan DM. Direct cost of surgically treated adult traumatic brachial plexus injuries. J Hand Surg. 2020;2(2):77–9.
10. Bucknor A, Huang A, Wu W, et al. Socioeconomic disparities in brachial plexus surgery: a national database analysis. Plastic Reconstruct Surg Glob Open. 2019;2(7):e2118.
11. Missouri Department of Social Services. https://dss.mo.gov/dssdiv.htm
12. Stonner MM, Keane G, Berlet L, Goldfarb CA, Pet MA. The impact of social deprivation and hand therapy attendance on range of motion after flexor tendon repair. J Hand Surg. 2022;47(7):655–61.
13. Yannascoli, SM, Stwalley, D, Saeed, MJ, Olsen, MA, Dy, CJ. A population-based assessment of depression and anxiety in patients with brachial plexus injuries. J Hand Surg Am 2018;43(12):1136-e1.
14. Brogan DM, Osei DA, Colorado BS, Sneag DB, Van Voorhis A, Dy CJ. Team approach: management of brachial plexus injuries. J Bone Joint Surg Rev. 2022;10(4):e21.
15. Dy CJ, Brogan DM, Lee SK, et al. The influence of psychosocial factors on disability and expected improvement before surgery for adult traumatic brachial plexus injury. J Hand Surg Am. 2023;
16. Narakas AO. The treatment of brachial plexus injuries. Int Orthop. 1985;9(1):29–36.
17. Choi PD, N CB, Mackinnon SE, Kline DG. Quality of life and functional outcome following brachial plexus injury. J Hand Surg Am. 1997;22:605–12.
18. Suroto H, Putra RA, Karimah A. Relationship between disability and pain to post-traumatic stress disorder, depression, and anxiety in patient with postoperative brachial plexus injury. Br J Neurosurg. 2021;35(3):254–8.
19. Novak CB, Anastakis DJ, Beaton DE, Mackinnon SE, Katz J. Biomedical and psychosocial factors associated with disability after peripheral nerve injury. J Bone Joint Surg. 2011;93(10):929–36.
20. Smolev ET, Rolf L, Zhu E, et al. "Pill pushers and CBD oil"—a thematic analysis of social media interactions about pain after traumatic brachial plexus injury. J Hand Surg Glob Online. 2021;3(1):36–40.
21. Maldonado AA, Kircher MF, Spinner RJ, Bishop AT, Shin AY. The role of elective amputation in patients with traumatic brachial plexus injury. J Plast Reconstr Aesthet Surg. 2016;69(3):311–7.
22. Landers ZA, Jethanandani R, Lee SK, Mancuso CA, Seehaus M, Wolfe SW. The psychological impact of adult traumatic brachial plexus injury. J Hand Surg Am. 2018;43(10):950–e1.
23. Hill JR, Lanier ST, Brogan DM, Dy CJ. Management of adult brachial plexus injuries. J Hand Surg Am. 2021;46(9):778–88.
24. Jena AB, Goldman D, Weaver L, Karaca-Mandic P. Opioid prescribing by multiple providers in Medicare: retrospective observational study of insurance claims. Br Med J. 2014;348
25. Morris MT, Daluiski A, Dy CJ. A thematic analysis of online discussion boards for brachial plexus injury. J Hand Surg Am. 2016;8(41):813–8.
26. Kim N, Matzon JL, Abboudi J, et al. A prospective evaluation of opioid utilization after upper-extremity surgical procedures: identifying consumption patterns and determining prescribing guidelines. J Bone Joint Surg Am. 2016;98(20):e89. https://doi.org/10.2106/jbjs.15.00614.
27. Brito S, White J, Thomacos N, Hill B. The lived experience following free functioning muscle transfer for management of pan-brachial plexus injury: reflections from a long-term follow-up study. Disabil Rehabil. 2021;11(43):1517–25.
28. Lieberdorfer A, Shivakumar N, Stonner MM, et al. Expectant management, tendon transfer, or nerve transfer surgery for radial nerve injury: a qualitative study exploring patient expectations, goals, and treatment experiences. J Bone Joint Surg Am. 2023;105(8):600–6. https://doi.org/10.2106/jbjs.22.01201.
29. Bowering KJ, O'Connell NE, Tabor A, et al. The effects of graded motor imagery and its components on chronic pain: a systematic review and meta-analysis. J Pain. 2013;14(1):3–13.
30. Stonner MM, Skladman R, Bettlach CLR, Kennedy C, Mackinnon SE. Recruiting hand therapists improves disposal of unused opioid medication. J Hand Ther. 2023;36(3):507–13.
31. Mancuso CA, Lee SK, Dy CJ, Landers ZA, Model Z, Wolfe SW. Expectations and limitations due to brachial plexus injury: a qualitative study. Hand. 2015;10(4):741–9.

Rehabilitation Guidelines for Specific Nerve Transfers: Scapulothoracic

Pectoralis Major to Spinal Accessory Nerve Transfer

Lorna C. Kahn

Background

Injury and subsequent palsy involving the spinal accessory nerve (SAN) can lead to severe shoulder pain, weakness, and difficulty with overhead activity [1]. The SAN innervates the trapezius muscle. This large, triangular muscle is composed of upper, middle, and lower fibers. Upper fibers elevate the shoulder, middle fibers retract the scapula, and lower fibers upwardly rotate it together with the upper fibers [2]. The trapezius is a scapulothoracic (ST) muscle that acts with the serratus anterior muscle to stabilize the shoulder proximally and rotate the scapula on the thorax to assist with arm elevation.

The trapezius is "the only muscle in the body that elevates the lateral tip of the scapula" [3]. Because of this, following injury to the SAN, the force of gravity and the unopposed antagonistic muscles influence the position of the shoulder, forcing it into depression, protraction, and excessive downward rotation [4]. This alteration in scapulothoracic kinematics leads to moderate to severe pain and weakness with arm elevation. Most notably, the individual will struggle with arm elevation in the frontal plane (glenohumeral abduction). During glenohumeral abduction, the middle trapezius creates a strong adduction (retraction) force on the scapula that contributes to and enables shoulder abduction [5]. Shoulder forward flexion is typically partially preserved if serratus anterior function is intact.

The trapezius muscle has an unusual innervation pattern that includes cranial nerve XI with some lesser contributions from C3 and C4. The spinal accessory nerve passes through the sternocleidomastoid muscle and becomes very superficial through the posterior triangle of the neck before extending along the posterior thorax. This makes it highly susceptible to injury and trauma, such as with impact from a lacrosse stick to the shoulder. It is also very susceptible to iatrogenic injuries from procedures within the posterior triangle of the neck such as lymph node biopsy and neck dissection for tumor excision [3, 6, 7].

When laceration of the SAN is identified, a direct repair or graft procedure is typically performed [8]. The SAN is a long nerve that extends along the upper back to reach the lower trapezius muscle fibers. If the injury to the nerve is very proximal in the neck, the chances of a repair or graft reaching the lower portion of the trapezius muscle in time are unlikely. In these situations, or when identification of the injury is delayed, distal nerve transfers are a good option to restore trapezius function. There are several donor options described in the literature. This chapter highlights the pectoralis donors. The pectoralis nerve has two branches. The lateral pectoralis nerve is considered advantageous for its location and high myelinated fiber count [9]. The medial branch is considered viable for its location as well.

Outcomes

There is a paucity of outcome data on the pectoralis-to-spinal accessory nerve transfer. In one case study utilizing the medial pectoral nerve as the donor, Novak and Mackinnon reported recovery of 90° of shoulder abduction at 13 months postoperatively and full abduction at a 3-year follow-up. Mild shoulder pain remained [10]. Maldonado and Spinner describe a series of two patients undergoing lateral pec to SAN. Two and a half years after surgery, one individual demonstrated full shoulder abduction with mild compensatory movement and mild winging. The second case had a 6-year follow-up at which time the patient demonstrated 160° of shoulder abduction with mild winging but no pain [9].

L. C. Kahn (✉)
Milliken Hand Rehabilitation Center, WashU Medicine,
St. Louis, MO, USA
e-mail: Kahn.lorna.c@wustl.edu

L. C. Kahn et al. (eds.), *Rehabilitation for Nerve Transfers of the Upper Extremity*,
https://doi.org/10.1007/978-3-031-92008-0_5

Surgical Description [11]

Microsurgical technique of Pectoralis Nerve to the Spinal Accessory Nerve Transfer

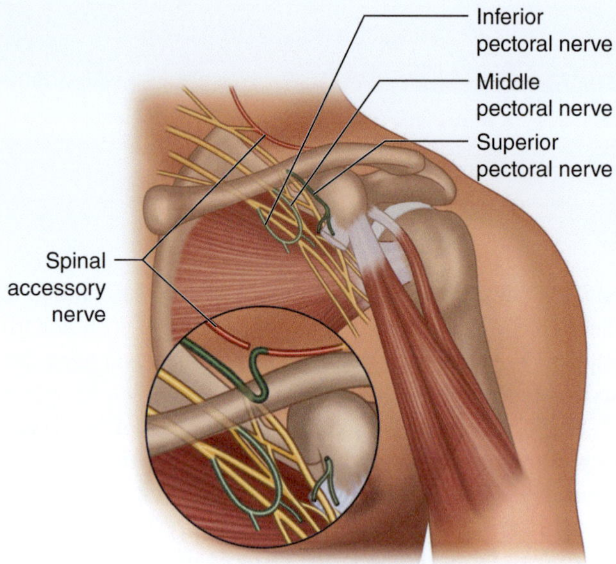

A transverse incision is made along the cephalad border of the clavicle. The platysma muscle is divided, and the omohyoid muscle is identified. While not necessary, it is helpful to preserve to omohyoid, as its trajectory is parallel to the course of the suprascapular nerve. The fat pad surrounding the brachial plexus is mobilized, and the upper trunk of the brachial plexus is identified. The upper trunk of the brachial plexus is identified and used as a guide to identify the C5 and C6 nerve roots more proximally. The C7 nerve root and its continuation of the middle trunk are identified, typically deep to the transverse cervical artery, which can be ligated at the surgeon's discretion. Internal neurolysis of the middle trunk into its posterior and anterior divisions is performed. A nerve stimulator is used to identify the division that primarily results in pectoral function. Further internal neurolysis of that division is performed to isolate a single fascicle that is both an appropriate size match for the spinal accessory nerve and predominantly results in pectoral function. The most medial aspect of the upper trapezius is released from the clavicle, allowing the surgeon to access the deep/posterior portion of the upper trapezius. The spinal accessory nerve is identified with the assistance of a handheld nerve stimulator, ensuring that the anesthesia team is not using any muscle paralytics. The spinal accessory nerve is then freed from the surrounding tissue, divided as proximally as possible, and transposed to meet the selected donor fascicle from the division of the middle trunk. Coaptation of the donor nerve to spinal accessory nerve is performed using microsurgical technique. It is important to note the relative rarity of this procedure and the importance of ensuring that sacrifice of a portion of the middle trunk does not substantially compromise the remaining upper limb.

Phases of Rehabilitation

Phase 1

Pre-op to 1/5 MMT in the Recipient Muscle

When the pectoralis nerves are involved as a donor or a recipient, it is imperative to see the operative note or discuss the case with the surgeon prior to starting therapy. In some cases, a tenotomy of the pectoralis major tendon is performed to access the nerves. The tendon is then repaired following the nerve transfer. While it is important to keep the region of the nerve transfer quiet for 2–3 weeks post-op, it is even more important not to stress the pectoralis major tendon repair to avoid additional impairment. In these cases, the individual should be placed in a shoulder immobilizer after surgery. They are typically seen in the physician's office 2–3 days later to have any drains or pain pumps removed. They may remove the immobilizer daily for hygiene, but precautions should be clearly outlined to avoid shoulder external rotation past neutral and abduction greater than 45° [12]. The distal strap of the sling should be loosened several times per day to allow the elbow to straighten to avoid ulnar nerve irritation. Protection of the pec repair (when applicable) with the shoulder immobilizer is recommended for 4 weeks [12]. When the pec tendon is not cut and repaired during the nerve transfer, an immobilizer or sling is recommended for the first 3 weeks to limit joint activity near the coaptation site and reduce the chance of developing edema or a seroma.

Positioning

Once the immobilizer or sling is discontinued, individuals will still benefit from some form of shoulder support. With a SAN palsy, the shoulder is likely to default to some degree of shoulder depression for many months. This position can lead to tremendous pain for many patients. Pain can originate from drag on the plexus, strain on the remaining muscles that are trying to work without the primary stabilizing forces supplied by the trapezius, and altered positioning of the glenohumeral joint with subsequent altered kinematics. Additionally, when the shoulder hangs in marked depression and scapular abduction, the denervated muscle is subject to significant and persistent stretch. This will put the patient at a disadvantage to adequately build force in the muscle as it reinnervates and attempts to contract [13].

Patients should be introduced to a variety of options to minimize overlengthening of the muscle and potentially altering the length and kinematics of the uninvolved shoulder muscles. Positioning with the arm supported in sitting with the arm on a table or pillow is the simplest option. When standing, a hip support device such as the type used by caretakers of infants/toddlers will provide a "shelf" to rest the arm on yet not cause patients to feel "closed in" as with a sling (Image 1). A standard sling is an option, but care must be taken to avoid developing GH joint restriction or pec tightness. If an individual is very active, a sling such as the Velpeau™ is recommended as it can be ordered with an immobilizing strap that comfortably stabilizes the arm to the body during activities such as running (Image 2). The Omotrain™ brace is also an option. It supports the weight of the arm with a snug sleeve and superiorly pulls the humerus closer into the glenoid. This allows for greater shoulder and elbow movement and is especially helpful as muscle function returns (Image 3).

Patient Education

Patient education is the main component of early therapy visits. Nerve transfer concepts are outlined, and donor-recipient nerves and functions are identified and frequently reviewed [13]. When setting realistic expectations, it is helpful to have a discussion of the anatomy and the length the nerve must grow following the transfer to reach the middle and lower trapezius. It may take a year before arm elevation is achieved in the frontal plane, and it may take more than 2 years to see the full outcome [9, 10]. Frequent reminders of this timeline will help to keep the individual motivated to continue with the motor reeducation program.

Passive range of motion (PROM) will be a rehabilitation priority in the second month following surgery. Three or four

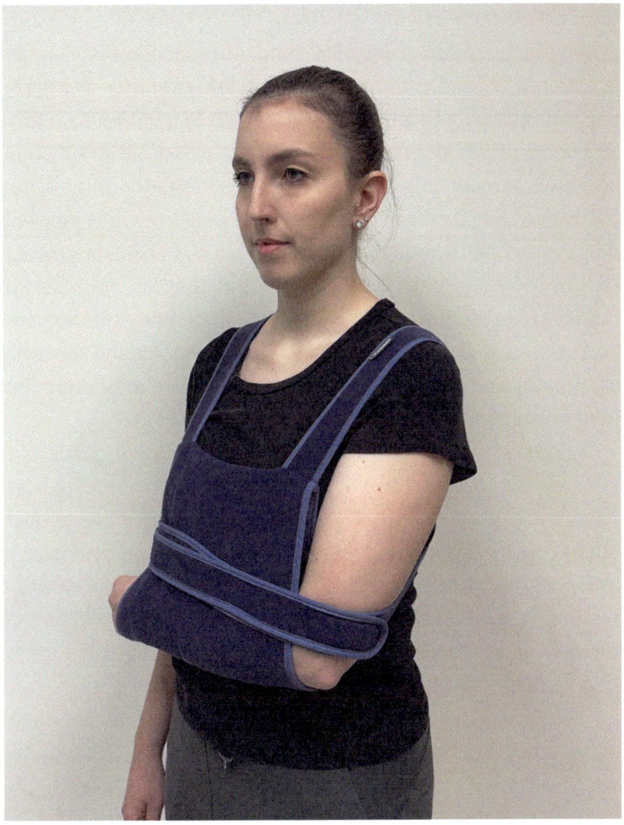

Image 2 The Velpeau® sling supports the weight of the arm and has 2 straps positioned over the shoulders to lessen the pull on the neck

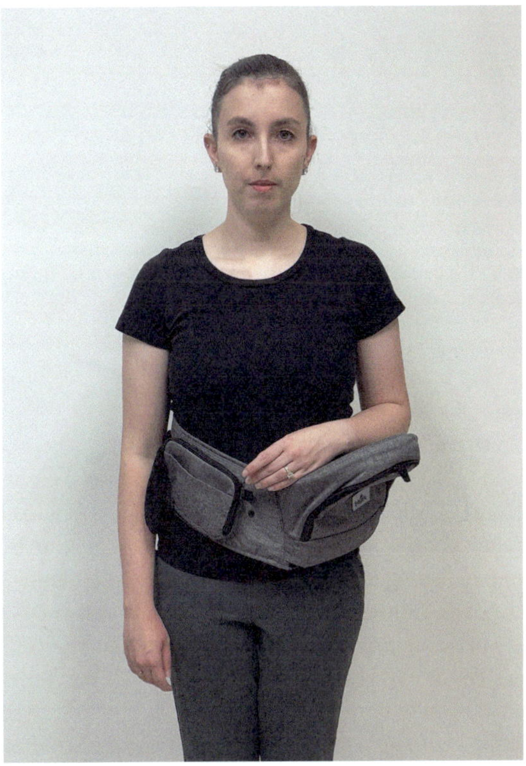

Image 1 To limit drag on the plexus and protect trapezius muscle length, a hip-based support such as those intended for toddlers and babies provides support to the arm

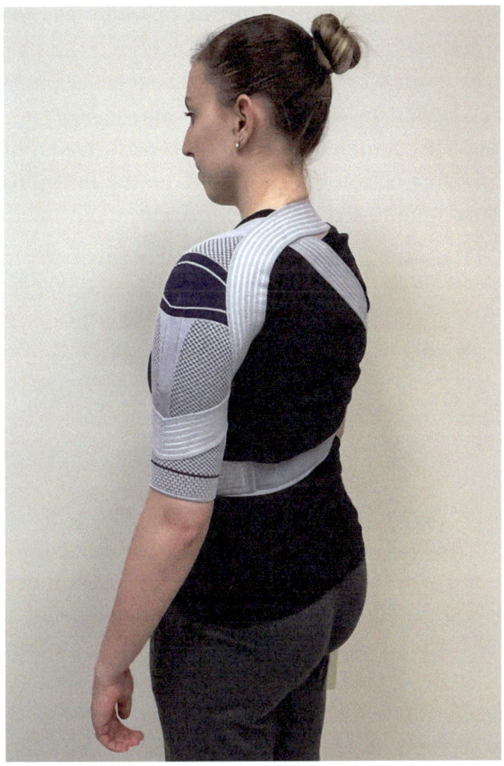

Image 3 The Omotrain® brace by Bauerfeind provides proximal support to the GH joint and scapula while allowing elbow and shoulder movement for those individuals with more arm function

weeks of immobilization will likely lead to some hypomobility of the glenohumeral joint. Heat modalities, gentle PROM, and active-assisted range of motion (AAROM) exercises should be performed until a functional range is met. In addition to supine and seated PROM exercises for the glenohumeral joint, some attention should be given to the scapulothoracic joint. If the patient has had the trapezius palsy for a long time, it is possible that the serratus muscle is excessively short. Persistent protraction of the scapula with a short serratus muscle can result in pain and length discrepancies in some glenohumeral muscles. Performing shoulder ROM in side-lying enables the therapist to monitor and passively assist the position of the scapula into upward rotation throughout the range (Image 4).

Edema management is rarely needed following this surgery if adequate positioning and behavioral modifications have been met. Kinesiotape™ may be helpful to reduce edema in the supraclavicular region where compression is not possible (Image 5). Scar massage is initiated once the wound is well healed. Therapists should avoid the use of metal scar tools in the region of neurotization to avoid irritation or injury to the fragile and superficial nerves.

The primary focus of phase one motor reeducation is donor activation [13]. The pectoralis major muscle is identified in the early visits with a focus on how this muscle is activated. The muscle is divided into clavicular and sternal portions. The upper/clavicular portion is innervated by the lateral pectoral nerve (LPN) with innervation arising from C5, 6, and 7 nerve roots. These upper fibers contribute to flexion and horizontal adduction, as with reaching for the opposite shoulder. The sternal portion is innervated by the C6, C7, C8, and T1 nerve roots. The lower fibers depress the shoulder and allow for horizontal adduction towards the opposite hip.

When a pec muscle/tendon repair is performed during the surgery, donor activation is **avoided for the first month**. In the second month, active pec motion or gentle isometrics are introduced. When the pec is not repaired, active and resisted donor activation may begin 3 weeks after surgery. Pairing of the active donor with passive recipient trapezius is initiated within the second postoperative month.

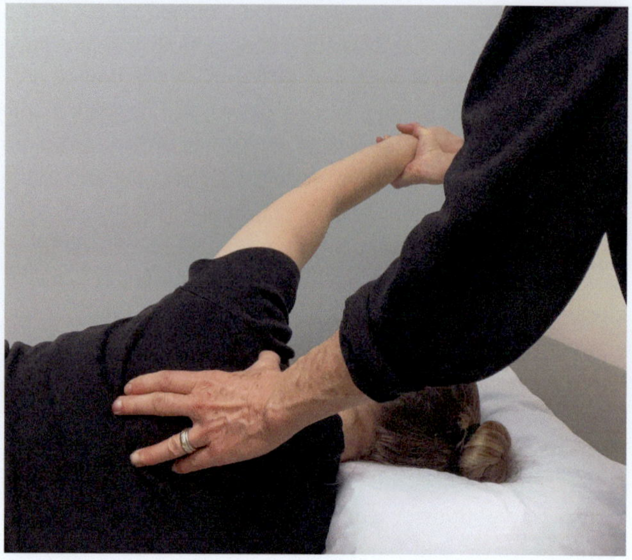

Image 4 Assisted shoulder ROM is demonstrated in side-lying with manual assist to the scapula into upward rotation

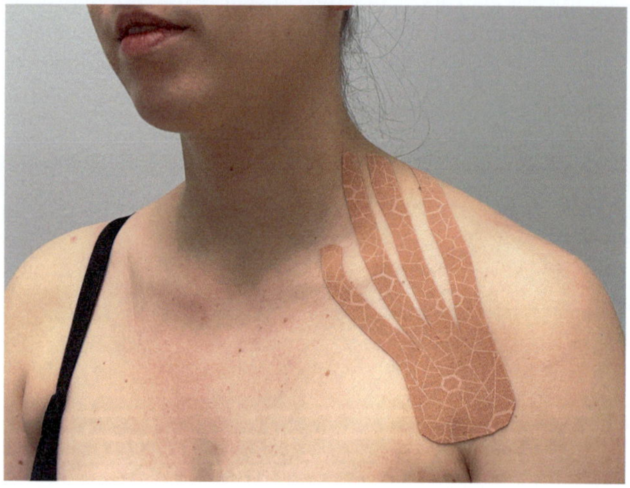

Image 5 Kinesiotape® may be used to reduce edema in the supraclavicular surgical region

Exercises

- ROM of Uninvolved Joints
  In supine or side-lying, shoulder PROM is performed by the therapist to regain any ROM lost during the immobilization period. If the pec has been cut to access the nerve transfer, this exercise should not begin until 4 weeks after surgery, and care should be taken not to injure the tendon repair [12]. Abduction and shoulder external rotation will put the greatest strain on the tendon repair. A home exercise program (HEP) highlighting PROM is vital to regaining passive motion, and compliance is encouraged. Seated table slides, supine dowel exercises, and pulleys are key components of a comprehensive PROM HEP (Image 6).
- Donor Activation
  A movement as simple as reaching across the body to touch the opposite shoulder or hip is discussed early on as a form of donor activation. Donor activation should be performed hourly. Resisted donor activation can be an isometric pec activation exercise. For example, with hands clasped in front of the chest, the patient presses the hands together. Hugging a large ball and pressing both hands into the sides of a large ball are other options for resisted donor/pec activation (Image 7). If the pec was cut/repaired during the nerve transfer, donor activation exercises should be delayed until 4 weeks postoperatively.
- Combined Donor with Passive Recipient Exercise
  If the patient can tolerate the prone position over a pillow, donor-recipient motor pairing can be achieved by pushing

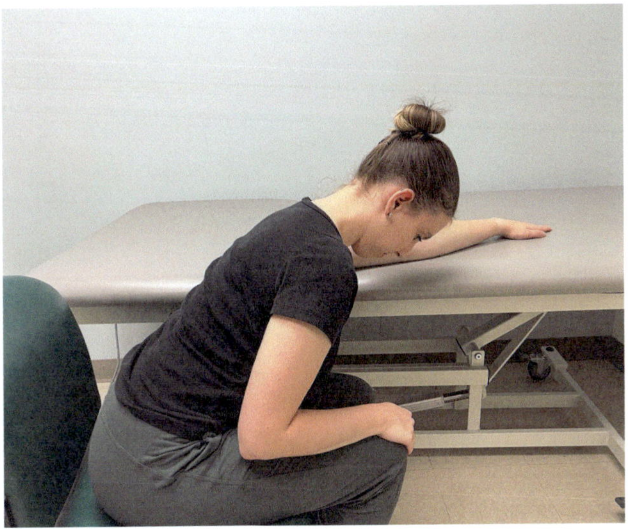

Image 6 Passive shoulder flexion is demonstrated. The patient is seated next to a table and slides the arm forward on the table while leaning forward

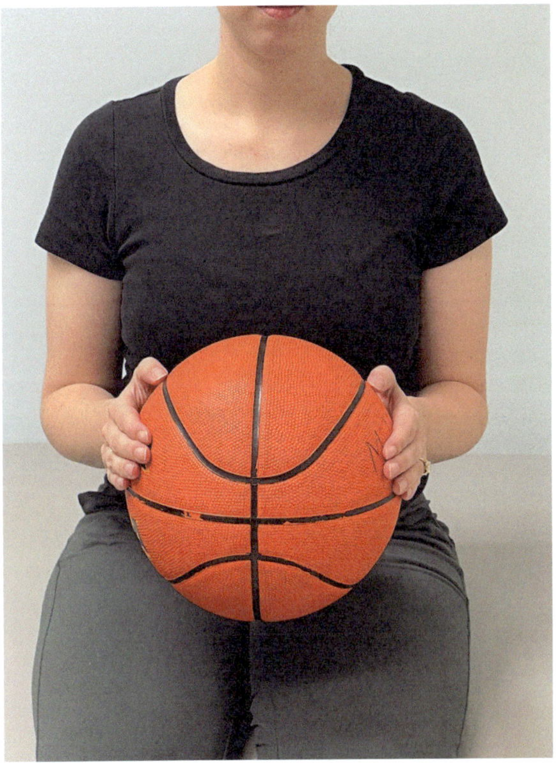

Image 7 Resisted pec donor activation is demonstrated with a basketball. The individual presses both sides of the ball medially to create pec muscle tension

down against the mat or floor (donor-pec activation) while sliding the arms forward to an overhead position. In the prone position, the effect of gravity is reduced, and the scapula is supported in a less abducted and depressed position than in sitting or standing. Initially, the therapist can hold the arm under the axilla and passively move the shoulder into elevation (towards the ear). At this time, some individuals may have developed a powerful, faulty movement pattern of shoulder depression using the latissimus muscle with efforts to elevate the arm, and it may take a great deal of counterforce and instruction to get the patient to relax the latissimus as the therapist attempts to passively shrug the shoulder (Image 8).

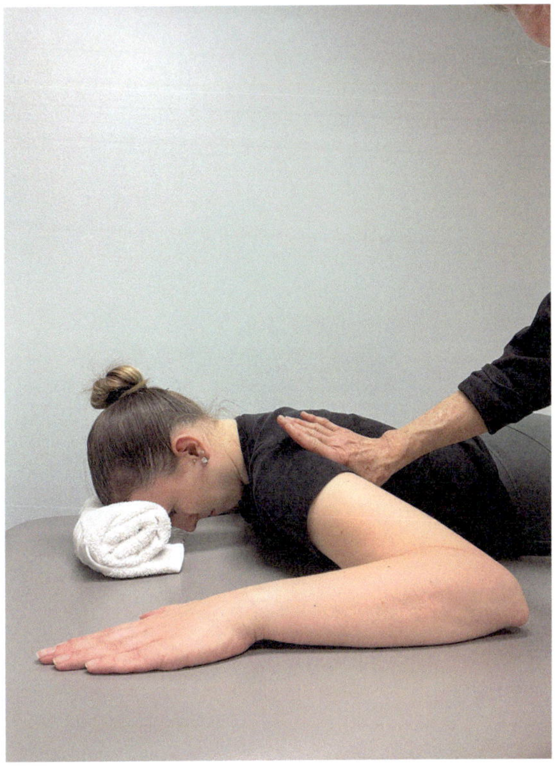

Image 8 Active donor with passive upper trapezius is demonstrated in prone. The individual presses against the table as the therapist passively shrugs the shoulder towards the ear

Alternatively, phase 1 rehabilitation for the middle and lower trapezius will require manually assisted passive scapular retraction and upward rotation during treatment sessions. Movement that combines active pec (donor) with passive middle trapezius (recipient) is performed in prone. The patient presses down on the table or ground and slides the arm forward while the therapist manually retracts and upwardly rotates the scapula (Image 9). The patient may also be positioned in side-lying with the involved arm over a large exercise ball. The patient presses down on the ball as he or she rolls the ball forward, passively moving the shoulder into flexion. The therapist may passively assist the movement of the scapula and shoulder in this position as well (Image 10).

Assessment of Recovery

Patients are typically anxious to see recovery. Evaluating recipient muscle recovery every month helps them better understand the nerve transfer and the rationale for their exercises. First, consider the path of the nerve through the top of the shoulder and distally along the scapula to the lower ribcage. The nerve

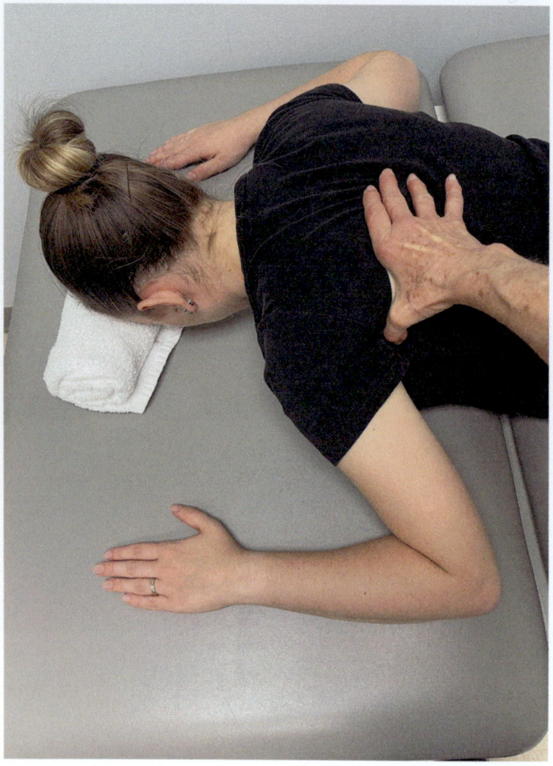

Image 9 Active donor with passive middle trapezius is demonstrated in prone. The therapist manually adducts/retracts the scapula as the individual presses into the table

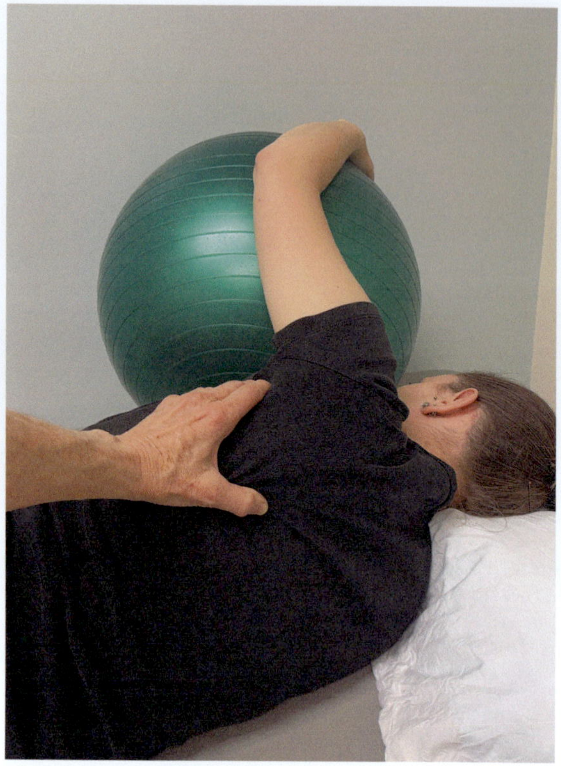

Image 10 Active donor with passive lower trapezius muscle exercise is demonstrated in side-lying. The involved arm rests on a large ball and pushes down while sliding it forward. The therapist manually assists the scapula into upward rotation

growth occurs in a proximal-to-distal direction, meaning the upper trapezius muscle will likely be the first to demonstrate signs of recovery, and the lower trapezius will be the last.

To assess the *upper* trapezius, position the patient in supine. Instruct them to reach across the body against the resistance of the tester's hand or against the opposite hand while asking them to shrug. Palpate along the top of the shoulder to the distal third of the clavicle (Image 11). To test the *middle* trapezius muscle, position the individual in prone and ask them to press into the mat to resist the donor while they retract the scapula bilaterally. Palpate between the spinous processes of the upper five thoracic vertebrae and the superior lip of the spine of the scapula (Image 12). This same position is used to assess for recovery of *lower* trapezius muscle, but the palpation will be between the lower thoracic vertebrae and the apex of the spine of the scapula [2] (Image 13).

Functional progress is also monitored with monthly, goniometric measures of active shoulder flexion and abduction in standing.

Therapy Frequency

The patient will likely need weekly or twice-weekly visits for at least 1–2 months to address PROM if the shoulder joint is significantly restricted. Once this is mostly resolved, and the individual demonstrates a clear understanding of all exercise instruction (including donor activation and donor-

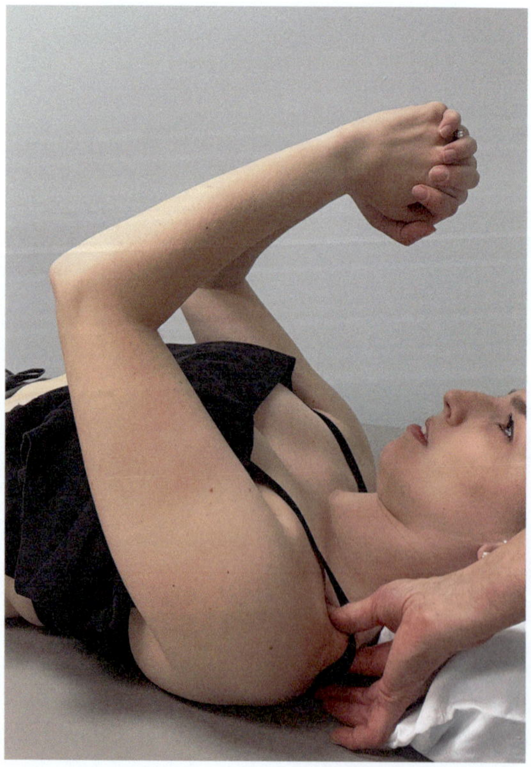

Image 11 Assessment of recovery of the upper trapezius muscle is assessed in supine. Horizontal adduction is resisted while palpating along the distal half of the clavicle for muscle tone or contraction

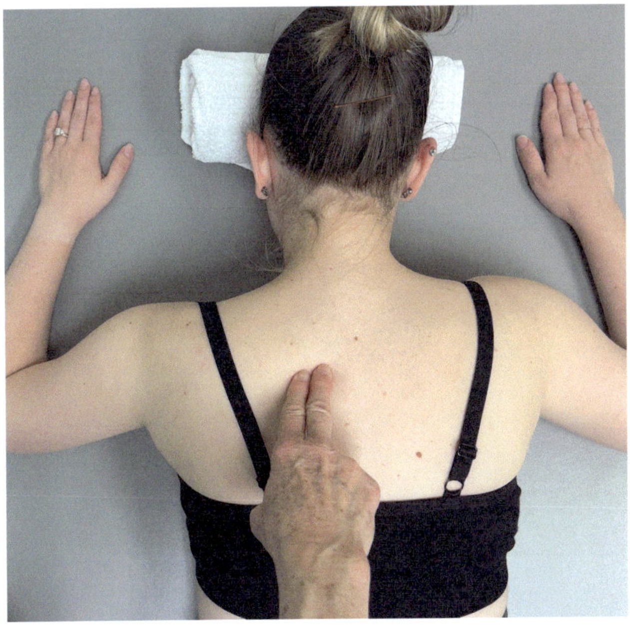

Image 12 Assessment of middle trapezius recovery is assessed in prone. The individual is instructed to resist the donor by pressing into the table as the therapist palpates between the spine of the scapula and the upper thoracic vertebrae

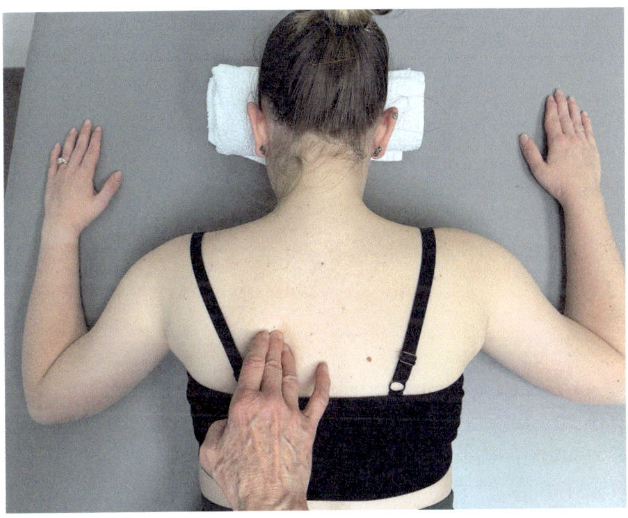

Image 13 Assessment of recovery in the lower trapezius fibers is performed in prone. As the individual presses into the table to activate the donor, the examiner palpates between the spine of the scapula and the lower thoracic vertebrae.

recipient muscle exercises), monthly (or twice monthly) visits should suffice.

Phase 2

2−/5 to 3/5 MMT in the Recipient Muscle

The trapezius muscle is essentially three muscle fiber groups, each with different but coordinating functions. Due to its length, the timing of recovery for each group will likely vary. The upper trapezius is the closest to the nerve transfer, so it will likely achieve each recovery phase before the more distal middle and lower divisions. Because the lower trapezius is the most distal, it will be at the greatest risk of having little or no recovery if the procedure was delayed for any reason. Progression of the motor reeducation program will therefore occur at different time points, but for simplicity's sake, all three will be described here together. Throughout most of this phase, all combined donor and recipient exercises will advance to active-assisted recipient movement and continue to be performed in supine, prone, and/or side-lying. This phase still necessitates scapular assistance from a therapist, friend, or caregiver.

Exercises

- Active Donor with Active-Assisted Recipient (Gravity-Minimized Plane)

Trapezius MMT = 2−/5 to 2/5

Upper Trapezius

In supine, instruct the patient to press their hands together while attempting to shrug. Assistance should be given to the shoulder by placing a hand in the axilla and pushing up, in the superior direction.

Middle Trapezius

In side-lying on the uninvolved side, support the involved arm manually or place it over a large ball. Have the individual press down to activate the pectoralis muscle while manually assisting the scapula to complete retraction (Image 14).

Middle and Lower Trapezius

In prone, instruct the patient to press into the mat while sliding the arms forward and outward ("V" position). Cues are given to retract and upwardly rotate the scapula. Manual assistance is given to complete this motion as needed (Image 15).

Upper Trapezius

In supine, the therapist manually positions the shoulder in end-range elevation while asking the patient to actively shrug bilaterally. Simultaneously, the patient presses his or her hands together for donor pec activation. The therapist releases the manual support as the patient attempts to independently maintain the shoulder shrug (Image 16).

Middle Trapezius

In prone with the elbows aligned with shoulders, instruct the patient to press his or her hands into the mat while attempt-

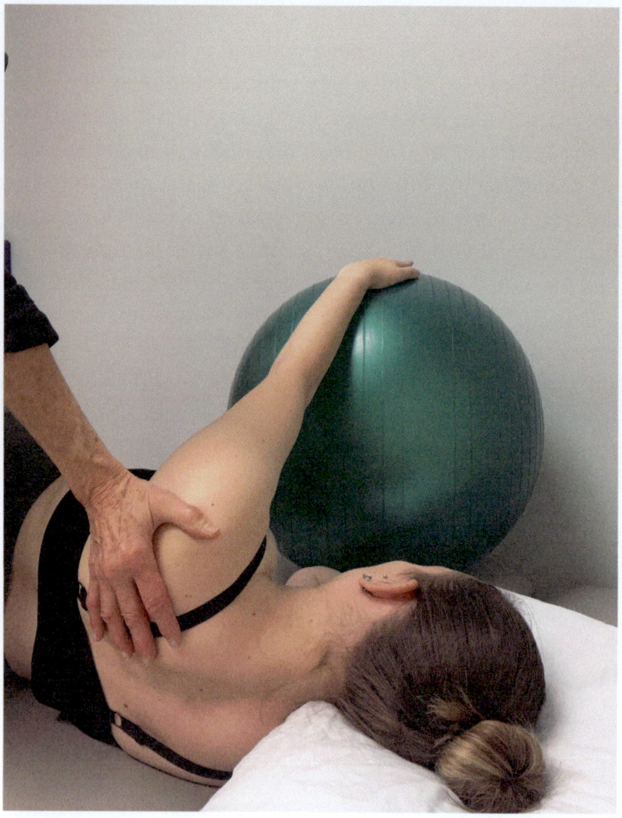

Image 14 Assisted scapular retraction/middle trapezius with donor pec activation is demonstrated in side lying with the arm resting on a large ball. While pressing into the ball to activate the pec muscle the patient is cued to retract the scapula while manual assistance is given to complete the motion

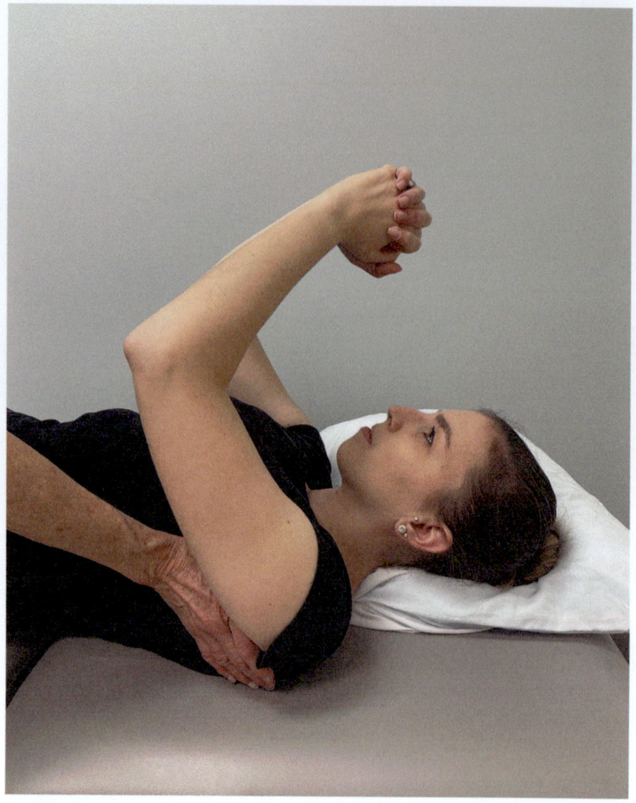

Image 16 "Place and hold" shoulder shrug is demonstrated in supine. The shoulder is placed in end range elevation/shrug while pressing their hands together to activate the donor. The individual is cued to try to maintain an end-range shrug (upper trap) as the assistance is removed.

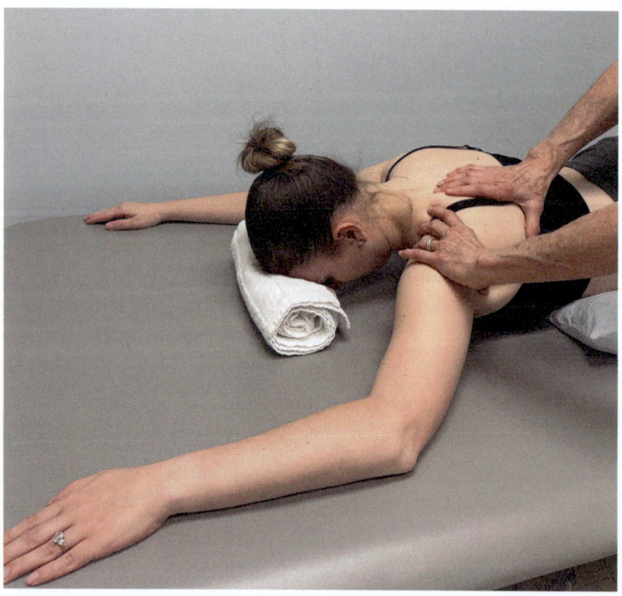

Image 15 Assisted middle and lower trapezius with donor activation is demonstrated in prone. As they slide the arms forward while pressing down on the table cues are given to move the scapula into retraction and upward rotation. The therapist may manually assist the scapula to complete this motion"Place and Hold" ExerciseTrapezius MMT = 2+/5

ing to raise the elbows. Manually assist the scapula into a retracted position. Release the manual support as the patient attempts to maintain this position (Image 17).

Lower Trapezius

In prone, the patient activates the donor by pressing down into the mat while sliding the arm forward. The therapist manually assists the scapula into full upward rotation and then releases the support as the patient attempts to maintain this position with pressure on the table (Image 18). This may also be performed in side-lying with the arm on a large exercise ball.

Upper Trapezius

In supine, the patient holds a small ball between the hands. Cues are given to press the hands together while he or she simultaneously shrugs the shoulders.

Middle Trapezius

Side-lying: The patient is seated with the involved arm on a shoulder height surface holding a taut resistance band (to resist the donor). The individual is cued to actively retract the scapula while maintaining tension on the pec

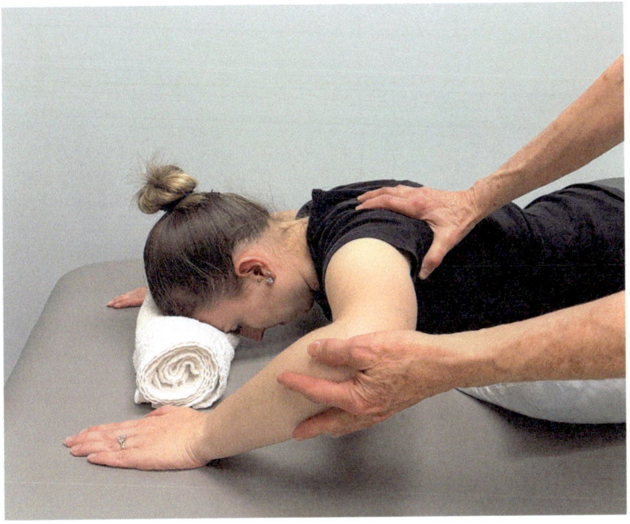

Image 17 "Place and hold" middle trapezius exercise is performed in prone with the palms on the table and the elbows aligned with the shoulders. The therapist manually assists the scapula into retraction while cueing the patient to press into the table and attempt to keep the elbows raised and the scapula retracted as the support is removed.

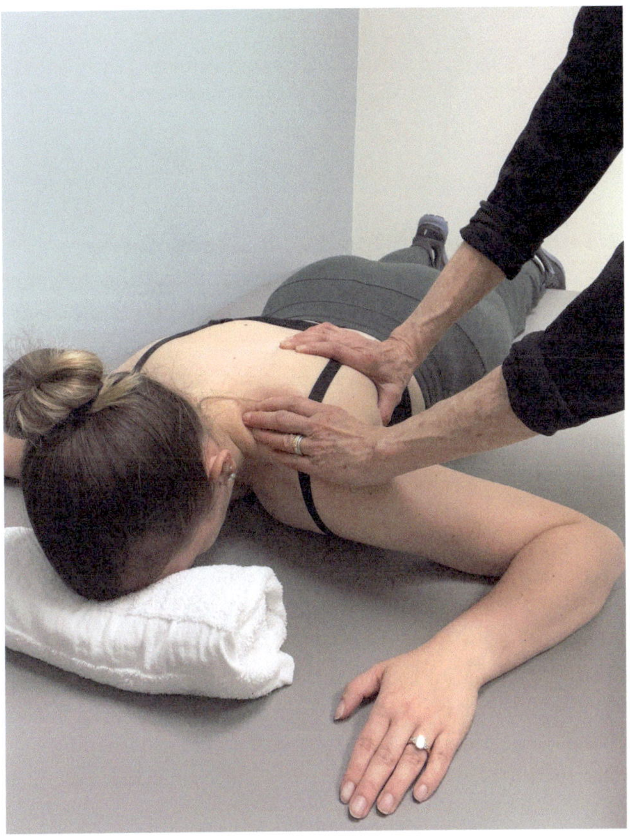

Image 18 "Place and hold" lower trap exercise is performed in prone. The individual is instructed to slide the arms forward while pressing into the mat. The scapula is manually placed in upward rotation then released while cues are given to attempt to maintain this positionActive (or Resisted) Donor with Active RecipientTrapezius MMT = 3−/5

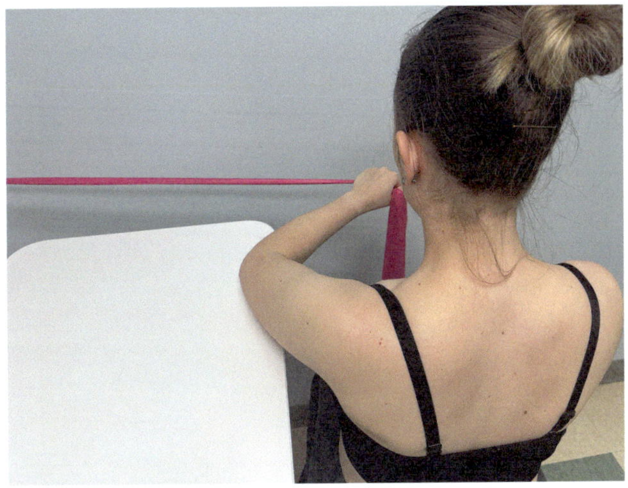

Image 19 Resisted donor with active middle trapezius muscle exercise is demonstrated in sitting with the involved arm at shoulder height. A taut resistance band is held to provide resistance to the donor pec muscle while actively retracting the scapula

(Image 19). Start with the shoulder in varying degrees of protraction to increase the distance the scapula will retract.

Lower Trapezius

Wall slides: In standing, the patient presses into a wall and slides the arms up into shoulder flexion (Image 20).

Upper Trapezius

In supine, place an empty container near the superior aspect of the shoulder. The patient attempts to move the container back by shrugging (Image 21). Consider simultaneously clasping hands together.

Middle/Lower Trapezius

By the end of phase 2, functional activities that incorporate donor and recipient function should be encouraged. For example, the patient stands holding a ball in both hands while reaching up and forward to place it on a shelf (Image 22).

Therapy Frequency

Given the complexity of exercises and the difficulty for patients to perform scapular assistance on their own, a frequency of once per week (or every other week) is ideal during phase 2. Given that this phase may last for a year or more, consideration should be given to the individual's financial and transportation constraints when making this determination.

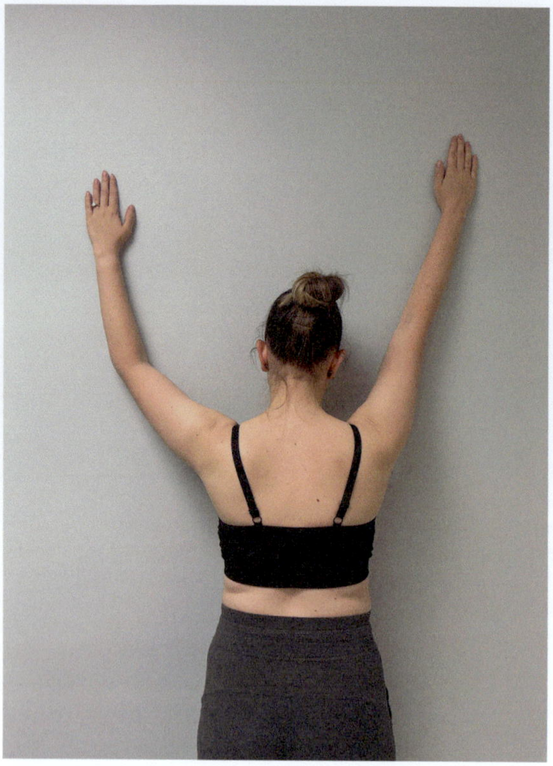

Image 20 Resisted donor with active lower trapezius muscle exercise is demonstrated in standing at a wall. The individual is cued to press into the wall while sliding the arms into flexion. Manual cues may be given to cue the scapula into full upward rotation

Functional Activity

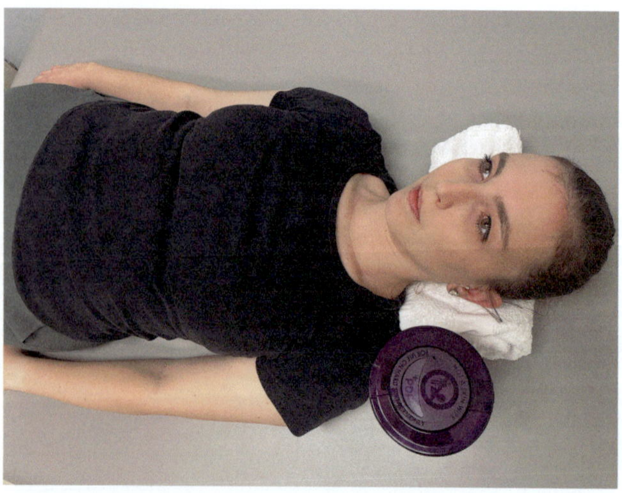

Image 21 In supine, the individual attempts to move the container by actively shrugging

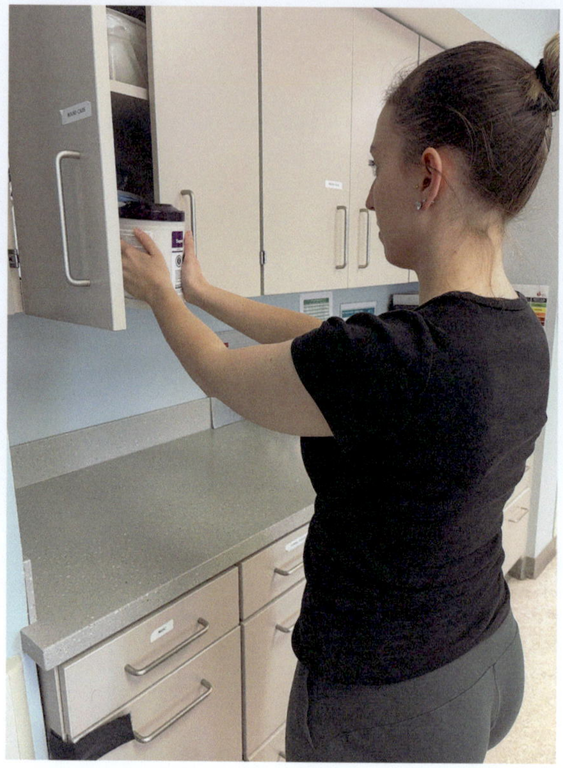

Image 22 Functional activities like placing items on a shelf with two hands encourages donor and recipient muscle activation.

Phase 3

3/5+ or Greater MMT in the Recipient Muscle

Once full scapular upward rotation and retraction are noted in a gravity-minimized plane, the exercise program expands to include exercises in seated and standing positions. At this time, active arm elevation should be significantly improved, and overhead activities are permitted. Fatigue will remain a limiting factor for many months at this point, and patients should be discouraged from using the arm overhead in a sustained or repetitive manner. The main concern is avoiding excessive fatigue in the muscle. Additionally, over-demand of the shoulder may result in cervical strain as patients attempt to substitute with cervical muscles.

Exercises

- Resistive Recipient Activity with Donor Contraction

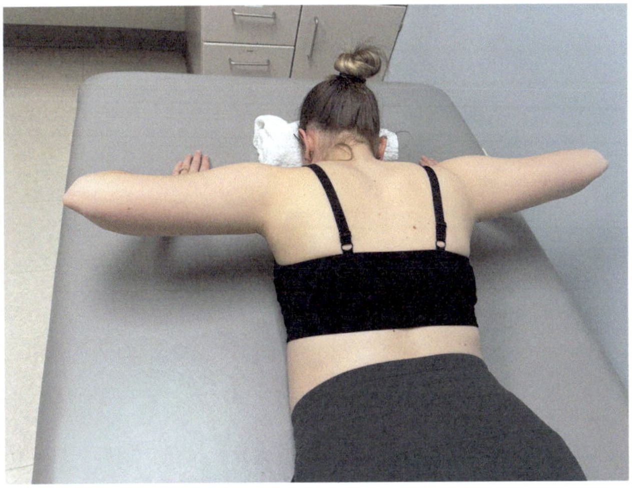

Image 23 Prone elbow raises with pressure into the mat provides resistance to the middle trapezius with donor activation.

Upper Trapezius

In sitting or standing, the patient presses the hands together while shrugging the shoulders against gravity towards his or her ears.

Middle Trapezius

In prone with the hands next to the patient's head (and the shoulder abducted to 90–95°), he or she presses down while raising the elbows with cues to retract the scapula (Image 23).

Lower Trapezius

In standing, the patient faces a wall with the elbows bent and both hands pressing into the wall with the ulnar aspect of the hands. The patient slides the arms overhead into a "V" or "Y" position while maintaining pressure on the wall. Cues are given to lift off the wall at end range (Image 24).

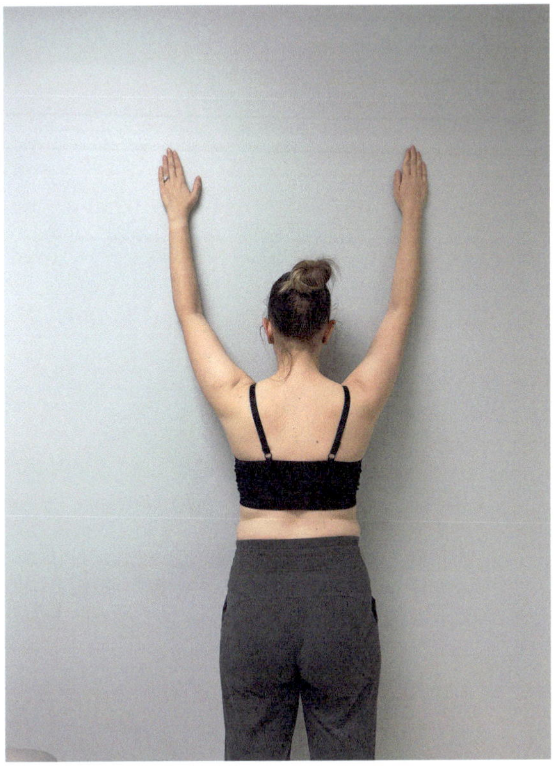

Image 24 Wall slides with a "lift off" is demonstrated for middle and lower trapezius strengthening. By instructing the person to press into the wall while sliding, greater donor assistance may be provided.Resistive recipient activity without donor contraction:As strength improves, donor muscle co-contraction will no longer be necessary

Upper Trapezius

The patient stands while holding a 1# weight in each hand while shrugging the shoulders.

Middle Trapezius

In prone, the patient is positioned with the arm off the edge of the mat with the elbow fully extended and the shoulder externally rotated (thumb up). The patient is instructed to raise the arm to the height of the mat at an angle of 95° of shoulder abduction. Cues are given to ensure that much of this motion is occurring with scapular retraction, not only with glenohumeral horizontal abduction. Light free weights may gradually be added to this exercise (Image 25).

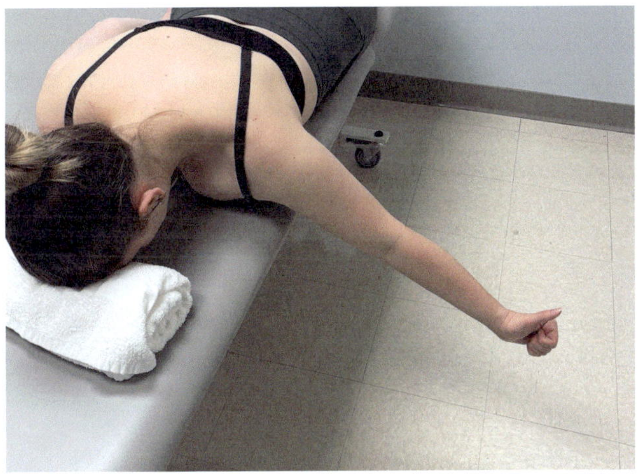

Image 25 Resisted middle trap without donor activation is demonstrated in prone with the arm off the table edge. The person is cued to keep the elbow straight and the shoulder externally rotated while raising the arm out to the side at approximately 90-95° of flexion.

Lower Trapezius

In prone, the patient is positioned with the arm off the edge of the mat, the elbow fully extended, and the shoulder externally rotated (thumb up). The patient is instructed to raise the arm to the height of the mat at an angle of 130° of shoulder abduction (Image 26). Light weight may gradually be added to increase the challenge.

Image 26 Resisted lower trap without donor activation is demonstrated in prone with the arm off the table edge. The person is cued to keep the elbow straight and the shoulder externally rotated while raising the arm forward and out (approximately 130°)

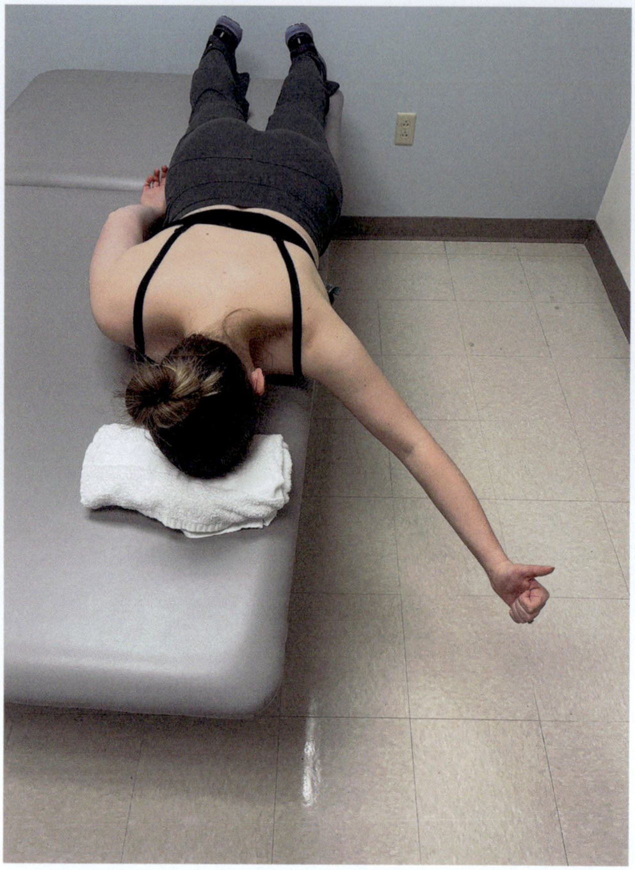

Therapy Frequency

With adequate compliance to the home exercise program, frequency of visits in phase 3 may be limited to once every 2–4 weeks with the expectation of continued slow recovery of strength, endurance, and function.

C7/Pectoralis nerve to Spinal Accessory nerve transfer

Nerve transfer overview					
Donor nerve	Donor action	Recipient nerve	Recipient action	Indications for functional restoration	Approximate months to functional movement
Lateral and/or medial pectoral nerves	Shoulder flexion and horizontal adduction	Spinal accessory nerve	Scapular elevation, retraction, and upward rotation	Loss of scapular stability from spinal accessory nerve palsy	Data not available

Information below are suggested guidelines. Precautions may vary according to surgeon preferences and patient factors

	Preoperative therapy	Early phase	Middle phase	Late phase
Criteria	Before surgery	0/5–1/5 MMT	2-/5 to 3/5 MMT	>3/5 MMT
Purpose of Phase	Educate and establish baseline function	Understand donor and recipient relationship	Consistently activate recipient	Strengthen recipient and separate from donor activation
Precautions	Prevent scapulothoracic and glenohumeral joint hypomobility	Avoid external rotation past neutral and abduction to 45° for the first 3 weeks post operatively. Support scapulothoracic and glenohumeral joint to minimize pain with scapular winging	Respect fatigue Exercises remain in gravity-minimized planes: supine, side-lying, or prone	Sitting and standing exercises are now permitted Avoid sustained overhead activities
Frequency of visits (considerations)	4–6 pre-op visits	1–2×/week until PROM is WNL and patient is independent with donor activation; then 1x monthly	1–2× per week to 1–2× per month based on shoulder or scapular hypomobility, patient needs and accurate, consistent demonstration of exercise program	1× every 1–2 weeks based on progress toward patient-specific goals
Orthosis considerations	To minimize pain and drag on the plexus, consider the Velpeau sling®, Omotrain® brace, or infant/toddler hip seat.	Full-time sling use for 2–3 weeks If a pec major tenotomy was performed, sling use for 4 weeks	Intermittent use of scapular and shoulder supports, such as the Omotrain®brace, Kinesiotape®, and low-profile sling options	NA
Interventions	PROM of the scapula: retraction, elevation, and upward rotation PROM of the glenohumeral joint	**Donor Activation**: Shoulder flexion and horizontal adduction **Donor-Recipient Pairing**: Isometric shoulder adduction combined with passive scapular elevation, retraction, and upward rotation	**Active/Resisted Donor with Active Assisted Recipient**: Gravity minimized plane: isometric horizontal adduction with therapist-assisted scapular elevation, retraction, and upward rotation **Place and Hold**: Gravity minimized plane: isometric horizontal adduction is coupled with therapist-assisted scapular elevation, retraction, or upward rotation. The support is removed and the patient attempted to maintain this each position	**Resisted Donor and Recipient**: Isometric horizontal adduction followed by scapular elevation in standing, scapular retraction in prone, and scapular upward rotation in standing (wall slides) **Resisted Recipient**: Standing shoulder shrugs with weights Prone (with arm off table edge) scapular retraction with arm raises at 95° of shoulder abduction and external rotation ("T" position) Prone scapular upward rotation with arm raises at 130° of shoulder abduction and external rotation ("Y" position)
Additional Interventions			Each exercise category will include 3 separate exercises for the upper, middle, and lower trapezius	Early phase 3 resistance includes the weight of the arm prior to adding weights or resistance bands

C7/Pectoralis Major to Spinal Accessory Nerve Transfer

Goal of Surgery: To provide stability to the scapula and improve ability to reach away from the body

Recipient Movement = scapular elevation, upward rotation, and retraction of the scapula

Recipient Muscles: Upper, middle, and lower trapezius

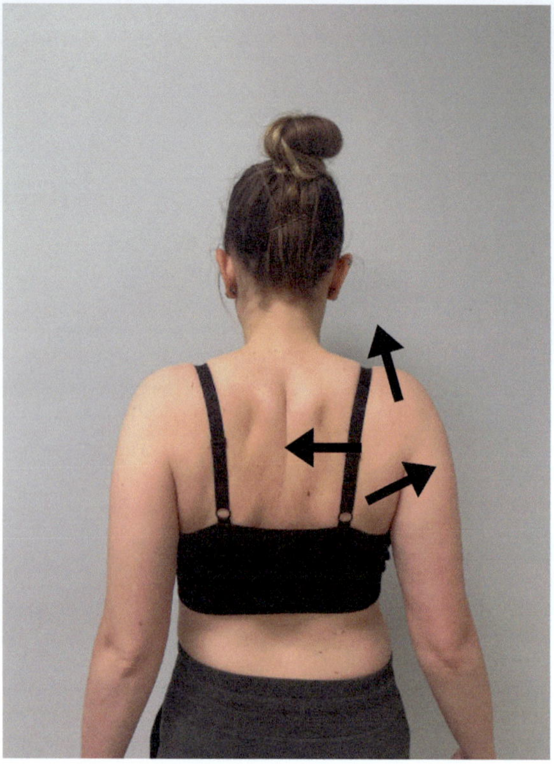

Donor Movement = Shoulder flexion and horizontal adduction

Donor Muscle: Pectoralis major muscle

Bring your arm toward the opposite hip

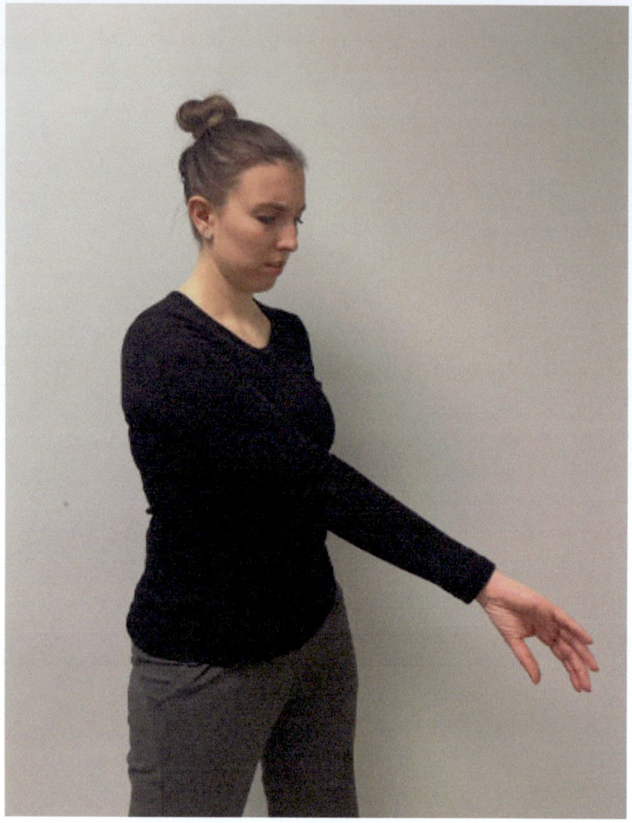

Phase 1 Pectoralis Major to Spinal Accessory Nerve Transfer Exercises:

☐ **Passive Range of Motion**

Table Slides: Sit with your arm supported on a table next to you.

- With your elbow straight, lean sideways toward the table pushing your arm away from you.

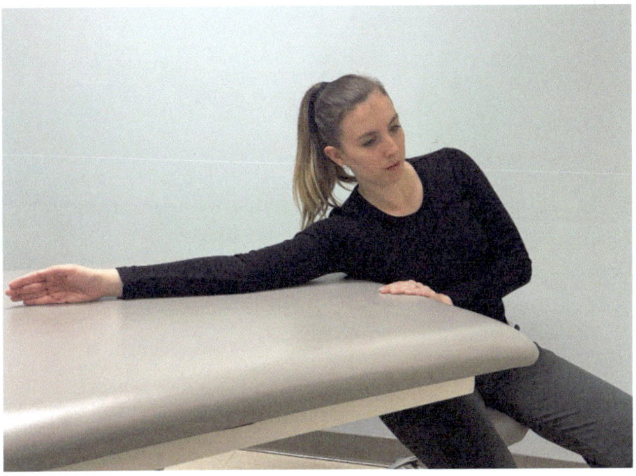

- Stretch your shoulder forward while keeping the arm supported on a table in front of you. Bend your body forward to obtain a deeper stretch.

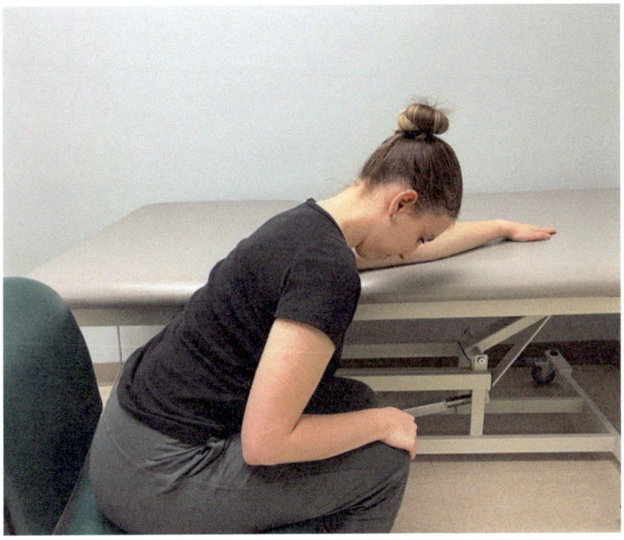

- ☐ **Active or Resisted Donor Movement**:
- Reach your arm across your body toward the opposite hip and hold 5 seconds.

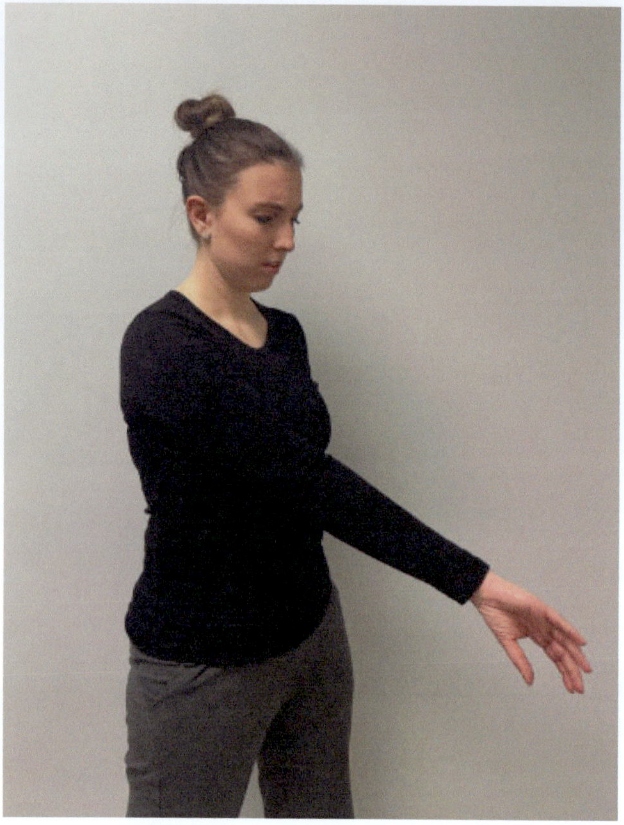

- Press your hands toward each other to activate your pecs. Hold 5 seconds, relax, and repeat.

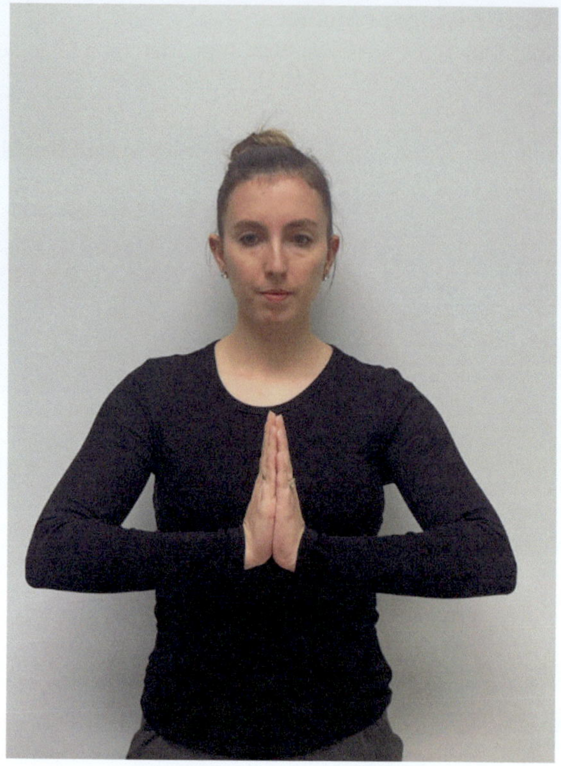

-

- ☐ **Combined Donor with Passive Recipient Exercise**

- *Upper Trapezius*: Lie on your stomach with your forehead supported on a rolled towel. Press your arm into the table while your friend or family member pushes your shoulder in an upward direction toward your ear.

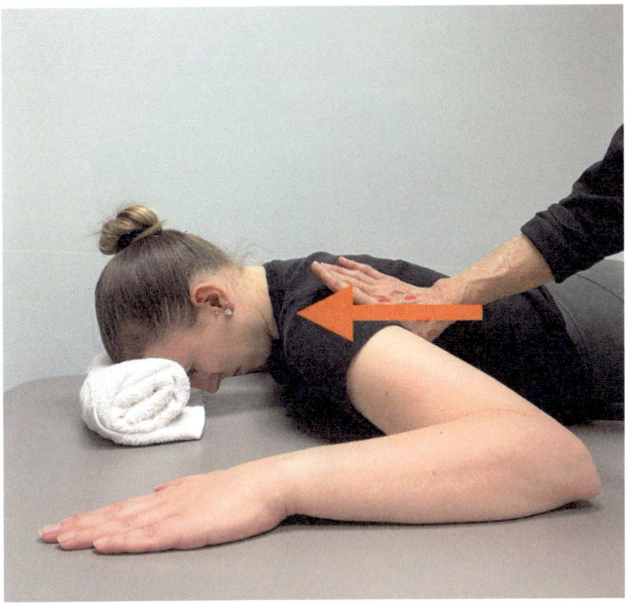

- *Middle Trapezius*: Lie on your stomach with your forehead supported on a rolled towel. Press your arm into the table while your friend or family member pushes your shoulder blade toward your spine.

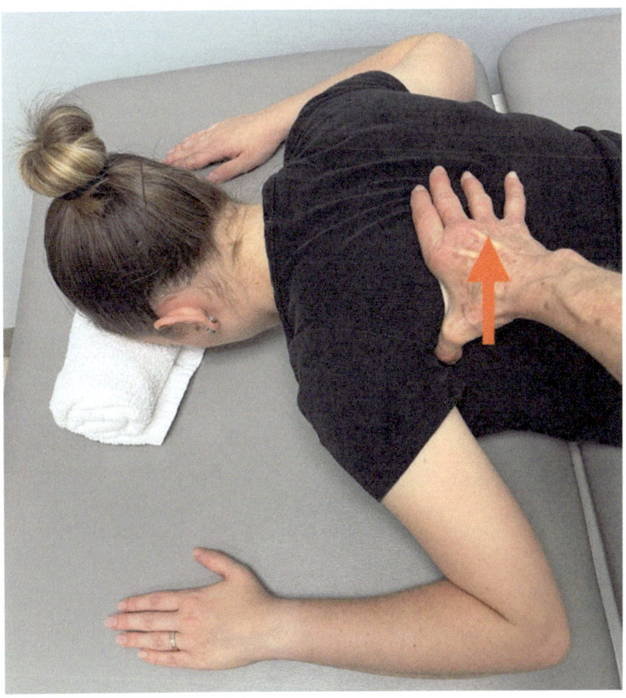

- *Lower Trapezius*: Lie on your uninjured side. Rest your arm on a large exercise ball. Push down on the ball while sliding the arm forward. Have your family member assist the bottom of the shoulder blade upward and outward.

Complete **10–15** repetitions, 3×/day as able

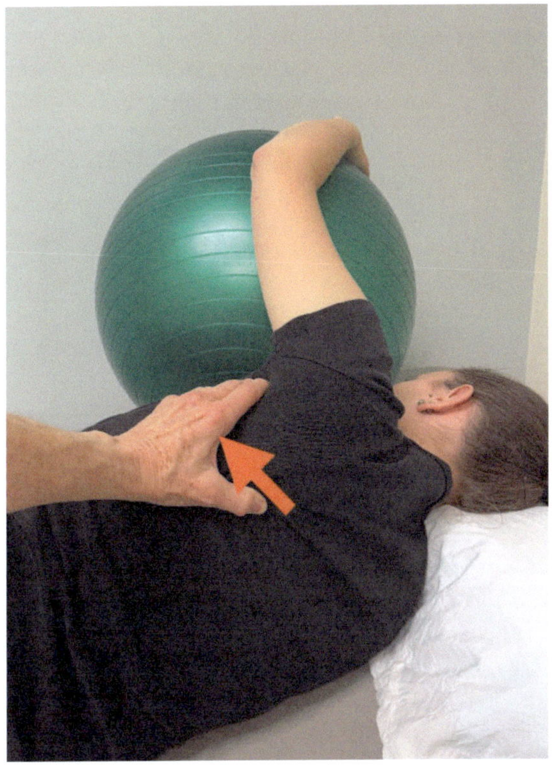

Phase 2 Pectoralis Major to Spinal Accessory Nerve Transfer Exercises

☐ **Active Donor + Active-Assisted Recipient**

- *Upper Trapezius*: Lie on your back with your hands clasped. Press your hands together as you elevate your shoulders up and overhead. Try to shrug your shoulders, and bring your shoulder close to your ear. Have your friend or family member place a hand under your arm, assisting the shoulder blade towards the ear.

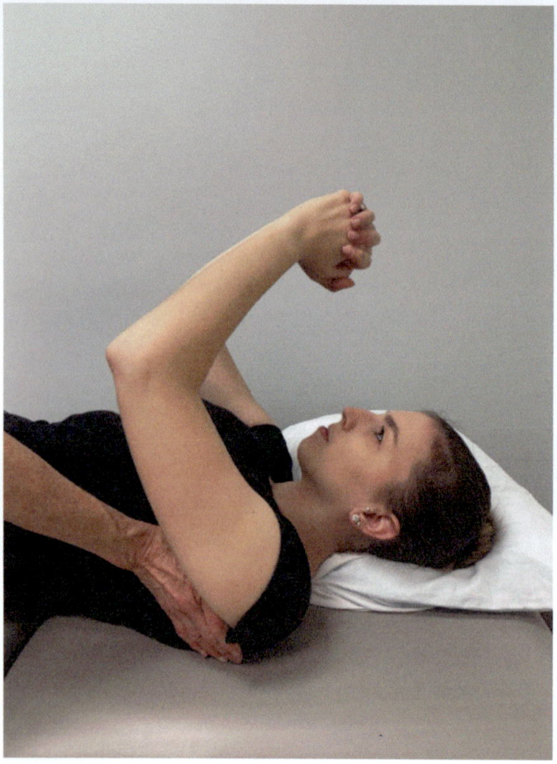

- *Middle Trapezius*: Lie on your uninjured side with your injured arm resting on a large exercise ball in front of you. Press into the ball while trying to pull your shoulder blade toward your spine. Have your friend or family member push the shoulder blade in to assist this motion.

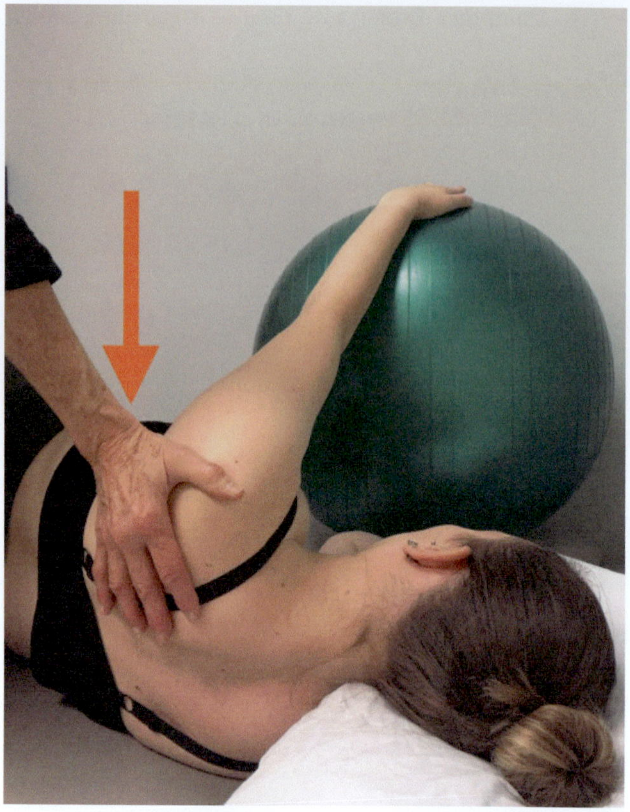

- *Lower Trapezius*: Lie on your stomach with your arms out to the side. Press down into the table as you simultaneously slide the arms forward. Try to think about squeezing your shoulder blades together as you do this. Have your friend or family member assist your shoulder blade with this motion (into retraction and upward rotation).

Complete 10 repetitions, 3 times per day

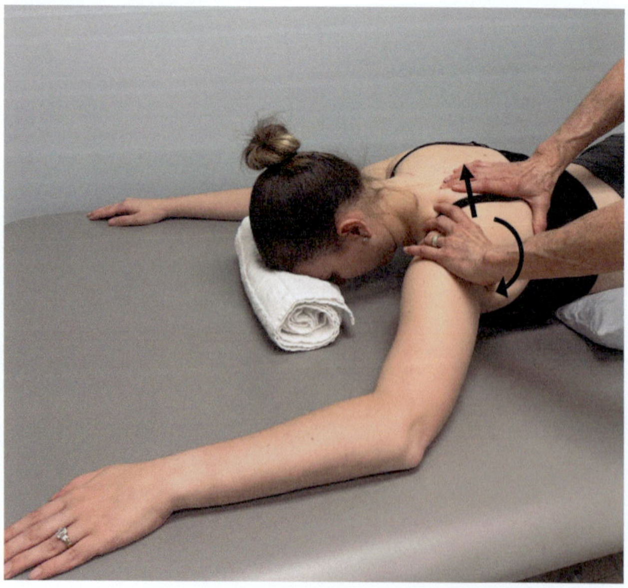

☐ "Place and Hold" Exercise

- *Upper Trapezius*: Lie on your back with your hands clasped. Press your hands together as your friend or family member pushes the shoulder in an upward direction (shoulder shrug). Try to maintain this shoulder shrug position as the assistance is removed.

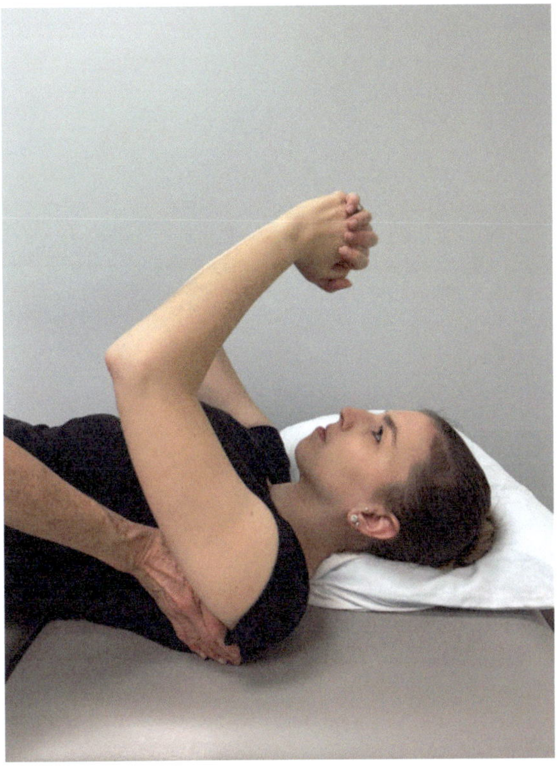

- *Middle Trapezius*: Lie on your stomach with your palms on the mat and your elbows at the level of your shoulders. Your friend or family member manually assists the shoulder blade toward the spine as you press into mat and raise your elbows. As your friend or family member removes the support, try to keep your elbows raised and shoulder blade retracted (toward the spine).

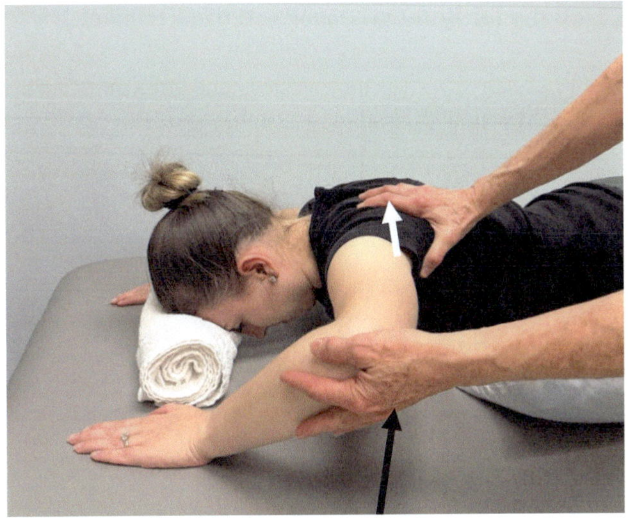

- *Lower Trapezius*: Lie on your stomach with your arms out to the side and elbows bent to 90°. Press into the mat while you slide your arm forward. Your friend or family member assists the shoulder blade upward and outward (scapular upward rotation). As this assistance is removed, try to maintain this position.

Complete 10 repetitions, 3 times per day

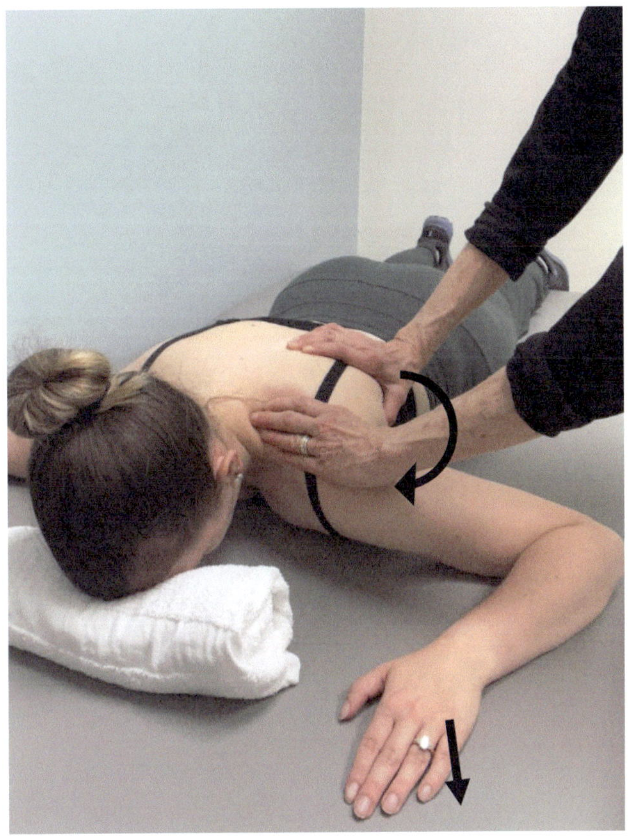

☐ **Active (or Resisted) Donor + Active Recipient**:

- *Upper Trapezius*: Lie on your belly and press down on the ground with both hands as you shrug your shoulders.

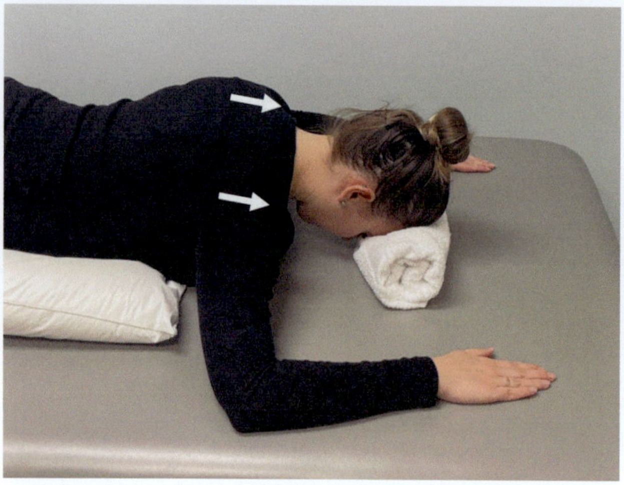

- *Middle Trapezius*: Sit with your arm supported on a table at shoulder height. Pull a resistance band toward the opposite side of the body while you try to bring your shoulder blade back toward the spine.

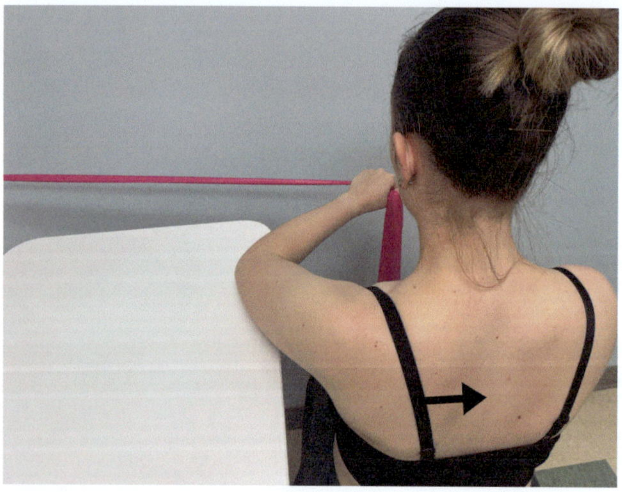

- *Lower Trapezius*: While standing at a wall, press your hands into the wall while sliding your arms upward.

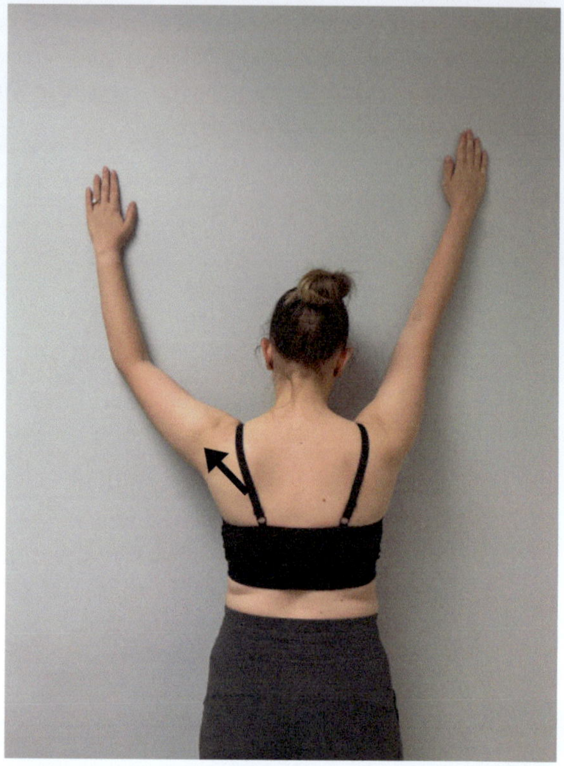

Phase 3 Pectoralis Major to Spinal Accessory Nerve Transfer Exercises:

☐ **Resisted Recipient Activity with Donor Contraction**:

- *Upper trapezius*: While seated or standing, press your hands together while shrugging the shoulders towards your ears.

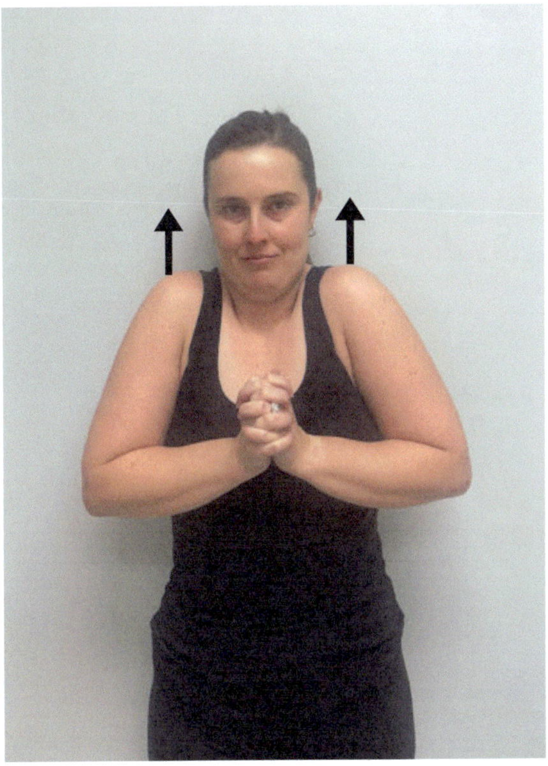

- *Middle Trapezius*: While lying on your stomach, press into the mat while you squeeze your shoulder blades together and raise your elbows. Hold 5 seconds, relax, and repeat.

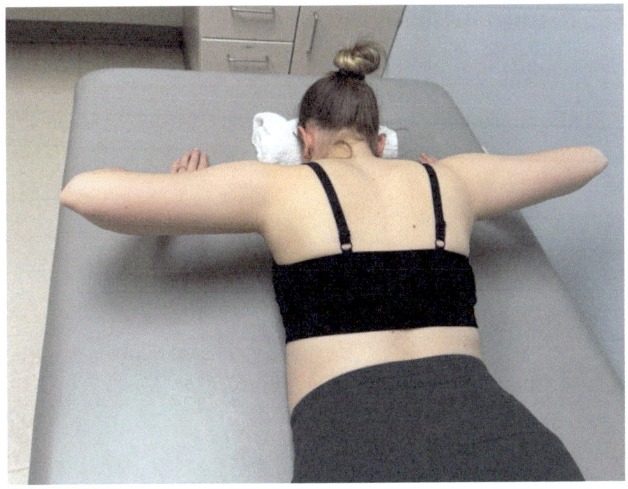

- *Lower Trapezius*: While standing at a wall, press your hands into the wall while sliding your arms upward. Once your arms are in a "V" position overhead, squeeze your shoulder blades together and lift your arms off the wall for 3-5 seconds.

Complete 10 repetitions, 3 times per day

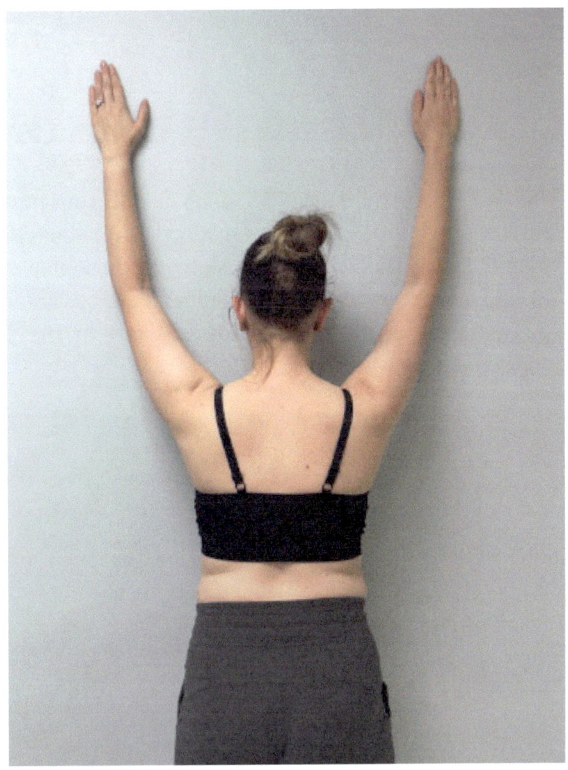

☐ **Resisted Recipient without Donor Contraction**:

- *Upper Trapezius*: Stand while holding ____ lb weights in your hands and shrug both shoulders. Hold 3-5 seconds, relax, and repeat.

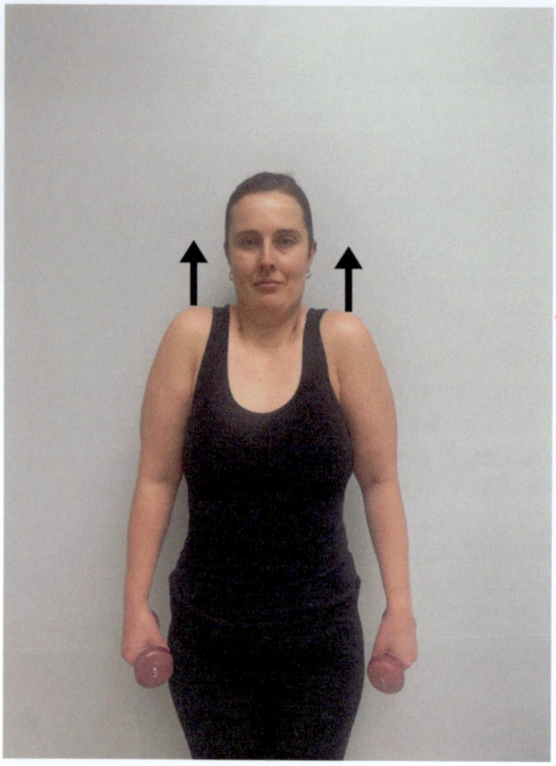

- *Middle Trapezius*: Lie on your stomach with your injured arm hanging off the edge of the mat/bed. With your elbow straight, rotate your shoulder away from you so that your thumb faces up. Squeeze your shoulder blade toward your spine while you lift the arm **up and out to the side** (approximately 90-95°).

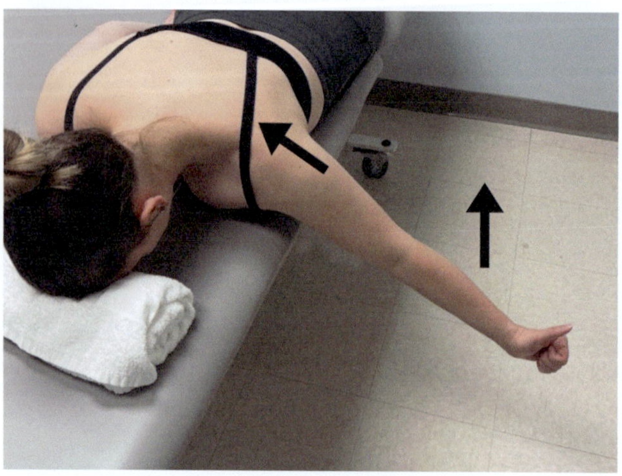

- *Lower Trapezius*: Lie on your stomach with your injured arm hanging off the edge of the mat/bed. With your elbow straight, rotate your shoulder away from you so that your thumb faces up. Raise your arm **up in front of you** (to approximately 130°) and hold 3–5 seconds.

Complete 10 repetitions, 3 times per day

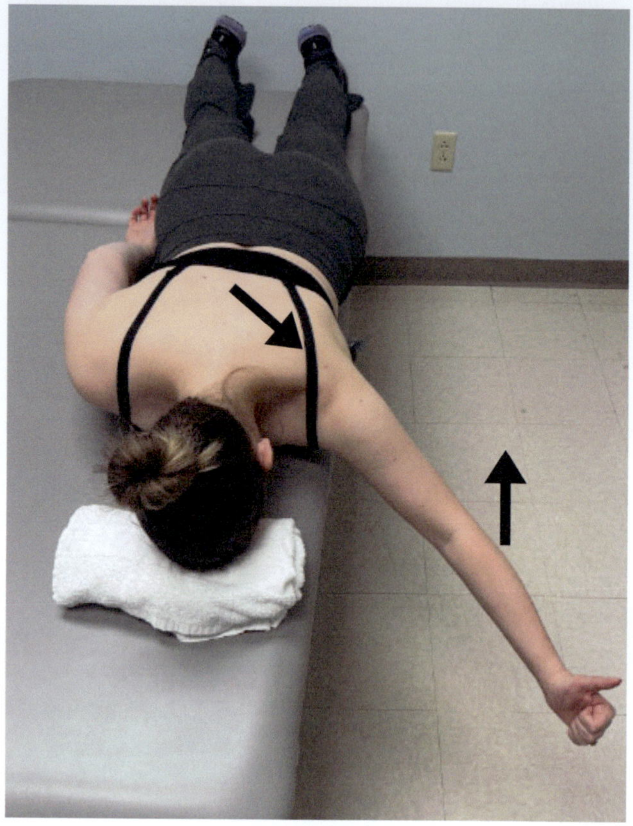

References

1. Macaluso S, Ross DC, Doherty TJ, Doherty CD, Miller TA. Spinal accessory nerve injury: a potentially missed cause of a painful, droopy shoulder. J Back Musculoskelet Rehab. 2016;29(4):899–904.
2. Kendall FP, McCreary EK, Provance PG, Rodgers MM, Romani WA. Muscles: testing and function with posture and pain, vol. 5. Baltimore, MD: Lippincott Williams & Wilkins; 2005. p. 1–100.
3. Safran MR. Nerve injury about the shoulder in athletes, part 2: long thoracic nerve, spinal accessory nerve, burners/stingers, thoracic outlet syndrome. Am J Sports Med. 2004;32(4):1063–76.
4. Neumann DA. Neumann kinesiology of the musculoskeletal system. Foundations for Rehabilitation; 2009.
5. Brunnstrom S. Muscle testing around the shoulder girdle: a study of the function of shoulder-blade fixators in seventeen cases of shoulder paralysis. JBJS. 1941;23(2):263–72.
6. Wu KY, Spinner RJ. Selective upper trunk posterior division fascicular nerve transfer for proximal spinal accessory neuropathy: illustrative case. J Neurosurg Case Lessons. 2023;6(9)
7. Mayer JA, Hruby LA, Salminger S, Bodner G, Aszmann OC. Reconstruction of the spinal accessory nerve with selective fascicular nerve transfer of the upper trunk. J Neurosurg Spine. 2019;31(1):133–8.
8. Bradley PJ, Ferlito A, Silver CE, Takes RP, Woolgar JA, Strojan P, et al. Neck treatment and shoulder morbidity: still a challenge. Head Neck. 2011;33(7):1060–7.
9. Maldonado AA, Spinner RJ. Lateral pectoral nerve transfer for spinal accessory nerve injury. J Neurosurg Spine. 2017;26(1):112–5.
10. Novak CB, Mackinnon SE. Treatment of a proximal accessory nerve injury with nerve transfer. Laryngoscope. 2004;114(8):1482–4.
11. Ye X, Shen YD, Feng JT, Xu WD. Nerve fascicle transfer using a part of the C-7 nerve for spinal accessory nerve injury. J Neurosurg Spine. 2018;28(5):555–61. https://doi.org/10.3171/2017.8.SPINE17582.
12. Manske RC, Prohaska D. Pectoralis major tendon repair post surgical rehabilitation. N Am J Sports Phys Therapy. 2007;2(1):22.
13. Kahn LC, Moore AM. Donor activation focused rehabilitation approach: maximizing outcomes after nerve transfers. Hand Clin. 2016;32(2):263–77.

Thoracodorsal Nerve to Long Thoracic Nerve Transfer

Lorna C. Kahn

Background

The long thoracic nerve (LTN) innervates the serratus anterior muscle. The nerve arises at the most proximal portion of the brachial plexus taking contributions from C5, C6, and C7 nerve roots prior to the formation of the upper and middle trunks of the plexus. It runs caudally along the rib cage innervating the multiple slips of the serratus muscle as they attach to ribs one through nine. The serratus muscle moves the scapula ventrally, also known as protraction. Along with the upper and lower trapezius muscles, the serratus anterior upwardly rotates the scapula during arm elevation and stabilizes the scapula on the thorax during shoulder movement [1]. When an upward rotator muscle is weak or absent, arm elevation is significantly limited. This relates to the 2/3:1/3 rule of scapulohumeral kinematics. To achieve full arm elevation, a combination of 120 degrees of glenohumeral joint motion and 60 degrees of scapular upward rotation is needed [1]. Classic presentation of long thoracic nerve palsy includes internal rotation and anterior tilt of the scapula, otherwise referred to as medial scapula winging. In addition to the loss of upward rotation, persistent winging of the scapula may result in subsequent shortening of the pec minor, deltoid, and supraspinatus muscles [1].

Functional loss associated with injury to the LTN includes decreased arm elevation (shoulder flexion more than abduction), inability to perform overhead functions, and difficulty lifting or carrying objects. Etiology of long thoracic nerve injuries includes closed-traction trauma often associated with overhead sports such as tennis, golf, gymnastics, and hockey. Additionally, isolated LTN injury or upper plexus trauma, viral plexitis, and compression (at the interscalene triangle or at the terminal muscle branches along the thorax) are implicated [2, 3]. Surgical decompression may suffice with compression injuries in cases where the point of compression can be identified [4]. Surgical reconstruction options typically aim to restrict winging of the inferior angle of the scapula with scapulopexy [5], muscle transfer, and scapulothoracic arthrodesis [6, 7]. These procedures may provide stabilization, but reinnervation of the serratus anterior muscle with restoration of scapular upward rotation is ideal. The thoracodorsal-to-long thoracic nerve transfer has been described as a viable option for this shoulder deficit, but the literature does not provide consensus for an ideal surgical management option.

The donor thoracodorsal nerve innervates the latissimus dorsi muscle. It is formed from nerve roots C6–C8 and branches off the posterior cord of the brachial plexus near the apex of the axilla. The latissimus dorsi muscle is a large, flat muscle that wraps around the posterior aspect of the rib cage from the lower back to the anterior shoulder. Most people associate the "lat" with the *pulling down* motion. This is considered shoulder extension, but the muscle also works in conjunction with the triceps, posterior deltoid, teres major, and sternal head of the pec major to provide shoulder extension as well as shoulder depression and adduction [1]. Contrary to the relative surgical ease of this transfer (given the close proximity of donor and recipient in the lateral thorax), motor reeducation can be challenging. The serratus anterior muscle plays a major role in shoulder flexion by providing scapular upward rotation with protraction. Conversely, the donor muscle aids the antagonistic movement of shoulder extension making for a less-than-synergistic transfer.

L. C. Kahn (✉)
Milliken Hand Rehabilitation Center, WashU Medicine, St. Louis, MO, USA
e-mail: Kahn.lorna.c@wustl.edu

L. C. Kahn et al. (eds.), *Rehabilitation for Nerve Transfers of the Upper Extremity*, https://doi.org/10.1007/978-3-031-92008-0_6

Surgical Description

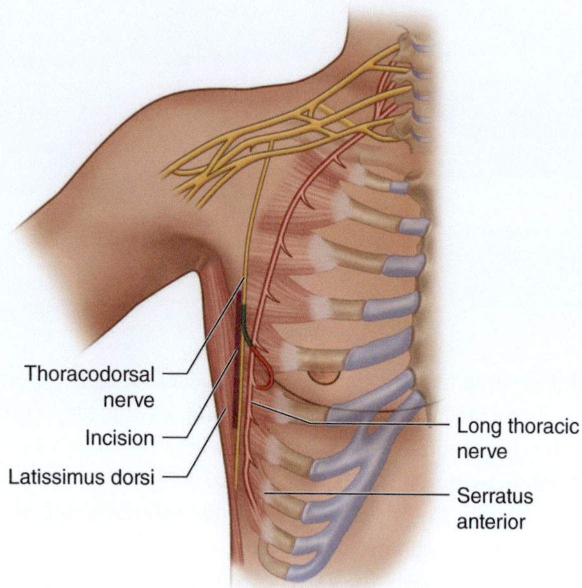

Microsurgical technique of thoracodorsal Nerve to the Long Thoracic Nerve

A longitudinal or oblique incision is made along the chest wall, near the mid-axial line and caudal to the axillary fold. The serratus anterior muscle is identified, and the long thoracic nerve is identified deep to the serratus muscle, closer to the axillary fold. A nerve stimulator is used to confirm absence of long thoracic nerve function, ensuring that the anesthesia team is not using muscle paralytics. The latissimus dorsi muscle is identified, and the anterior and posterior branches of the thoracodorsal nerve are identified. Both branches are stimulated with a nerve stimulator to confirm function, ensuring that the anesthesia team is not using muscle paralytics. Assuming similar response in each branch, the surgeon selects the donor branch based on the length obtained during dissection. The donor branch from the thoracodorsal nerve is divided distally and transposed to meet the long thoracic nerve, which is divided proximally. Coaptation of a branch from the thoracodorsal nerve to the long thoracic nerve is performed using microsurgical technique.

Outcomes

Uepairojkt et al. published a study of five patients with upper plexus injuries including a winged scapula, who underwent reconstruction including TD-to-LTN transfer [8]. Spinal accessory nerve (SAN) to triceps and suprascapular nerve (SSN) to axillary nerve transfers were also performed at the same time. At a mean follow-up of 28 months, all five recovered serratus function. Complete resolution of scapula winging was reported in two of the five and partial resolution in the remaining three. The authors describe the results for two as excellent, two as good, and one as fair. Shoulder abduction and external range of motion were included as outcome measures, and the mean abduction arc was 134° [8]. No measure of shoulder flexion is mentioned. Ray et al. described resolution of scapular winging with recovery of full shoulder elevation following a double-nerve transfer involving TD to LTN for the distal portion of the serratus muscle and pec/C7 for the proximal aspect [9]. In 2002, a case report by Novak and Mackinnon described this nerve transfer in isolation in one teenage male. Follow-up at 6.5 years (the patient failed to return prior to this) revealed no scapular winging, full shoulder ROM, and no functional limitations relating to the donor or recipient muscles [10].

Phases of Rehabilitation

Phase 1

Preoperative to 1/5 MMT in the Recipient Muscle

A period of rest for the involved arm is encouraged for the first 2–3 weeks following surgery. Depending on the surgeon's preference, this may include use of a shoulder immobilizer or sling to limit the potential for seroma formation. The patient should limit shoulder movement to 45 degrees of shoulder elevation to allow just enough for axillary hygiene. Some surgeons advocate showering in the first week with no use of the involved arm. Elbow, wrist, and hand active range of motion (AROM) should be initiated during this time to limit postoperative edema and stiffness in the hand and arm.

Formal therapy may commence following the rest period. The initial focus is to re-establish passive range of motion (PROM) of the shoulder complex. This includes both glenohumeral motion and scapulothoracic motion. Scar management is generally not needed but should be assessed. When present, edema in the wound site may be managed with gentle massage, lymphedema massage, and sports taping techniques that reduce edema.

Attention should be given to the trapezius strength. Many people generally have postural weakness in the trapezius muscles. During the period of absence of the serratus anterior muscle strength, it becomes more important to improve trapezius strength to bolster scapular stability and provide some scapular upward rotation.

Patient education is focused on the pertinent anatomy. Donor and recipient muscles are identified, and their muscle actions are explained. Simple donor activation exercises should be initiated within the first month. Timelines for recovery are introduced, and an explanation of the motor recovery monitoring is described [9, 11].

Exercises

- ROM of Uninvolved Joints
  The shoulder is likely to be the primary joint with hypomobility following the first few postoperative weeks due

to reduced activity and sling use. Any prolonged period of scapular winging preoperatively may also cause the pec minor, deltoid, and supraspinatus muscles to become short. This may be addressed with passive stretches performed manually by the therapist or a family member. Lying on a foam roller (along the length of the 36-inch roller from head to tailbone) will provide some pec minor and anterior deltoid stretch (Image 1). Manually stabilizing the scapula may be required to adequately stretch all three heads of a tight deltoid.

- Donor Activation

Activation of the latissimus dorsi muscle involves shoulder extension with adduction. This may be performed in prone, sitting, and/or standing. For example, the patient stands with his or her back to a wall and extends the shoulder by pressing the hand backwards into the wall while keeping the arm in shoulder adduction (Image 2).

- Combined Donor with Passive Recipient Exercise
  While seated with hands clasped and both arms on a table, the patient presses down on the table to resist the latissimus donor while sliding the arms forward into shoulder flexion with the assistance of the uninvolved hand. The therapist assists by grasping the scapula and moving it into protraction with upward rotation along the thorax (Image 3).

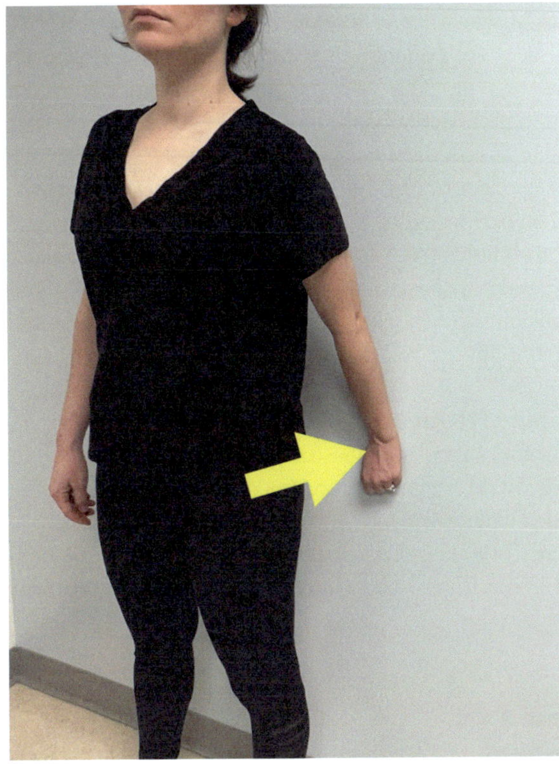

Image 2 Donor activation involves resisting the latissimus dorsi muscle. In standing this is achieved by reaching back into shoulder extension with some adduction against a wall

Assessment of Recovery

Assessment of motor recovery of the serratus anterior muscle is performed at each monthly visit. This can be assessed in sitting, side-lying, or standing. Position the patient seated facing a table or elevated mat at shoulder height. The serratus muscle inserts along the lateral aspect of ribs 1–8 (9) and can be palpated along the lateral thorax anterior to the scapula. The patient presses the arm down into the table (in the direction of shoulder extension) to activate the donor latissimus muscle while having the patient slide the arm into shoulder flexion. Palpation close to the scapular border on the rib cage during this action will reveal a muscle contraction in the ser-

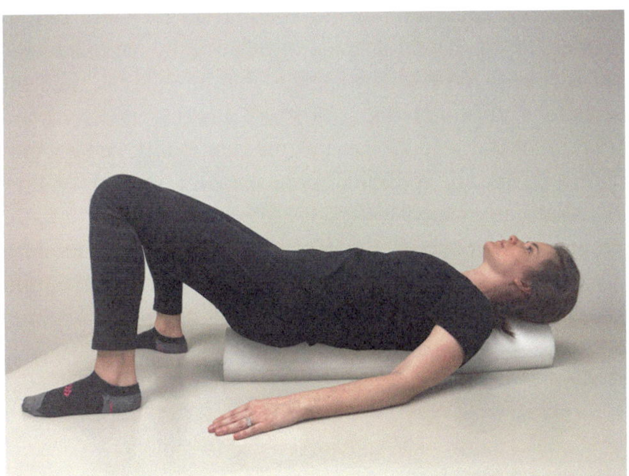

Image 1 Lying on a foam roller enables the individual to achieve some passive stretch to the pec minor muscle

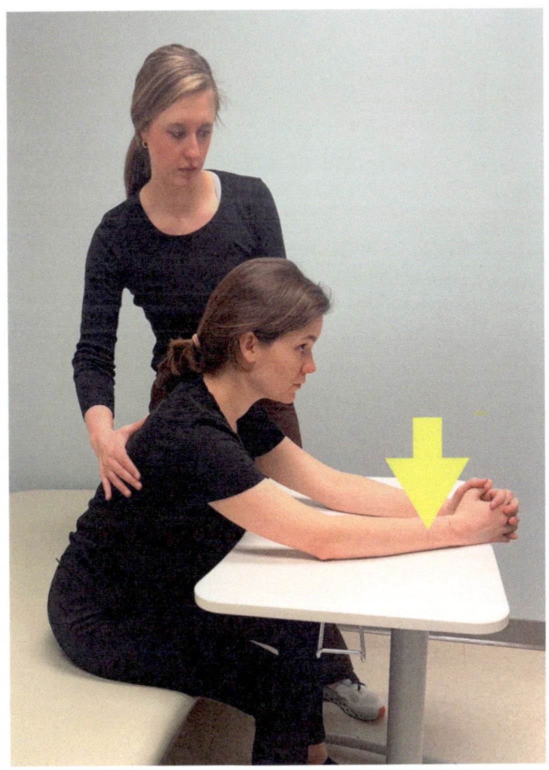

Image 3 To combine *resisted* donor with *assisted* recipient movement, the individual rests the arms on a table with hands clasped. Pressing down into the table provides latissimus resistance as the arm slides along the table into passive flexion. When possible, the therapist will passively protract the scapula

ratus muscle when it is reinnervated. In standing, the therapist faces the patient and places their wrist/forearm on the therapist's shoulder with the elbow straight. The patient is cued to press down on the shoulder to activate the latissimus muscle as the therapist palpates along the lateral/posterior rib cage, anterior to the scapula (Image 4). Assessment can also be performed in side-lying on the uninvolved side. The therapist holds the involved arm against their trunk and cues the patient to press the arm into the direction of shoulder extension while palpating the rib cage and observing for any scapular upward rotation (Image 5).

Therapy Frequency

Frequency of visits in phase 1 will vary based on individual's needs, ROM limitations, and his or her ability to perform the needed exercises. Once PROM is addressed, and the patient can perform the exercises accurately, frequency is decreased to 1x/month until some activation is noted in the serratus muscle.

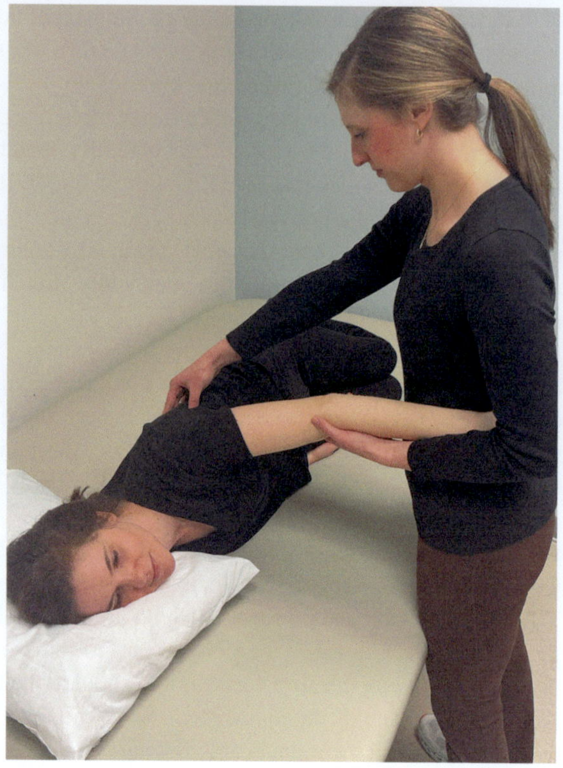

Image 5 To assess for recovery of the serratus muscle in side-lying, the assessor supports the involved arm and provides resistance to shoulder extension while palpating along the rib cage anterior to the scapula

Phase 2

2−/5 to 3/5 MMT in the Recipient Muscle

Once activation of the serratus anterior muscle is noted, exercises are advanced from passive to active assisted with active (or resisted) donor movement. The challenge of this nerve transfer becomes evident as the two antagonist movements are actively combined. During this phase, the exercises can be performed in sitting, supine, side-lying, and/or prone. For example, in sitting, a pulley can be used to provide assisted shoulder flexion. To attain co-contraction with the donor/latissimus, the uninjured hand pulls down and the patient is cued to limit the speed of the injured arm moving up by resisting the upward pull (Image 6).

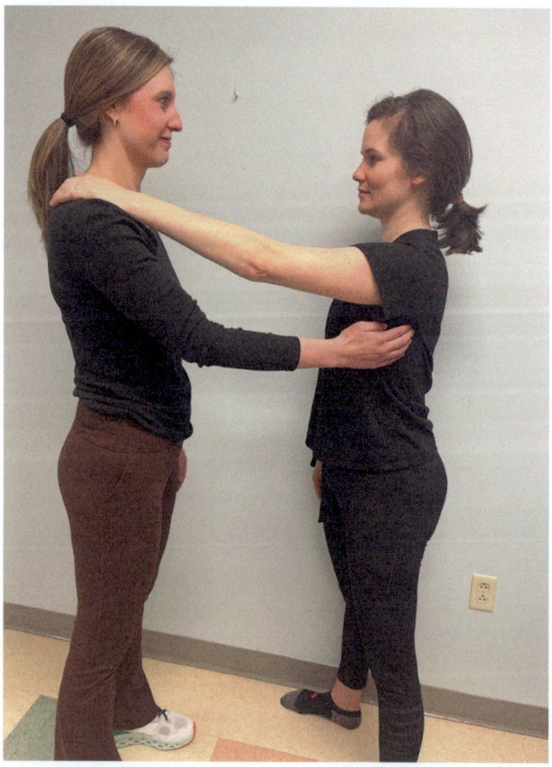

Image 4 To assess for recovery of the serratus muscle in standing, the arm is placed on the assessor's shoulder. As he or she presses the arm into the shoulder to activate the donor latissimus, the assessor palpates along the ribs anterior to the scapula

Periscapular, and specifically middle and lower trapezius muscle, strengthening should continue to be addressed, as needed, to support the scapula while awaiting recipient muscle recovery. When the trapezius muscle is weak, and the serratus is not functioning for many months, the downward rotators of the scapula, such as the rhomboids, can become short and add to the limitation in scapular upward rotation. By providing manual assistance to scapular protraction, the therapist is not only aiding in serratus motor reeducation but also correcting the rhomboid length as well. During this phase, some patients may benefit from therapy visits every 1–2 weeks if their insurance allows.

Exercises

- Active Donor with Active-Assisted Recipient

$$\text{Serratus Anterior MMT} = 2-/5 \text{ to } 2/5$$

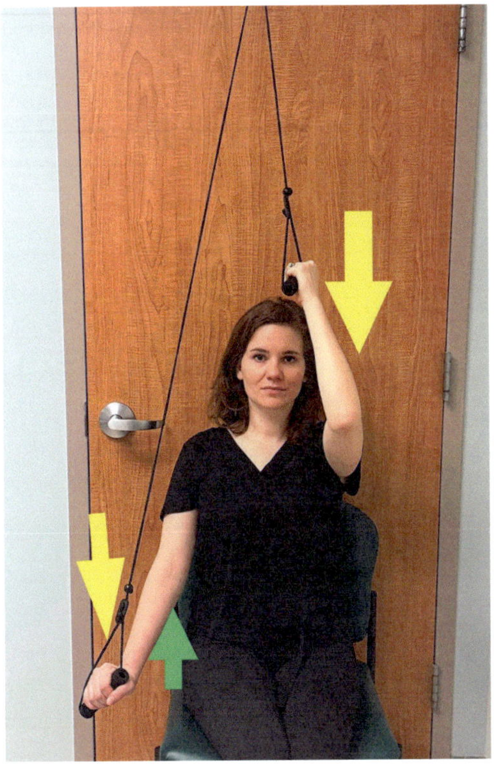

Image 6 A pulley is used to provide resisted donor latissimus (extension) movement with assisted shoulder flexion

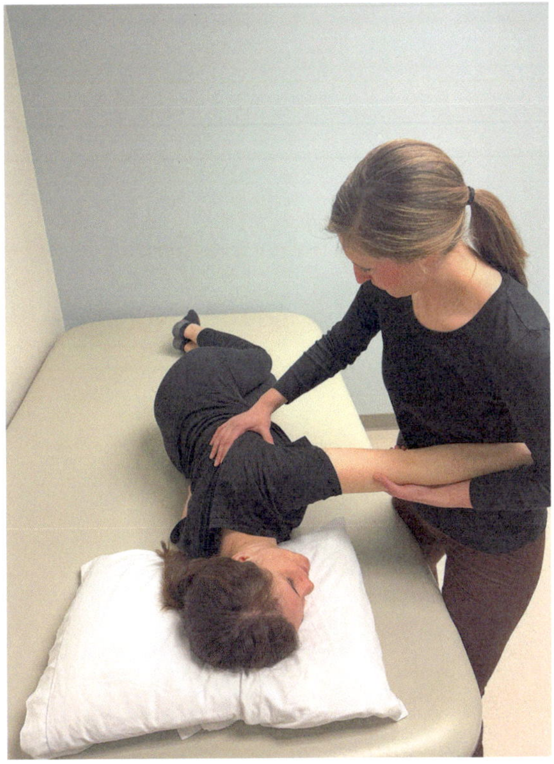

Image 8 "Place and hold" serratus exercises are demonstrated in side-lying. The therapist provides resistance to the donor (shoulder extension) against her waist while manually placing the scapula into available protraction. The placement/assistance is removed, and the individual is cued to maintain this protracted position of the scapula

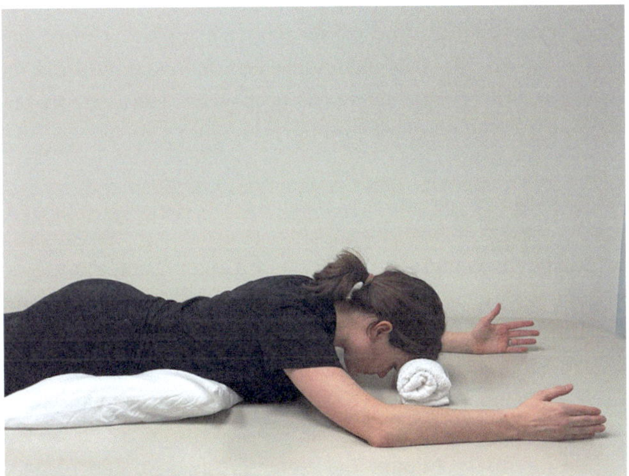

Image 7 During phase 2, assisted recipient exercises may be performed in prone over pillows. The individual presses down into the mat while sliding the arms into flexion. The therapist may assist the scapula into protraction when available

With the patient in prone (gravity-minimized plane) on a mat over pillows, he or she slides the arms forward (into shoulder flexion) while pushing down on the mat (Image 7). Pressure can be applied to the posterior upper arm while the patient slides the arm forward to cue for additional donor/latissimus resistance. Manual assistance may be provided from the therapist to the scapula to aid with upward rotation.

- "Place and Hold"

  $$\text{Serratus Anterior MMT} = 2+/5$$

  In side-lying on the uninvolved side, the therapist holds the affected arm with one hand and provide resistance to the latissimus by having the patient press into the therapist's abdomen while guiding the arm into forward flexion. With the opposite hand, the therapist can guide the scapula into protraction and upward rotation and ask the patient to attempt to maintain the scapula in this position once support is released (Image 8).
- Active Donor with Active Recipient

  $$\text{Serratus Anterior MMT} = 3-/5$$

  As serratus strength increases, wall slides may be introduced. Although this is technically an antigravity position, the wall provides support and assistance. With the ulnar aspect of the hands on the wall, the patient slides the arm up a wall into a "V" position. For added donor resistance, the therapist can place his or her hand under the elbow to provide a cue for resisting the latissimus donor (pulling down) while sliding up the wall, co-contracting the donor and recipient muscles (Image 9). This promotes scapular upward rotation with shoulder flexion.

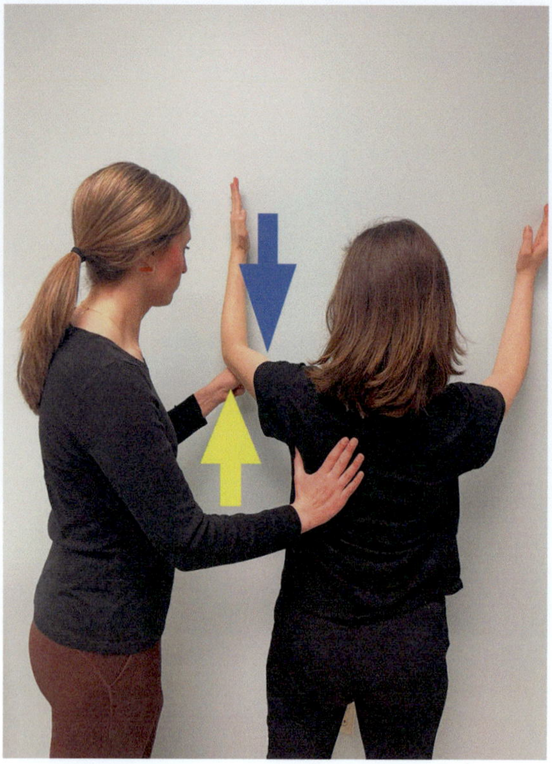

Image 9 Wall slides are demonstrated with passive resistance to the donor latissimus. The therapist places a fist under the elbow to resist shoulder extension while simultaneously encouraging active shoulder flexion with assisted scapular protraction

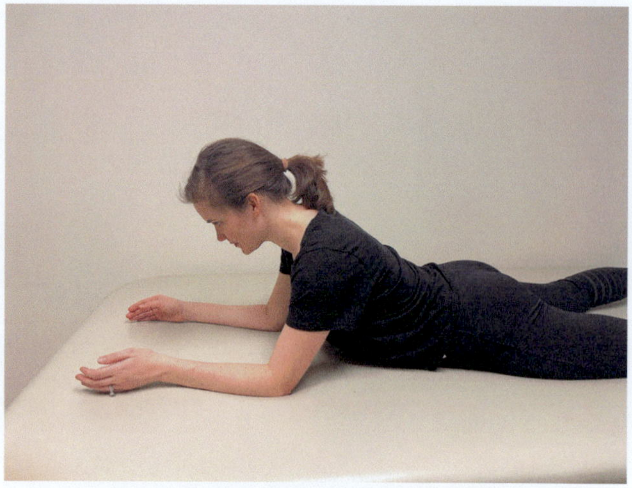

Image 10 Active serratus protraction is demonstrated with resistance while prone on elbows

Functional Activity

With the arm on a table or a raised mat, the patient can slide the arm forward while cueing for scapular protraction as he or she attempts to reach an object that is placed at a distance.

Therapy Frequency

The patient may attend therapy once a week, depending on the specific needs of the individual. If he or she has joint limitations or is struggling to learn the new motor control pattern, weekly therapy is warranted.

Phase 3

3+/5 or Greater MMT in the Recipient Muscle

In the authors' experience, an MMT grade higher than 3+/5 is not typically achieved following this transfer, at least not in the first 2 years that they are followed. To achieve a 3+ or greater, the inferior angle should protract to the midline of the thorax and take some resistance in a direction of retraction at the same time as resistance is applied to the arm at 90+ degrees of flexion. As overhead reaching improves, individuals should be advised to avoid strenuous lifting in the frontal/sagittal plane unless the scapula remains well seated on the thorax (no winging). Excessive lifting, especially overhead, can lead to substitutions that create stresses on the cervical spine.

Exercises are carefully graded to resist the serratus muscle. In phase 3, reaching overhead into full flexion is initially performed with close monitoring of the scapula position. Once adequate movement and stability are demonstrated, light resistance may be added to shoulder flexion exercises. During this phase, the exercises should require less manual input from the therapist. The frequency of visits may be decreased to one time every 2 weeks, based on the individual's needs.

Exercises

- Resistive Recipient Activity with Donor Contraction
  The patient is prone on the elbows with the hips on the floor (Image 10), which places demand on both the donor latissimus and the recipient serratus anterior muscles. As this becomes easier, the patient may attempt a plank position and gradually increase the hold time based on the ability to maintain the scapula against the thorax. Additionally, prone on elbows with alternating arm slides (Image 11) will challenge the serratus both with forward sliding and with weight-bearing while the opposite arm is sliding.
- Resistive Recipient Activity Without Donor Contraction
  Standing shoulder flexion without wall support is the ultimate goal of this surgery. Once patients can achieve this without scapular winging and without support, they may be challenged to use light free weights (starting with 1#) or light theraband. Functionally, patients should be encouraged to reach and place items on an overhead shelf with cues to maintain good scapular control.

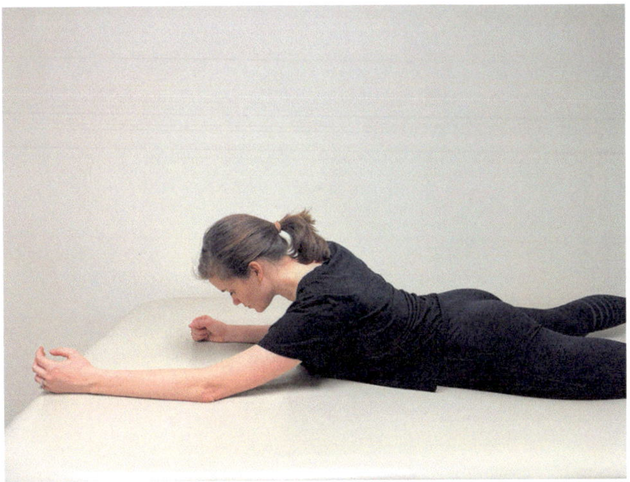

Image 11 Alternating arm slides into shoulder flexion while prone on elbows is demanding for the reinnervating serratus muscle. One must maintain the scapula against the ribcage while moving the opposite hand forward. This increases the demand on the statically positioned arm

Therapy Frequency

During this phase, the exercises are easier to complete without manual participation from the therapist. Once the patient can demonstrate the home exercise program (HEP) accurately, appointments should be scheduled every 2 weeks to advance the program. Once goals are completed, patients may be discharged to an HEP with the understanding that their momentary strength may be acceptable, but their endurance for repetitive activities may take many years to regain.

Thoracodorsal to Long Thoracic Nerve Transfer

Nerve transfer overview					
Donor nerve	Donor action	Recipient nerve	Recipient action	Indications for functional restoration	Approximate months to functional movement
Thoracodorsal nerve	Shoulder extension, internal rotation, adduction	Long thoracic nerve	Scapular protraction (assists with shoulder flexion)	Long thoracic nerve palsy	12 months [12]

Information below are suggested guidelines. Precautions may vary according to surgeon preferences and patient factors

	Preoperative therapy	Early phase	Middle phase	Late phase
Criteria	Before Surgery	0/5–1/5 MMT	2-/5 to 3/5 MMT	>3/5 MMT
Purpose of phase	Educate and establish baseline function	Understand donor and recipient relationship	Consistently activate recipient	Strengthen recipient muscle
Precautions	Prevent hypomobility of the glenohumeral and scapulothoracic joints, with special attention to the downward rotators (pec minor, latissiumus dorsi, and rhomboids)	Shoulder immobilizer or sling the first 3 weeks Limit shoulder elevation to 45° in the first 3 weeks	Respect fatigue and prevent dominance of scapular downward rotators	Avoid anti-gravity or resisted shoulder flexion until consistent 3/5 MMT is achieved. Note that not all patients achieve 3/5 strength
Frequency of visits (considerations)	2–3 pre-op visits May increase if PROM limitations exist	1–2×/week until PROM is WNL and patient is independent with donor activation; then 1-2× monthly	1× per week to 1× per month based on patient needs and accurate, consistent demonstration of exercise program	1× every 1–2 weeks based on progress toward patient-specific goals
Orthosis considerations	Support devices to decrease pain with scapular winging, including the Omotrain® brace, an infant/toddler hip support, or Kinesio®-tape	Full-time sling support for the first 3 weeks. OK to remove for hygiene and for AROM of the elbow	Resume support devices to decrease pain with scapular winging, including the Omotrain® brace, an infant/toddler hip support, or Kinesio®-tape	NA
Interventions	PROM for scapular protraction, scapular upward rotation, and glenohumeral motion	**Donor Activation:** Shoulder extension and adduction **Donor-Recipient Pairing**: Shoulder extension (± adduction) combined with passive scapular protraction ± shoulder flexion	**Active/Resisted Donor with Active Assisted Recipient:** The patient is seated with the arm supported on a table. He or she presses downward into a ball (latissimus donor) in the direction of shoulder flexion. The contralateral hand (or another person) assists the scapula further into upward rotation **Place and Hold**: The patient is side-lying, and passive scapular protraction is performed with the shoulder supported in mid -range flexion. The patient presses the arm into the therapist's body in the direction of shoulder extension. The patient attempts to maintain this scapular position as the support is removed **Active Donor with Active Recipient:** Wall slide: The injured arm is supported on a wall with the opposite fist pressing up on the injured elbow to cue the donor. The patient creates resistance in the donor/lat, limiting the speed of arm as it slides up the wall into flexion	**Resisted Donor and Recipient:** While prone on the elbows, the patient arches the upper back, protracting the scapula and holds this position **Resisted Recipient:** While supine and holding a light weight, the arm is in 90 degrees of flexion. The patient protracts the scapula, lifting the shoulder off the mat
Additional interventions			Phase 2 exercises should initially be in a gravity-minimized plane and then at the wall with support Exercises should aim to make the movement easier on the recovering serratus: sliding the arm on a cloth, on a ball, up a wall, or with the assistance of a friend or therapist	In the beginning of phase 3, resistance should first be achieved through the weight of the arm against gravity. Weights or bands may be introduced later, if appropriate

During all phases it is essential to continue cortical reorganization, psychological and psychosocial interventions, progress to incorporate donor/recipient with ADL's

Thoracodorsal to Long Thoracic Nerve Transfer

Goal of Surgery: Restore the ability to control the shoulder blade and allow for stability during shoulder motion

Recipient Movement = Scapular protraction (assists with shoulder flexion)

Recipient Muscle: Serratus Anterior
Recipient Nerve: Long Thoracic Nerve

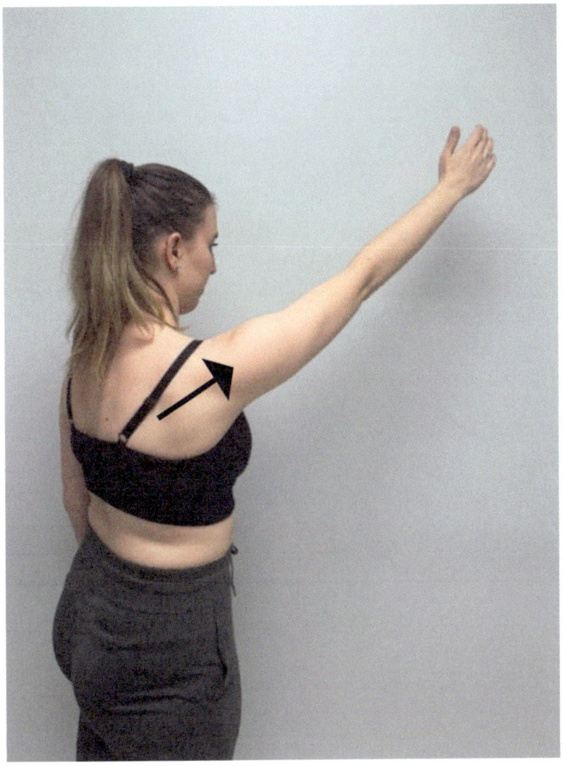

Push shoulder blade forward as the arm moves up

Donor Movement = Shoulder extension and adduction

Donor Muscle: Latissimus dorsi
Donor Nerve: Thoracodorsal nerve

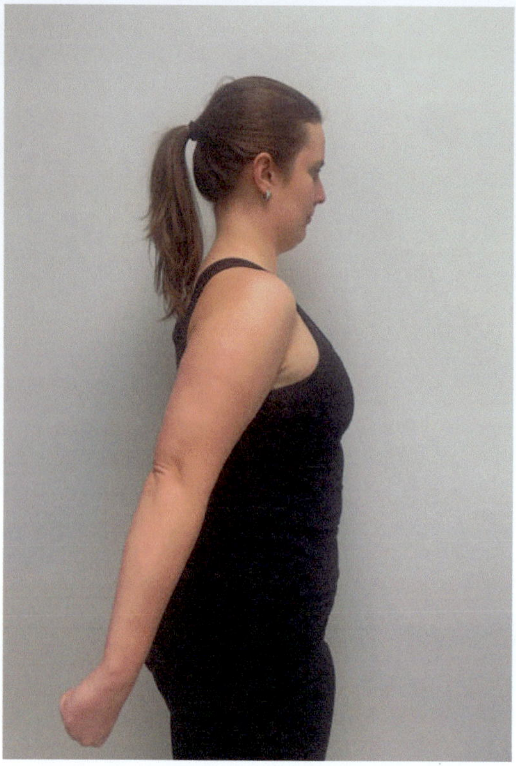

Bring shoulder back and in

Phase 1 Thoracodorsal to Long Thoracic Nerve Transfer Exercises

☐ **Passive Range of Motion:**
Complete the exercises 3–5 repetitions, 2–3 times per day.

- While lying on your back, your family member or friend will cup your shoulder blade and gently glide it in an outward and upward direction.

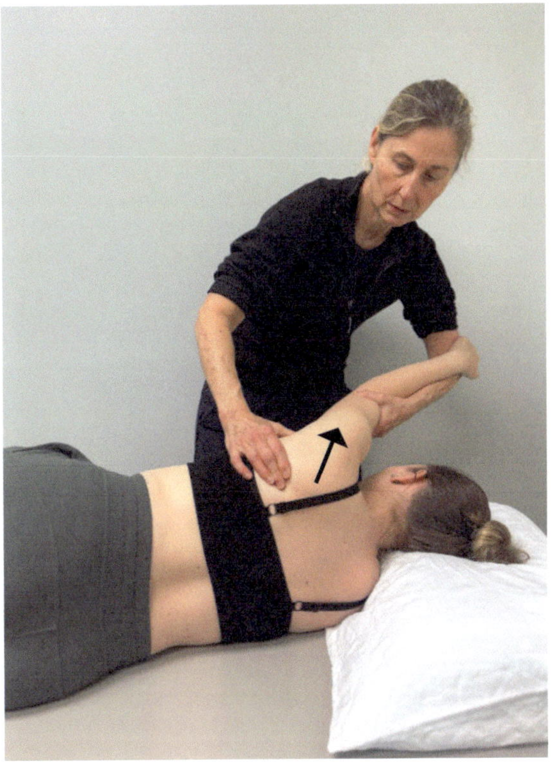

- In this same position, your family member or friend will press your entire shoulder downward and outward to stretch your chest muscle (pectoralis minor).

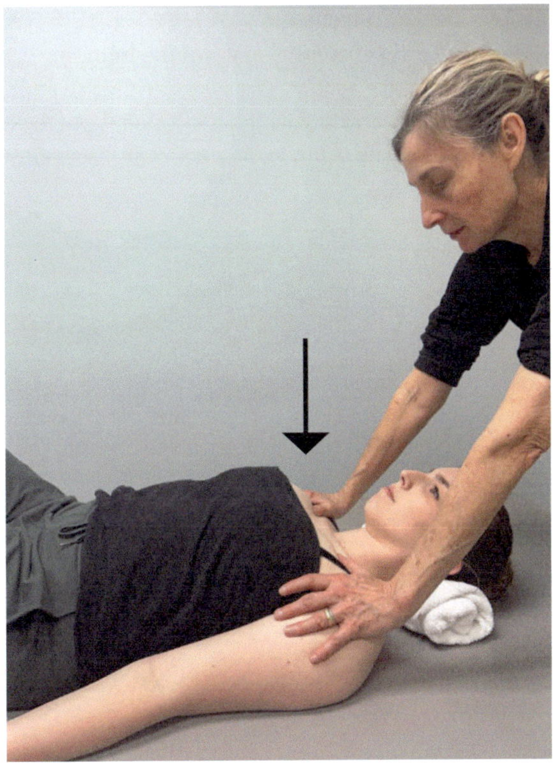

- Lie on a foam roller positioned vertically along the middle of your back. Keep your arms resting comfortably at your side, your knees bent, and your feet resting on the floor. Relax and hold this position for 3–5 min to gently feel a stretch across your chest

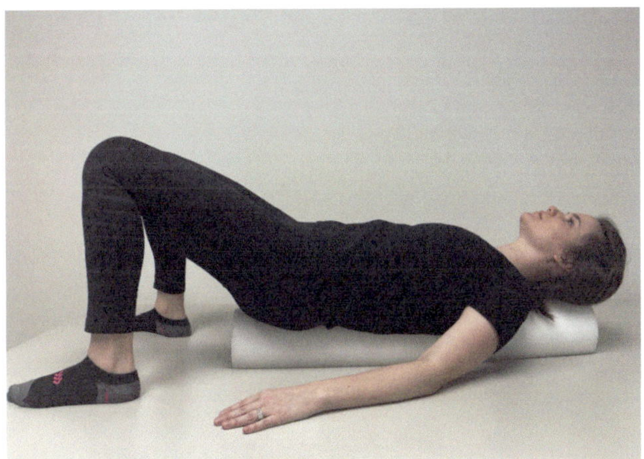

☐ **Active Donor Movement:**
Complete 10 repetitions every waking hour.

- Begin by standing with your back to a wall. With the palm of your hand facing behind you, press your fist against the wall. Keep your shoulders relaxed and down as you complete the movement. Relax and repeat.

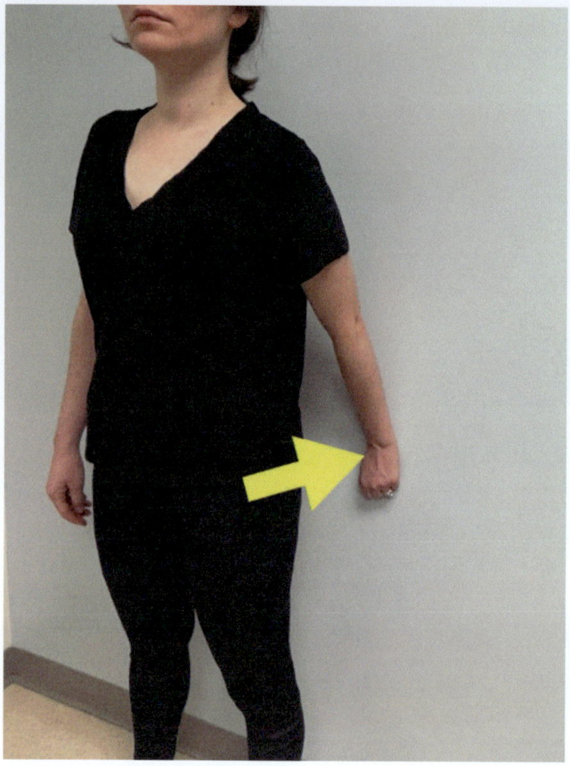

☐ **Active (or Resisted) Donor + Passive Recipient Movement:**

Complete 10 repetitions, 2–3 times per day.

- Begin by sitting at a table with both hands clasped before you. Press down on the table with your injured arm as your other arm helps slide it forward. A family member or friend can help by cupping your shoulder blade and gently guiding it forward as your arm moves forward.

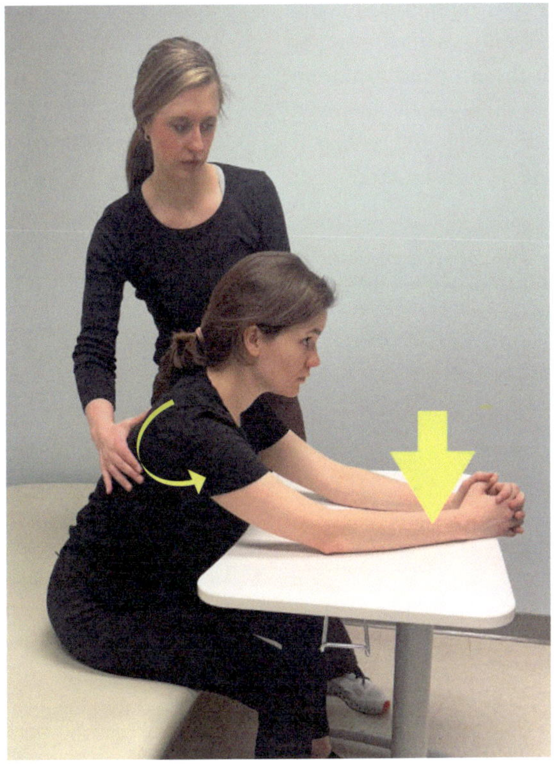

Phase 2 Thoracodorsal to Long Thoracic Nerve Transfer Exercises

☐ **Active Donor + Active-Assisted Recipient Movement: Complete these exercises 1–10 repetitions, 2–3 times per day.**

- Begin by sitting on a chair with a pulley system anchored on a door behind you. Start with your injured arm down and your other arm above you. Pull down with your uninjured arm to create resistance to the involved arm, and attempt to control this resistance by allowing the involved arm to raise very slowly. You are essentially pulling it down a bit while slowly allowing it to raise over your head.

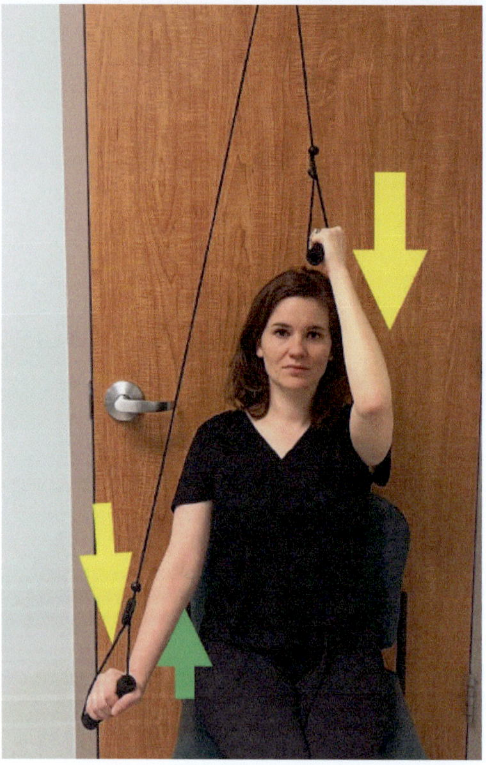

- Sit in front of a table with your arm resting a soft, medium-sized ball. Push down on the ball and roll your arm forward, allowing your shoulder to move forward as well. Maintain the pressure as you roll it back to the starting position. Relax and repeat.

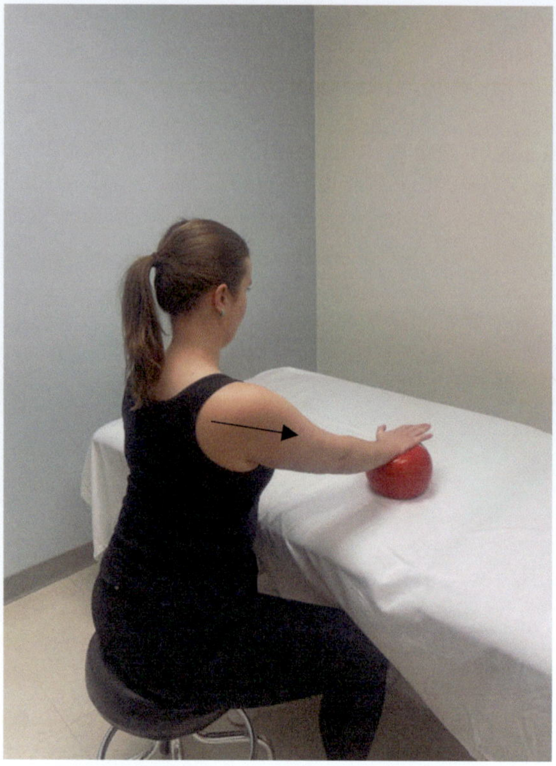

- Lie on your stomach with a rolled towel supporting your forehead. Press your arms into the mat or floor as you slide your arms forward. **A friend or family member may assist your shoulder blades into an forward and outward direction.**

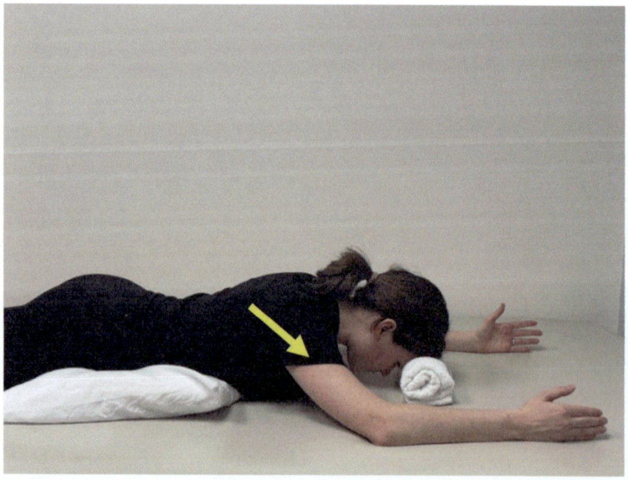

☐ **"Place and Hold" Exercise**
Complete <u>1–10</u> repetitions, <u>2–3</u> times per day.

- Lie on your side with a friend or family member supporting your arm by his or her side. Press your arm into your friend as he or she assists your shoulder blade into an forward and outward direction (protraction). Try to maintain this position of the shoulder as the support is removed. Hold 5 seconds, relax, and repeat.

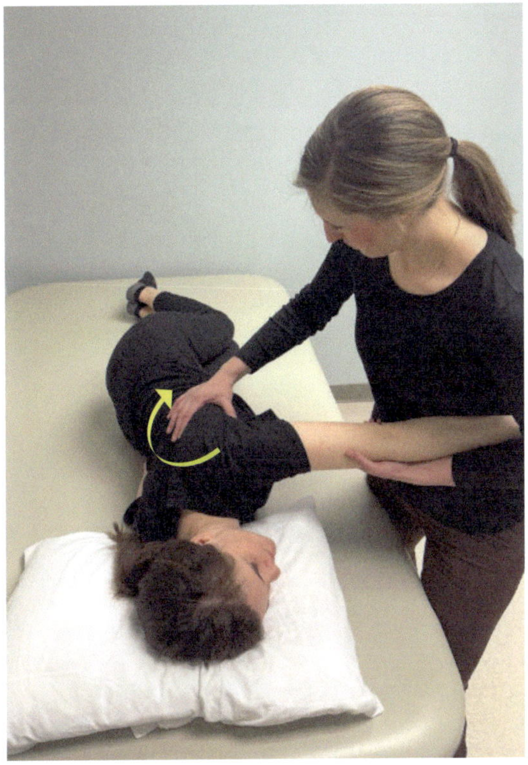

☐ **Active Donor + Active Recipient**

Complete these exercises 1–10 repetitions, 2–3 times per day.

- Wall Slides: Stand with the pinky sides of your hand on a wall. Press your opposite fist just above your elbow on the injured arm in an upward direction. Attempt to create resistance in your donor muscle (downward motion) by limiting the speed of your arm movement as you slide the arm overhead very slowly. You should feel the scapula rotating with less winging.

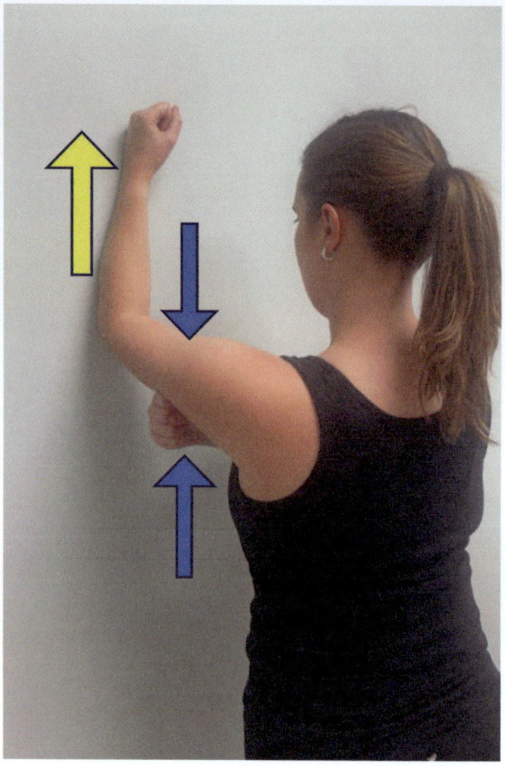

Phase 3 Thoracodorsal to Long Thoracic Nerve Transfer Exercises

Complete these exercises 1–10 repetitions, 2–3 times per day.

☐ **Resisted Donor + Resisted Recipient Movement:**

- Prone Press Up on Elbows: Begin this exercise lying on your stomach and resting on your elbows. Push up on your elbows and bend your back upward (arch). Hold this position while keeping your shoulder blades engaged. Keep your hips in contact with the floor throughout the exercise.

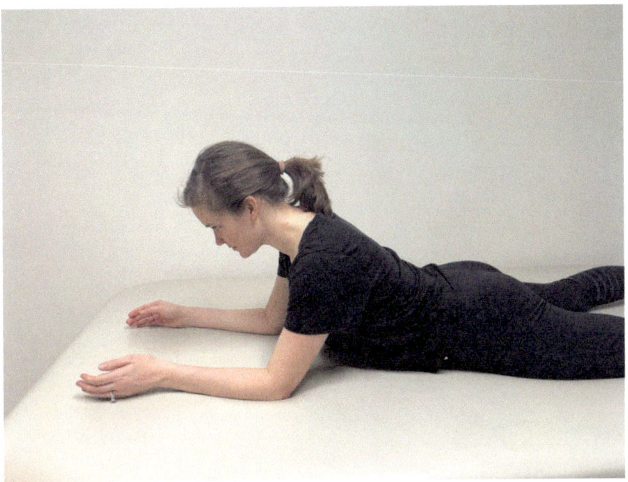

- Prone on Elbows with Alternating Arm Slides: Lie on your stomach propped on your elbows. Slowly slide one arm forward as you think about your shoulder blade, keeping it engaged. Bring your arm back to the starting position and complete the same with your other arm.

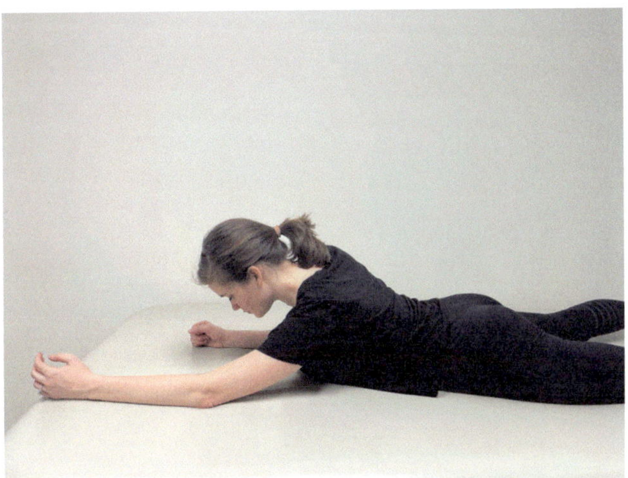

- Plank: Lie on your stomach propped on your elbows. Engage your upper back and abdominal muscles as you lift your hips and legs into a plank position. Keep your elbows under your shoulders and hold the position as long as your shoulder blades remain engaged.

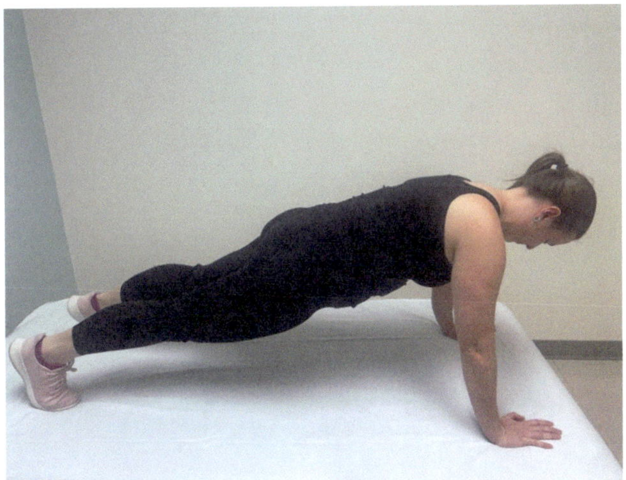

☐ **Resistive Recipient Movement**

- Single Arm Punch : Lie on your back while holding a light weight in your hand. Raise your arm towards the ceiling. Keeping your elbow straight, punch your arm toward the ceiling, raising your shoulder off the ground.

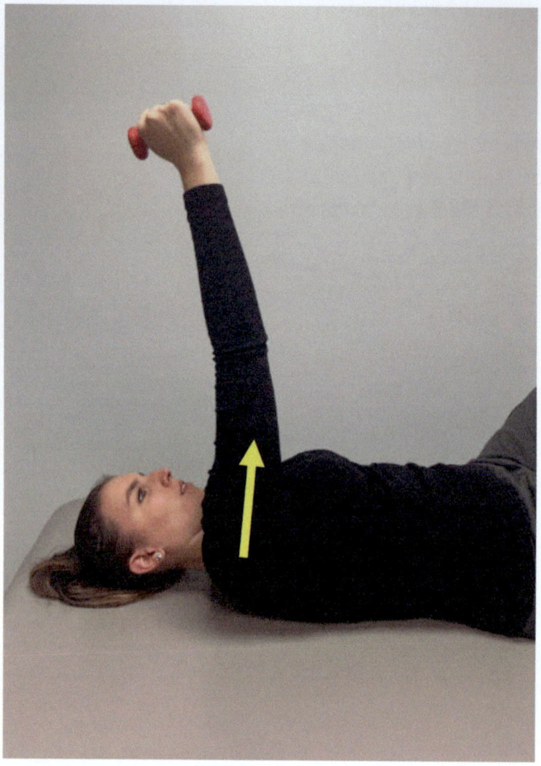

- Wall Push "Up and Out": Begin with your arms supported on a wall in front you at shoulder height. First lean slightly into the wall. Then push yourself away from the wall by rounding your upper body and pulling your shoulder blades apart. (Think about "arching" your upper back.) Then, allow your body to lean toward the wall relaxing your shoulder blades slowly as they come together.

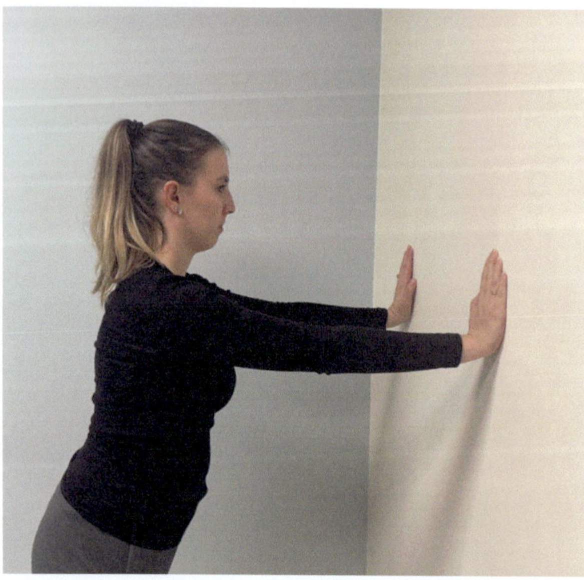

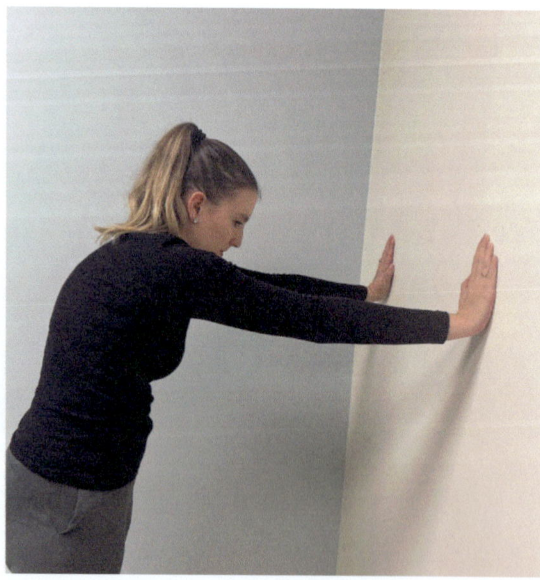

- Dynamic Hug with Resistance Band: While standing, hold the ends of a resistance band wrapped around your mid back. Reach forward with your arms as if hugging a beach ball, then slowly return to the starting position and repeat.

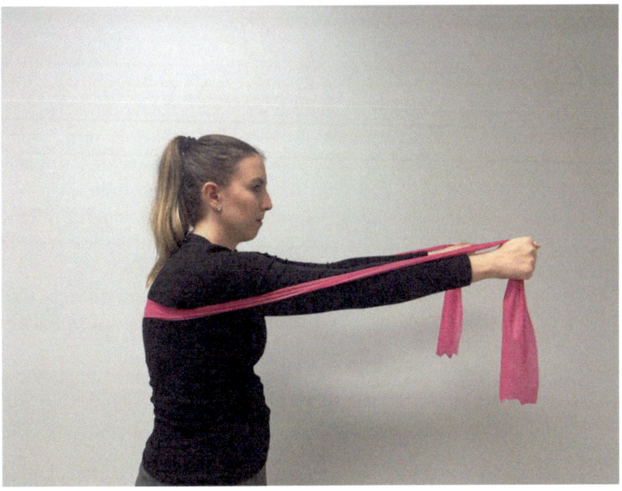

References

1. Neumann DA. Kinesiology of the musculoskeletal system-e-book: foundations for rehabilitation. Elsevier Health Sciences; 2016.
2. Safran MR. Nerve injury about the shoulder in athletes, part 2: long thoracic nerve, spinal accessory nerve, burners/stingers, thoracic outlet syndrome. Am J Sports Med. 2004;32(4):1063–76.
3. Maire N, Abane L, Kempf JF, Clavert P. Long thoracic nerve release for scapular winging: clinical study of a continuous series of eight patients. Orthop Traumatol Surg Res. 2013;99(6):S329–35.
4. Pinder EM, Ng CY. Scratch collapse test is a useful clinical sign in assessing long thoracic nerve entrapment. J Hand Microsurg. 2016;8(02):122–4.
5. Leechavengvongs S, Jiamton C, Uerpairojkit C, Malungpaishorpe K, Witoonchart K, Poonotoke P. Polyester tape scapulopexy for chronic upper extremity brachial plexus injury. J Hand Surg Am. 2015;40(6):1184–9.
6. Warner JJ, Navarro RA. Serratus anterior dysfunction. Clin Orthop Relat Res. 1998:139–48.
7. Chalmers PN, Saltzman BM, Feldheim TF, et al. A comprehensive analysis of pectoralis major transfer for long thoracic nerve palsy. J Shoulder Elbow Surg. 2015;24(7):1028–35.
8. Uerpairojkit C, Leechavengvongs S, Witoonchart K, Malungpaishorpe K, Raksakulkiat R. Nerve transfer to serratus anterior muscle using the thoracodorsal nerve for winged scapula in C5 and C6 brachial plexus root avulsions. J Hand Surg Am. 2009;34(1):74–8.
9. Ray WZ, Pet MA, Nicoson MC, Yee A, Kahn LC, Mackinnon SE. Two-level motor nerve transfer for the treatment of long thoracic nerve palsy: case report. J Neurosurg. 2011;115(4):858–64.
10. Novak CB, Mackinnon SE. Surgical treatment of a long thoracic nerve palsy. Ann Thorac Surg. 2002;73(5):1643–5.
11. Kahn L, Moore A. Donor activation focused rehabilitation approach: maximizing outcomes after nerve transfers. Hand Clin. 2016;32(2):263–77.
12. Hill JL, Turner LC, Jones RD, Jimulia DT, Miller C, Power DM. The stages of rehabilitation following motor nerve transfer surgery. J Musculoskelet Surg Res. 2019;3:60.

Intercostal Nerves to Long Thoracic Nerve Transfer

Jennifer Q. Farrar

Background

The long thoracic nerve (LTN) derives from cervical nerve roots of C5, C6, and C7 at the most proximal aspect of the brachial plexus [1, 2]. It provides innervation to the serratus anterior muscle [1]. The serratus anterior protracts the scapula, upwardly rotates the scapula, and provides stability for glenohumeral joint motion. When the muscle is denervated or weak, stability is compromised, and this results in what is commonly referred to as scapular winging [1–3].

Active forward flexion of the shoulder beyond 90 is typically more limited by this instability pattern than abduction beyond 90° [4]. The loss of strength and stability with reaching that results from long thoracic nerve palsy makes it difficult for people to perform functional activities including self-care.

Surgical interventions for LTN palsy may include a nerve transfer to restore motor innervation and function in the serratus anterior muscle. Donor options for this include the intercostal nerves. The intercostal nerves innervate the intercostal muscles, which are responsible for accessory breathing, contributing to inspiration and expiration. Additionally, they are considered postural muscles as they aid in trunk rotation and flexion [5, 6]. Intercostal nerves have been demonstrated to be effective donors for several nerve transfers in the realm of brachial plexopathies without resultant pulmonary deficits [7, 8].

Surgical Description

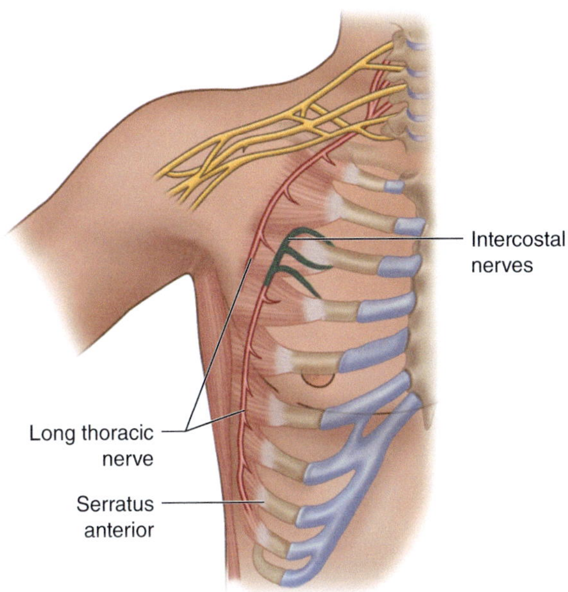

Microsurgical technique of Intercostal nerves to long thoracic nerve transfer

J. Q. Farrar (✉)
Vanderbilt Health Belle Meade Clinic, Vanderbilt University Medical Center, Nashville, TN, USA
e-mail: jennifer.q.farrar@vumc.org

L. C. Kahn et al. (eds.), *Rehabilitation for Nerve Transfers of the Upper Extremity*,
https://doi.org/10.1007/978-3-031-92008-0_7

An inframammary incision is made along the chest wall. The ribs (typically the third through fifth ribs, although there is variability in which ribs are selected) and intercostal muscles are exposed. The serratus anterior muscle is identified, and the long thoracic nerve is identified deep to the serratus muscle, closer to the axillary fold. A nerve stimulator is used to confirm absence of long thoracic nerve function, ensuring that the anesthesia team is not using muscle paralytics. For each rib, the intercostal nerve is identified, typically using a handheld nerve stimulator to facilitate. It is important to ensure that the anesthesia team is not using any muscle paralytics. The intercostal nerves are dissected free from the surrounding tissue as distal as possible (towards the sternum). Usually, two intercostal nerves are used for a nerve transfer to the serratus anterior. The donor intercostal nerves are divided distally and reflected proximally, often being passed through the slips of the serratus anterior muscle. The recipient's long thoracic nerve is divided proximally. Coaptation of the intercostal nerves to the long thoracic nerve is performed using microsurgical technique.

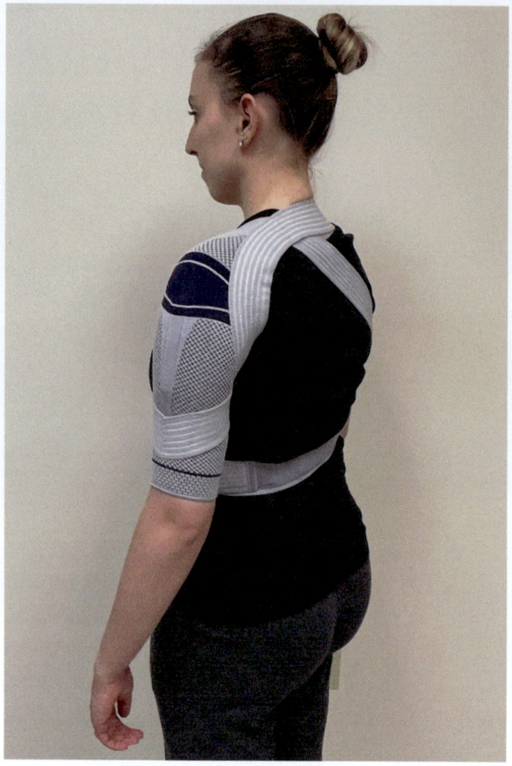

Image 1 An Omotrain® brace by Bauerfeind is used to provide support and may reduce pain in the limb with LTN palsy

Outcomes

The literature currently lacks outcomes for this nerve transfer. An anatomic feasibility study performed in 2017 confirmed the potential for this transfer from a surgical perspective [1], but there are no functional outcomes to share at this time.

Phases of Rehabilitation

Phase 1

Preoperative to 1/5 MMT in the Recipient Muscle

Because scapular mechanics are quite complex, preoperative therapy is often helpful to discuss the surgery, expectations, and glenohumeral and scapular anatomy.

Following surgery, patients are typically seen after 2 weeks. The patient is evaluated in the therapy clinic and instructed in proper arm positioning, recovery timelines, and motor reeducation exercises [9]. Measures of donor and recipient muscle strength are taken in the first month to establish baseline shoulder function. ROM of the shoulder is typically limited post-op to protect the coaptation of the transfer. The therapist may inquire about respiratory status to note any changes, but this is not expected following ICN transfers.

A sling or shoulder immobilizer is typically used for the first three postoperative weeks to rest the coaptation site and limit seroma formation [10, 11]. If the patient is experiencing pain associated with the scapular winging, options for arm support that are less confining than a sling should be discussed. An Omotrain® shoulder support (Image 1), a hip-based arm support (such as a Babymust® or Tushbaby®), and/or Kinesiotape® can provide support to the arm and may reduce associated pain.

Scar management begins once the patient's sutures have been removed and the steri-strips have fallen off. Patients are instructed to massage the scar for 5 minutes 2–3 times each day to limit adhesions to the chest wall.

Exercises

- ROM of Involved and Uninvolved Joints
  Patients are educated on the importance of preserving passive range of motion (ROM) of the shoulder in order to prevent joint restriction. Monitoring ROM of the entire limb is typically unnecessary in isolated LTN injuries but may be relevant with a more involved brachial plexus injury. Attention should also be paid to the scapulothoracic range. When the serratus is absent, and the lower trapezius is unable to provide the necessary scapular upward rotation, the unopposed antagonist muscles can become stiff and short [12]. Manually performing scapular upward rotation (with or without shoulder flexion) will help to maintain appropriate length in the downward rotators including the latissimus dorsi and rhomboids (Image 2). The pectoralis minor muscle is also likely to shorten. To address this, instruction is given to a family member or friend to passively stretch the anterior shoulders in a

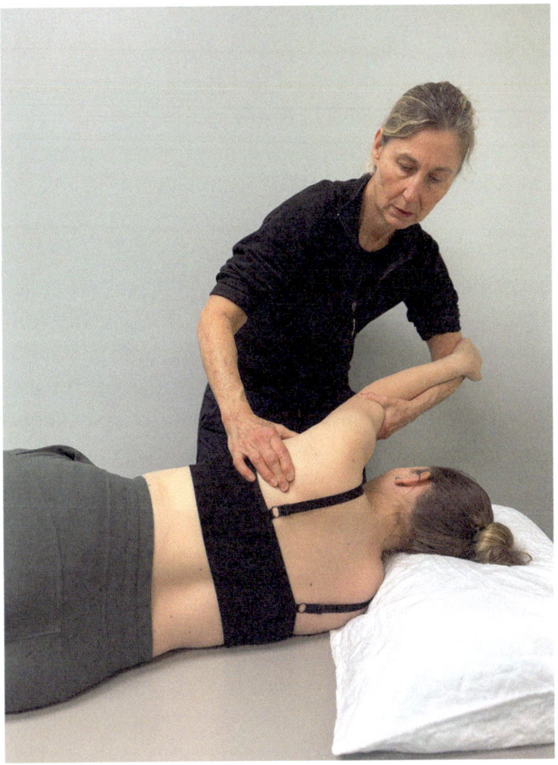

Image 2 Manually assisted scapular protraction and upward rotation is demonstrated in side lying. Maintaining this motion helps to prevent shortening in the unopposed muscles

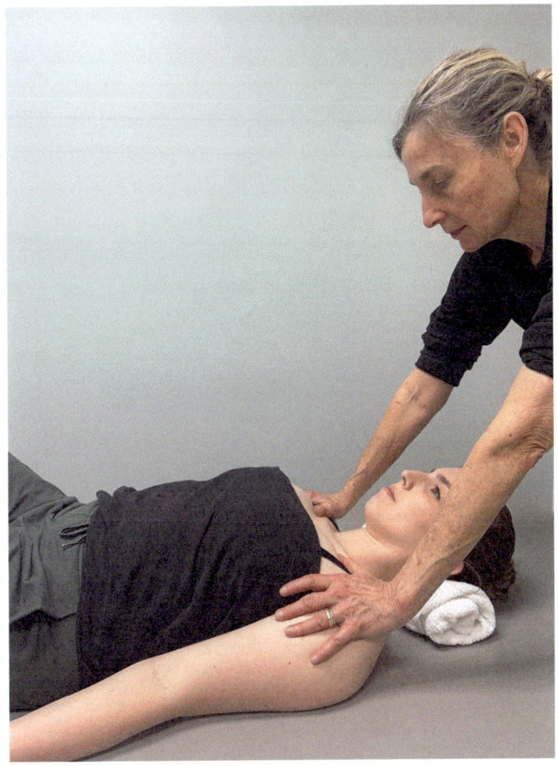

Image 3 Passive stretch to the pectoralis minor muscle is demonstrated in supine. Pressure is applied in a downward and outward direction

downward and outward direction while the patient is supine (Image 3). Lying supine on a 36" foam roller (placed longitudinally along the spine) will achieve some level of pectoralis minor stretch as well.

Passive ROM to the shoulder is initially avoided during the first 3–4 weeks to prevent tension on the nerve transfer site. After 3 weeks, shoulder PROM is introduced if needed. It is important for therapists to confirm any restrictions set by the surgeon regarding this. Coaptations involving intercostal nerves may be limited in length and therefore require limited shoulder ROM beyond 90° [13].

- Donor Activation

  Motor reeducation begins with a general discussion of the donor and recipient muscles and their functions. The intercostal muscles are not the typical donor muscle; they are muscles of respiration that are controlled by the central nervous system (CNS). Numerous studies of their efficacy and function have been performed to better understand their utility as a donor for nerve transfers. Cortical plasticity plays a large role in the CNS's ability to adapt to the intercostal nerves' new function [14]. Functionally, the actions of the donor intercostal muscles include inhalation, exhalation, coughing, trunk flexion, and trunk rotation [5, 6]. A study by Chalidipong et al. demonstrated that in nerve transfers to restore elbow flexion using ICN donor nerves, trunk flexion elicited greater response in the recipient muscle than forced respiration [6]. One may then assume that this information would translate to other nerve transfers that utilize intercostal nerves as donors. Donor activation may therefore be performed with trunk flexion in sitting or supine. Patients are instructed to perform a partial trunk curl (with or without forced exhalation) on an hourly basis (Image 4).

- Combined Donor with Passive Recipient Exercise

  In phase 1 of motor recovery, co-contraction of the donor with passive recipient activity is achieved with the shoulder supported in forward flexion. For example, with the arm resting on a table or over a large exercise ball, the patient exhales while flexing the trunk and sliding the arm forward into flexion (Image 5a). If possible, they should attempt to reach across their chest with the uninvolved hand and passively pull the involved scapula forward into protraction (Image 5b).

  Throughout phases 1 and 2, it is helpful to re-establish serratus length and scapular function by performing passive scapula protraction and upward rotation with the patient in side lying on the uninvolved side (Image 6). Additionally, instruction in periscapular muscle strengthening to preserve shoulder stability is important. The middle and lower trapezius muscles aid in scapular stabilization and upward rotation and should be emphasized early on in the rehabilitation program.

Assessment of Recovery

During monthly therapy visits, donor activation, donor-recipient co-contraction exercises, and assessment of recipient function are performed. The serratus anterior muscle can be difficult to palpate. With the patient positioned in sitting or supine, the arm is supported in shoulder flexion to 90°, and instruction is given to activate the donor muscle by flexing the trunk and forcefully exhaling. The therapist simultaneously palpates along the lateral border of the scapula where the muscles originate from the lateral aspects of the upper 8–9 ribs (Image 7). A positive tender sign may be noted in the muscle by 6 months [15]. A realistic timeframe to expect a palpable muscle contraction following this transfer is 9 months. Functional movement of the serratus, anterior muscle, however, may take 18 months [15].

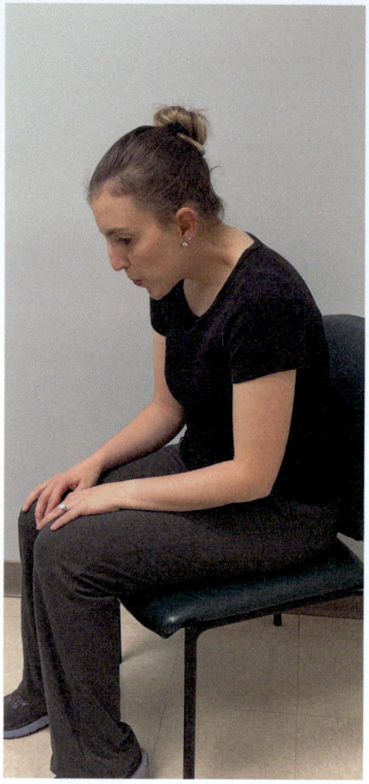

Image 4 Donor activation is demonstrated in sitting with forced expiration while flexing the trunk

Therapy Frequency

Frequency of therapy in phase 1 is very patient-dependent. If the shoulder joint is hypomobile, or the patient struggles with the motor reeducation concepts, one time per week may be required in the initial months. Once the patient demonstrates a clear understanding of the donor-recipient concepts for motor reeducation, and shoulder ROM is improved, monthly visits may commence.

Phase 2

2−/5 to 3/5 MMT in the Recipient Muscle

In phase 2, the patient will continue to perform the motor reeducation exercises with forced exhalation and trunk flexion but will advance to incorporating more active and active-assisted shoulder protraction.

Exercises

- Active Donor with Active-Assisted Recipient
  Serratus Anterior MMT = 2−/5 to 2/5
  The patient continues to perform donor-recipient co-contraction exercises of forced exhalation and trunk flexion with active-assisted scapular protraction. In sitting, the affected arm is supported on an exercise ball or table. If using a table, the arm may sit on top of a slick cloth or an arm skate for ease of movement [9]. The patient flexes the trunk and shoulder, while assistance is provided to the scapula by the therapist or, when possible, with their

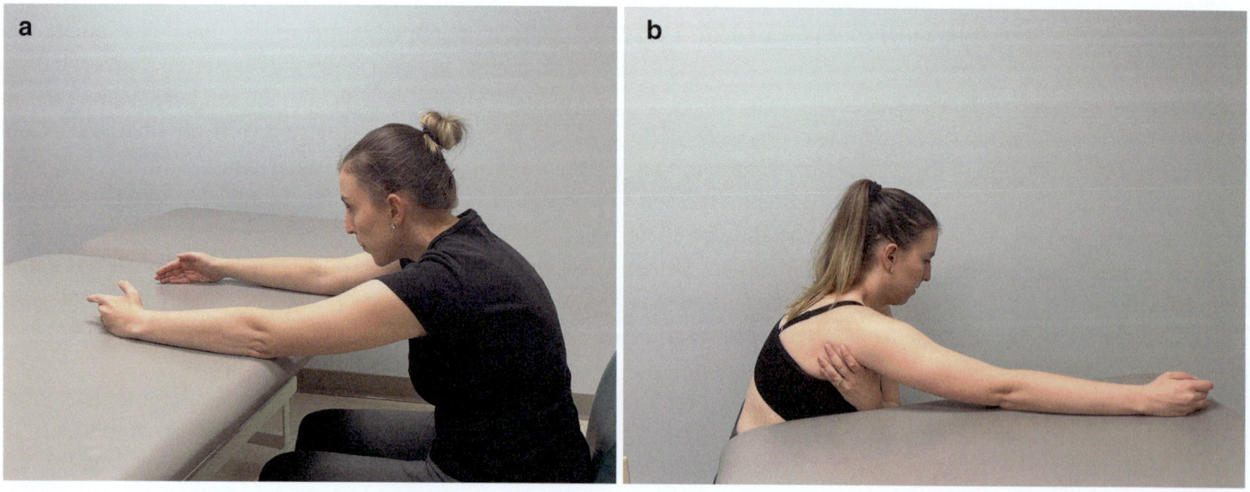

Image 5 (**a**) Combined donor activation with passive recipient pairing is demonstrated with the arm on a table. The individual is instructed to forcefully exhale and flex the trunk while sliding the arm forward, flexing the shoulder. (**b**) If possible, patients are instructed to grasp the scapula with the opposite hand to aid in passive scapular protraction

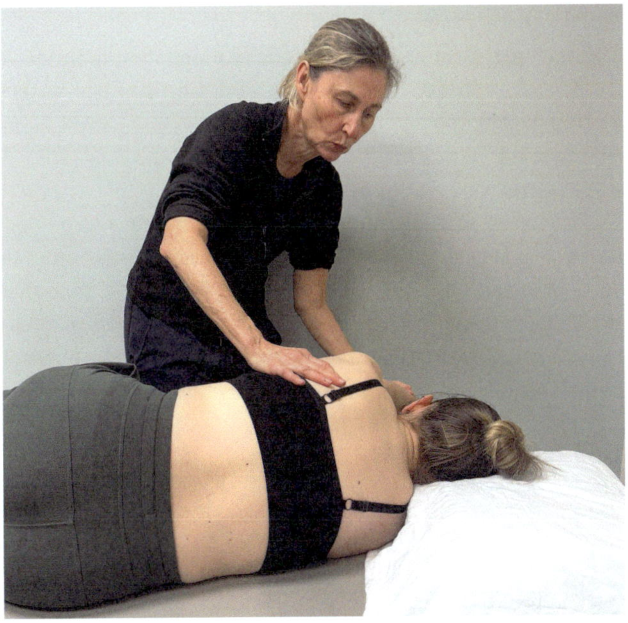

Image 6 During clinic visits the therapist may provide passive scapular protraction and upward rotation with the individual in side lying. Instructions are given to actively flex the trunk and exhale at the same time

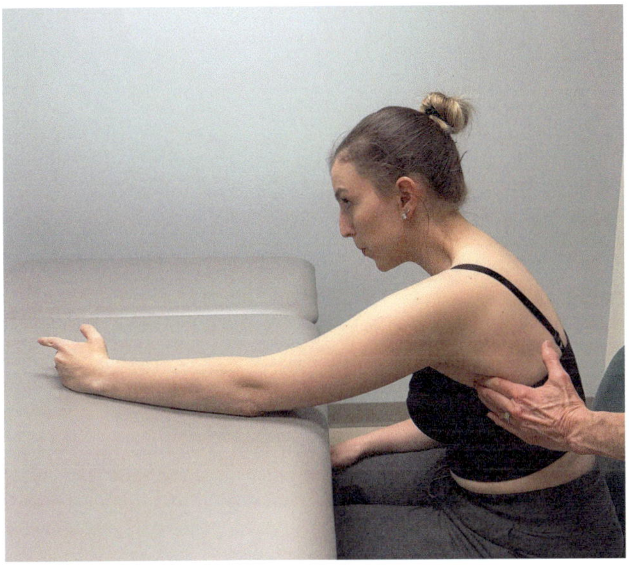

Image 7 Monitoring for recovery of the recipient serratus anterior muscle function is demonstrated in sitting with the arm supported in shoulder flexion. As the individual forcefully flexes the trunk and exhales the therapist palpates along the lateral aspect of the ribs, anterior to the lateral edge of the scapula

opposite hand (Image 8). Instruction may be given to a family member to assist with this. The patient is encouraged to complete ten repetitions three or more times each day, as able.

In side lying (a gravity-minimized plane), the therapist may resist trunk flexion while the patient reaches into active shoulder flexion over an exercise ball. The therapist assists the scapula to end-range upward rotation, as

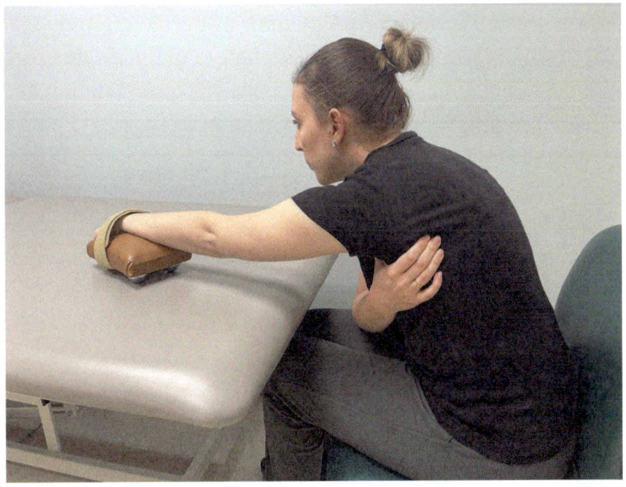

Image 8 Pairing the donor and recipient continues in sitting. The individual attempts active shoulder flexion on an arm skate while actively protracting the scapula. The motion is completed by manually assisting the scapula with the opposite hand

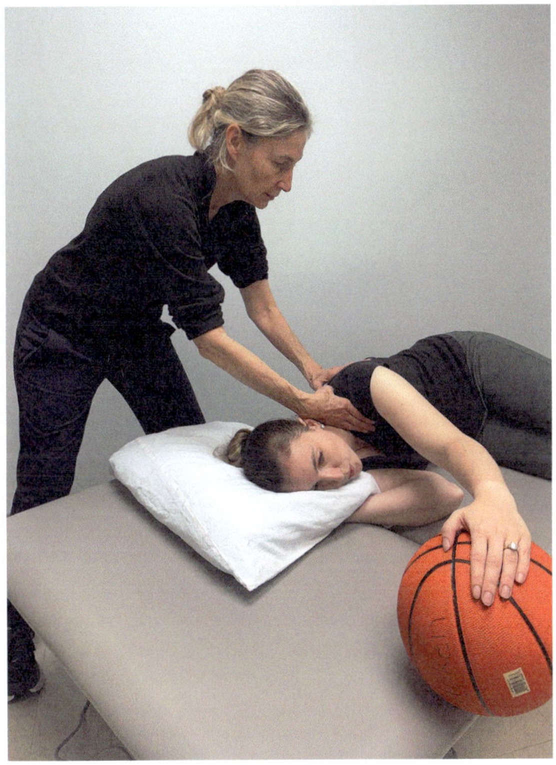

Image 9 Pairing the donor and recipient is demonstrated in side lying with the affected arm on a large ball. The individual actively flexes the trunk against resistance provided by the therapist while sliding the arm forward into flexion with manual scapular assist into upward rotation and protraction

needed, and instructs the patient to do so with the contralateral hand (Image 9).

- "Place and Hold"

  Serratus Anterior MMT = 2+/5

  As the patient continues to regain muscle strength, a "place and hold" exercise may be performed. This is achieved by passively placing the affected arm into flexion with full scapular protraction using the contralateral hand. The patient is cued to attempt to maintain this protracted position (with simultaneous forced exhalation and active trunk flexion) when the hand is removed.

- Active Donor with Active Recipient
  Serratus Anterior MMT = 3−/5
  As the patient progresses from a 3−/5 to a 3/5 MMT level, exercises are completed against gravity in supine or standing at a wall. With both hands resting on a wall, the individual is instructed to slide them up the wall, flexing the shoulder with arms parallel and simultaneously exhaling and flexing the trunk. Holding a cloth in the hand may reduce friction and assist the motion up the wall (Image 10).
- Functional Activity
  The therapist may demonstrate ways to simulate the donor-recipient action by having patients flex their trunk to reach, retrieve, and drop an item into a waste basket (Image 11).

Assessment of Recovery

Evaluation of serratus muscle recovery continues to be performed on a monthly basis. The patient's arm is supported in 90 degrees of shoulder flexion on the therapist's shoulder. While the patient flexes the upper trunk and exhales forcefully, the therapist palpates along the lateral rib cage, anterior to the scapula where the muscle inserts into ribs 5–9.

Therapy Frequency

The patient may attend therapy once or twice a week during this time.

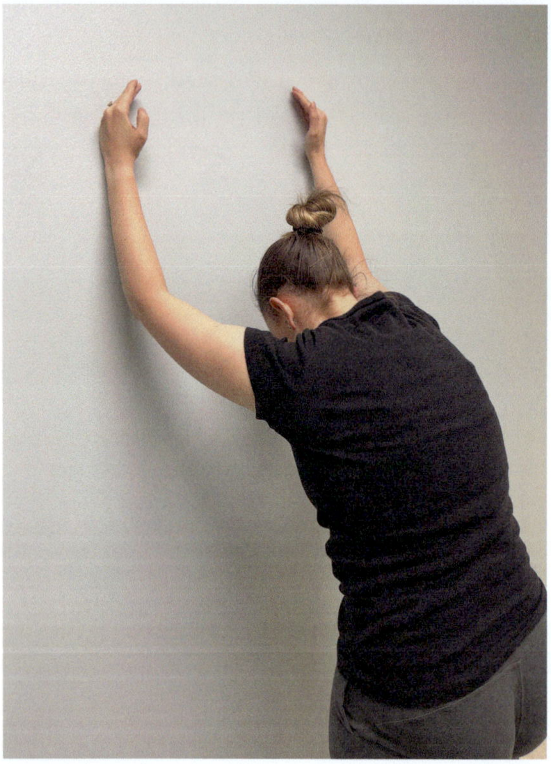

Image 10 Wall slides are performed to demonstrate exercises against gravity that combine donor trunk flexion with shoulder flexion

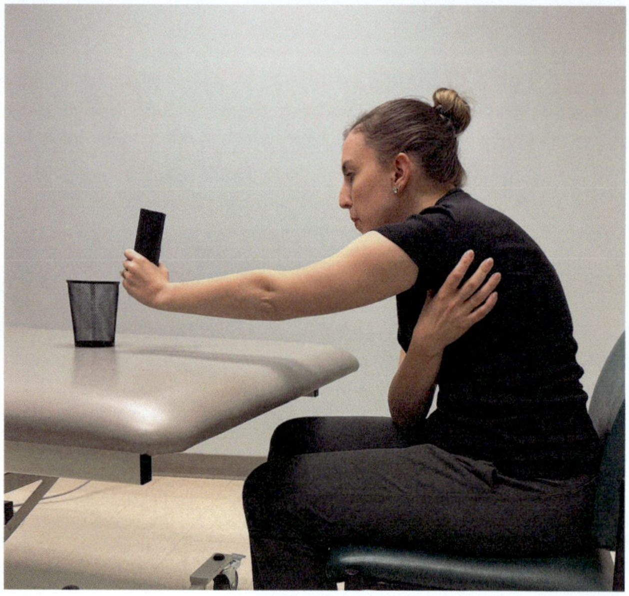

Image 11 A functional task that involves both donor and recipient action is demonstrated with reaching for an object with shoulder flexion and assisted scapular protraction, retrieving it, and dropping it in a waste basket

Phase 3

3+/5 MMT in the Recipient Muscle

If the patient reaches phase 3, the patient will not only be able to work against gravity but also with light resistance. The patient will continue to perform the combined forced exhalation and trunk flexion with active scapular protraction. Positioning for exercises may include sitting, standing, and supine and should incorporate movement through the full range of the shoulder with some object or weight. *However, in the beginning of phase 3, the weight of the arm against gravity is considered enough resistance for early "strengthening" of the serratus anterior and shoulder complex.*

Given the lack of outcomes in the literature, it is difficult to set realistic expectations following this nerve transfer. In general, the patient should be advised that their maximal outcome may ultimately take 2–3 years to achieve.

Exercises

- **Resistive Recipient Activity with Donor Contraction**
  In a standing, light resistance is introduced with shoulder elevation while monitoring the scapula to make sure that it moves along the thorax without winging. Resistance with arm elevation can take the form of manual resistance from the therapist, light resistance bands, or a free weight. Simultaneous donor activation with forceful exhalation, trunk rotation, or a standing trunk flexion-crunch is performed with light resistance to shoulder flexion. Bilateral arm flexion is encouraged. Functional activities that promote scapular protraction are encouraged such as pushing items away from him or her along a table. Compensatory movements should be avoided, such as contralateral side bending of the torso and anterior tilting of the scapula with forward rounding of the shoulder (Image 12).
- **Resistive Recipient Activity Without Donor Contraction**
  As the muscles continue to strengthen, the patient may be advanced to completing active scapular protraction but without forced exhalation or active trunk flexion. This separation can take well over a year to achieve and may ultimately take 2–3 years to regain functional strength. The patient may continue to show the strongest activation when the donor and recipient muscles are co-activated. Wall push-ups may be introduced to de-emphasize the assistive intercostal contribution, with caution to ensure that scapular winging does not occur.

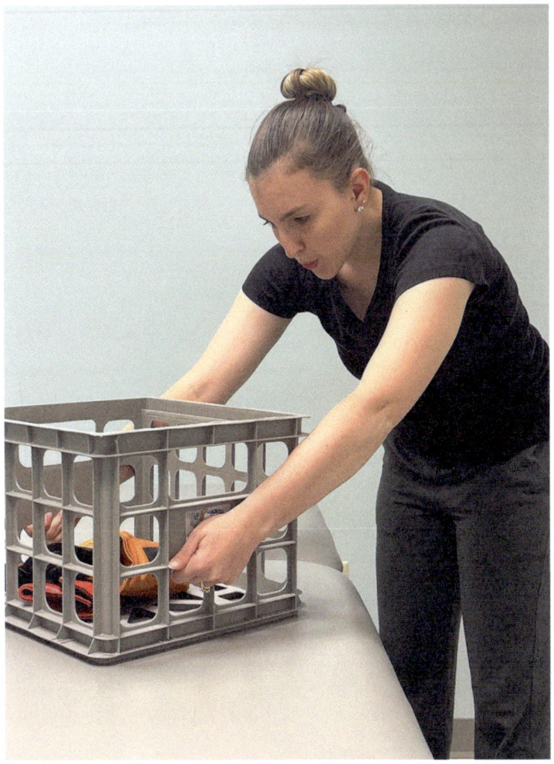

Image 12 Pushing a heavy item along a table with cues for scapular protraction with trunk flexion is introduced in Phase 3 to encourage functional tasks that promote serratus anterior strength

Therapy Frequency

Therapy is recommended 1–2 times a month during this phase, when possible.

Intercostal nerves to the Long thoracic nerve transfer

Nerve transfer overview					
Donor nerve	Donor action	Recipient nerve	Recipient action	Indications for functional restoration	Approximate months to functional movement
Intercostal nerves	Trunk flexion, trunk rotation, inspiration, and expiration	Long thoracic nerve	Scapular protraction (assists with shoulder flexion)	Long thoracic nerve palsy	Approximately 18 months [1, 15]

Information below is suggested guidelines. Precautions may vary according to surgeon preferences and patient factors

	Preoperative therapy	Early phase	Middle phase	Late phase
Criteria	Before Surgery	0/5–1/5 MMT	2-/5 to 3/5 MMT	>3/5 MMT
Purpose of phase	Educate and establish baseline function	Understand donor and recipient relationship	Consistently activate recipient	Strengthen recipient muscle
Precautions	Prevent hypomobility of the glenohumeral and scapulothoracic joints, with special attention to the downward rotators (pectoralis minor, latissiumus dorsi, and rhomboids)	Avoid end-range passive shoulder ROM in the first 4 weeks after surgery (surgeon specific) In some cases if the length of the transfer is limited, allowable ROM will be more restricted	Respect fatigue and prevent dominance of scapular downward rotators	Avoid anti-gravity or resisted shoulder flexion until consistent 3/5 MMT is achieved. Note that not all patients achieve 3/5 strength
Frequency of visits (considerations)	1–2 pre-op visits May increase if PROM limitations exist	1–2×/week until PROM is WNL and patient is independent with donor activation; then 1–2× monthly	1× per week to 1× per month based on patient needs and accurate, consistent demonstration of exercise program	1× every 1–2 weeks based on progress toward patient-specific goals
Orthosis considerations	Support devices to decrease pain with scapular winging, including the Omotrain® brace, an infant/toddler hip support, or Kinesio®-tape	Full-time sling support for the first 3–4 weeks. May remove for hygiene	Resume support devices to decrease pain with scapular winging, including the Omotrain® brace, an infant/toddler hip support, or Kinesio®-tape	NA
Interventions	PROM for scapular protraction, scapular upward rotation, and glenohumeral motion	**Donor Activation:** Primarily trunk flexion and exhalation. Others include trunk rotation and cardiovascular exercise to encourage inspiration and expiration **Donor-Recipient Pairing**: Exhalation and trunk flexion combined with passive scapular protraction ± shoulder flexion	**Active/Resisted Donor with Active Assisted Recipient:** Patient is either seated with the arm supported on table OR side-lying with arm supported on a large ball. Exhalation and trunk flexion is performed with active shoulder flexion. The contralateral hand (or therapist) assists the scapula further into upward rotation **Place and Hold**: Passive scapular protraction is performed with the shoulder supported in mid range flexion. The patient exhales, flexes the trunk, and attempts to maintain this position as the scapular support is removed **Active Donor with Active Recipient:** Wall slide: With both arms supported against a wall, exhalation and trunk flexion is performed as the arms slide up the wall into flexion and scapular protraction	**Resisted Donor and Recipient:** While supine holding a resistance band, the patient performs an upper body "crunch" while flexing the shoulder **Resisted Recipient:** While supine and holding a light weight, the arm is in 90 degrees of flexion. The patient protracts the scapula, lifting the shoulder off the mat
Additional interventions				In the beginning of phase 3, resistance should first be achieved through the weight of the arm against gravity. Weights or bands may be introduced later, if appropriate

During all phases it is essential to continue cortical reorganization, psychological and psychosocial interventions, and progress to incorporate donor/recipient with ADL.

Intercostal Nerve to Long Thoracic Nerve Transfer

Goal of Surgery: Restore the ability to control the shoulder blade and allow for stability during shoulder motion.

Recipient Movement = Scapular protraction (assists with shoulder flexion)

Recipient Muscle: Serratus Anterior

Recipient Nerve: Long Thoracic Nerve

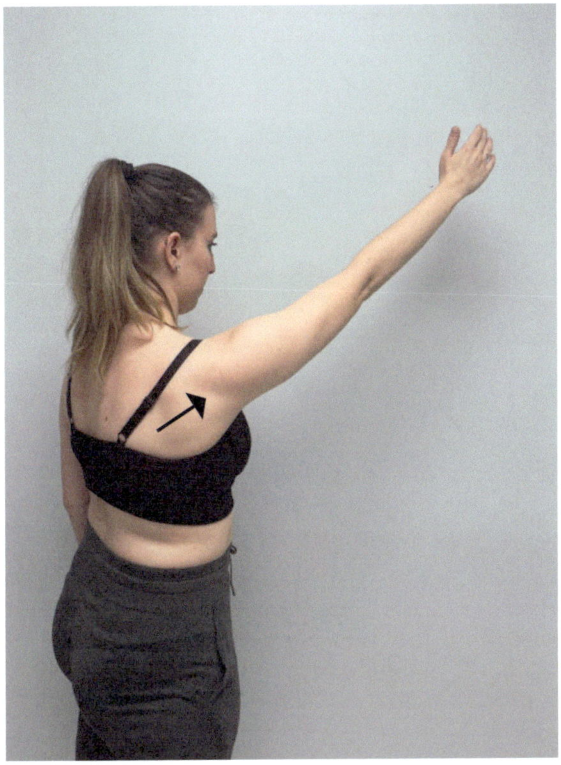

Push shoulder blade forward as the arm moves up

Donor Movement = Exhalation, Inhalation, and Trunk Flexion

Donor Muscle: Intercostal muscles

Donor Nerve: Intercostal nerves (3rd, 4th, 5th and 6th)

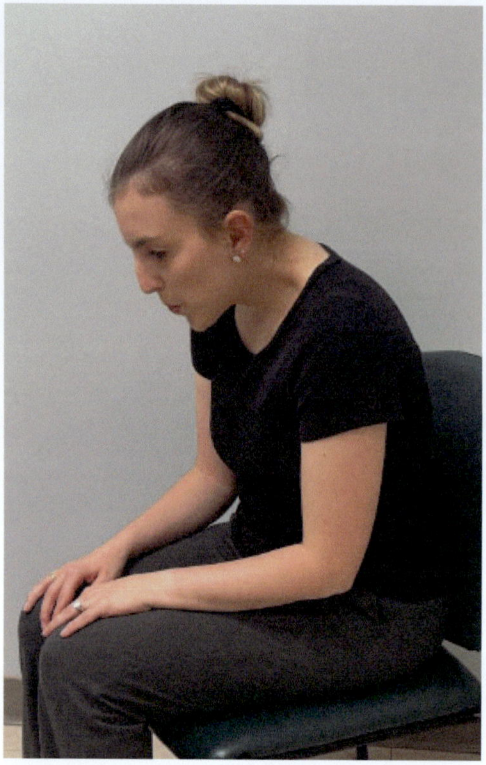

Bend upper body forward and breathe out forcefully

Phase 1 Intercostal to Long Thoracic Nerve Transfer Exercises

☐ **Passive Range of Motion:**

Complete the below exercises 3–5 repetitions, 2–3 times per day.

- While lying on your side, a family member or friend will cup the bottom of your shoulder blade and gently glide it in an forward and upward direction.

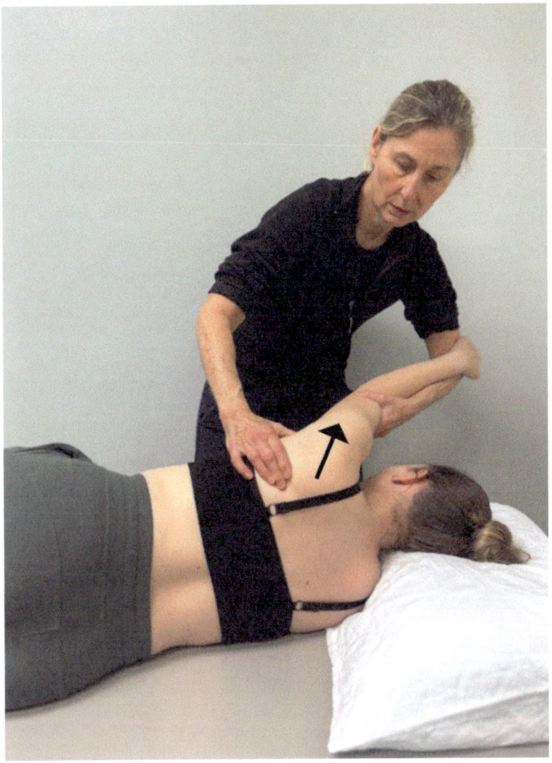

- While lying on your back, a family member or friend will guide your entire shoulder downward and outward to stretch your chest muscle (pectoralis minor).

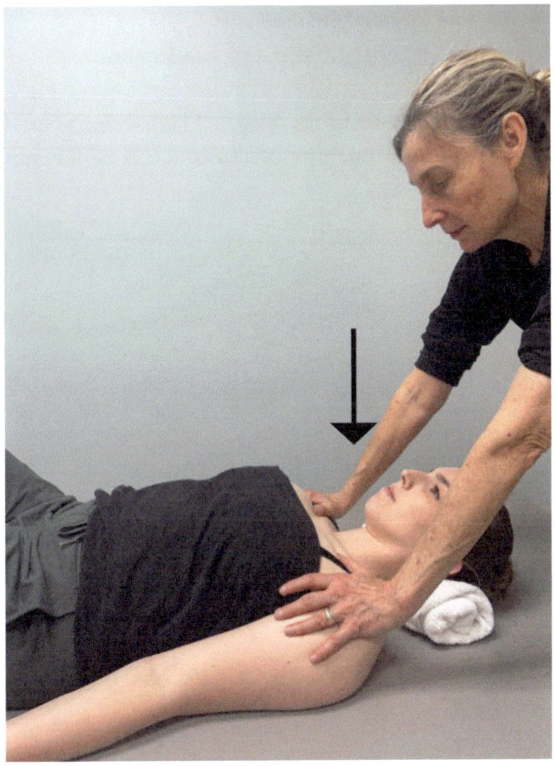

- Stretch your shoulder forward while keeping the arm supported on a table in front of you. Bend your body forward to obtain a deeper stretch.

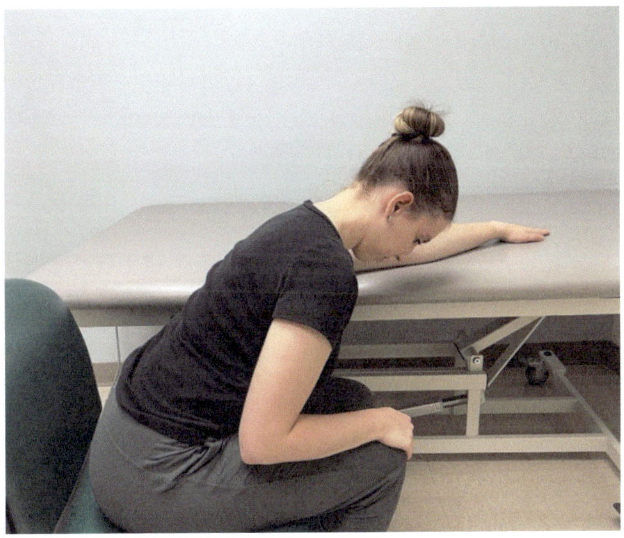

☐ **Active Donor Movement:**
Complete 10 repetitions every waking hour.

- While seated, take a big breath. Then, bend your trunk forward as you forcefully breathe out. (This may also be performed lying in bed by performing a partial sit-up while exhaling.)

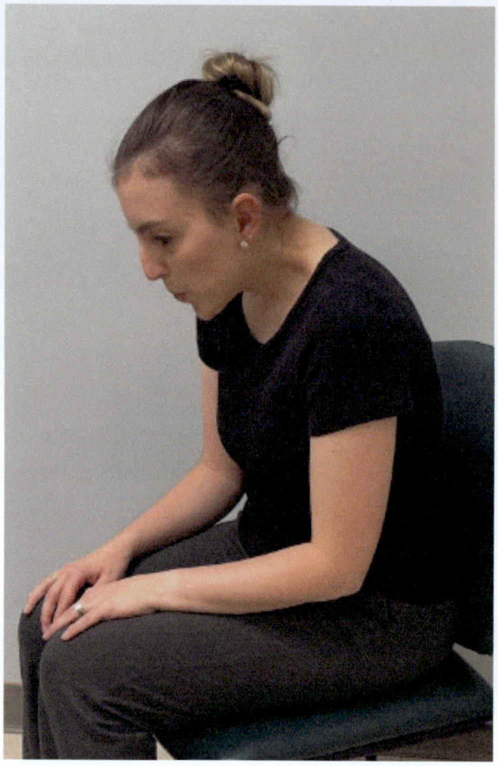

☐ **Active Donor + Passive Recipient Movement: Complete one or both of the below exercises 10 repetitions, 2–3 times per day.**

- Sit facing a table with both arms supported out in front of you. First take a big breath in. As you breathe out, lean forward as you try to stretch your arm farther away.

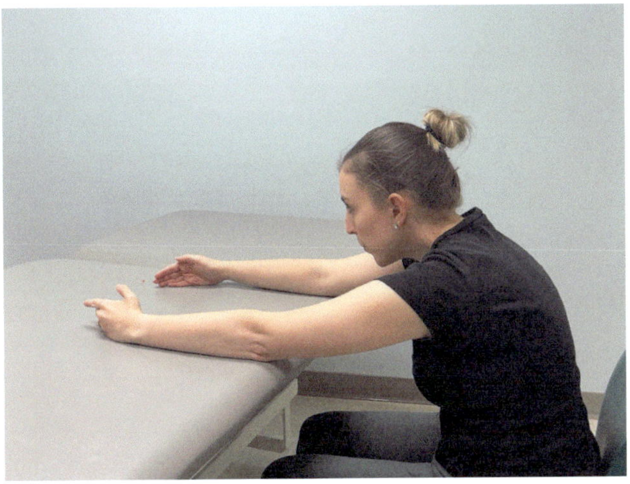

- Lie on your uninjured side. Take a big breath in, and as you breathe out, bend your trunk forward. At the same time, your therapist, friend, or family member will cup your shoulder blade and rotate it away from the spine as he or she supports the arm forward.

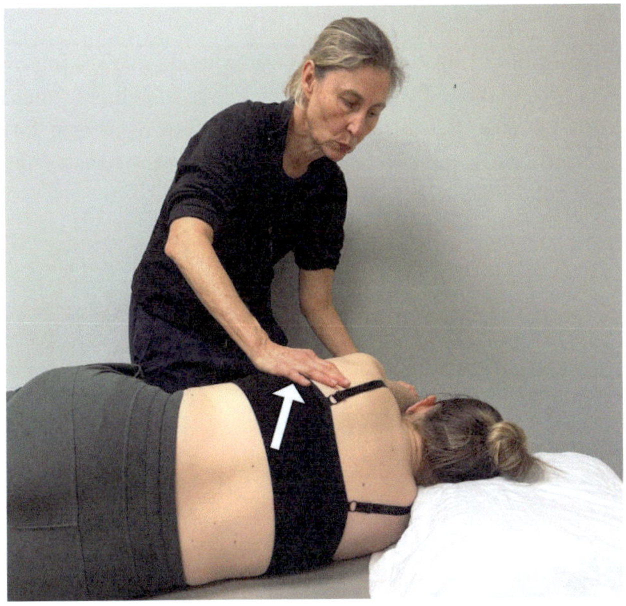

Phase 2 Intercostal Nerve to Long Thoracic Nerve Transfer Exercises

☐ **Active Donor + Active-Assisted Recipient Movement: Complete the below exercises 1–10 repetitions, 2–3 times per day.**

- Sit while facing a table with your injured hand resting on a slick cloth or arm skate. The shoulder and elbow should be by your side. Breathe out, try to slide your arm forward, and, if possible, use your opposite hand to assist the shoulder blade forward.

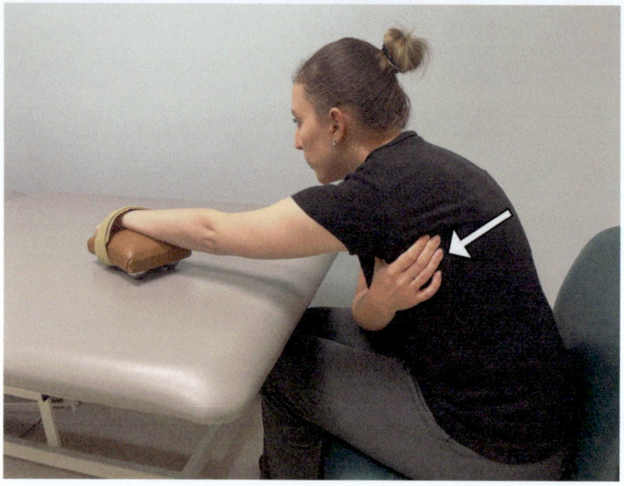

- Lie on your uninjured side with your injured arm resting on a ball. Curl your trunk forward as you forcefully breathe out and roll the ball forward. Your therapist may help pull and rotate the shoulder blade around your trunk.

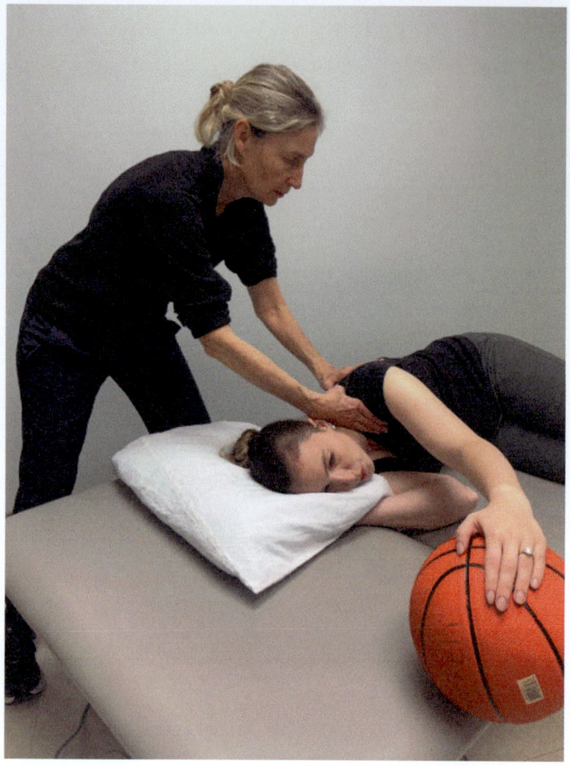

□ "Place and Hold" Exercise

- Start with your arm supported in front you. Use your opposite hand (or your therapist's hand) to assist your shoulder blade forward, around your trunk. Forcefully exhale, let go of your shoulder blade, and try to maintain your arm out in front of you without support.

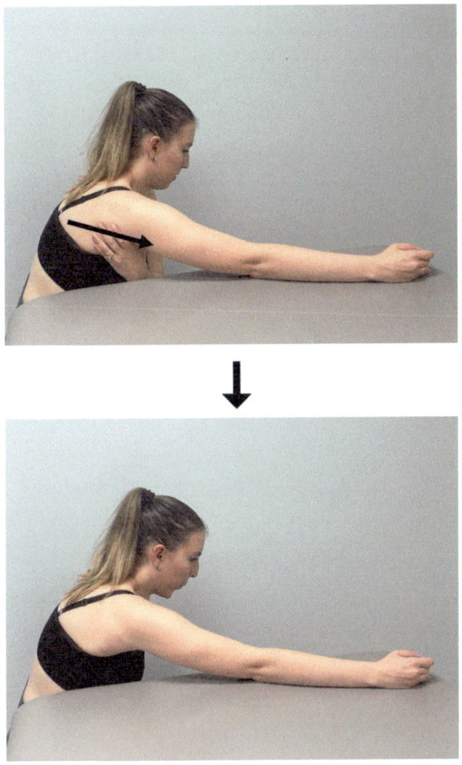

☐ **Active Donor + Active Recipient**

- Begin with your arms supported on a wall in front you at shoulder height. Exhale forcefully, lean into the wall, and then push your body away from the wall by rounding your upper back and pulling your shoulder blades apart. Then slide the arms overhead as far as they will go. Relax, slide the arms back to the starting position and repeat.

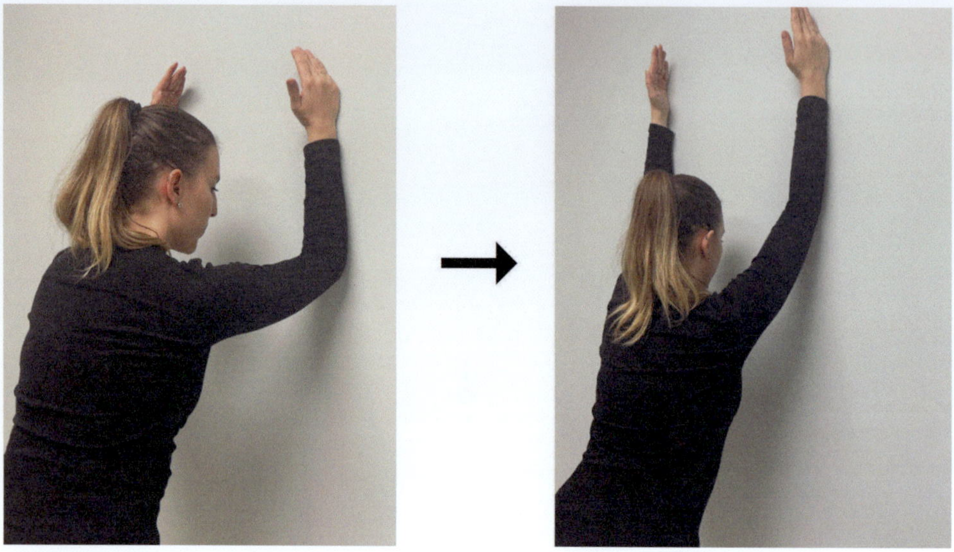

Phase 3 Intercostal Nerve to Long Thoracic Nerve Transfer Exercises

Complete these exercises 1–10 repetitions, 2–3 times per day.

☐ **Resisted Donor + Resisted Recipient Movement:**

- Begin in a standing position. As you exhale and/or bend your trunk forward, slowly lift both arms up in front of you. Use the wall for assistance if you feel your shoulder blade "winging."

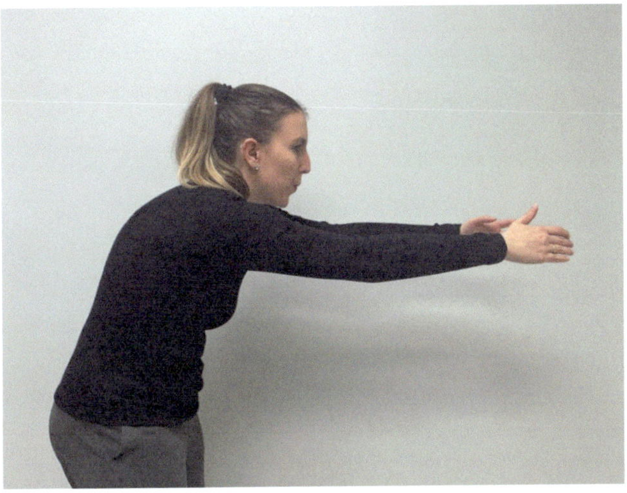

- Lie on your back with a resistance band anchored around your foot. Do an abdominal crunch while you reach your arm up and overhead.

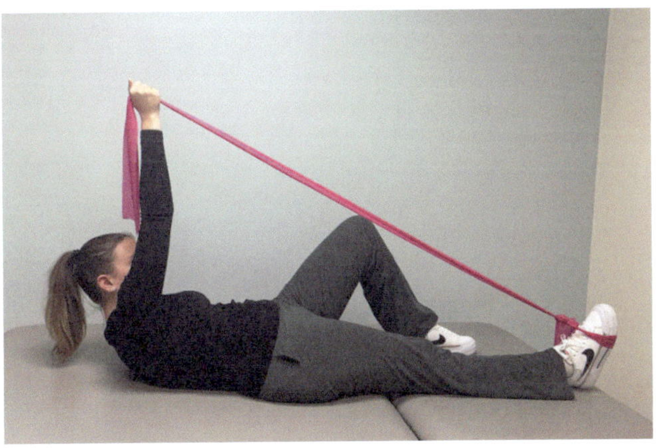

- Lie on your back with resistance band wrapped around your back and the ends held in both hands. Reach your arms up towards the ceiling while rounding your upper back and exhaling.

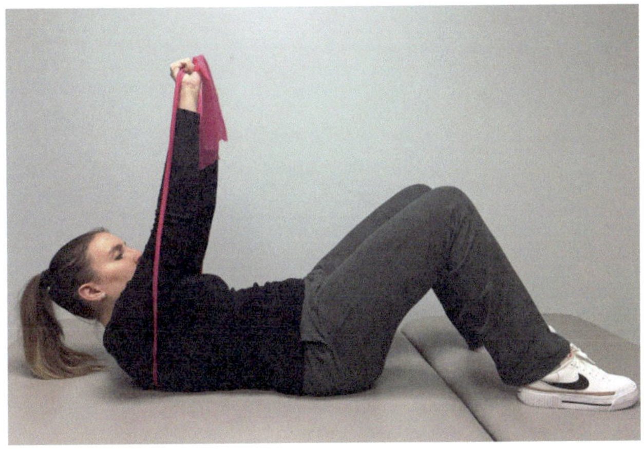

☐ **Resisted Recipient Movement**

- Begin lying on your back while holding a dumbbell in your hand. Raise your arm towards the ceiling. Keep your elbow straight and punch your arm toward the ceiling, raising your shoulder off the ground.

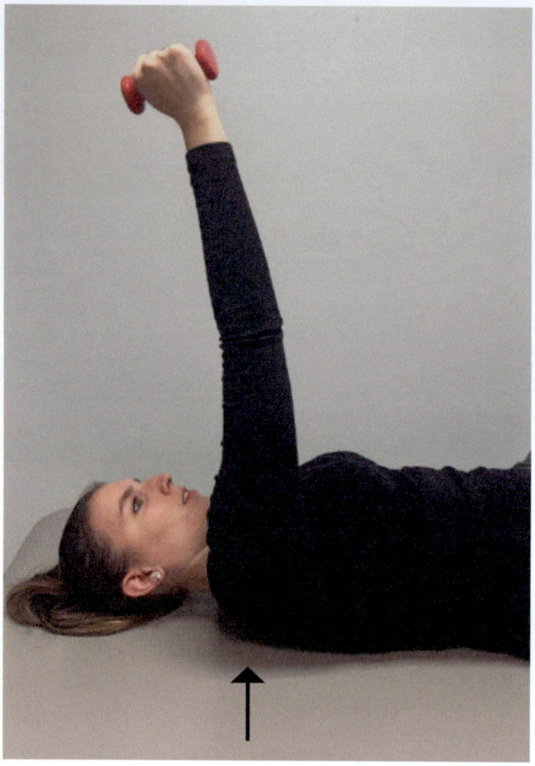

- Wall Push "Up and Out": Begin with your arms supported on a wall in front of you at shoulder height. First lean slightly into the wall. Then push yourself away from the wall by rounding your upper body and pulling your shoulder blades apart. Think about "arching" your upper back. Then, allow your body to lean toward the wall as your shoulder blades slowly come together.

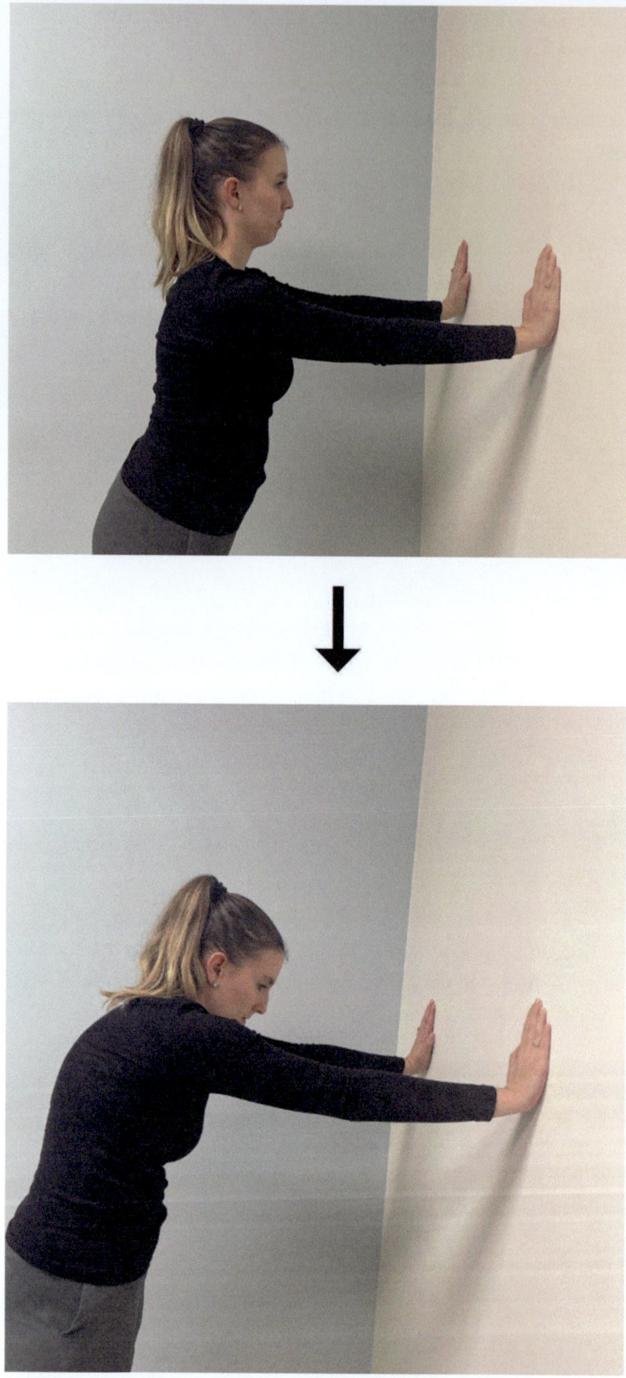

- Dynamic Hug with Resistance Band
  While standing, hold the ends of a resistance band wrapped around your mid back. Reach forward with your arms as if hugging a beach ball, then slowly return to the starting position and repeat.

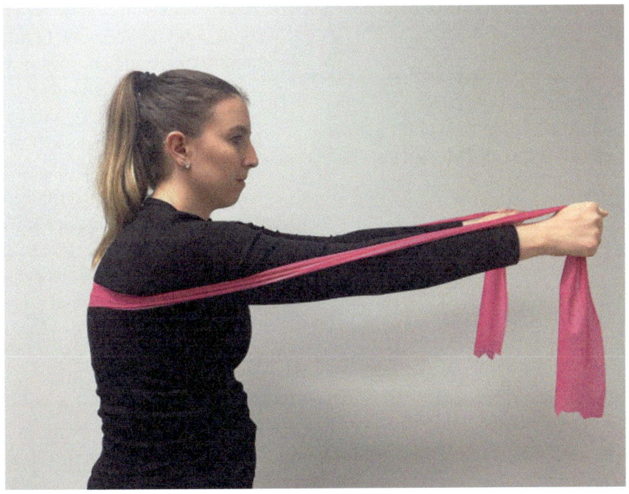

References

1. Louis RG Jr, Whitesides JD, Kollias TF, Iwanaga J, Tubbs RS, Loukas M. Intercostal nerve to long thoracic nerve transfer for the treatment of winged scapula: a cadaveric feasibility study. Cureus. 2017;9(11)
2. Chan K, Lee SK. Surgical management of adult traumatic brachial plexus injures. In: Osterman AL, Skirven TM, Fedorczyk JM, Amadio PC, Feldscher SB, Shin EK, editors. Rehabilitation of the hand and upper extremity. 7th ed. Elsevier Mosby; 2020.
3. MacKenzie A. Restoration of function after adult brachial plexus injury. In: Osterman AL, Skirven TM, Fedorczyk JM, Amadio PC, Feldscher SB, Shin EK, editors. Rehabilitation of the hand and upper extremity. 7th ed. Elsevier Mosby; 2020.
4. Novak CB, Mackinnon SE. Surgical treatment of a long thoracic nerve palsy. Ann Thoracic Surg. 2002;73(5):1643–5.
5. Kawai H. Intercostal nerve transfer. Brachial Plexus Palsy Singapore: World Scientific; 2000. p. 161–236.
6. Chalidapong P, Sananpanich K, Klaphajone J. Electromyographic comparison of various exercises to improve elbow flexion following intercostal nerve transfer. J Bone Joint Surg (Br Vol). 2006;88(5):620–2.
7. Chalidapong P, Sananpanich K, Kraisarin J, Bumroongkit C. Pulmonary and biceps function after intercostal and phrenic nerve transfer for brachial plexus injuries. J Hand Surg. 2004;29(1):8–11.
8. Giddins GEB, Kakkar N, Alltree J, Birch R. The effect of unilateral intercostal nerve transfer upon lung function. J Hand Surg: Br Eur Vol. 1995;20(5):675–6.
9. Kahn L, Moore A. Donor activation focused rehabilitation approach: maximizing outcomes after nerve transfers. Hand Clin. 2016;32(2):263–77.
10. Wahegaonkar AL, Doi K, Hattori Y, Addosooki AI. Technique of intercostal nerve harvest and transfer for various neurotization procedures in brachial plexus injuries. Tech Hand Upper Extremity Surg. 2007;11(3):184–94.
11. Vetter M, Charran O, Yilmaz E, et al. Winged scapula: a comprehensive review of surgical treatment. Cureus. 2017;9(12)
12. Neumann DA. Kinesiology of the musculoskeletal system-e-book: foundations for rehabilitation. Elsevier Health Sciences; 2016.
13. Maldonado AA, Kircher MF, Spinner RJ, Bishop AT, Shin AY. Free functioning gracilis muscle transfer versus intercostal nerve transfer to musculocutaneous nerve for restoration of elbow flexion after traumatic adult brachial pan-plexus injury. Plast Reconstruct Surg. 2016;138(3):483e–8e.
14. Dahlin LB, Andersson G, Backman C, Svensson H, Björkman A. Rehabilitation, using guided cerebral plasticity, of a brachial plexus injury treated with intercostal and phrenic nerve transfers. Front Neurol. 2017;8:72.
15. Hill JL, Turner LC, Jones RD, et al. The stages of rehabilitation following motor nerve transfer surgery. J Musculoskelet Surg Res. 2019;3(60)

Rehabilitation Guidelines for Specific Nerve Transfers: Glenohumeral

Spinal Accessory Nerve to Axillary Nerve Transfer

Jennifer Q. Farrar

Background

The axillary nerve innervates the deltoid and teres minor muscles. These muscles are responsible for shoulder abduction, flexion, and external rotation, all of which are necessary when performing reaching activities, such as grooming, showering, and household management. Injury to this nerve occurs from both trauma and iatrogenic causes. Additionally, an injury to the upper trunk of the brachial plexus (cervical roots 5 and 6) may result in loss of shoulder function. Surgical reconstruction options for the restoration of axillary nerve function may include the spinal accessory to axillary nerve transfer. A lower branch of the spinal accessory nerve, which innervates the middle and/or lower trapezius muscles, is used as the donor. Therefore, performing scapular depression and retraction in combination with shoulder abduction is encouraged to activate the recipient axillary nerve, as it reinnervates the deltoid and teres minor muscles [1–4]. It is important to note that the mid and lower trapezius muscles are important stabilizers to the scapula. If their strength is downgraded by this transfer, shoulder function will be affected even if the deltoid muscle recovers significant strength.

Surgical Description

A transverse incision is made along the cephalad border of the clavicle. The platysma muscle is divided. The most medial aspect of the upper trapezius is released from the clavicle, allowing the surgeon to access the deep/posterior portion of the upper trapezius. The spinal accessory nerve is identified with the assistance of a handheld nerve stimulator, ensuring that the anesthesia team is not using any muscle paralytics. The spinal accessory nerve is then freed from the surrounding tissue and divided as distally as possible. A separate incision is made in the deltopectoral interval. The pectoralis major insertion is detached from the humerus, ensuring that it can be reattached at conclusion of the procedure. The pectoralis major muscle is elevated. The posterior cord is then identified adjacent to the anterior aspect of the glenohumeral joint. The axillary nerve is then dissected at the distal aspect of the subscapularis muscle. Intraoperative stimulation is used to confirm that the axillary nerve is not functioning, and the axillary nerve is then neurolyzed from the posterior cord as proximally as possible and divided. The divided spinal accessory nerve branch is transposed to

J. Q. Farrar (✉)
Vanderbilt Health Belle Meade Clinic, Vanderbilt University Medical Center, Nashville, TN, USA
e-mail: jennifer.q.farrar@vumc.org

L. C. Kahn et al. (eds.), *Rehabilitation for Nerve Transfers of the Upper Extremity*,
https://doi.org/10.1007/978-3-031-92008-0_8

meet the axillary nerve. Coaptation of the spinal accessory nerve to the axillary nerve is performed using microsurgical technique, acknowledging the potential need for an intercalary nerve autograft to avoid tension on the coaptation.

Outcomes

The spinal accessory to axillary nerve transfer is considered a "moderately good" surgical alternative to the spinal accessory to suprascapular nerve transfer to restore abduction. Spinner and colleagues from the Mayo Clinic found that patients who underwent spinal accessory to axillary nerve transfer obtained 60% functional recovery compared to an 80% recovery in individuals who had a spinal accessory to suprascapular transfer [2]. Functional recovery was defined as a manual muscle test (MMT) grade 3/5 or higher. The authors describe range of motion outcomes as follows: 60 degrees of shoulder abduction, 45 degrees of shoulder flexion, and no external rotation [2]. Samard et al. found that in eight patients treated with spinal accessory to axillary nerve transfer, the first sign of motor recovery was after 8–15 months, and recovery plateaued after 15–24 months [5]. There are few existing papers documenting outcomes for this specific transfer.

Phases of Rehabilitation

Phase 1

Pre-op to 1/5 MMT in the Recipient Muscle

Preoperative

At the preoperative therapy visit, baseline motor and sensory testing is performed for bilateral upper extremities. Manual muscle testing (MMT) should include the upper, middle, and lower trapezius muscles; the sternocleidomastoid muscle; all three heads of the deltoid muscle; as well as other periscapular, elbow, and rotator cuff muscles. Patient education begins with a discussion of postoperative expectations, behavioral modifications based on social support, recovery timelines, and an overview of nerve transfer training concepts [4].

Postoperative

Postoperative therapy should begin 2–4 weeks following surgery or whenever the postoperative immobilization period ends. Patients will typically arrive at therapy in a sling or shoulder immobilizer to adequately rest and protect the surgical site. It is imperative to review the operative note to confirm whether or not the pectoralis major muscle insertion was detached and repaired as this will delay movement of the shoulder joint and may require a longer protection time frame. A pectoralis major muscle repair typically requires 4 weeks of protection positioned in shoulder internal rotation and 0–45 degrees of shoulder abduction [6]. Patients may remove the shoulder support for hygiene and elbow ROM. Once the protective period is over, continued need for shoulder support is based on patient discomfort and any potential glenohumeral (GH) joint subluxation. Supporting the arm in standing and sitting will protect the length of the denervated muscle, especially in individuals with suprascapular nerve involvement (upper trunk lesions) while awaiting deltoid reinnervation [4, 7]. Options for supporting the GH joint in the absence of a deltoid muscle include the GivMohr® sling, OmoTrain® sling (Image 1), and/or a standard sling.

Exercises

- Donor Activation
  Nerve transfer training begins with an explanation of the donor and recipient muscles, along with the motions that activate them. The donor muscle is the trapezius muscle, more specifically the middle and/or lower trapezius. Therefore, donor activation exercises involve scapular retraction and depression. The patient should be instructed to pull the shoulder blade "back and down" (Image 2) 10–20 repetitions every hour.
- Combined Donor with Passive Recipient Exercise
  The recipient deltoid muscle contributes to shoulder flexion, abduction, and extension (anterior, middle, and posterior heads). Throughout phase 1, pairing the donor and recipient muscles requires full passive assistance to the deltoid muscle. This is best performed in a gravity-lessened plane. For example, in supine, passive shoulder abduction is achieved with a dowel and verbal cues to retract and depress the scapula. The contralateral hand holds the dowel and assists the involved arm into passive abduction (Image 3). In prone, the therapist can manually abduct the shoulder while the patient retracts the scapula (Image 4). Those with a structurally and neurologically intact rotator cuff muscles will have an easier time with this.

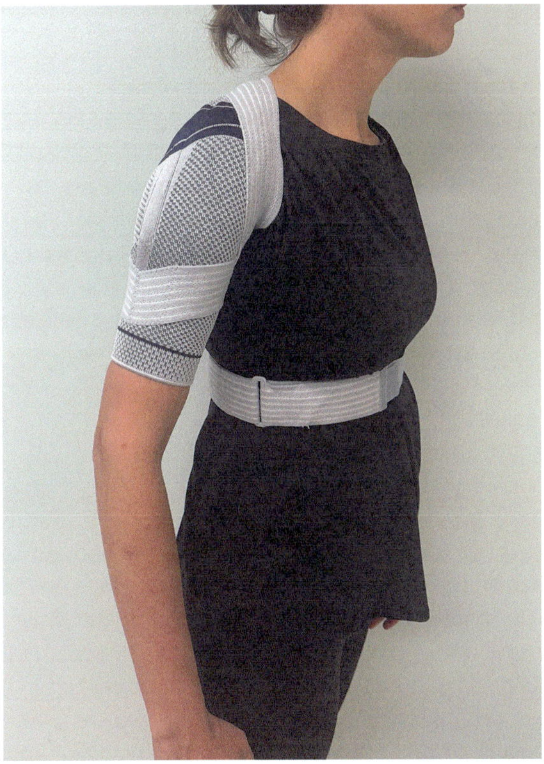

Image 1 The Omotrain® brace by Bauerfeind is an example of an option that provides support to the glenohumeral joint in the absence of the deltoid muscle

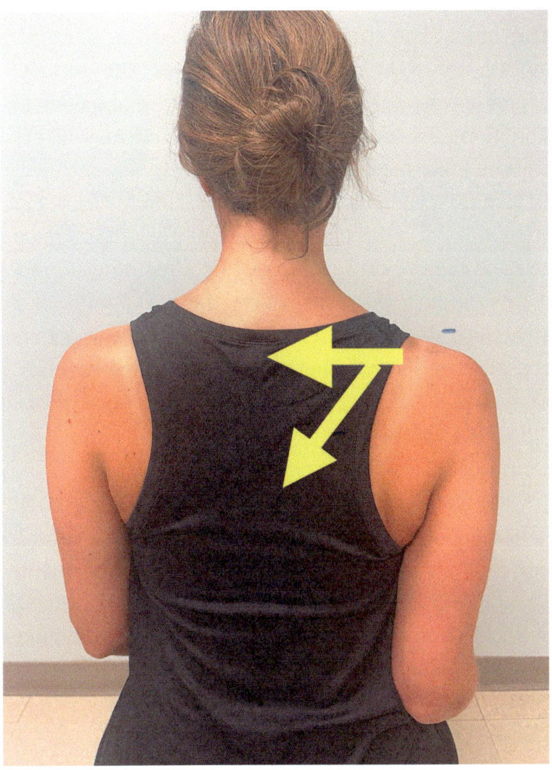

Image 2 Individuals are instructed to activate the donor muscles frequently by retracting and pulling the scapula down

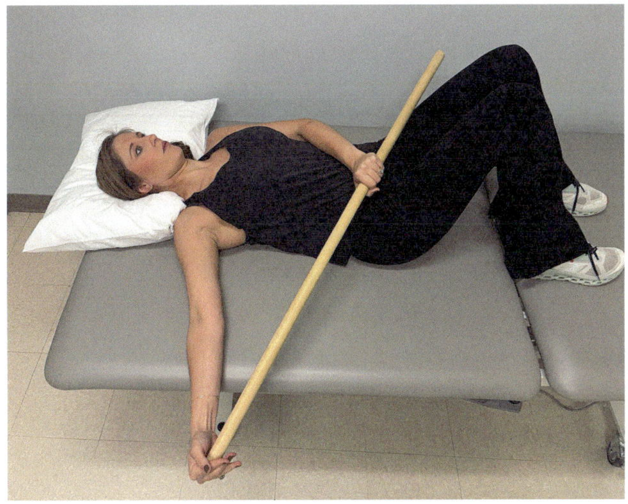

Image 3 In phase 1, active donor with passive recipient exercise is demonstrated in supine with a dowel rod to provide passive shoulder abduction while the patient retracts and pulls the scapula down

- ROM of Uninvolved Joints
  Active (AROM) and passive (PROM) range of motion of the shoulder, elbow, wrist, forearm, and digits are encouraged to prevent joint contractures. In the setting of a complete brachial plexus lesion, PROM is prioritized, and the patient is instructed to move each joint through the full available range ten times, three to five times each day [8]. Other considerations include periscapular muscle strengthening to preserve shoulder stability, including serratus anterior muscle strengthening if the long thoracic nerve is intact.

Assessment of Recovery

Co-contraction of the trapezius muscle while attempting to activate the deltoid should ultimately elicit a response in the recipient deltoid. If the nerve transfer included the entire axillary nerve, one would expect the earliest response to be in the posterior deltoid muscle. Initially, this may be perceived by a positive tender sign, in which pinching the recipient muscle produces pain and tenderness in the muscle [9, 10]. The posterior deltoid receives the first branch of axillary nerve innervation before the middle and anterior heads, so the posterior shoulder is palpated during this assessment (Image 5). The examiner should instruct the patient to strongly retract the scapula while attempting to abduct and extend the shoulder. In the later stages, deltoid function should be assessed in a gravity-lessened plane. During phase 1, positioning is less important; the expectation is simply to feel tension in the muscle. Care should be taken to isolate the long head of the triceps, which can also extend the shoulder as its muscle contraction may be misinterpreted for the posterior deltoid.

Frequency of Visits

Therapy typically begins 2–4 weeks following the nerve transfer surgery. Patients may attend therapy once a week

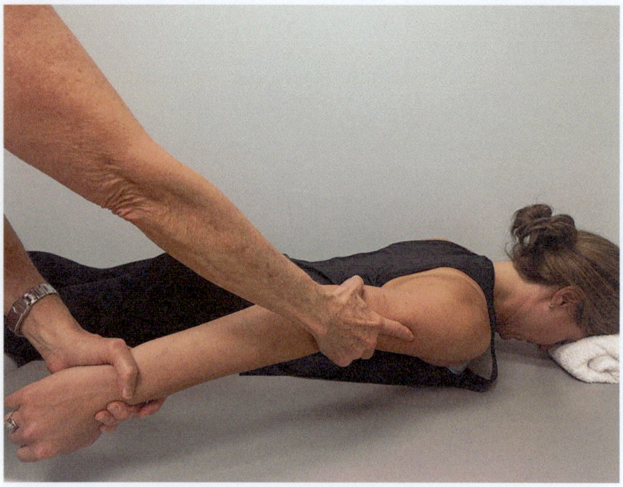

Image 4 Active donor and passive recipient exercise may also be performed in prone to encourage greater scapular input with passive shoulder abduction provided by the therapist

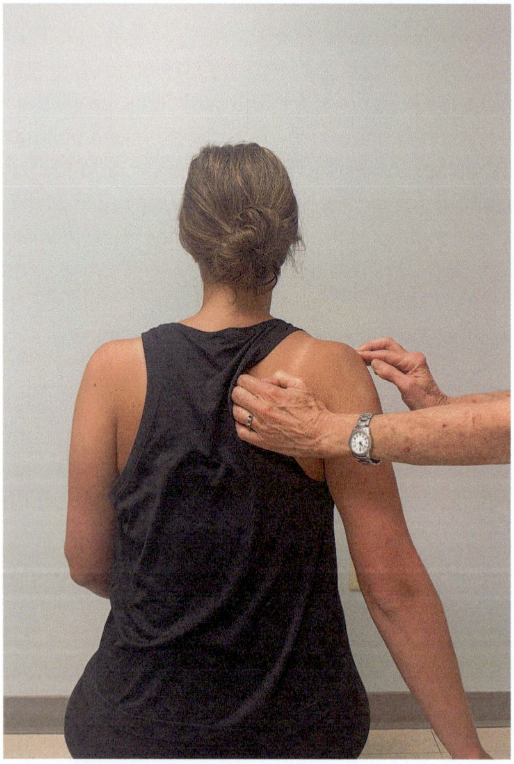

Image 5 To assess recovery following this nerve transfer, the deltoid muscle is palpated while the patient is cued to retract and depress the scapula. Typically, a muscle twitch is first felt in the posterior aspect of the recipient muscle

until any postoperative edema and upper extremity joint restrictions are resolved. At that time, they should be able to identify donor and recipient functions and demonstrate an understanding of nerve transfer exercises so that monthly therapy visits should suffice.

Phase 2

2–/5 to 3/5 MMT in the Recipient Muscle

In phase 2, the patient will continue to perform donor activation exercises of active scapular retraction and depression throughout the day. Combined donor-recipient exercises will advance from passive to active-assistive shoulder abduction in gravity-lessened or -assisted ranges. To improve ease of movement for the neurologically weak but recovering deltoid, an arm skate, slick fabric, or exercise ball may be used to assist early shoulder movement [4].

Exercises

- Active Donor with Active-Assisted Recipient
  Deltoid MMT = 2–/5 to 2/5
  Once the deltoid demonstrates active joint movement, exercises are advanced to include active-assisted movement in a gravity-lessened plane. In sitting, the patient may rest the injured hand/arm onto a large exercise ball. Instruction is given to lean towards the injured arm while depressing and retracting the scapula, attempting to move the ball away from the side into shoulder abduction (Image 6). The therapist may assist with holding and moving the ball in the early stages.
  Additionally, the patient may sit with the arm on a table or mat raised to shoulder height with the shoulder positioned in flexion. The patient retracts and depresses the scapula while attempting to slide the arm into horizontal abduction. The patient may also be positioned supine with the arm on a skate or slick fabric, which will assist with motion by reducing friction. He or she retracts and depresses the scapula while attempting shoulder abduction along the mat (Image 7). Assistance may be given to complete the motion, as needed.
  In supine, a cane or dowel may be used to assist shoulder abduction with the unaffected arm. The patient is cued to activate the donor trapezius while attempting to independently abduct the arm along the mat—with as much assistance that is needed from the cane. The patient will complete ten repetitions of the exercises several times each day.
- "Place and Hold"
  Deltoid MMT = 2+/5
  As the patient continues to regain muscle strength, a "place and hold" exercise may be performed. The affected arm is passively positioned into some degree of shoulder abduction while standing. The patient then attempts to actively hold it in abduction while simultaneously depressing and retracting the scapula.
- Active Donor with Active Recipient
  Deltoid MMT= 3–/5
  As deltoid strength improves to a 3/5 MMT level, exercises may be completed against gravity: in a standing, sit-

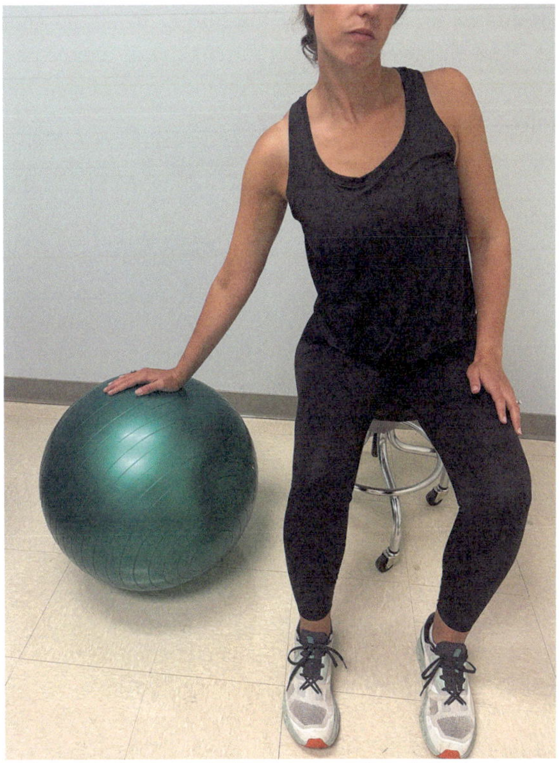

Image 6 In phase 2, co-contraction of donor and recipient exercises includes active-assisted shoulder abduction provided by leaning into a large exercise ball as the patient retracts the scapula

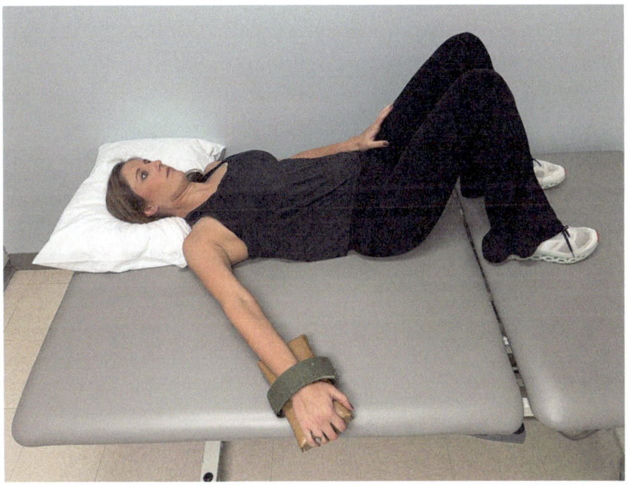

Image 7 An arm skate is used to assist active motion of the shoulder in a gravity-lessened plane while the patient is cued to activate the donor middle and lower trapezius muscles by retracting and pulling the scapula down

ting, or side-lying position (on the unaffected arm/shoulder). The patient is also instructed in wall slides—either with both hands clasped or holding a towel to assist the affected arm up the wall (Image 8).

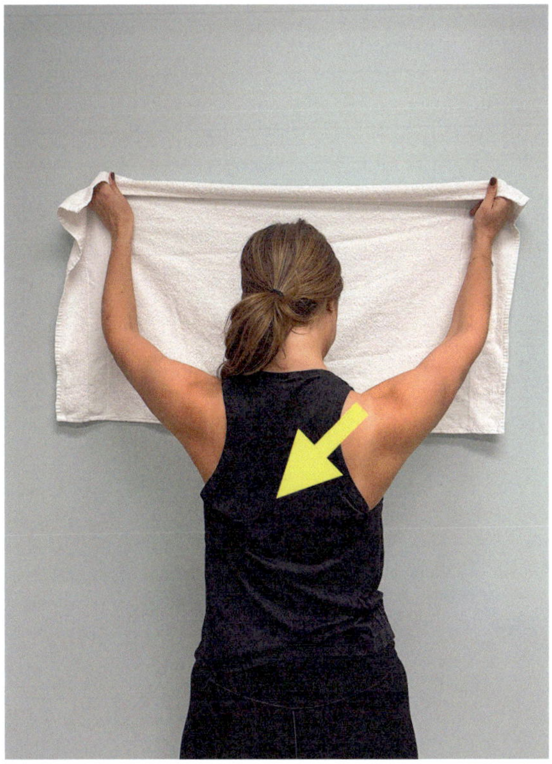

Image 8 Active donor with active recipient exercise is demonstrated at a wall with hands on a towel to improve ease of sliding up the wall. Cues are given to retract and depress the scapula to co-contract the donor muscles

Functional Activity

Simulation of self-care activities such as washing the axillary area, applying deodorant, or donning a shirt can be incorporated into the exercise routine. Patients need to remember to first co-contract the trapezius simultaneously with the deltoid. Other functional activities that may diversify the exercise program include retrieving an object such as a hairbrush or a cup from a countertop (Image 9). Active abduction to reach and grab the handle of a laundry basket and/or folding towels may also incorporate functional activities (if elbow function is intact).

Assessment of Recovery

Assessment of recipient function is performed during monthly therapy visits and determines the appropriate exercise program and frequency of therapy visits. The therapist palpates the deltoid (all three heads separately) while cueing the patient to strongly retract the scapula and attempt to abduct and extend the shoulder. Measuring the degrees of shoulder abduction during assessments provides quantifiable progress towards specific goals for deltoid recovery progress and aids with patient motivation (Image 10).

Frequency of Visits

The patient may attend therapy anywhere from once a week to once a month during this time. This will vary based on

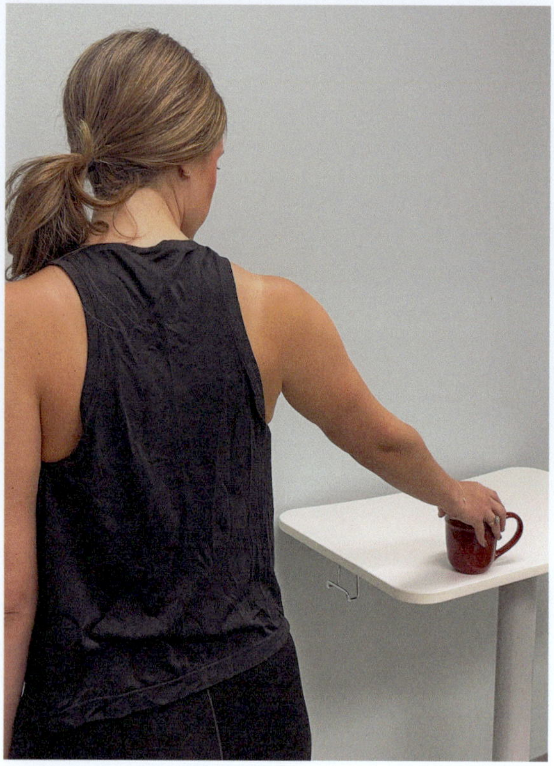

Image 9 Functional activities that promote active recipient/deltoid action combined with donor scapular retraction are demonstrated. Here the patient is shown to retract the scapula while abducting the shoulder to place a mug on a table

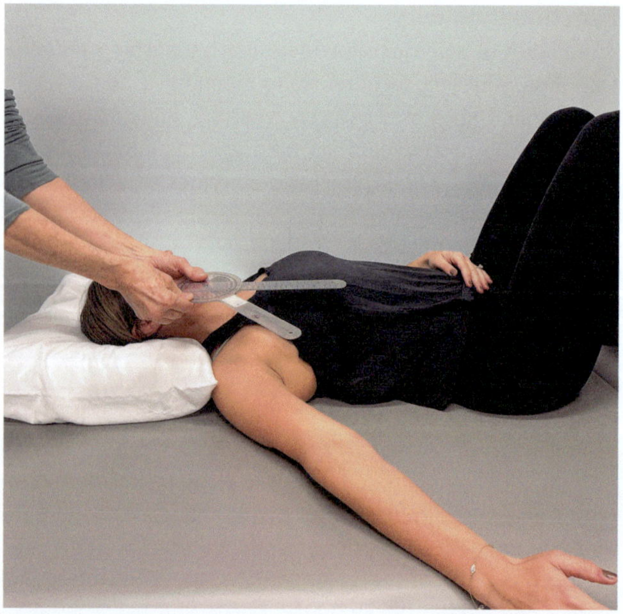

Image 10 During phase 2, monitoring objective measures of deltoid recovery can be achieved with goniometric measures of active shoulder abduction in supine and standing while cueing the individual to retract and depress the scapula

the needs of the patient and the ability to attend therapy visits. The importance of consistent home exercises performed multiple times per day should be reviewed during therapy visits.

Phase 3

3+/5 MMT in the Recipient Muscle

Phase 3 exercises include shoulder abduction against gravity and may advance to include resistance exercises when appropriate. The patient will continue combined movements of scapular retraction and depression with shoulder abduction until adequate strength is developed in the deltoid to reduce the need for donor contribution. Isolated and functional exercises in seated, standing, and prone positions are incorporated into the home exercise programs. Resistance may initially be introduced with small functional items such as a cell phone and progress to resistance bands and free weights. Keep in mind that 3+/5 deltoid strength is not attained by all individuals undergoing this transfer.

Exercises

- Resistive Recipient Activity with Donor Contraction
  The patient may perform standing shoulder abduction with light weights (or cuff weights if the patient lacks hand function) (Image 11). The therapist should monitor the shoulder movement to avoid compensatory movement strategies, such as contralateral side bending of the torso, excess upper trapezius contraction (shoulder hiking), or excess pectoralis major contribution which pulls the shoulder into more flexion than abduction.
- Resistive Recipient Activity Without Donor Contraction
  As the deltoid function improves, attempts may be made to separate donor and recipient muscle actions. But this is not necessary with this transfer due to the synergistic nature of the donor/trapezius being a scapular stabilizer for shoulder motion. The patient may continue to show the strongest activation when the donor and recipient muscles are co-activated.

Frequency of Visits

The patient may attend therapy anywhere from once a week to once a month, depending on the needs of the individual. Patients may benefit from more frequent visits if they have joint limitations, pain, periscapular muscle imbalance, and nerve sensitivity and/or they require higher-level activities for strength and endurance.

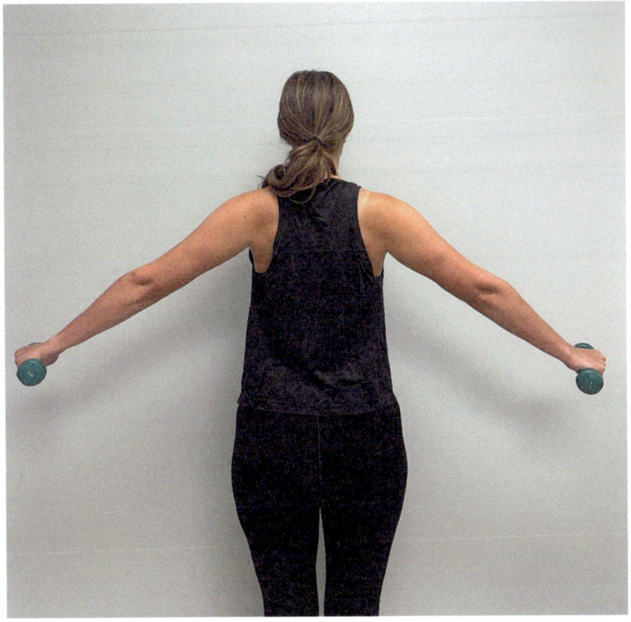

Image 11 Resisted deltoid exercises are added, as able, in phase 3 when the patient demonstrates the ability to abduct to 90° against gravity. The amount of weight should be minimal at first with care to avoid substitution patterns

Spinal accessory to Axillary nerve transfer

Nerve transfer overview					
Donor nerve	Donor action	Recipient nerve	Recipient action	Indications for functional restoration	Approximate months to functional movement
Spinal accessory nerve	Scapular retraction and depression	Axillary nerve	Shoulder abduction (primary) Shoulder flexion and external rotation (secondary)	Restore ability to reach overhead and away from the body	Data not available

Information below are suggested guidelines. Precautions may vary according to surgeon preferences and patient factors.

	Preoperative therapy	Early phase	Middle phase	Late phase
Criteria	Before surgery	0/5 to −1/5 MMT	2-/5 to 3/5 MMT	>3/5 MMT
Purpose of Phase	Educate and establish baseline function	Understand donor-recipient relationship Activate donor: scapular retraction and depression	Consistently activate recipient muscle	Strengthen recipient muscle
Precautions	NA	Sling and post-operative dressings for 2 weeks after surgery If the pec major was repaired, the shoulder should be immobilized for 4 weeks	Avoid high intensity exercise Minimize fatigue and force placed on the weak recipient deltoid	Resistive exercise should not be performed before the deltoid demonstrates 3/5 MMT Avoid fatigue with resistance training
Frequency of visits (considerations)	1–2 visit(s); more if PROM limitations are present	1×/week until PROM is restored, and the patient is independent with the HEP Decrease to 1×/month based on progress	1× per month unless patient requires more guidance If additional nerve transfers were performed, more frequent therapy is warranted	1× per month
Orthosis considerations	Sling for comfort	Sling for the first 2 weeks After 2 weeks, additional shoulder support is encouraged to minimize glenohumeral subluxation: Givmohr® sling, Omotrain® brace, or a standard sling	Continue a shoulder support as needed to protect the length of the denervated deltoid	NA
Interventions		**Donor activation:** Scapular retraction and depression 10× every hour **Donor-recipient pairing:** Scapular retraction and/or depression with passive shoulder abduction 10–20 reps, 6–8×/per day	**Active/Resisted Donor with Active Assist Recipient:** Scapular retraction with active-assisted shoulder abduction is performed in a gravity minimized plane **Place and Hold:** The shoulder is supported in abduction on an elevated surface. The patient retracts the scapula, slides the arm off and attempts to hold it in abduction	**Resisted Donor and Recipient:** Resisted shoulder abduction (and/or external rotation) while retracting the scapula. Resistance can be in the form of bands, dumbbells, or cuff weights **Resisted Recipient Without Donor Contraction:** Not recommended with this nerve transfer due to the synergistic and assistive nature of the donor trapezius muscle
Additional intervention considerations			Respect fatigue	Initially focus on high frequency, low resistance exercises

During all phases it is essential to continue cortical reorganization, psychological and psychosocial interventions, and progress to incorporate donor/recipient with ADL

Spinal Accessory to Axillary Nerve Transfer

Goal of Surgery: To restore ability to reach overhead

Recipient Muscle Movement = Shoulder abduction (primary), flexion, and external rotation

Recipient Muscle: Deltoid muscle

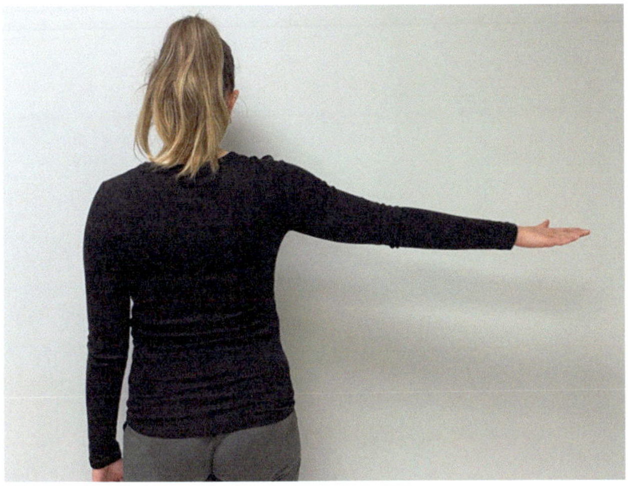

Bring arm out to the side (abduction)

Donor Movements = Scapular retraction and depression
Donor Muscles: Middle and lower trapezius

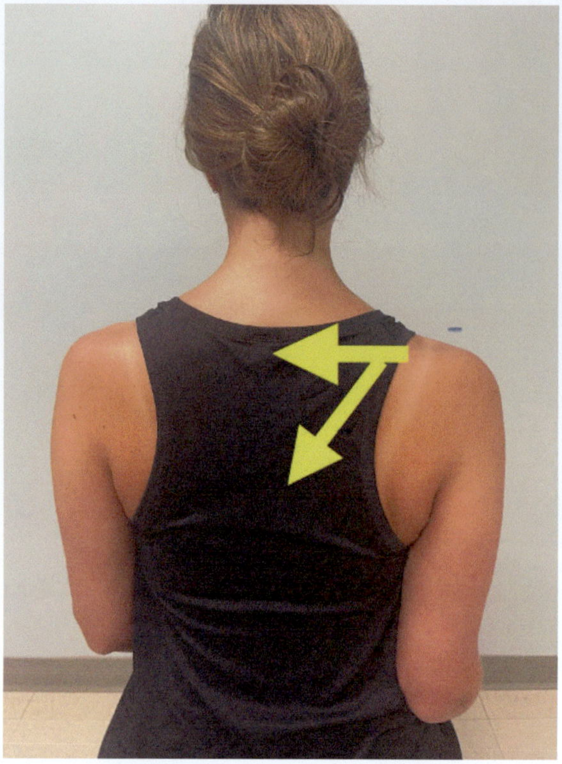

Phase 1 Spinal Accessory to Axillary Nerve Transfer Exercises

☐ **Active or Resisted Donor Movement:**

☐ Sit with your arm resting by your side. Pull your shoulders back by pinching your shoulder blades together as you keep your shoulders down. Hold this position for 3–5 seconds, rest, and repeat.

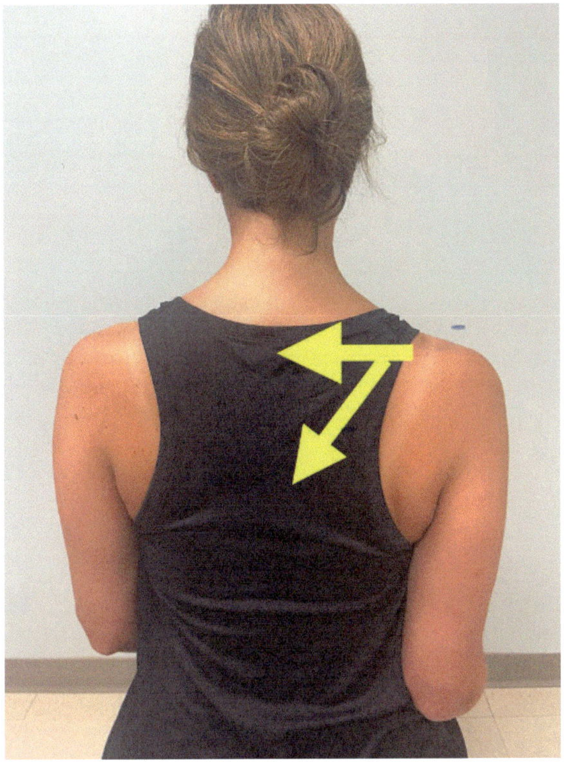

Complete 10 repetitions every hour

☐ **Combined Donor with Passive Recipient Exercise:**

- While lying on your back, hold one end of a dowel, cane, or stick with your injured arm. Use your unaffected arm to guide the dowel and move your arm directly out to the side of your body as you pinch your shoulder blades together and keep your shoulders down.

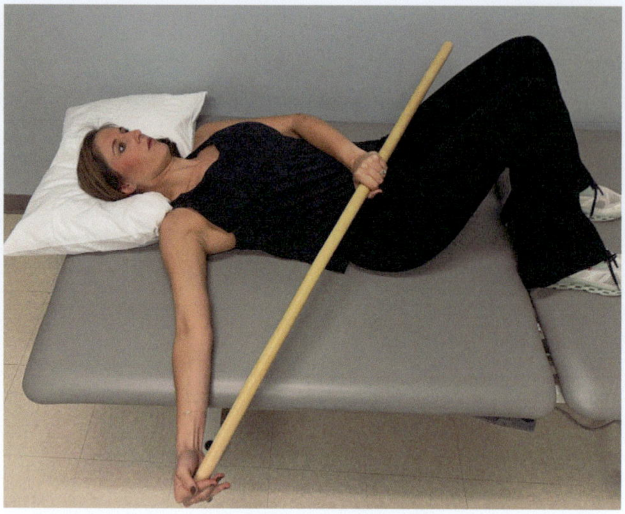

Complete 10–15 repetitions, 3–5 times per day

Phase 2 Spinal Accessory to Axillary Nerve Transfer Exercises

☐ **Active Donor + Active-Assisted Recipient:**

- Sit next to a large exercise ball. Squeeze your shoulder blade "back and down" as you roll the ball away from you. Try to move your arm to the side with the ball assisting the movement.

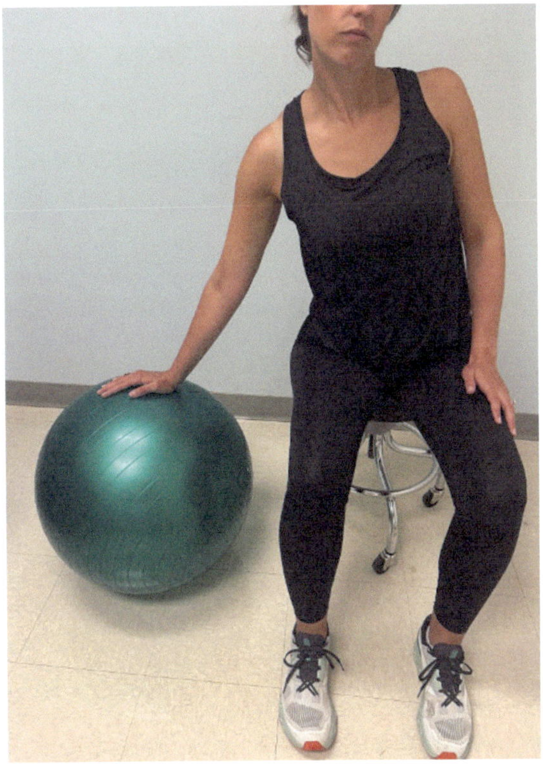

- Sit next to a table with your arm resting on a towel in front of you. Slide your arm to the side as you pull your shoulders back and down. Return to the starting position by sliding your arm in front of you and repeat.

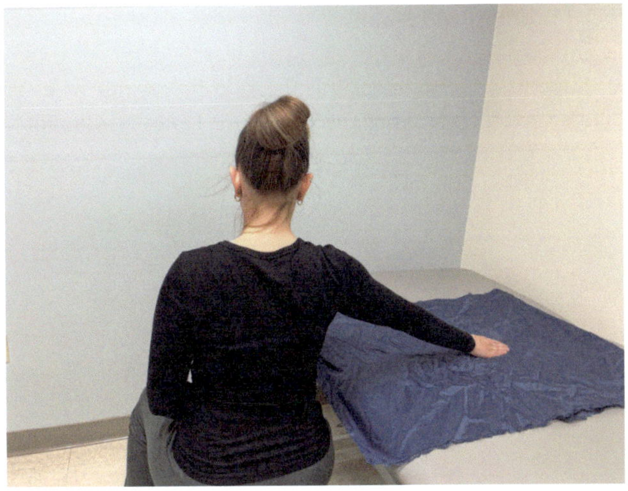

- Lie on your back with your arm by your side. Squeeze your shoulder blades together while you bring the arm out to the side. You may use a slick surface or an arm skate to help this movement.
  - You may also hold a dowel or stick. First try to move the shoulder on your own and then push with the unaffected arm until your injured arm slides all the way out to the side.

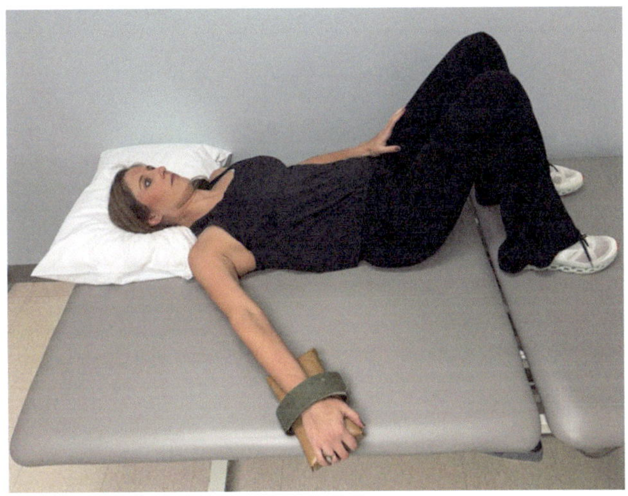

☐ **"Place and Hold"**

- Support your shoulder out the side by resting it on an elevated surface. Slide the arm off the table and attempt to hold it in place for a count of 5 seconds, then slower lower the arm. Relax and repeat.

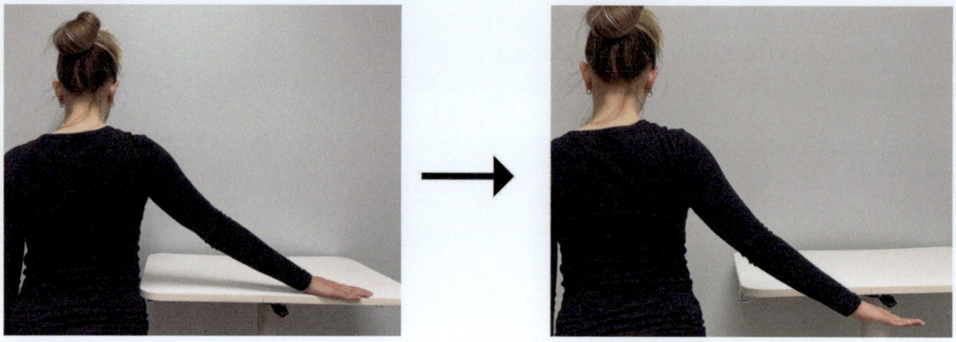

Complete 10–15 repetitions, 3–5 times per day

☐ **Active Donor + Active Recipient Movement:**

- Stand facing a wall with both hands pressed on a towel in front of you. Pull your shoulder back and down by pinching your shoulder blades together as you slide your arm diagonally up on the wall.

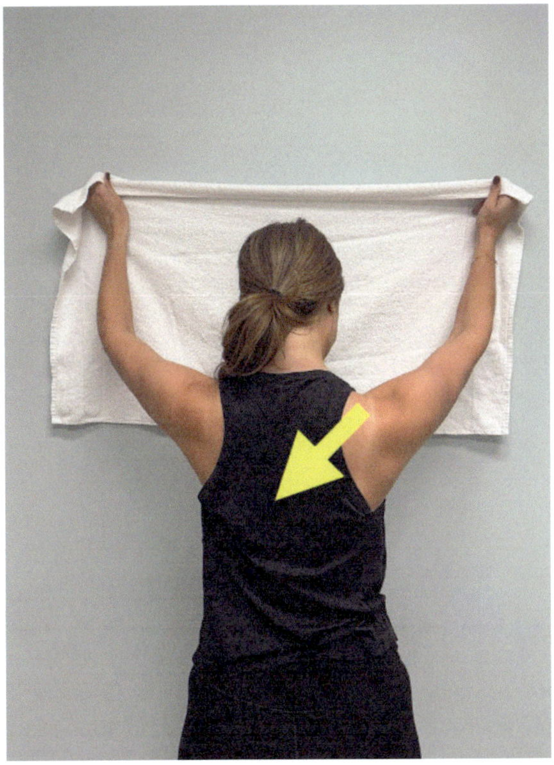

- Lie on your stomach with your arm resting by your side. Squeeze the shoulder blades back and down. Try to do a "reverse snow angel" by bringing the arm out to the side.

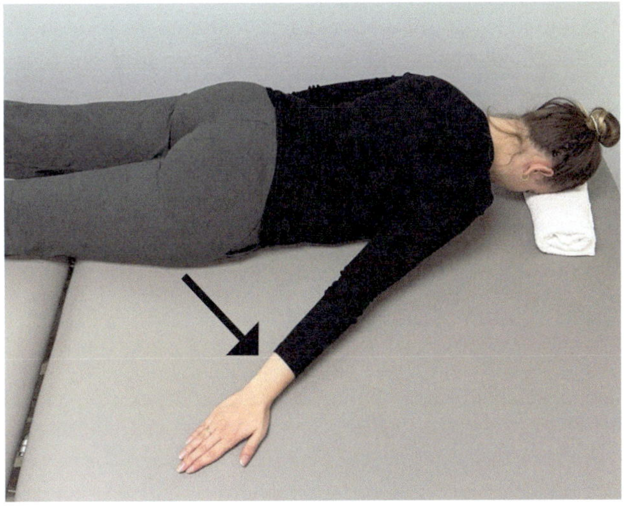

Complete 10–15 repetitions, 3–5 times per day

Phase 3 Spinal Accessory to Axillary Nerve Transfer Exercises

☐ **Resisted Recipient Activity with Donor Contraction:**

- Hold light weights in both hands and squeeze your shoulder blades "back and down." Bring your arms out to the side as high as you can. Do 10 slow repetitions, relax, and repeat. Try to avoid "hiking" the shoulders up toward your ear.

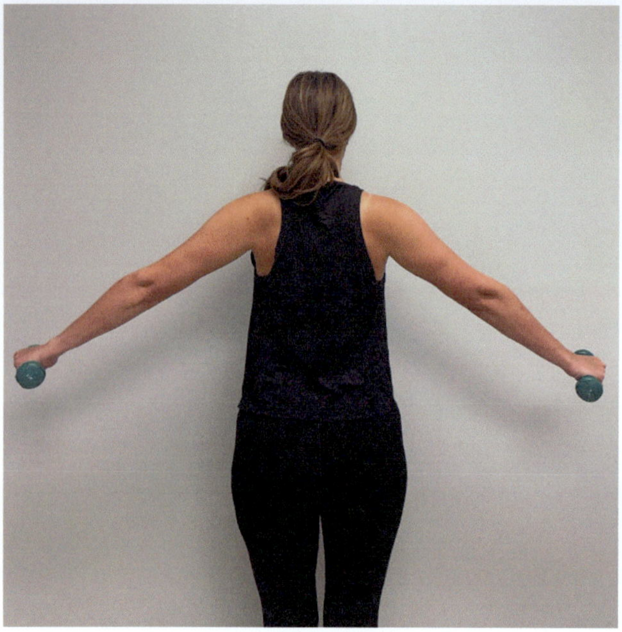

- Hold a therapy band with the opposite end anchored under your foot. Squeeze your shoulder blade "back and down" as you bring the arm up and out to the side. Hold 3–5 seconds, relax, and repeat.

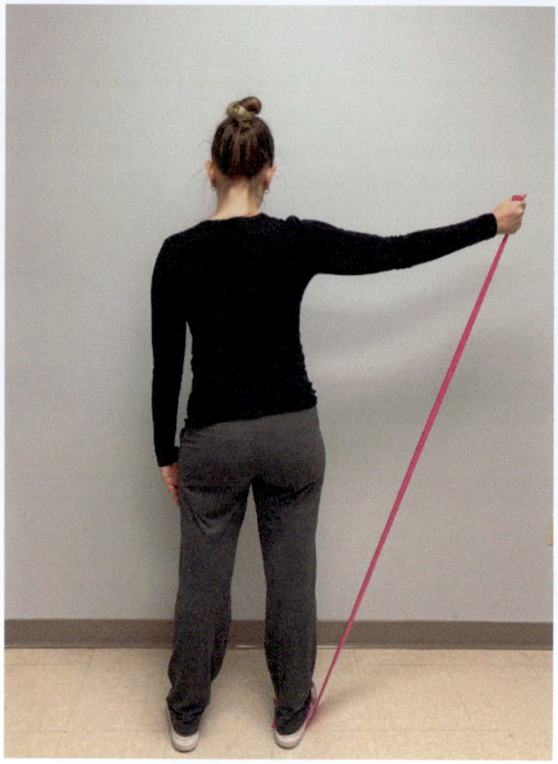

Complete 10 repetitions, 3 times per day

☐ **Resisted Recipient without Donor Contraction:**

- Not recommended for this nerve transfer due to the assistive and synergistic nature of the donor trapezius and deltoid recipient muscles.

References

1. Rohde RS, Wolfe SW. Nerve transfers for adult traumatic brachial plexus palsy (brachial plexus nerve transfer). HSS J. 2007;31(1):77–82.
2. Songcharoen P, Wongtrakul S, Spinner RJ. Brachial plexus injuries in the adult. Nerve transfers: the Siriraj Hospital experience. Hand Clin. 2005;21(1):83–9.
3. Chan K, Lee SK. Surgical management of adult traumatic brachial plexus injures. In: Osterman AL, Skirven TM, Fedorczyk JM, Amadio PC, Feldscher SB, Shin EK, editors. Rehabilitation of the hand and upper extremity. 7th ed. Elsevier Mosby; 2020.
4. Kahn L, Moore A. Donor activation focused rehabilitation approach: maximizing outcomes after nerve transfers. Hand Clin. 2016;32(2):263–77.
5. Samard M, Rasulić L, Gruji D, Mili B. Results of nerve transfers to the musculocutaneous and axillary nerves. Neurosurgery. 2000;46(1):93–103.
6. Manske RC, Prohaska D. Pectoralis major tendon repair postsurgical rehabilitation. N Am J Sports Phys Ther. 2007;2(1):22.
7. Kahn LC, Stonner MM, Dy CJ. Key concepts for nerve transfer rehabilitation after surgical reconstruction for brachial plexus and peripheral nerve injuries. J Hand Surg. 2023;
8. MacKenzie A. Restoration of function after adult brachial plexus injury. In: Osterman AL, Skirven TM, Fedorczyk JM, Amadio PC, Feldscher SB, Shin EK, editors. Rehabilitation of the hand and upper extremity. 7th ed. Elsevier Mosby; 2020.
9. Chuang DCC, Yeh MC, Wei FC. Intercostal nerve transfer of the musculocutaneous nerve in avulsed brachial plexus injuries: evaluation of 66 patients. J Hand Surg. 1992;17(5)
10. Lee EY, Karjalainen TV, Sebastin SJ, Lim AY. The value of the tender muscle sign in detecting motor recovery after peripheral nerve reconstruction. J Hand Surg. 2015;40(3):433–7.

Radial Nerve Branch to the Triceps to Axillary Nerve Transfer

Lorna C. Kahn

Background

The axillary nerve branches off the posterior cord (C5–6) of the brachial plexus to innervate the anterior, middle, and posterior deltoid and teres minor muscles. Axillary nerve injuries result in weakness of glenohumeral abduction, flexion, extension, and external rotation. There are two branches of the axillary nerve. The anterior branch innervates the anterior and middle deltoid, and the posterior branch innervates the posterior deltoid and teres minor muscles. The posterior branch also provides sensory branches to the proximal lateral arm. The most common nerve transfer to restore axillary nerve function is the triceps-to-axillary nerve transfer. Typically, this nerve transfer occurs at the trunk of the axillary nerve prior to the branching, but there are instances when only transferring into a single branch is possible. Axillary nerve injuries often result in neuropraxia, which recovers over time. For severe nerve injuries (Sunderland 3–5) [1], the prognosis for deltoid muscle recovery diminishes when there is a delay in accurate diagnosis of more than 6–12 months [2, 3].

The teres minor muscle externally rotates the humerus, which provides clearance between the greater tuberosity and the acromion during abduction. If the axillary nerve injury is associated with an upper plexus injury, including suprascapular nerve dysfunction, it is important to restore some external rotation force by reinnervating the teres minor as well as the deltoid when the nerve transfer is performed.

The triceps brachii muscle has three heads: medial, lateral, and long. The medial and lateral heads attach on the shaft of the humerus and provide extension torque at the elbow. The origin of the long head is on the infraglenoid tubercle of the scapula making it a two-joint muscle that contributes to both elbow and shoulder extension. If the long head is used as the donor, then shoulder extension should be included in the motor reeducation program.

Shoulder abduction is primarily associated with deltoid function, but abduction torque at the glenohumeral joint is produced by equal contributions from the supraspinatus and deltoid muscles [4]. If the deltoid is injured or denervated, the supraspinatus *may* be capable of fully abducting the shoulder but with diminished torque. This is how some axillary nerve injuries can be missed. The reverse is not true. When the supraspinatus is significantly torn, ruptured, or denervated, full abduction is typically impossible due to changes in the kinematics of the glenohumeral joint. If both supraspinatus and deltoid muscles are injured, shoulder abduction cannot be attained. Therefore, it is important to ascertain the structural integrity of the rotator cuff when treating an axillary nerve injury to ensure realistic goal setting.

There are many potential sources of injury to the axillary nerve. About half of all infraclavicular injuries to the brachial plexus involve the axillary nerve. Other sources include: [2, 5, 6]

- Trauma, especially that which involves anterior shoulder dislocation
- Blunt trauma as seen with contact sports, such as rugby and football
- Brachial plexus neuritis
- Quadrangular space syndrome
- Iatrogenic injury relating to total shoulder or reverse total shoulder replacement surgery
- Space-occupying lesions related to compression
- Hyperextension of the shoulder

L. C. Kahn (✉)
Milliken Hand Rehabilitation Center, WashU Medicine, St. Louis, MO, USA
e-mail: Kahn.lorna.c@wustl.edu

L. C. Kahn et al. (eds.), *Rehabilitation for Nerve Transfers of the Upper Extremity*, https://doi.org/10.1007/978-3-031-92008-0_9

Surgical Description

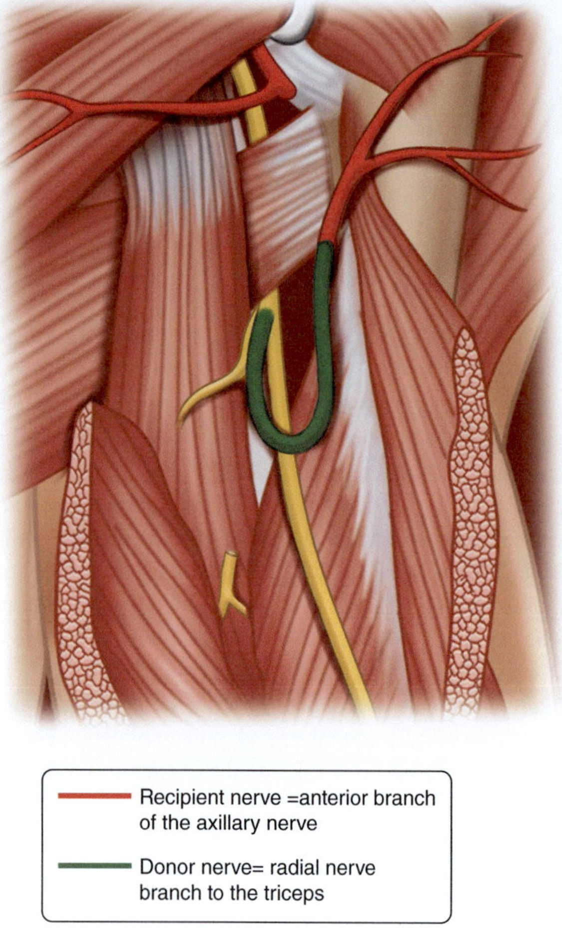

Microsurgical technique Triceps Branch of the Radial Nerve to the Axillary Nerve

Triceps-to-axillary nerve transfer is typically performed from a posterior approach, providing the advantage of performing the coaptation closer to the recipient muscle. A longitudinal incision is made along the posterior brachium, beginning just cephalad to the posterolateral corner of the acromion and continuing to the mid-brachium. The interval between the posterior deltoid and triceps is identified. It can be helpful, but not necessary, to identify the posterior cutaneous branch from the axillary nerve, which can be used as a guide to the axillary nerve proper. Retracting the posterior head of the deltoid, the quadrangular space is exposed. Being sure to preserve the circumflex humeral artery and its branches, the anterior and posterior branches of the axillary nerve are identified. Surgeons may choose to preferentially target the anterior branch of the axillary nerve, as it more consistently provides innervation to the anterior and middle heads of the deltoid. A nerve stimulator is used to confirm that the axillary nerve is not functioning, ensuring that the anesthesia team is not using any muscle paralytics. The surgeon then exposes the radial nerve in the triangular interval, identifying branches from the radial nerve to the triceps. The selection of a donor nerve from the lateral, long, or middle heads of the triceps is based on surgeon preference. The donor nerve is dissected distally, and before dividing it, a handheld nerve stimulator is used to confirm response only in the triceps (and not in the wrist or fingers). The donor triceps branch is divided distally to meet the anterior branch of the axillary nerve, which is divided proximally. Coaptation of the triceps branch from the radial nerve to the anterior branch of the axillary nerve is performed using microsurgical technique.

Outcomes

Outcomes for triceps-to-axillary nerve transfers vary from fair to excellent. However, some studies describe that 25% of patients fail to achieve a 3/5 manual muscle testing (MMT) grade. Factors that affect outcomes in isolated axillary nerve injuries include delay in timing of surgery, patient age, and increased body mass index (BMI) [5]. Leechavengvongs et al. described "useful functional recovery" in seven out of seven patients with an average of 124 degrees of shoulder abduction achieved [7]. All participants were noted to take some resistance against abduction. Krauss et al. described outcomes for 49 patients who underwent triceps-to-axillary nerve transfer. At their final follow-up, 64.6% achieved MMT grade 3/5 or better. Just over 87% of those with isolated axillary nerve injuries recovered greater strength with a median MMT grade of 4.25. For those with a plexus-related injury, a median MMT grade of 3 was achieved at the final visit [8].

Phases of Rehabilitation

Phase 1

Preoperative to 1/5 MMT in the Recipient Muscle

Preoperative

Prior to surgery, baseline measures of upper extremity (UE) range of motion (ROM), MMT strength grading of donor and recipient muscles, and axillary nerve sensation are evaluated. Particular attention is given to examination of the rotator cuff as this will play a role in the recovery of arm elevation.

Treatment at this stage includes shoulder/UE passive ROM, active and resistive exercises for uninvolved muscles, and, if needed, pain management. No braces or orthotics are required unless there is a positive sulcus sign, which is often seen with upper trunk injuries. An OmoTrain® brace is a good option for individuals with humeral head subluxation to support the weight of the arm (Image 1). If the patient cannot tolerate the tight fit of the OmoTrain®, Kinesio® taping may be a useful, temporary option (Image 2) to provide a superior pull of the humerus and minimize drag on the axillary nerve. The authors have recently started using a hip support such as the BABYMUST® (Image 3), designed for mothers of infants or toddlers to support the weight of the child, for upper plexus patients to support the weight of the arm.

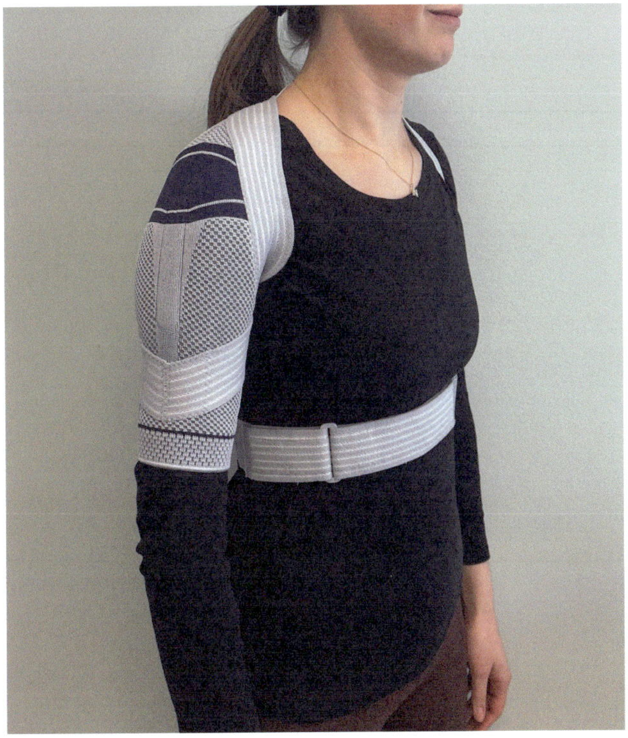

Image 1 The Omotrain brace by Bauerfeind is recommended for patients pre-operatively and post operatively to support the weight of the arm and limit glenohumeral subluxation

Postoperative

For the first 2–3 weeks after surgery, the patient may be placed in a shoulder immobilizer to protect the nerve transfer and prevent seroma formation by limiting activity. Wound care is specific to each surgeon. Therapists should consult their corresponding surgeons regarding wound care preferences. A tight-fitting brace such as the OmoTrain® is not recommended for the first month postoperatively due to its compressive nature and the risk of edema in the early phase. Active and passive ROM of the elbow, wrist, and hand are encouraged. Lifting, holding, or exerting force through the arm should be avoided for the first month. Once sutures are removed, scar massage may begin to limit adherence to the underlying soft tissue.

Exercises

- ROM of Shoulder
  Following the initial rest period of 2 weeks, passive and active-assisted shoulder ROM are initiated. Patients are instructed in supine dowel exercises for flexion, abduction (Image 4), and external rotation. In a seated position, table slides also provide a safe form of self-administered passive ROM (Image 5). If the patient develops postoperative adhesive capsulitis, joint mobilization and passive ROM exercises become the focus of treatment in addition to formal nerve transfer training.
- Donor Activation
  Once postoperative wound healing and joint ROM have been addressed, the concepts of motor reeducation are introduced. Donor muscle activation in the form of active and isometric triceps exercises is initiated as early as 2 weeks from surgery. This can be as simple as sliding a hand along the thigh towards the knee (requiring elbow extension) or pushing a tight fist into the contralateral palm in a downward direction to create tension in the triceps muscle (Image 6). In supine, pressingc the hand into the bed will also activate the triceps. If the patient can support the shoulder in flexion with the opposite hand while supine, active elbow extension against gravity provides a more challenging form of donor activation.
- Combined Donor with Passive Recipient Exercise
  To combine donor and recipient muscle activity, the patient is instructed in active or resisted elbow extension with passive shoulder elevation. To achieve this, two options are described:

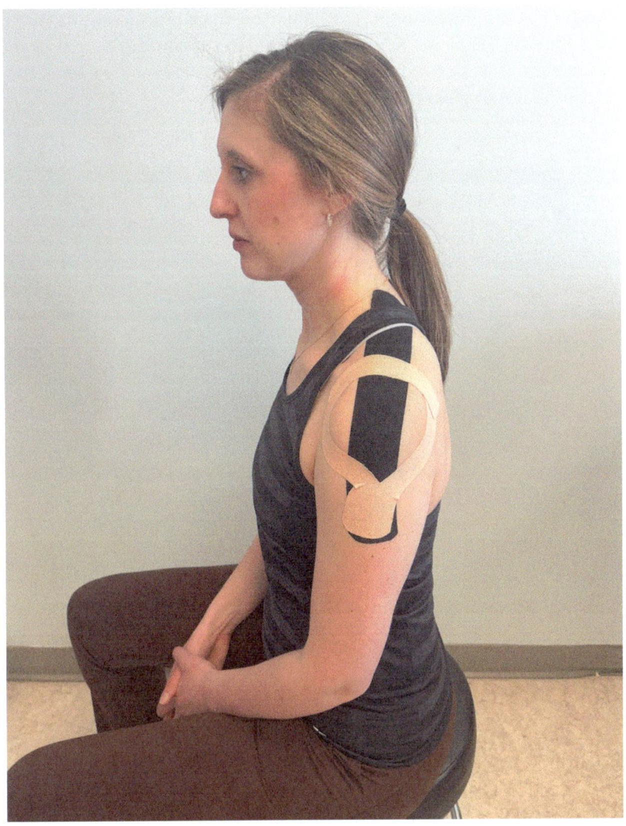

Image 2 Taping the shoulder with athletic tape such as Kinesio Tape® is an alternative to bracing but must be changed every three days. Some individuals may not tolerate tape due to skin sensitivity

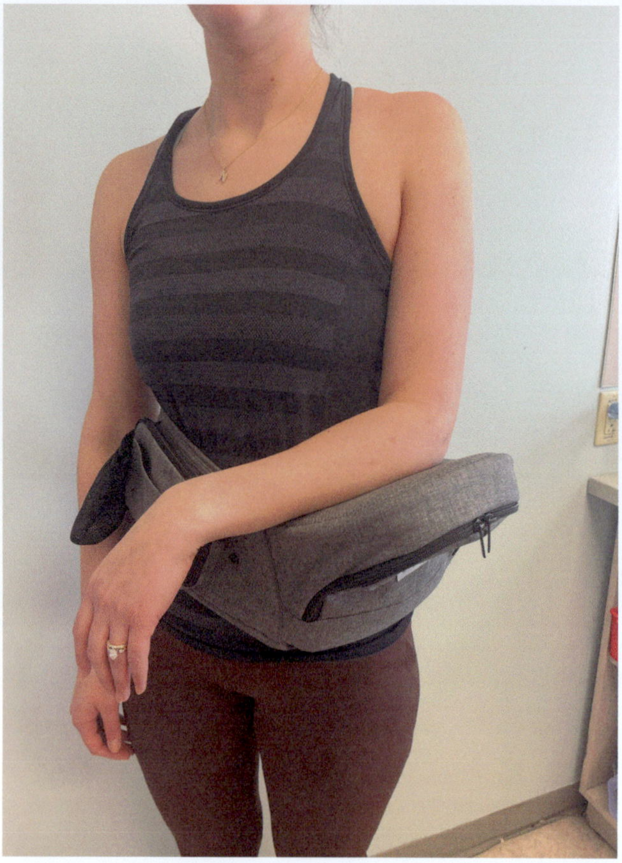

Image 3 A hip-based support, originally designed to support an infant or toddler on the parent's hip, can be used to support the weight of the injured arm if lack of proximal strength leads to drag on the plexus and/or contributes to glenohumeral subluxation

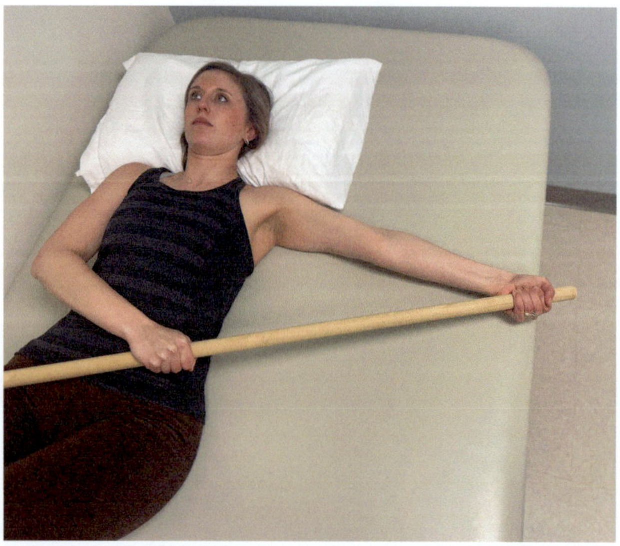

Image 4 In Phase 1, shoulder PROM exercises are demonstrated as shown here with the patient lying supine using a dowel to abduct the arm

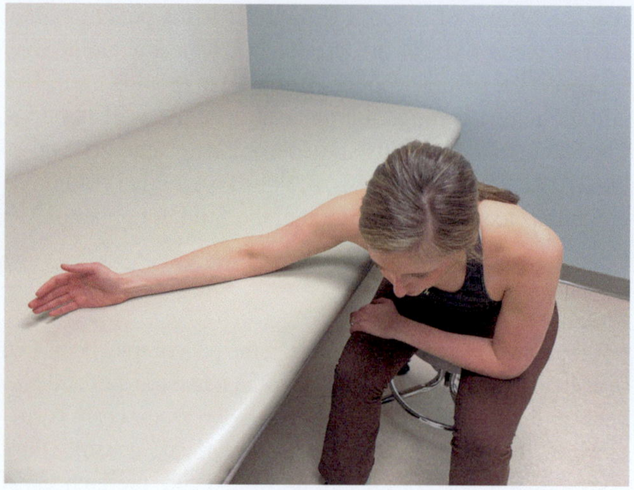

Image 5 Shoulder PROM can also be achieved in sitting, with the arm supported on a table for table slides

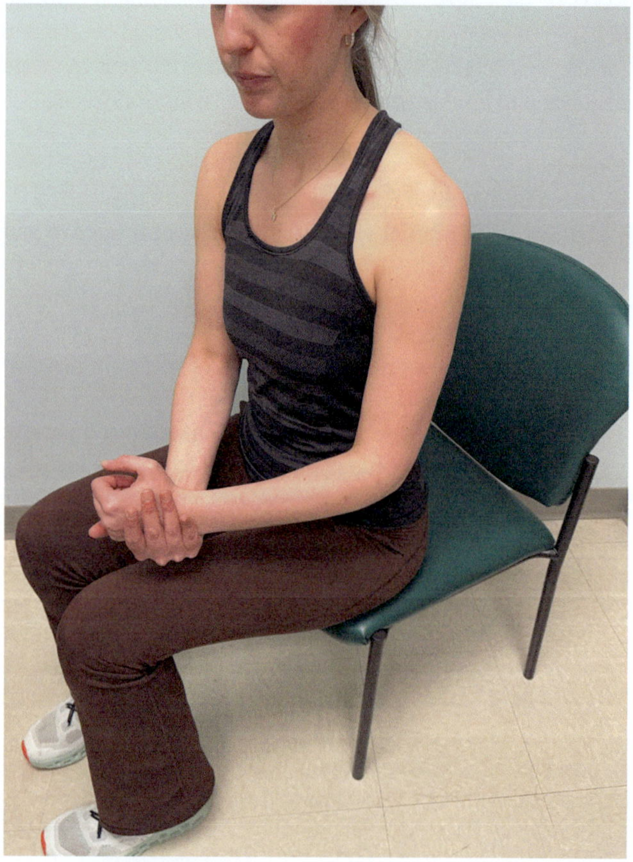

Image 6 Isometric donor activation of the triceps muscle is achieved by pushing the involved fist into the opposite hand in a downward direction

- Sitting on a chair next to a large exercise ball: Press down on the ball with the elbow in extension and lean out to allow the shoulder to passively abduct (Image 7). Note that the patient should not be positioned on a stool as illustrated in the image.
- Supine: Hold a dowel with the hands at either end. Slide the injured arm into shoulder abduction with the assistance of the uninvolved hand while cueing the patient to maintain elbow extension.

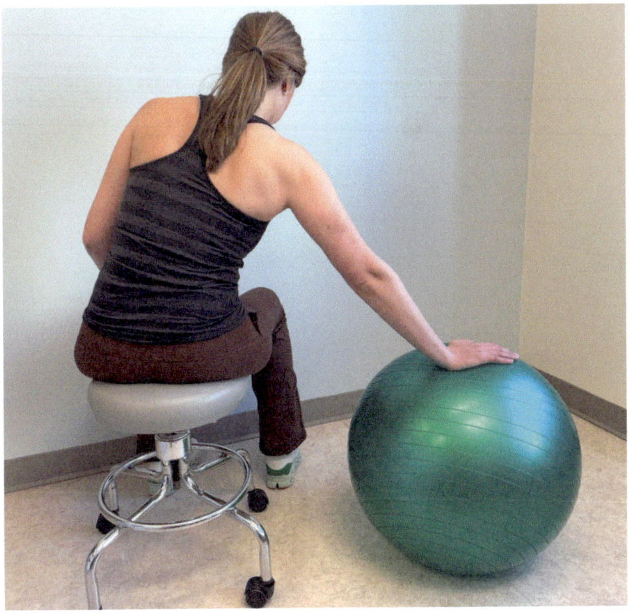

Image 7 Active donor with passive recipient exercises can be performed using a large ball. The individual is instructed to press down on the ball to activate the triceps while leaning forward or to the side to passively flex and abduct the shoulder

Assessment of Recovery

Assessment of recipient function is performed during monthly therapy visits to capture the earliest sign of a twitch response in the deltoid and teres minor muscles. To do this, the therapist resists the triceps muscle while palpating the deltoid muscle (Image 8). If the nerve transfer includes all branches of the axillary nerve, then the therapist should start by palpating along the posterior head of the deltoid. The nerve travels from posterior to anterior, so the posterior deltoid will likely register a response before the middle or anterior heads. The therapist needs to be precise with palpation skills due to the relatively close location of the long head of the triceps to the posterior deltoid in this area. It is generally active with shoulder abduction and extension, and may be misinterpreted for the posterior deltoid.

Therapy Frequency

Frequency of visits will vary with the needs of the patient. If passive ROM is relatively normal and the patient demonstrates an understanding of basic donor and combined donor-recipient exercise concepts, monthly visits should be adequate. During the monthly visits, joint ROM, edema, and general function of the UE are assessed. Donor and recipient concepts should be continuously reviewed.

Phase 2

2−/5 to 3/5 MMT in the Recipient Muscle

Once a twitch is noted, patients should be monitored for deltoid contraction, and movement of the shoulder in gravity-minimized planes will make any movement easier to perform. Adding a nylon sleeve or a skate under the arm to reduce frictional force will also enhance early movement. Exercises should be demonstrated, and patients should be encouraged to perform these with limited repetitions.

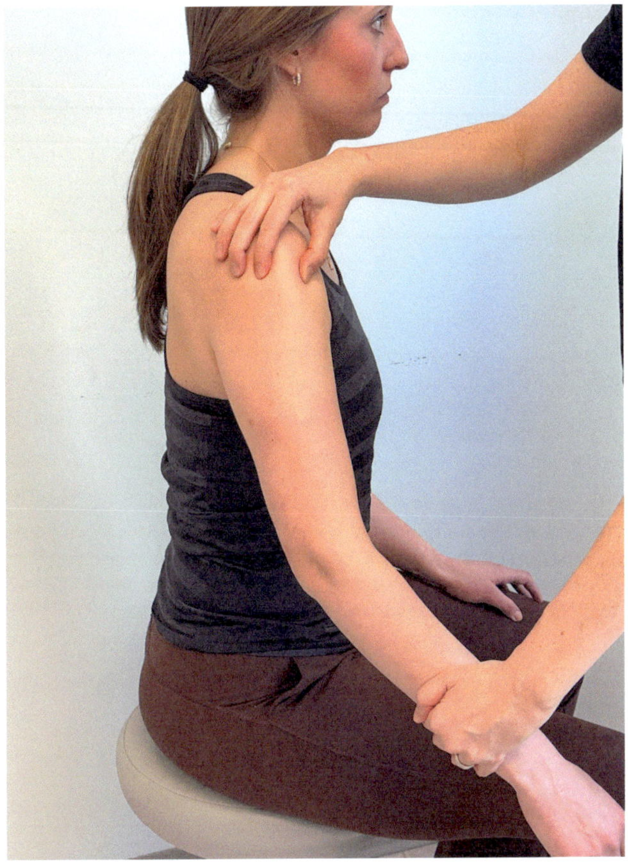

Image 8 Assessment of recovery is performed by palpating the deltoid muscle while resisting the triceps muscle

Exercises

- Active Donor with Active-Assisted Recipient Deltoid/Teres Minor MMT=2−/5 to 2/5

  Supine chest press: The patient is supine with a wand or dowel in both hands, and a "chest press" is completed by actively extending the elbows against gravity while performing *assisted* shoulder flexion to 90° (Image 9). Note that although this is largely recruiting pectoralis major, the anterior deltoid is also involved.

  Seated ball push: The patient can be seated with the hand on an exercise ball. He or she presses into the ball while moving it midway between shoulder extension and abduction to isolate the posterior fibers of the deltoid.

  Pillow slides: While supine with the arm on a pillow (with slick nylon over it), the patient tenses the triceps while sliding the arm out (into abduction) and off the pillow so gravity may assist the movement (Image 10).

  Donor resistance: A resistance band can be attached above a door jamb, as shown below. The patient holds the

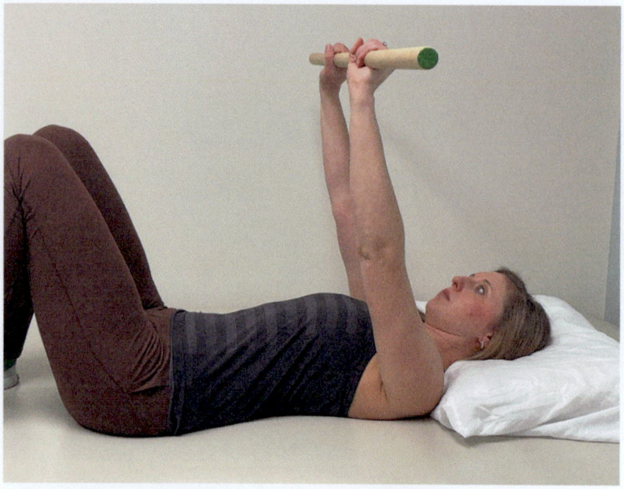

Image 9 Active donor with active-assisted recipient exercises are demonstrated in supine, holding a dowel, and performing a "chest press" by extending the elbows (donor- triceps) while flexing the involved shoulder with the aid of the uninvolved arm

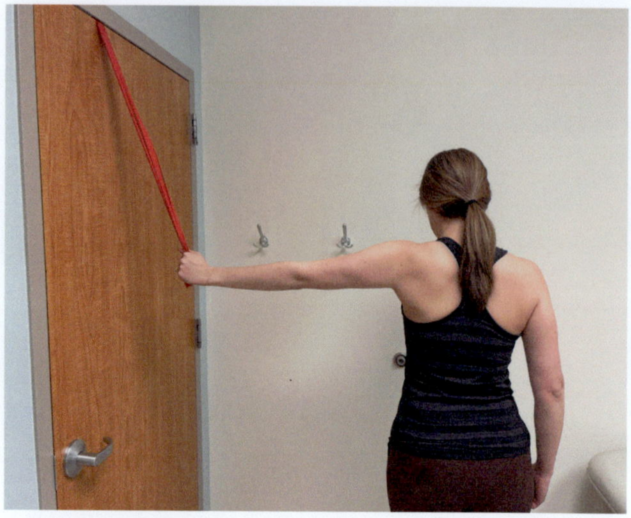

Image 11 By pulling down on a stiff therapy band while maintaining elbow extension, the arm will be assisted into elevation as the downward pull is released

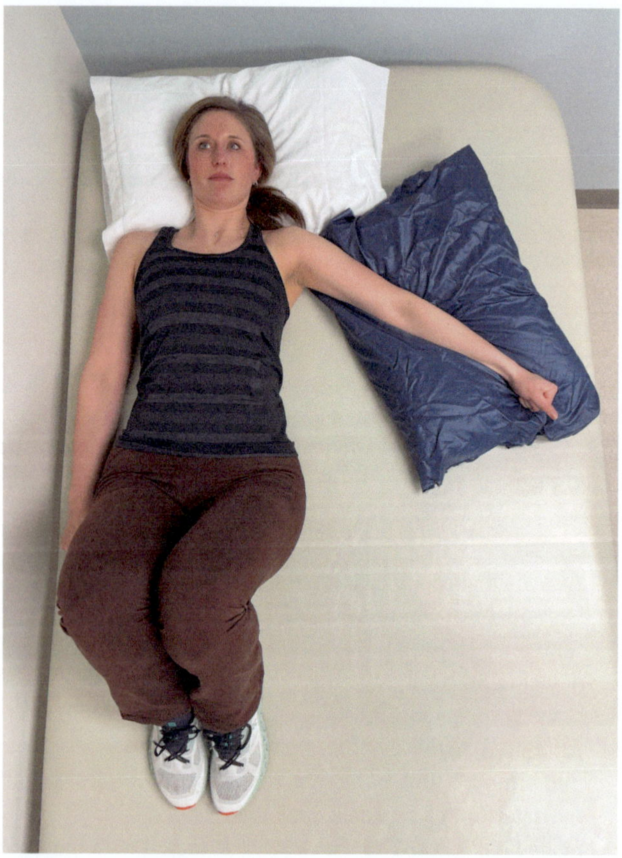

Image 10 Active donor with active-assisted recipient muscle exercises may be achieved with the individual lying supine with the involved arm on a slick pillow. Firmly maintaining the elbow in extension, the individual is instructed to abduct the shoulder off the pillow so gravity may assist the movement

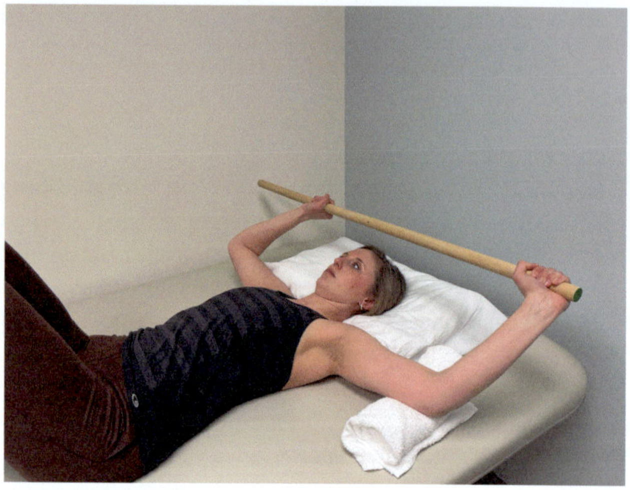

Image 12 To strengthen the teres minor with donor activation, the individual is instructed to externally rotate the shoulders with both arms using a dowel while pulling outward on the dowel to activate or tense the donor triceps

band up high, placing the shoulder in flexion, and pulls it down and up while maintaining elbow extension. If the band is strong, it will rebound, assisting in raising the arm forward as the downward tension is released. The stiffer the band, the more it will propel the arm forward and up. The patient can also pull the band down and *out* to help with abduction (Image 11). Pulleys may also be used for assisted arm elevation with clear instructions to include elbow extension to involve the donor triceps.

Supine external rotation: The patient is supine holding a wand or dowel bilaterally with shoulders in 90° of abduction. A towel is placed just proximal to the elbows for support. Starting from full internal rotation, the patient performs bilateral external rotation, so the dowel ends overhead. The patient can simultaneously perform isometric elbow extension with cues to pull outward on the dowel (triceps donor activation) (Image 12).

- "Place and Hold" Exercise
  Deltoid/Teres Minor MMT = 2+/5
  In standing, sitting, or side lying, the patient abducts the shoulder as far as possible with the elbow in extension. The therapist then takes the weight of the arm and assists it into greater abduction while asking the patient to hold the abduction range as the therapist releases support.
- Active Donor with Active Recipient
  Deltoid/Teres Minor MMT = 3−/5 to 3/5
  Reverse snow angel: In prone, the patient will automatically activate the triceps donor (and latissimus dorsi) to lift or move the arm while the deltoid remains weak. Additionally, higher demand is placed on the posterior deltoid for abduction in this position. The patient slides the shoulder into abduction with as little assistance as needed from the therapist. A slick surface or arm skate under the arm will improve ease of movement (Image 13).
  If the patient has an isolated axillary nerve injury, active and resisted rotator cuff and periscapular strengthening exercises are appropriate throughout phases 2 and 3 of therapy. Supraspinatus exercises may need to be modified to avoid antigravity positions for some time if the patient does not demonstrate adequate pre-injury strength.

Functional Activity

Functional activities may include holding, reaching, or placing a ball in varying angles of shoulder, flexion, abduction, and extension. The therapist can manually resist the donor triceps as the patient reaches to increase activation in the recipient muscle. Tossing a ball with elbow extension may also be attempted. Additionally, holding a golf club or tennis racquet and swinging it will create some momentum, assisting shoulder abduction as the patient is cued to maintain elbow extension. Any activity that combines donor and recipient movement but does not overwhelm the deltoid would be appropriate if it is performed with limited frequency.

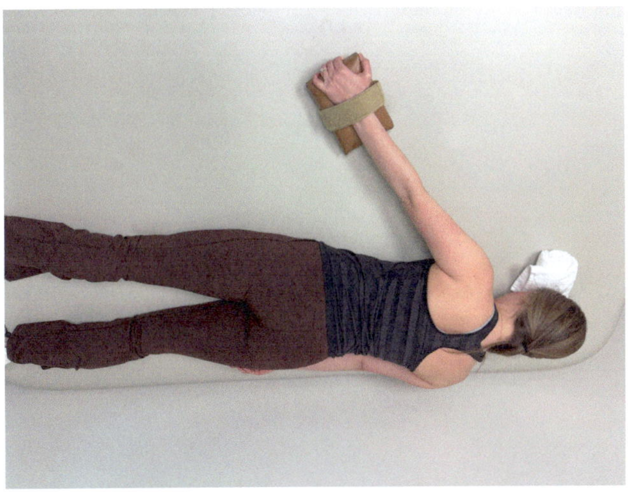

Image 13 The "reverse snow angel" exercise promotes triceps activation as the individual is instructed to slide the arm into abduction while maintaining full elbow extension

Assessment of Recovery

Assessment of recipient function should be monitored at each therapy session. The therapist should resist the triceps while palpating the deltoid muscle, with care to isolate each head as the patient attempts flexion, abduction, and extension. Phase 2 evaluation depends on the degree of shoulder active ROM achieved and whether performed in an antigravity or gravity-minimized plane. To monitor subtle changes throughout phase 2, goniometric measures of shoulder abduction should be taken while the donor triceps is activated. The examiner should not apply resistance to the recipient muscle until full active ROM against gravity is achieved, which would be considered 90° for the deltoid (3/5 MMT).

Therapy Frequency

The frequency of visits in phase 2 depends on the needs of the patient.

Unless passive joint restrictions are still being addressed, no more than one time per week is necessary. If patients are compliant with their home exercise program, one to two times per month will usually suffice.

Phase 3

3+/5 MMT in the Recipient Muscle

Once the patient demonstrates the ability to actively abduct the shoulder to 90° against gravity, the program advances to the strengthening phase. Note that 90° is considered full motion regarding deltoid function in isolation. Keep in mind that endurance will remain low for a long time. Therefore, an exercise program that challenges the deltoid muscle and teres minor for short sessions with limited repetitions is ideal during the onset of this phase.

Younger patients who are compliant with their exercises often demonstrate larger pectoralis and periscapular muscles as these tend to compensate for the lack of deltoid function. Monitoring for excessive scapulothoracic motion is important when measuring shoulder flexion and abduction as the 2/3 to 1/3 principle of glenohumeral to scapulothoracic motion [4] is often altered by this substitution to accommodate deltoid weakness [9]. Substitution patterns may present with excessive scapular elevation, scapular anterior tilt and/or downward rotation, and spinal extension with attempted GH motion. If this is not corrected, measurements of arm elevation may be inaccurate.

Exercises

- Resistive Recipient Activity with Donor Contraction
  During the beginning of phase 3, the weight of the arm is often adequate resistance for early strengthening.
  - Active shoulder flexion and abduction are performed in standing or side lying with cues to tense the triceps donor. The patient may advance to holding light weights as tolerated (Image 14), but the therapist should monitor for substitution patterns to avoid advancing strengthening before the individual has adequate strength to do so. Often, the substitution includes excess upper trapezius and excess scapular upward rotation. Patients should abduct and/or flex the shoulder only to 90° without substitution before advancing.
  - Wall push-ups are another good option that activates both the triceps and the anterior deltoid. Weight-bearing through the wall provides resistance to both donor and recipient muscle groups.
  - Wall slides are performed with the ulnar side of the hands resting on the wall. The patient is instructed to press the hands into the wall to tense the triceps, straightening the elbows as the arms slide up the wall to form a "V." The hands then slide down the wall, and the exercise is repeated (Image 15).
  - Resistance can be added to both donor and recipient muscles with resistance band exercises in supine. With shoulders flexed to 90° and elbows extended, resisted horizontal abduction is performed (Image 16).
- Resistive Recipient Activity without Donor Contraction
  Resistive recipient activity without donor contraction is gradually introduced if it does not require substitution of the periscapular and shoulder elevation muscles, such as the levator scapula and upper trapezius, which may irritate the cervical spine. In standing, a resistance band is used to provide resistive shoulder abduction without the assistive action of the donor triceps by maintaining the elbows in some degree of flexion (Image 17).

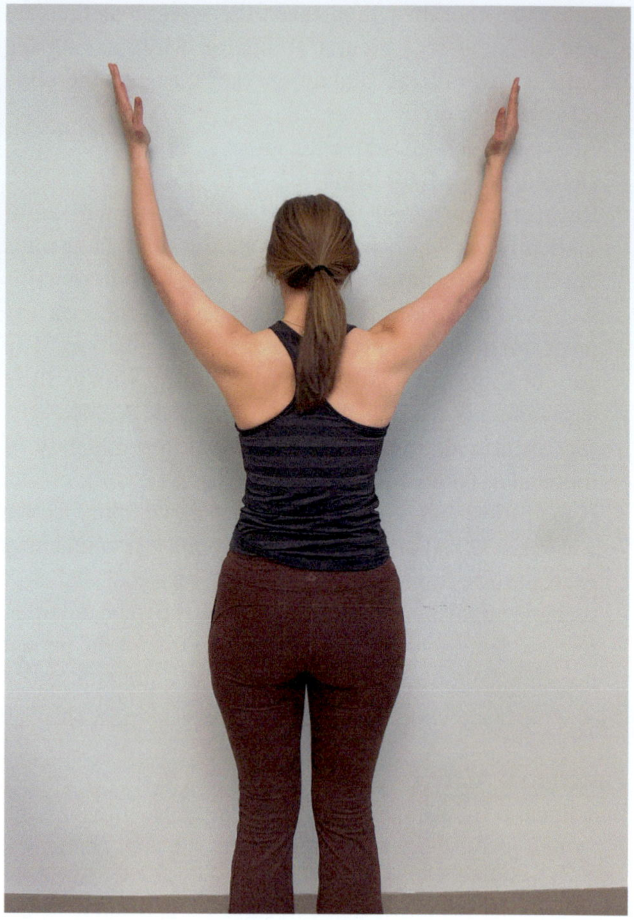

Image 15 Wall slides are a good introduction to anti-gravity exercises. As the individual slides both arms up a wall into a "V" position the triceps are activated. To increase the challenge, patients may attempt to lift the hands off the wall when they fully extend the elbows

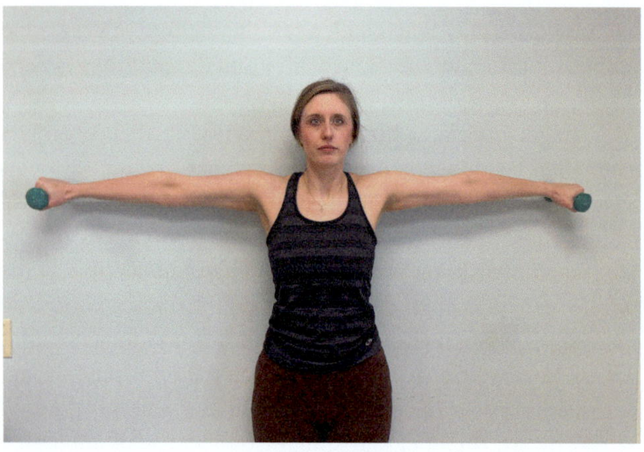

Image 14 In phase 3, light weights are introduced for strengthening the deltoid. Initially, this is performed with co-contraction of the donor triceps as demonstrated here. Abduction and flexion are initially limited to 90°

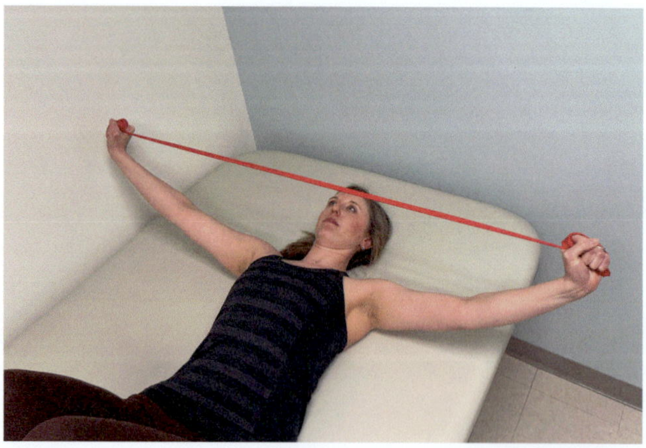

Image 16 Resisted donor with resisted recipient muscle exercises can be performed with resistance bands in supine. Holding a band with both hands with the shoulders flexed to 90° and elbows extended, the individual is instructed to perform resisted horizontal abduction by pulling the band apart

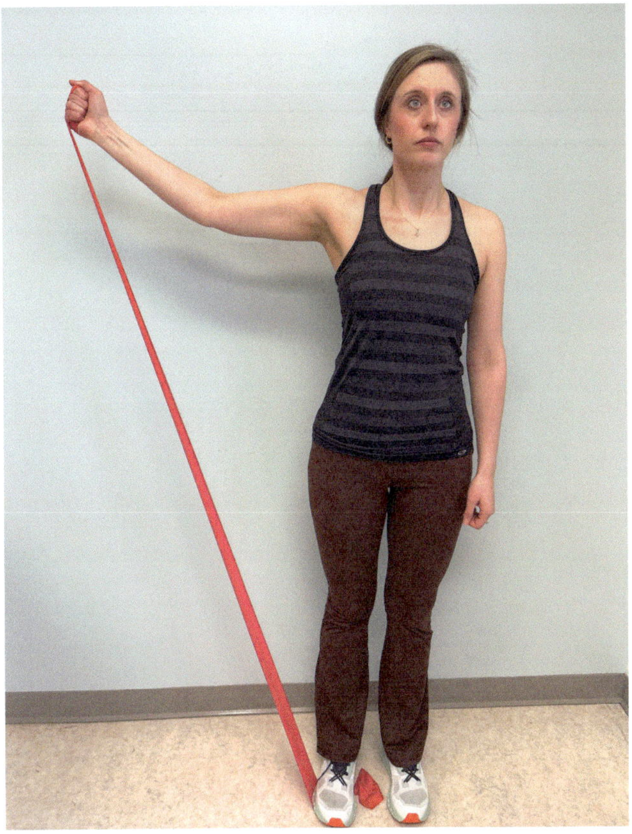

Image 17 Resisted deltoid exercise without the contribution of the donor triceps is achieved by maintaining the elbow is some degree of flexion while resisting shoulder flexion or abduction with a resistance band

Therapy Frequency

Frequency of visits in phase 3 depends on patient needs. Not all patients reach this phase, and many of them are young and athletic. If they are working with a trainer to return to their sport or activity, monthly therapy visits may suffice. For others who need the supervision and explicit guidance, two visits per month are recommended. This phase may last an additional year, and endurance will be last to return.

Triceps branch of the Radial Nerve to Axillary Nerve Transfer

Nerve transfer overview					
Donor nerve	Donor action	Recipient nerve	Recipient action	Indications for functional restoration	Approximate months to functional movement
Radial nerve to the triceps brachii	Elbow extension	Axillary nerve	Shoulder abduction (primary) Shoulder flexion and external rotation (secondary)	Restore ability to reach overhead and away from the body	12 months [5, 7, 10]

Information below are suggested guidelines. Precautions may vary according to surgeon preferences and patient factors

	Preoperative therapy	Early phase	Middle phase	Late phase
Criteria	Before surgery	0/5 to −1/5 MMT	2-/5 to 3/5 MMT	>3/5 MMT
Purpose of Phase	Educate and establish baseline function	Understand donor-recipient relationship Activate donor: elbow extension	Consistently activate recipient muscle	Strengthen recipient muscle
Precautions	NA	Sling/immobilizer for 2 weeks after surgery	Avoid high intensity exercise Minimize fatigue and force placed on the weak recipient deltoid	Resistive exercise should not be performed before the deltoid demonstrates 3/5 MMT Avoid fatigue with resistance training
Frequency of visits (considerations)	1–2 visit(s); more if PROM limitations are present	1×/week until PROM is restored, and the patient is independent with the HEP Decrease to 1×/month based on progress	1× per month unless patient requires more guidance If additional nerve transfers were performed, more frequent therapy is warranted	1× per month
Orthosis considerations	Sling for comfort	Sling for the first 2 weeks After 4 weeks, additional shoulder support is encouraged to minimize glenohumeral subluxation: Givmohr® sling, Omotrain® brace, or a standard sling	Continue a shoulder support as needed to protect the length of the denervated deltoid	NA
Interventions		**Donor Activation:** Isometric or active elbow extension 10× every hour **Donor-Recipient Pairing:** Elbow extension with passive shoulder abduction 10–20 reps, 6–8×/per day	**Active/Resisted Donor with Active Assist Recipient:** Elbow extension with active-assisted shoulder abduction is performed in a gravity minimized plane **Place and Hold:** The arm is manually placed in shoulder abduction and elbow extension. The patient attempts to maintain this position against gravity when the support is removed	**Resisted Donor and Recipient:** Resisted shoulder abduction (and/or flexion or external rotation) while maintaining elbow extension. Resistance can be in the form of bands, dumbbells, or cuff weights **Resisted Recipient Without Donor Contraction:** Resisted shoulder abduction (and/or flexion or external rotation) with the elbow in mid-range flexion
Additional intervention considerations			Respect fatigue	Initially focus on high frequency, low resistance exercises. Strengthen the rotator cuff, as able

During all phases it is essential to continue cortical reorganization, psychological and psychosocial interventions, and progress to incorporate donor/recipient with ADLS

Triceps to Axillary Nerve Transfer

Goal of Surgery: Restore the ability to raise the arm away from the body in all directions.

Recipient Movement = Shoulder abduction (primary), flexion, external rotation, and extension

Recipient Muscle: Anterior, Middle, and Posterior Deltoid and Teres Minor

Recipient Nerve: Axillary Nerve

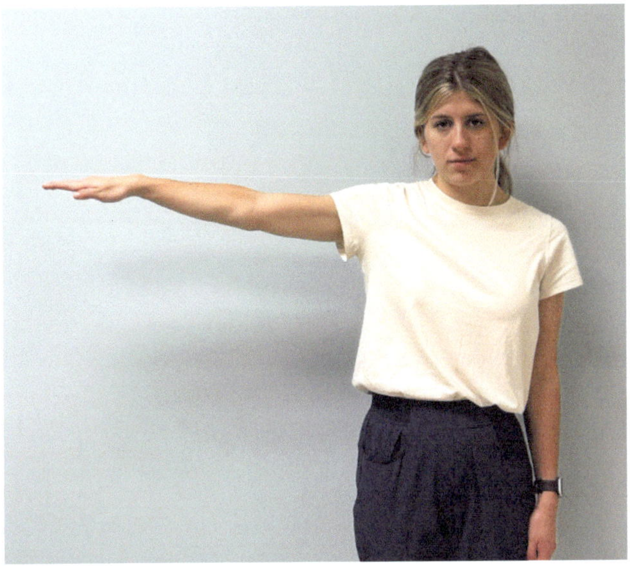

Raise arm out to the side (shoulder abduction)

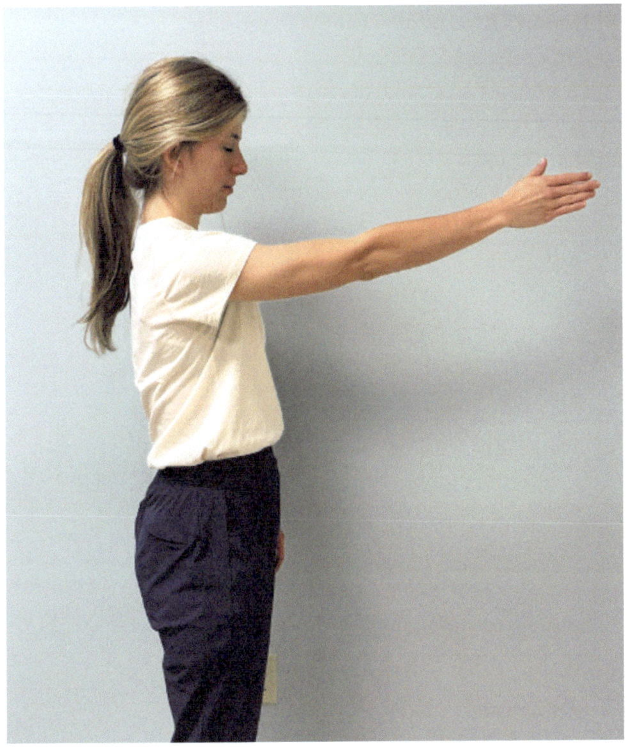

Raise arm in front of you (shoulder flexion)

Donor Movement = Elbow extension
Donor Muscle: Triceps
Donor Nerve: Radial Nerve

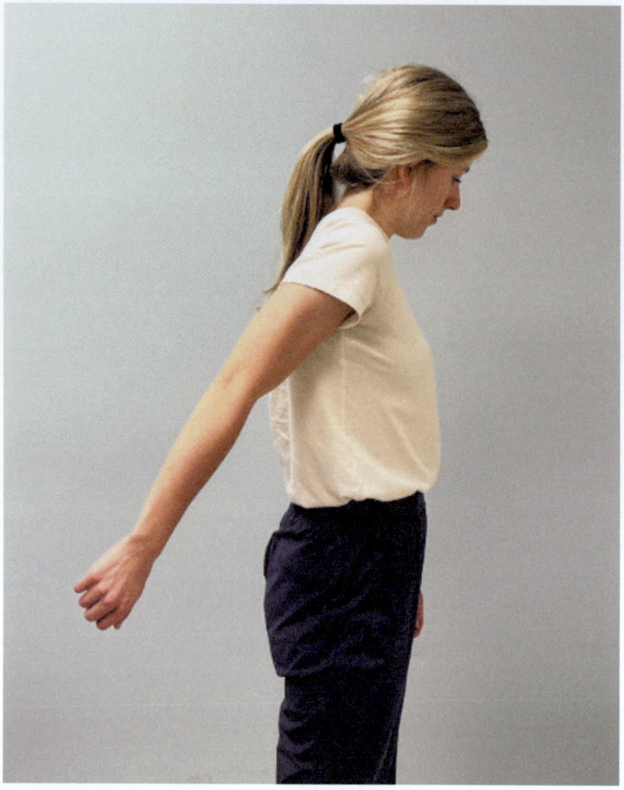

Extend the elbow

Phase 1 Triceps to Axillary Nerve Transfer Exercises

☐ **Passive Range of Motion:**

Complete the below exercises 3–5 repetitions, 2–3 times per day.

Table Slides: Sit with your arm supported on a table next to you. Place a towel under your arm.

1. With your arm straight, lean forward pushing the towel forward along the table.

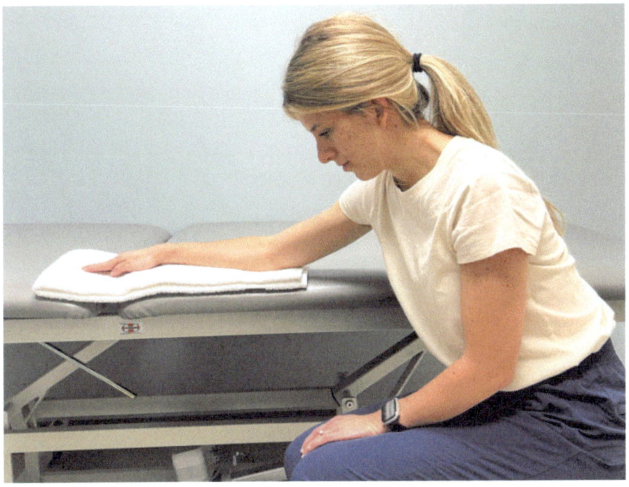

2. With your arm straight, lean sideways toward the table pushing the towel out to the side across the table.

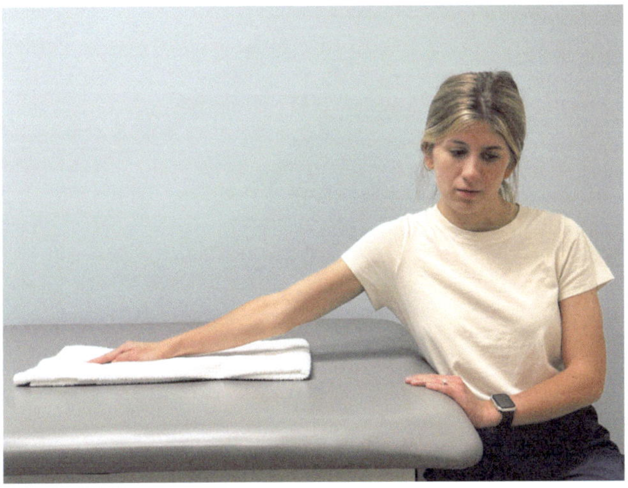

3. With your arm out to the side and elbow bent, lean forward.

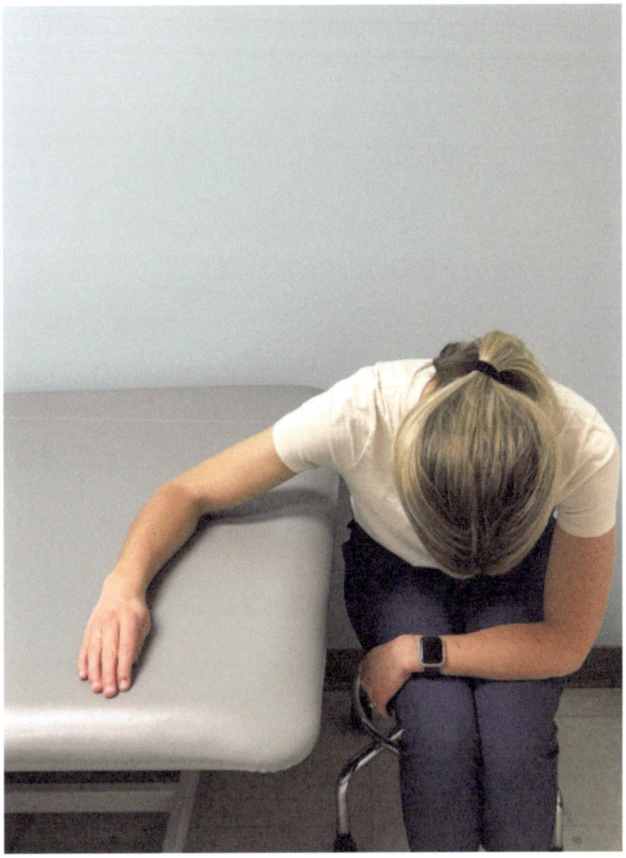

☐ **Active or Resisted Donor Movement:**

1. While seated, rest your hand on your thigh. Straighten your arm by slowly sliding your hand toward your knee. Return to the start position and repeat.

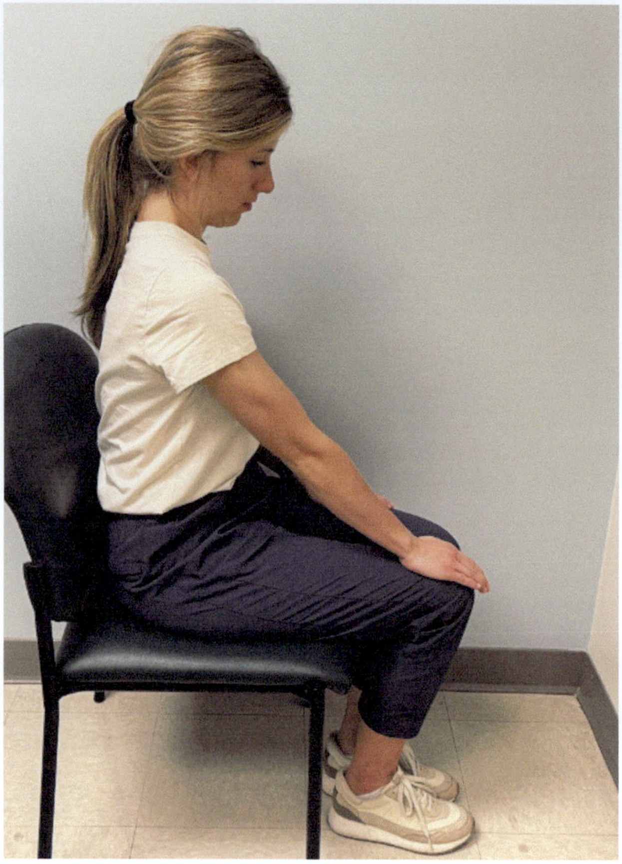

Complete 10 repetitions, every waking hour

2. Lying on your back, raise your arm forward to the ceiling using your other hand to support your upper arm. Keep your shoulder still, only move your elbow as you straighten your arm toward the ceiling. Lower the arm back to the start position and repeat.
   - You may use a pound weight to complete this exercise when recommended by your therapist.

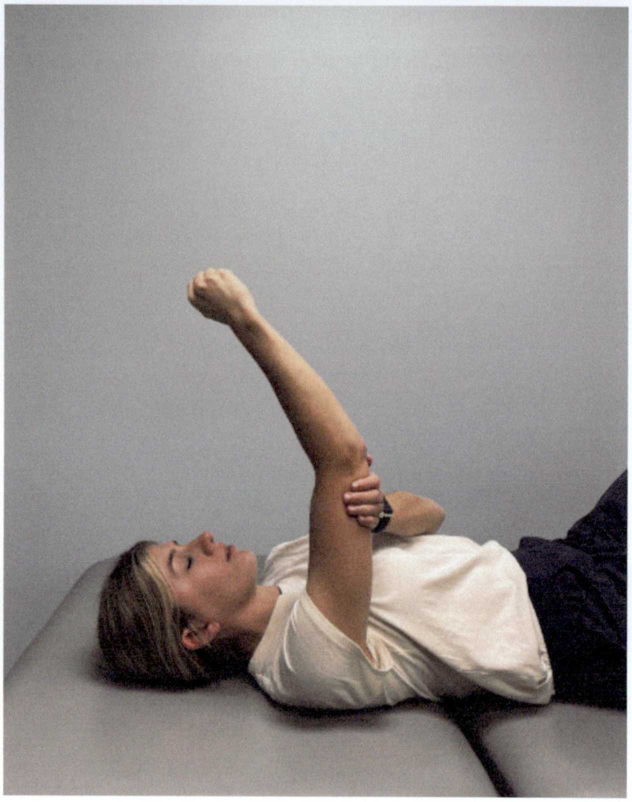

Complete 10 repetitions, 2–3 times per day

☐ **Isometric Donor Activation:**

Complete one of the below exercises 10 repetitions, 3 times per day.

- With elbow bent, make a fist and rest it on the palm of your other hand. Press your fist down into the palm of your other hand to resist this movement.
- Hold for 5 seconds. Relax and repeat.

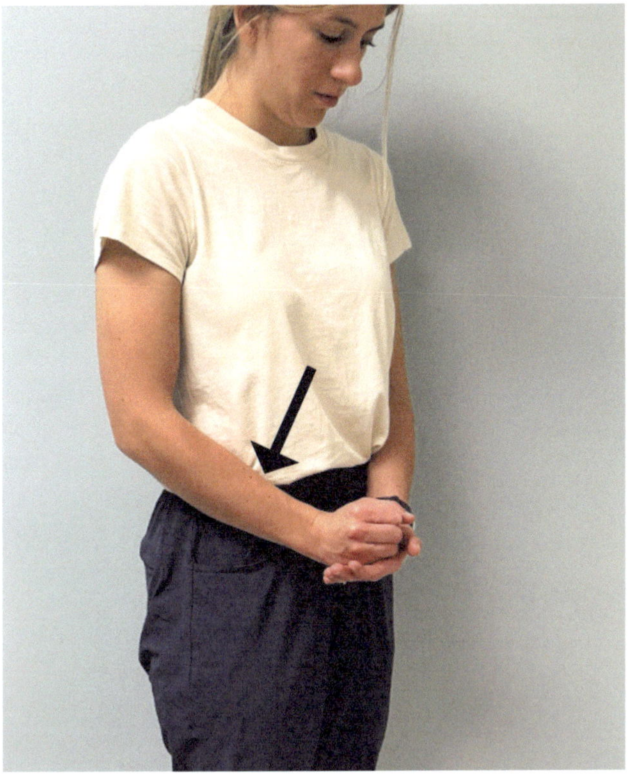

☐ **Active Donor + Passive Recipient Movement: Complete one or both exercises <u>10</u> repetitions, <u>2–3</u> times per day.**

1. Lying on your back, hold a dowel or stick with hands at either end. Keeping your involved elbow straight, use the opposite arm to push the dowel out to the side, assisting your arm as it slides away from your body. Try to avoid arching your back.

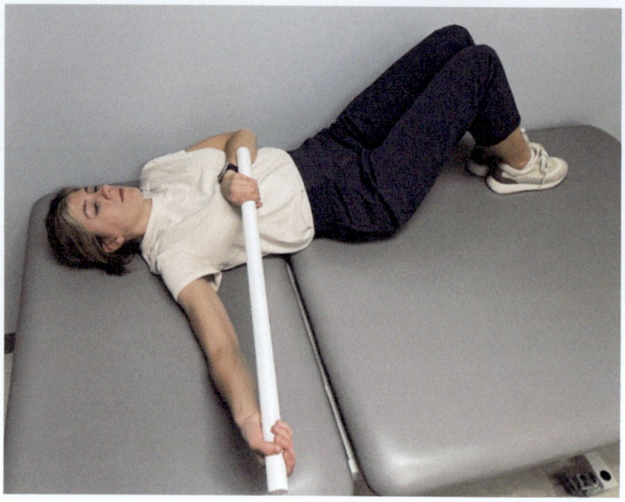

2. Lying on your back, clasp your hands together (or support your forearm with your other hand). Keeping your elbow straight, use your other hand to help raise your arm forward, toward the ceiling.

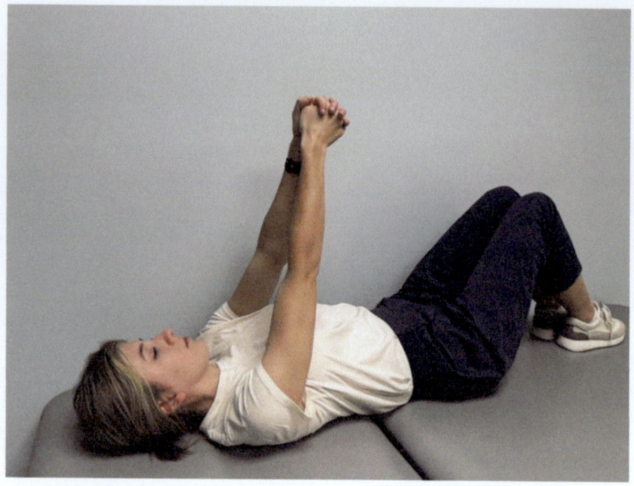

Phase 2 Triceps to Axillary Nerve Transfer Exercises

☐ **Active or Resisted Donor + Active-Assisted Recipient Movement:**

Complete the below exercises 1–10 repetitions, 2–3 times per day.

Only complete the exercises approved by your therapist.

1. Chest Press: Lying on your back, hold a dowel rod or stick with both hands. Push the stick towards the ceiling by straightening your elbowss.

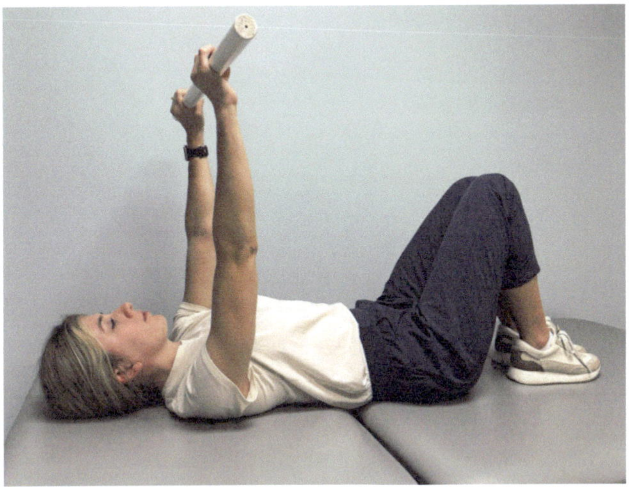

2. Pillow Slides: Lying on your back with your involved arm supported on a pillow, straighten your elbow while you slide your arm out to the side, off the pillow.

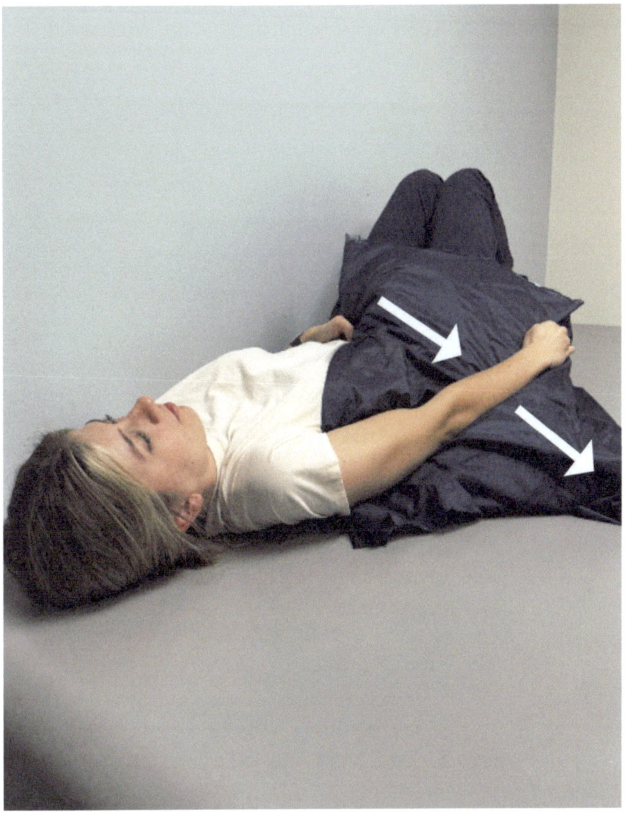

3. Theraband Pulls: Tie a knot at the end of a resistance band and secure it at the top of a door. Hold the band up high (with assistance from the opposite hand) so it creates enough tension to keep your arm comfortably in front of you. Pull the resistance band down until you reach the side of your hip. Straighten your elbow as you allow the resistance band to raise your arm forward, assisting your shoulder muscles to bring it back to the starting position.
   - You may also complete this exercise by pulling the band down and *out to the side*.

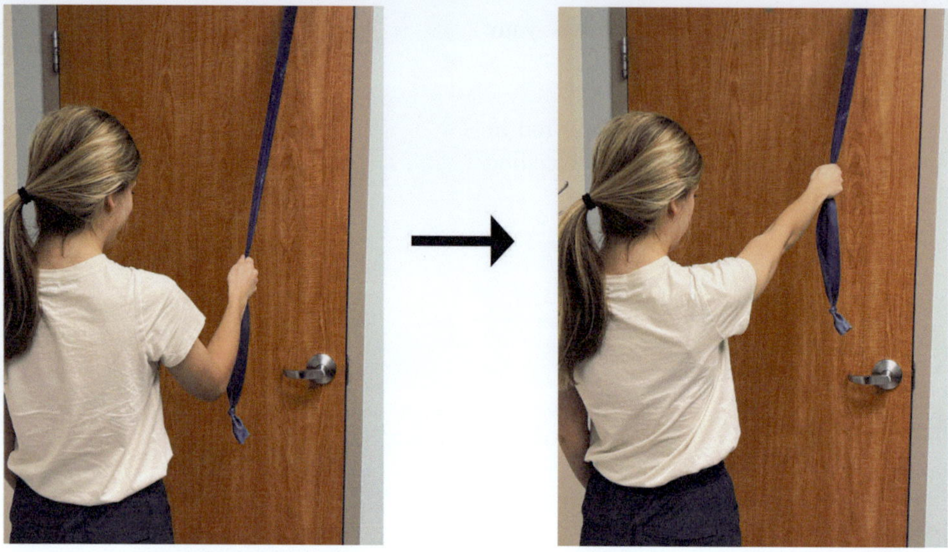

4. Ball Pushes: Sit on a chair with a large exercise ball next to you. Push your hand into the ball keeping your elbow completely straight. Then, lean out to the side, allowing the ball to roll and assist your shoulder out to the side.

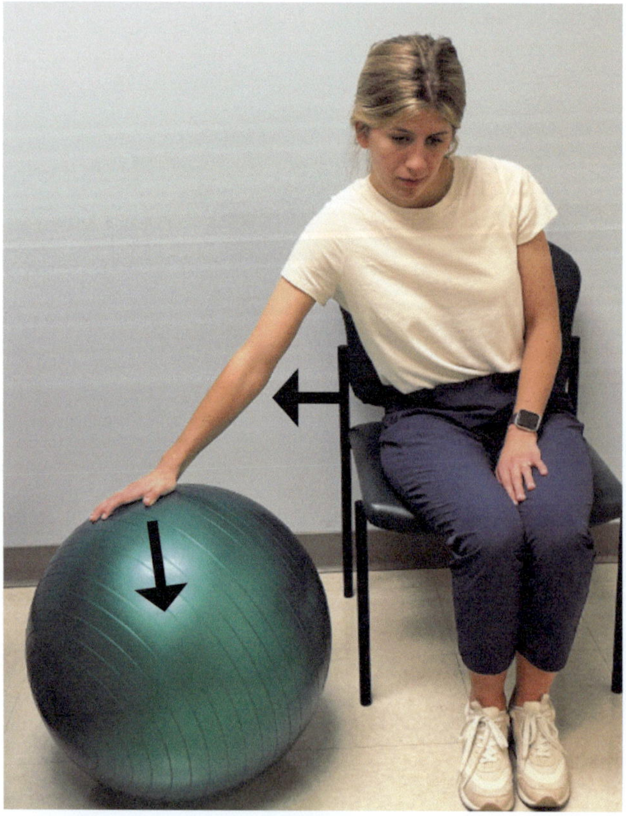

Phase 3 Triceps to Axillary Nerve Transfer Exercises

☐ **Resisted Donor + Recipient Movement:**

Complete the below exercises 1–10 repetitions, 2–3 times per day.

Only complete the exercises approved by your therapist.

1. Stand with both arms resting at your sides. Keeping your elbows straight, raise both arms out to the side. Lower them back down. Avoid shrugging your shoulders during this exercise. You may also complete the same exercise but raise your arms forward instead of out to the side.
   - You may use a weight when recommended by your therapist.

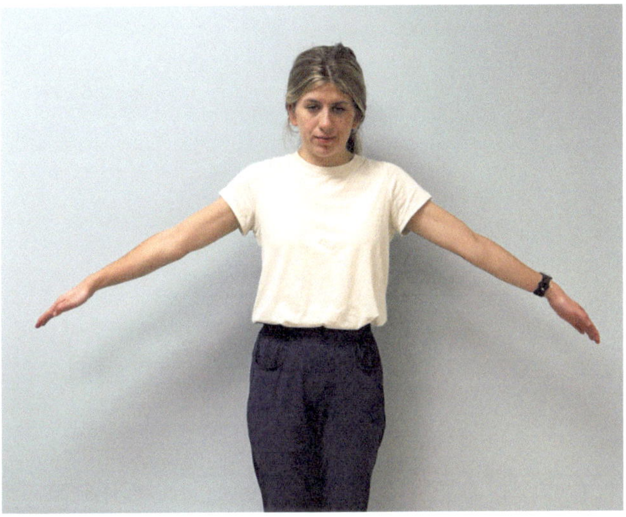

2. Wall Push-Ups: Place both hands flat on a wall at shoulder height with the elbows bent. Lean toward the wall, bending the elbows. Straighten both arms to push yourself away from the wall.

   Return to the starting position.

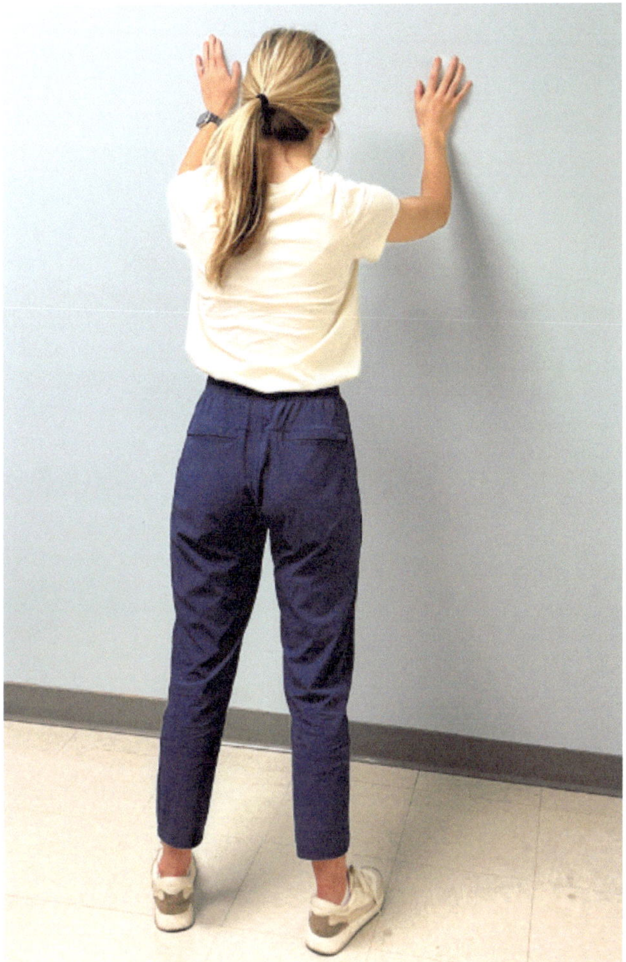

3. Wall Slides: Stand facing a wall. Place the pinky finger side of both hands on the wall at shoulder level with your elbows bent. Slide your arms up the wall to form a "V." Lower arms back to the start position.
   - Start using the weight of the arm against gravity before using a resistance band.

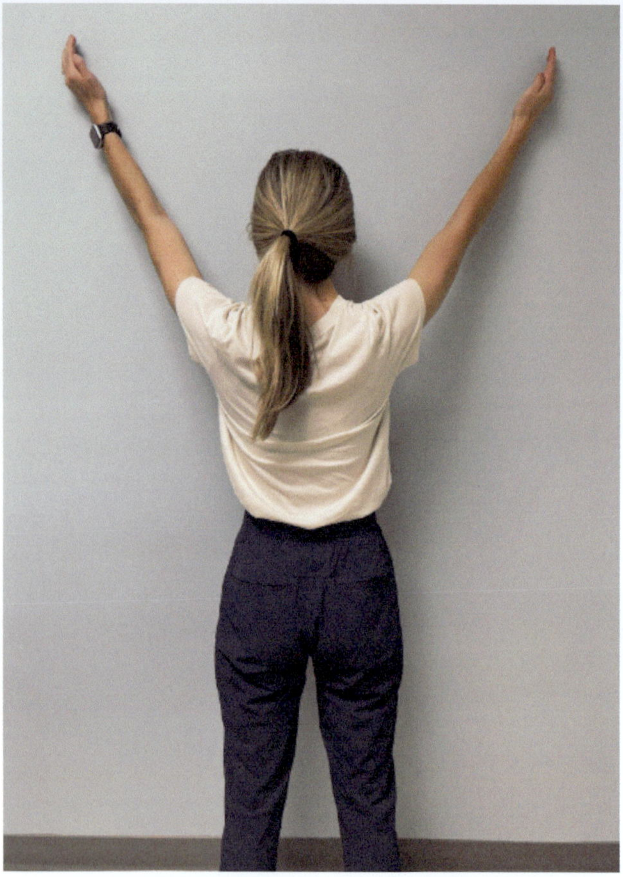

4. Lying on your back, hold a resistance band with hands at either end and arms straight toward the ceiling. Pull your hands apart against the resistance of the band, until you are in the shape of a "T." Return to the starting position.

Complete 5–10 repetitions, 2–3 times per day.

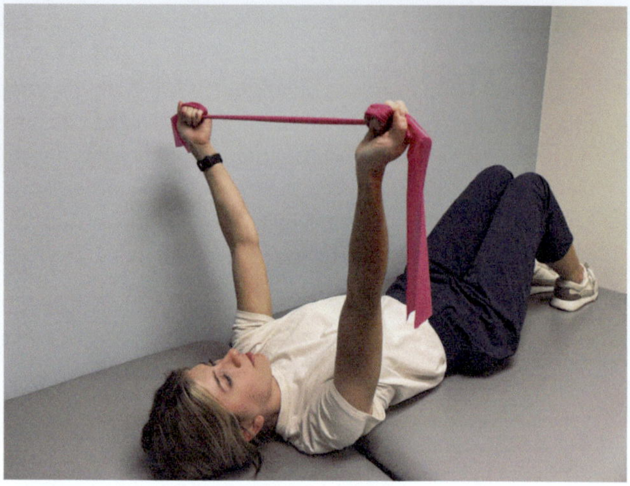

☐ **Isometric Recipient Activation:**

Stand next to a wall with your elbow bent to 90°. Place a towel between your forearm and the wall. Gently press your arm out to the side, into the wall. Hold for 5 seconds. Relax and repeat.

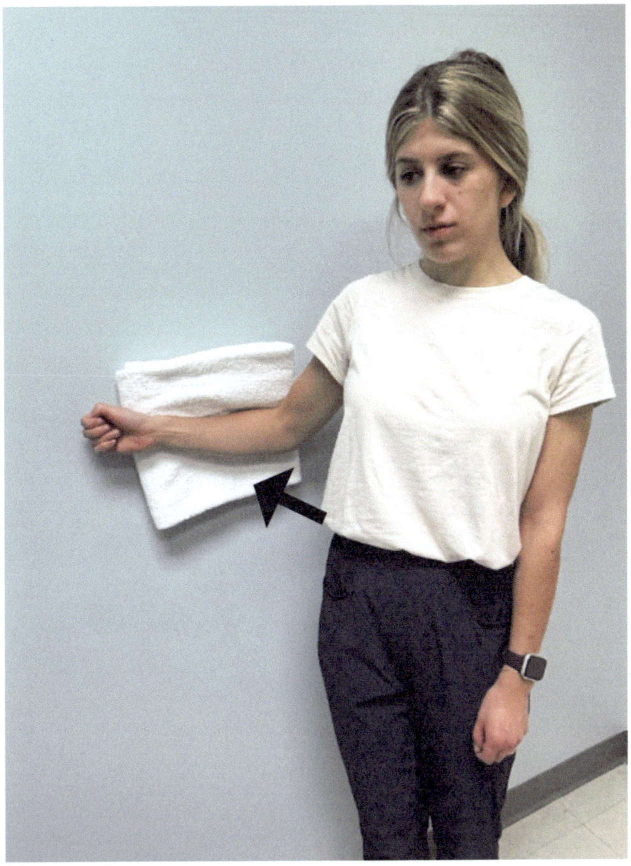

☐ **Resisted Recipient Movement:**

Complete the below exercises 5-10 repetitions, 1-2 times per day.

- While holding _____ pound weights, bend your elbows to 90° and raise your arm out to the side to shoulder level. Slowly lower your arm and return to the start position. Repeat. Avoid shrugging your shoulder during this exercise.

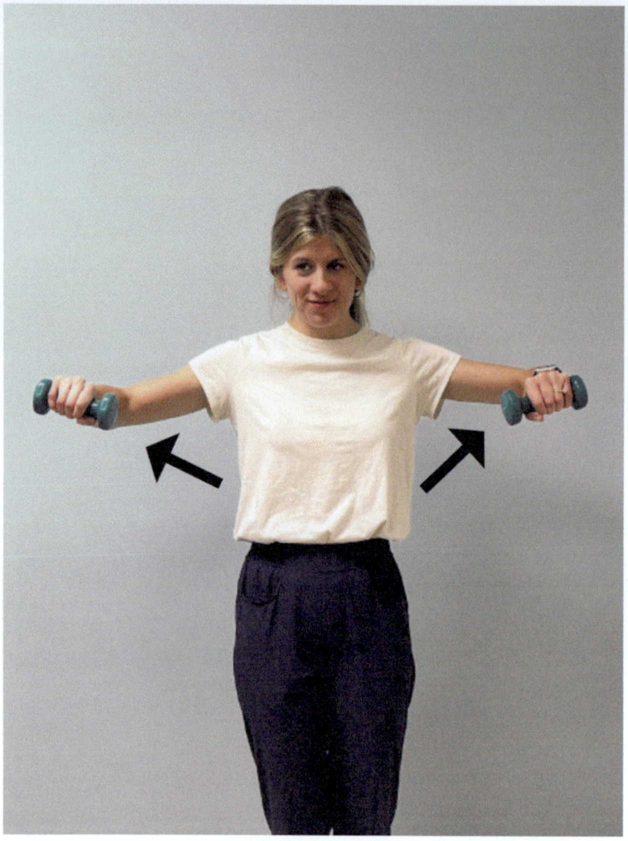

References

1. Sunderland S. A classification of peripheral nerve injuries producing loss of function. Brain. 1951;74(4):491–516.
2. Hems TEJ, Mahmood F. Injuries of the terminal branches of the infraclavicular brachial plexus: patterns of injury, management and outcome. J Bone Joint Surg Br. 2012;94(6):799–804.
3. Sakellariou VI, Badilas NK, Mazis GA, et al. Brachial plexus injuries in adults: evaluation and diagnostic approach. Int Scholar Res Notices. 2014:1–9.
4. Neumann DA. Kinesiology of the musculoskeletal system-e-book: foundations for rehabilitation. Elsevier Health Sciences; 2016.
5. Lee JY, Kircher MF, Spinner RJ, Bishop AT, Shin AY. Factors affecting outcome of triceps motor branch transfer for isolated axillary nerve injury. J Hand Surg. 2012;37(11):2350–6.
6. Mitchell JJ, Chen C, Liechti DJ, Heare A, Chahla J, Bravman JT. Axillary nerve palsy and deltoid muscle atony. J Bone Joint Surg Rev. 2017;5(7):e1.
7. Leechavengvongs S, Witoonchart K, Uerpairojkit C, Thuvasethakul P. Nerve transfer to deltoid muscle using the nerve to the long head of the triceps, part II: a report of 7 cases. J Hand Surg. 2003;28(4):633–8.
8. Krauss EM, Noland SS, Hill EJ, Jain NS, Kahn LC, Mackinnon SE. Outcome analysis of medial triceps motor nerve transfer to axillary nerve in isolated and brachial plexus–associated axillary nerve palsy. Plast Reconstruct Surg. 2022;149(6):1380–90.
9. Crosbie J, Kilbreath SL, Hollmann L, York S. Scapulohumeral rhythm and associated spinal motion. Clin Biomech. 2008;23(2):184–92.
10. Hill JL, Turner LC, Jones RD, Jimulia DT, Miller C, Power DM. The stages of rehabilitation following motor nerve transfer surgery. J Musculoskelet Surg Res. 2019;3:60.

Medial Pectoral Nerve to Axillary Nerve Transfer

Elizabeth Westland

Introduction

The deltoid muscle plays a vital role in shoulder abduction and stability. It works synergistically with the supraspinatus muscle of the rotator cuff to produce abduction. The first 30 degrees of shoulder abduction is initiated by the supraspinatus muscle, followed by synchronous function of both the supraspinatus and deltoid muscles to achieve full abduction [1]. Together, these muscles provide stable motion away from the body, enabling functional overhead reaching. The deltoid also assists in stability of the shoulder through relationships with other muscles via force couples. Loss of deltoid function therefore alters the mechanics of the shoulder girdle complex and can lead to loss of stability and functional reaching.

The deltoid muscle is innervated by the axillary nerve (AXN). The axillary nerve arises from nerve roots of C5 and C6. Injury at various levels of the brachial plexus can result in damage of the axillary nerve; these locations include the upper trunk, posterior division, posterior cord, or terminal branch of the axillary nerve. The axillary nerve has an anterior branch and a posterior branch. The anterior portion innervates the anterior and middle deltoid with the posterior branch innervating the posterior deltoid, teres minor, and sensation to the proximal lateral shoulder and arm [1].

There are a variety of mechanisms of injury that may result in axillary nerve damage. Infraclavicular injuries have a high incident of damage to the axillary nerve [2]. High-velocity injuries such as motorcycle accidents, blunt trauma, ballistic injuries, iatrogenic injury (most often related to total shoulder replacement or reverse total shoulder replacement), and anterior shoulder dislocation are also frequently associated with axillary nerve injury [2, 3].

Surgical options to improve deltoid function following axillary nerve injury include a variety of nerve transfers. Included among these is the transfer of the medial pectoral nerve (MPN) to the axillary nerve. The MPN is often spared in upper plexus injuries, making it a viable donor for the deltoid muscle. Arising from the nerve roots of C8 and T1, the MPN travels through the anterior division of the lower trunk and ultimately branches off the medial cord of the brachial plexus to innervate the pectoralis minor muscle and co-innervate the sternal head of the pectoralis major muscle. The pectoralis major contributes to shoulder flexion, internal rotation, and cross-body adduction. The pectoralis minor muscle is responsible for scapular protraction and depression and assists in inspiration with the insertion fixed [1, 3–5].

Surgical Description

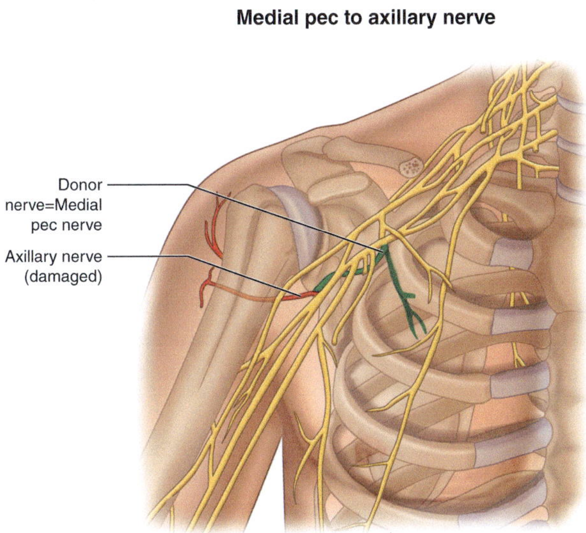

E. Westland (✉)
Athletico Physical Therapy/ Hand Therapy, Saint Louis, MO, USA

L. C. Kahn et al. (eds.), *Rehabilitation for Nerve Transfers of the Upper Extremity*,
https://doi.org/10.1007/978-3-031-92008-0_10

An incision is made in the deltopectoral interval. The pectoralis major insertion is detached from the humerus, ensuring that it can be reattached at conclusion of the procedure. The pectoralis major muscle is elevated, taking care to preserve the nerve branches entering its undersurface (deep aspect). The pectoralis minor tendon is released from the coracoid. The cord-level brachial plexus is identified within the fat pad deep to the pectoralis minor. Typically, the lateral cord is the first to be identified, and branches from the lateral cord to the pectoralis major are visualized, the function of which is confirmed with a handheld nerve stimulator. It is important to ensure that there are no muscle paralytics being used by the anesthesia team. Occasionally, the surgeon may choose a donor branch coming off the medial cord of the brachial plexus. The posterior cord is then identified adjacent to the anterior aspect of the glenohumeral joint. The axillary nerve is dissected at the distal aspect of the subscapularis muscle. Intraoperative stimulation is used to confirm that the axillary nerve is not functioning, and the axillary nerve is then neurolyzed from the posterior cord and divided proximally. The selected donor nerve from the pectoralis major is then dissected as distally as possible, divided, and transposed to meet the recipient axillary nerve. Coaptation of the pectoralis major branch to the axillary nerve is performed using microsurgical technique.

Outcomes

Outcomes for MPN-to-AXN transfer vary from poor to excellent. A systematic review compared outcomes for this nerve transfer ($n = 46$) to reconstruction with a graft of the axillary nerve in posttraumatic, isolated axillary nerve injuries [6]. The authors found that 87% of the patients who underwent MPN-to-AXN transfer achieved a manual muscle testing (MMT) grade of 3/5 or better strength in the deltoid muscle. Seventy-four percent (74%) of patients achieved 4/5 deltoid strength. Ray et al. described excellent results (MMT 5/5) in 50% of patients in his eight-case series [7]. Two individuals achieved good (MMT 4/5) results, one fair (MMT 3/5), and one poor (MMT 0–1/5) result. The authors of these studies report that they were surprised that age and timing of surgery were not as predictive of outcomes as they originally surmised.

Phases of Rehabilitation

Phase 1

Preoperative to 1/5 MMT of the Recipient Muscle

Preoperative

Preoperative assessment includes baseline measurements of shoulder range of motion (active AROM and passive PROM), donor and recipient muscle strength, evidence of a sulcus sign, and lateral arm sensation. All three heads of the deltoid should be assessed for atrophy and strength. A description of gross shoulder kinematics including glenohumeral (GH) and scapulothoracic (ST) ratios [1] would be helpful when discussing surgery, rehabilitation, and expectations with the patient. When the deltoid muscle is absent or weak, shoulder movement often occurs with excessive scapulothoracic motion and minimal glenohumeral motion.

Recovery and maintenance of shoulder PROM are prioritized in the preoperative period. Pain management includes behavioral modifications such as positioning to avoid drag on the plexus and overlengthening of the deltoid muscle. Use of a sling or OmoTrain® brace is encouraged for these reasons as well as to improve comfort.

Patient education includes postoperative precautions, healing timelines, and expected outcomes. Donor and recipient muscle names and functions are introduced, and donor activation exercises may be initiated [8, 9]. Active and resistive exercises can be performed with all uninvolved muscles.

Postoperative

Precautions

If the pec muscle was taken down and repaired to access pertinent anatomy for the nerve transfer, it is imperative to protect this muscle-tendon repair for **4** weeks [10]. Accidental tear to this muscle-tendon repair could result in further loss of shoulder function. A shoulder immobilizer or a sturdy sling is recommended to maintain a position of shoulder adduction and internal rotation during this time. The elbow is typically flexed but may come out of the immobilizer frequently to extend the elbow and prevent ulnar nerve irritation. If the pec muscle was not taken down, then following the first **2** weeks after surgery, elevation of the arm should remain limited to 90° in both shoulder flexion or abduction for several weeks. Access to the operative note is especially important in this transfer to determine which approach was used and how much protection is needed.

Surgical sites are often closed with staples, sutures, or glue. Wound care preferences will be physician specific, and it is important to be in contact with the surgeon regarding these preferences as needed to appropriately instruct and educate the patient. Postoperative precautions include adherence to sling use and avoidance of shoulder elevation above 90° for 2 weeks. The patient is seen for their first postoperative visit with their surgeon around 2–3 weeks after surgery. Postoperative therapy should begin at this time.

At the first postoperative therapy visit, A/PROM and sensation measurements of the shoulder are taken, and assessment of donor and recipient muscle function is noted. A large part of this visit should be spent reviewing education given preoperatively. If the patient did not have any preoperative therapy, it is important to then educate the patient on expectations, healing timelines, expected outcomes, postoperative precautions, and donor activation [9]. Shoulder and arm ROM is initiated (specifics outlined below). Following removal of sutures/staples, scar massage is initiated. This can help with decreasing adherence to underlying tissues while also providing desensitization to this area. The patient should be encouraged to touch and look at their arm, as some patients may be fearful or anxious about the postoperative appearance of their arm.

Exercises

- Passive Range of Motion
  It is important to passively range the shoulder to decrease soft tissue and capsular tightness as the patient awaits muscle reinnervation. For most patients, passive self-mobilization of the shoulder is difficult. Some good options for shoulder PROM include door pulleys, supine dowel exercises, and table slides into flexion and scaption. For table slides, the patient should sit in a chair facing a table that is just below or at shoulder height. The patient will place his or her arms on the table and use his or her body weight to passively move the arm into flexion or scaption. Caregivers can also be instructed in supine PROM to assist in both regaining and maintaining joint mobility.
- Donor Activation
  There are several methods to "flood the donor" by engaging the pec muscle throughout the day. The pec contributes to shoulder internal rotation, horizontal adduction, and flexion. Isometrics may be performed for any or all these actions.
  Seated horizontal adduction: Patients may sit with their arms in front of them and their fingers interlocked. They are instructed to press their hands together for isometric pec activation. Patient should be instructed in 3–5-s holds before relaxing. They may squeeze a ball between their hands for added challenge (Image 1).
  Standing shoulder internal rotation: Patients may stand in a doorframe, facing the doorframe with their elbow flexed at their side. With a towel roll in hand, the patient pushes the towel roll into the doorframe in the direction of internal rotation (Image 2).
  Standing shoulder flexion: The patient stands in front of a wall with his/her shoulder adducted and elbow slightly flexed. A towel roll is placed between the wall and the patient's fist, and he or she pushes the towel into the wall in the direction of shoulder flexion and adduction (Image 3).
- Combined Donor with Passive Recipient Exercise
  Once the patient is proficient with frequent donor activation, donor activation is paired with passive ROM of the recipient muscle. This strengthens the new neural pathway and enhances cortical reorganization [11]. Examples include the following:
  Supine pec press: With the patient supine holding a dowel in both hands, a chest press is performed by extending the elbows while flexing the shoulders to 90°. Instructing the patient to press the hands towards each other while raising the dowel (isometric adduction) may create greater demand on the pec muscle (Image 4).
  Side-lying pec press: The patient lies on the uninvolved side with a large exercise ball in front of him or her.

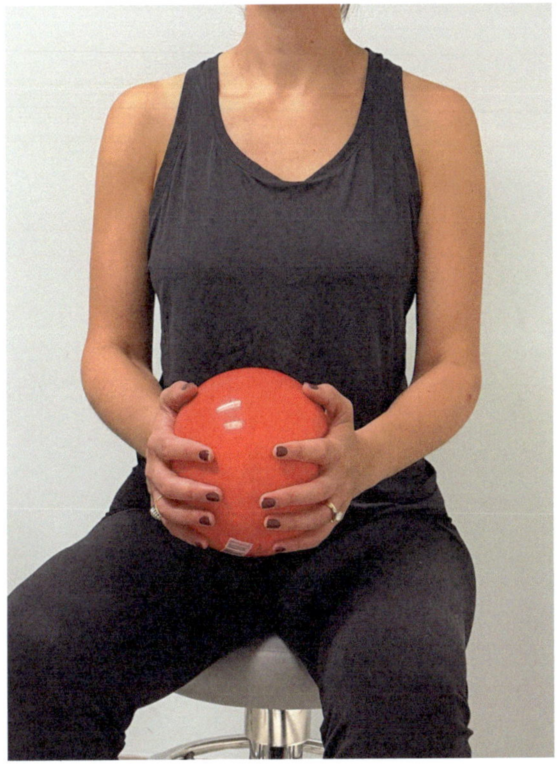

Image 1 Donor activation is performed with isometric pec muscle activation by instructing the individual to press a ball between his or her hands

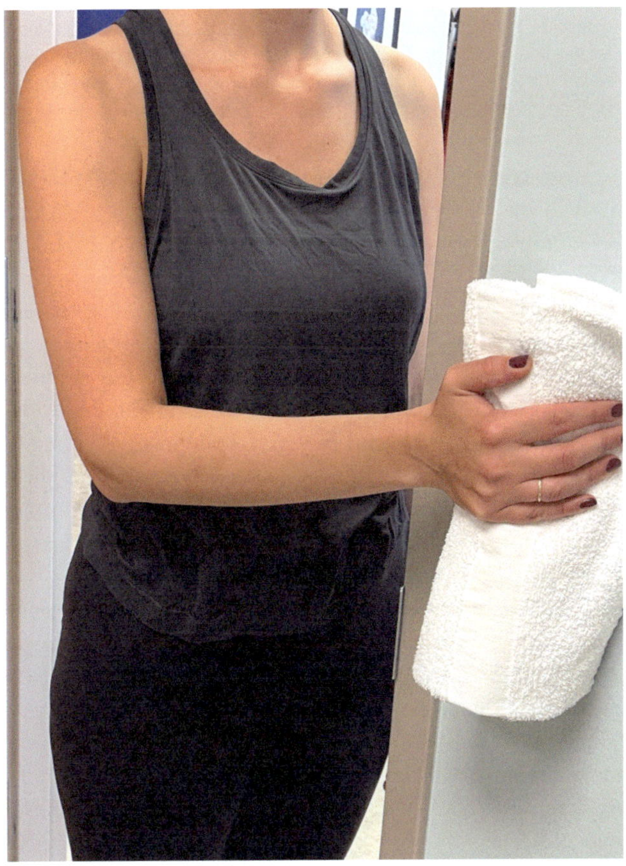

Image 2 Donor activation is achieved with isometric shoulder internal rotation by instructing the individual to stand in a door frame and press into the direction of internal rotation

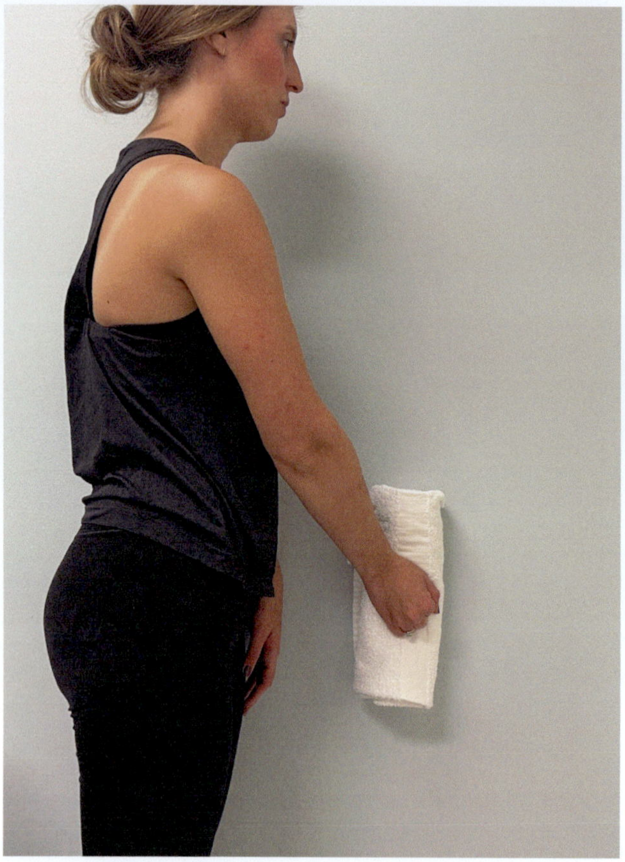

Image 3 Isometric pectoralis exercise is also achieved with shoulder flexion and adduction. The patient stands in front of a wall holding a folded towel and is instructed to press into the wall in the direction of shoulder flexion and adduction

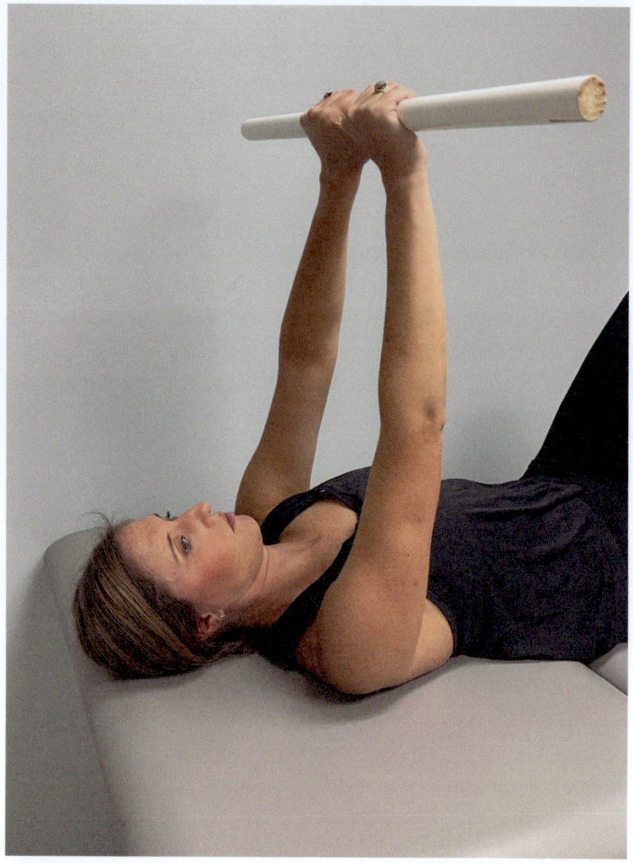

Image 4 In Phase 1, combined active (or resisted) donor with passive recipient exercise is achieved with a supine chest press. Cues to grasp and isometrically push the hands towards the center of the dowel (shoulder adduction) while raising it will create greater donor response

Instruction is given to press down on the ball while sliding it in the direction of shoulder flexion. Gravity and ball rolling will assist the recipient movement (Image 5).

Assessment of Recovery

Routine strength and ROM measurements of the recipient deltoid, donor pectoralis major, and other affected muscles and joints provide helpful pre- and postoperative comparisons. The therapist should assess recipient MMT strength at least monthly to assess for signs of deltoid and teres minor recovery. Appropriate therapeutic exercises and changes to home instructions will then be made.

To evaluate for deltoid muscle return, the arm is manually supported in sitting or supine. Resistance is applied to the arm in the direction of horizontal abduction, and the patient is instructed to resist this motion to activate the donor/pec. Simultaneously, the patient is cued to attempt to move the shoulder into abduction, flexion, and/or extension. When the axillary nerve is coapted proximally to capture both anterior and posterior portions, one would expect to see the initial response in the posterior head of the deltoid as the nerve travels in a posterior-to-anterior direction. Palpation is performed along the acromion to palpate for a twitch of deltoid muscle response (Image 6). If the axillary nerve branch to the teres minor was included in the nerve transfer, palpation is also made along the lateral border of the scapula. The examiner should monitor for substitution from the supraspinatus muscle throughout this assessment. If a trace muscle response is present in the recipient muscle, assess the patient in supine and measure any active abduction in this gravity-lessened position.

Therapy Frequency

Frequency of visits in this phase will vary greatly with the needs of each individual patient. Factors to consider when determining the frequency of visits should include patient anxiety, understanding of precautions, understanding of basic donor and donor/recipient exercise concepts, wound closure/swelling, and insurance limitations. If patients have limitations in passive ROM and/or have difficulty grasping basic donor and donor/recipient exercise concepts, they should be seen once or twice a week. Once the patient has near-full PROM, normal wound closure, and a good understanding of basic donor and donor/recipient exercise concepts, the frequency of visits is reduced to one to two times per month.

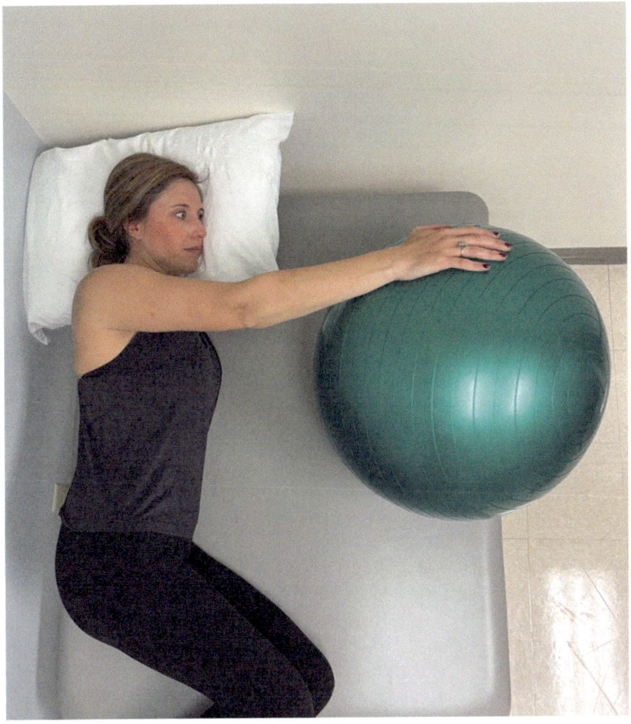

Image 5 In side-lying, passive shoulder flexion is achieved with the help of gravity and a large exercise ball. Pressing on the ball in the direction of shoulder adduction will activate the donor/pec, and the ball will roll forward into flexion

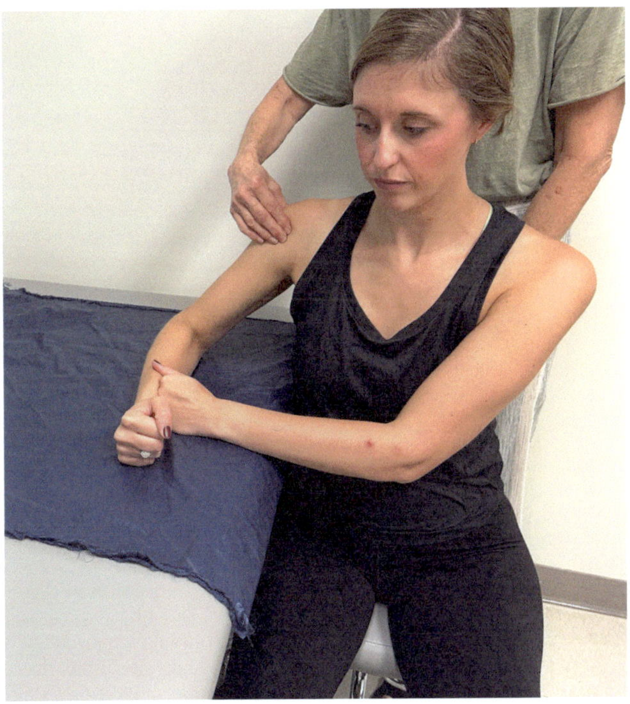

Image 6 Early monitoring for recipient deltoid recovery is performed by palpating along the acromion for a deltoid response while the patient resists the arm in the direction of horizontal adduction while he or she is cued to attempt shoulder extension, abduction or flexion

Phase 2

2−/5 to 3/5 MMT in the Recipient Muscle

Once a twitch is elicited in the deltoid muscle and the patient can demonstrate some movement through a gravity-minimized plane, phase 2 of therapy is initiated. At this point in recovery, the primary focus is to encourage active ROM and active-assisted ROM in a position that is easy for the recipient/deltoid. The patient will be able to achieve more motion in a gravity-lessened position. Activities and exercises are devised to improve the connection between the donor and recipient muscles with an increased focus on coupling or co-contracting. Donor activation should continue in this phase. Without deltoid function, the patient will often substitute with the upper trapezius muscle to perform activities of daily living (ADLs) and attempt to move the arm away from the body. It is important to make the patient aware of these substitution patterns and avoid overuse of the upper trapezius. Avoiding such biomechanical faults will promote activation of the deltoid. If the patient is still wearing a sling for comfort, he or she may be weaned at this time (always consult with MD about discontinuation of sling or orthosis). The OmoTrain® shoulder brace may provide better longitudinal support than the sling and does not interfere with elbow function (Image 7).

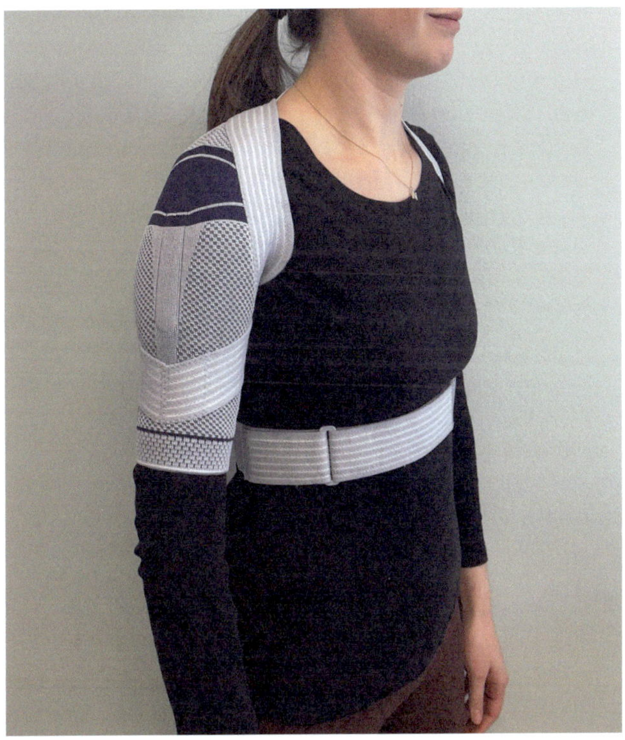

Image 7 The Omotrain™ brace is recommended to provide longitudinal support to the involved arm and shoulder, thus minimizing glenohumeral subluxation and pain. Use of this brace will discourage distal humeral subluxation (positive sulcus sign) and support the weight of the arm without blocking elbow function

Precautions

Once the pec muscle is fully recovered from the surgical repair, no precautions are necessary for individuals with isolated axillary nerve injuries. If other nerve transfers were performed, consult other chapters (along with the patient's surgeon) to ensure that all precautions are maintained.

Exercises

- Active Donor with Active-Assisted Recipient
  Deltoid MMT = 2−/5 to 2/5
  Once the patient demonstrates partial movement of the deltoid in a gravity-minimized plane, phase 2 exercises may begin. Exercise examples include the following:
  Supine chest press: The patient may continue the chest press described in phase 1. However, this differs from phase 1 where deltoid motion was purely passive. In phase 2, active-*assisted* shoulder flexion is achieved with some contribution from the recovering deltoid.
  Table slides: The patient is seated with the elbow flexed and the forearm supported on a table. The patient pushes his or her hand into their uninvolved hand in the direction of shoulder internal rotation while attempting to slide the elbow in the direction of shoulder flexion or abduction. The opposite hand also assists with these motions.
  Side-lying shoulder flexion: The patient is side-lying on the unaffected shoulder, and the contralateral arm assists the involved arm forward to 90 degrees of flexion with slight internal rotation. A large foam wedge with a downward slope could be used to assist with the movement as needed to make it gravity-assisted or gravity-minimized active-assisted ROM (Image 8). The patient simultaneously performs isometric pec activation while the arm slides into flexion.
  Behind-the-back internal rotation: The patient holds a dowel behind their back, parallel to the floor just at hip level with both hands. Instruction is given to push his or her fists isometrically towards the center of the dowel to activate the pec while attempting to raise both elbows in the direction of shoulder abduction (Image 9).
  Ball squeezes: With an inflatable ball between the hands, the patient squeezes into the ball and then attempts to raise the arm into shoulder flexion. This may be performed first in supine and eventually in standing (Image 10).
- "Place and Hold" Exercise
  Deltoid MMT = 2 + /5
  With the patient in side-lying on the uninvolved side, the involved arm is passively placed in shoulder abduction at 90°. The therapist slowly releases the arm, and the patient attempts to hold that position while the therapist resists the pec muscle (palm to arm to resist horizontal adduction).
- Active Donor with Active Recipient
  Deltoid MMT = 3−/5 to 3/5

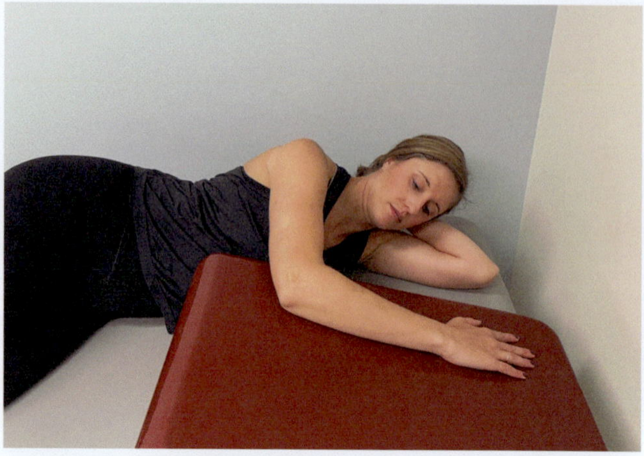

Image 8 Position the patient in side-lying with the arm supported on a foam wedge, as shown. A nylon cloth may be added to reduce friction. The patient presses into the wedge to activate the pec donor muscle as he or she attempts to slide the arm forward into shoulder flexion with the assistance of gravity

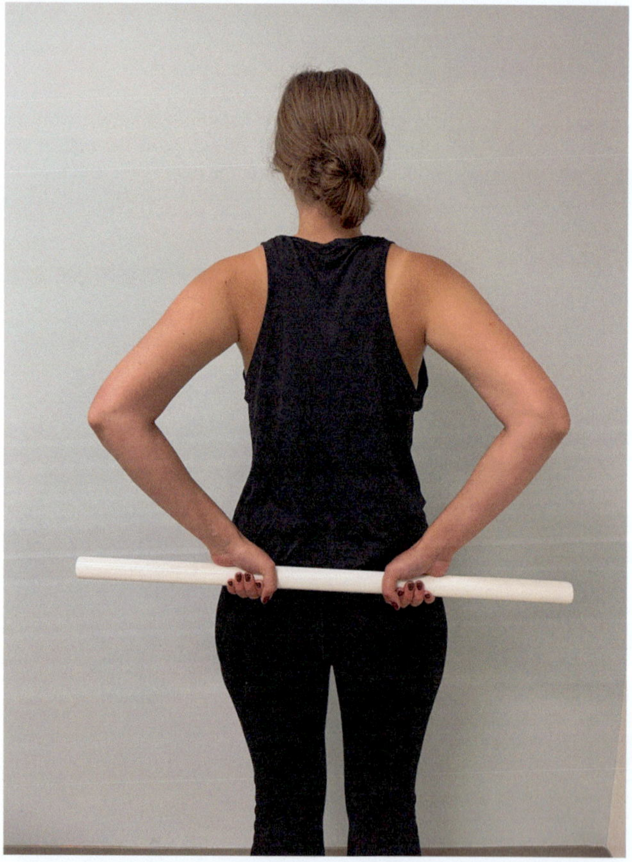

Image 9 Combined donor and assisted recipient/deltoid movement is demonstrated with a dowel behind the back. The individual is instructed to grasp and press inward (internal rotation and adduction) while attempting to raise the elbows with the assist of the uninvolved arm

Once the patient demonstrates >50% ROM of the deltoid in a gravity-minimized plane, he or she can perform antigravity recipient exercises. Examples may include the following:

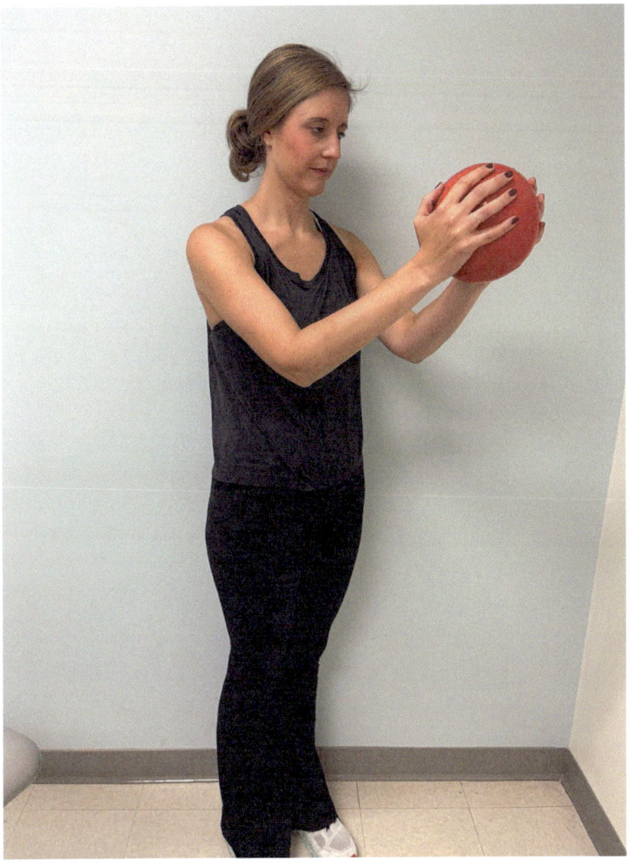

Image 10 Active donor with active recipient motion is demonstrated in standing holding a ball between the hands to activate the donor pec muscle. While pressing the hands into the ball, both shoulders flex forward

Side-lying wall slide: The patient is positioned in side-lying on the uninvolved side, facing a wall. The hand presses into the wall holding a washcloth to reduce friction. Cues are given to press into the wall (pec donor activation) while attempting to slide the arm up the wall into shoulder abduction (Image 11).

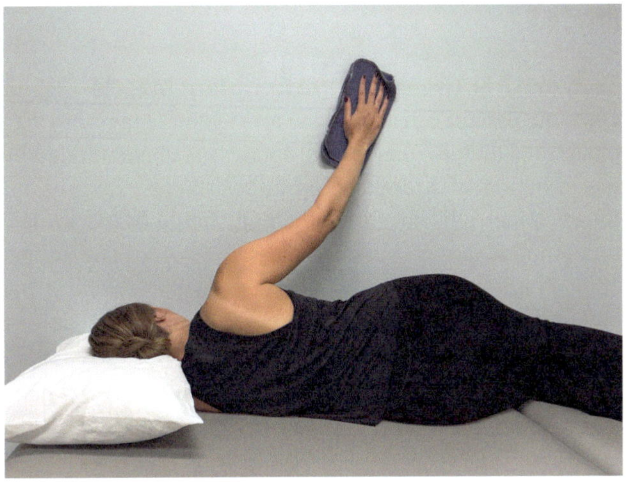

Image 11 Active deltoid with donor resistance is performed in side-lying on the unaffected side facing a wall. The individual is instructed to press into the wall for pec activation while sliding up the wall into shoulder abduction

- Functional Activity

  Patients should be encouraged to perform daily tasks that require shoulder flexion or abduction while isometrically contracting the pec muscle. For example, when lying in bed on the uninvolved side and facing the side of the bed, the patient reaches across the body for an object on a side table, such as a cup or book.

Therapy Frequency

Frequency of therapy appointments in phase 2 depends on patient needs. If the patient has not achieved full PROM in all planes, one to two times per week is appropriate. Treatment can decrease to once or twice per month if the patient has achieved full passive motion, has a good understanding of donor-recipient activation, and demonstrates compliance of the home exercise program.

Phase 3

3+/5 MMT or Greater in the Recipient Muscle

Once the patient can abduct the arm against gravity to 90°, phase 3 of therapy may begin. Phase 3 is characterized by the initiation of strengthening or resistance exercises for the recipient muscle. Strengthening should be performed to a point of fatigue but not excessive fatigue. The patient and therapist should respect fatigue by acknowledging that endurance recovery is very slow and allow the deltoid muscle adequate rest and time to recover from each exercise [8]. Endurance limitations will be present up to 2 years. As the deltoid muscle develops strength in time, substitution patterns will continue. The therapist should instruct the patient how to recognize these faulty movement patterns and correct them. This typically happens if the exercise exceeds the capacity of the recovering deltoid. It is therefore important to avoid advancing a strengthening program too quickly. Not all patients will achieve this level.

Exercises

- Resisted Recipient with Donor Contraction
  Strengthening begins with co-contraction of the donor pec. This will contribute to greater force production in the deltoid muscle. Examples may include the following:
  Wall push-ups: The patient stands and places his or her hands on a wall with elbows extended and shoulders flexed to 90°. Performing a push-up requires resisted pec activation and anterior deltoid function. Raising the height of the hands will increase the demand of the deltoid (Image 12).
  Side-lying shoulder flexion and abduction: In side-lying on the uninvolved side, the patient flexes or abducts the shoulder to 90° against the resistance of a therapy band. To include the donor pec, the patient resists horizontal adduction with the opposite hand while performing resisted flexion and/or abduction (Image 13).
- Resisted Recipient Activity Without Donor Contraction
  Once the patient demonstrates reliable strength in the recipient deltoid muscle, he or she may begin to de-emphasize the donor pec as necessary.
  Supine horizontal abduction: In supine with shoulders flexed to 90° holding a resistance band in each hand, the patient horizontally abducts bilaterally against the resistance of the band and then slowly returns to the starting position (Image 14). This action biases the posterior deltoid.
  Standing shoulder flexion and abduction: The patient raises his or her arms into shoulder flexion while holding light weights (1/2 pound to 1 pound) or a light resistance band. The same exercise can be performed in shoulder abduction. Special attention should be placed on minimizing upper trapezius substitution.

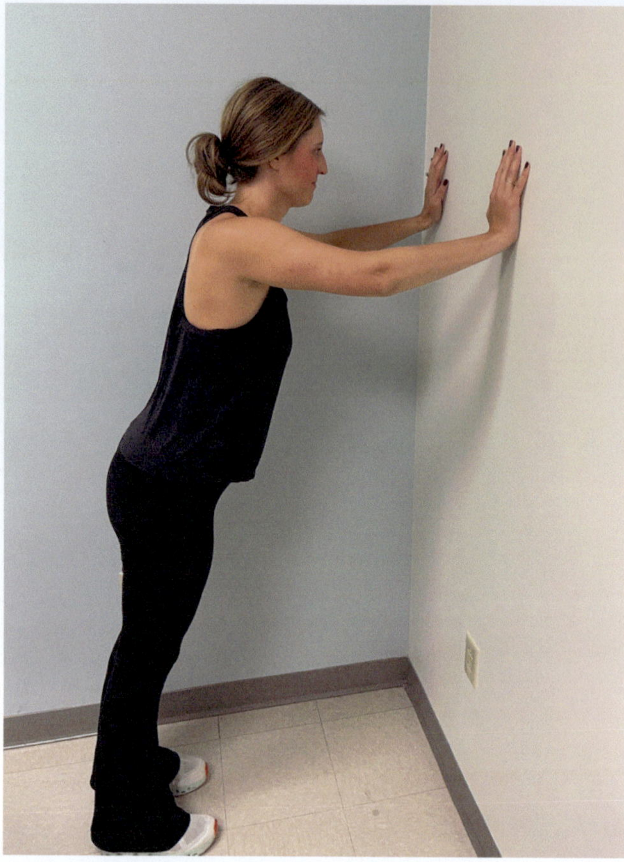

Image 12 In Phase 3, strengthening of the deltoid may be achieved with resisted donor as demonstrated with wall push-ups

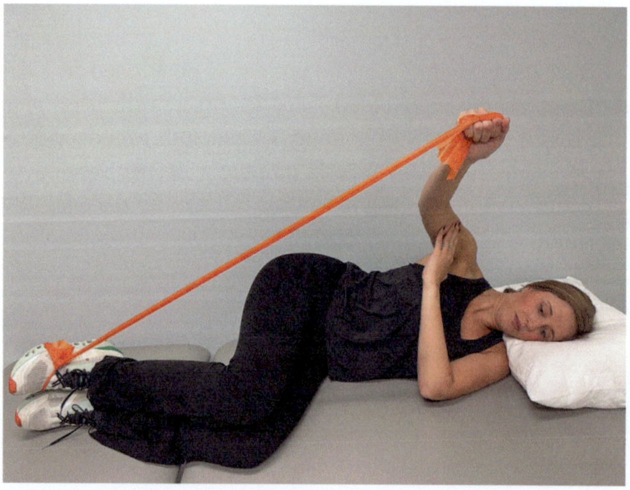

Image 13 A resistance band is used for deltoid strengthening in side-lying. The opposite hand provides resistance to the donor pec by resisting horizontal adduction while raising the arm into shoulder abduction against the resistance of the band

Therapy Frequency

Frequency of visits in phase 3 remains patient dependent. Younger, athletic patients often benefit from once a month, while other patients may require more supervised therapy

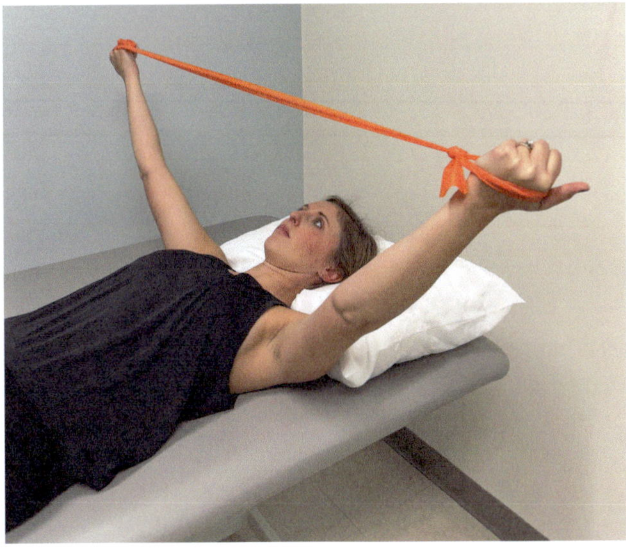

Image 14 Deltoid strengthening without donor activation is performed in supine. Holding a therapy band in both hands, resistance is applied to the posterior deltoid as the arm pulls into horizontal abduction

instruction by maintaining weekly or bimonthly therapy sessions. During this time, a large focus should be on independence with activities and working towards functional patient goals. Strength and endurance can take more than 2 years to recover, so it is important to promote independence while educating the patient that they will need to continue a strengthening routine long after formal therapy has ended.

Pec to axillary nerve transfer

Nerve transfer overview					
Donor nerve	Donor action	Recipient nerve	Recipient action	Indications for functional restoration	Approximate months to functional movement
Medial pectoral nerve to the pectoralis major (sternal portion)	Shoulder adduction and internal rotation (and partial flexion) Patients with axillary nerve palsy often lack flexion so donor activation via adduction and internal rotation is prioritized	Axillary nerve	Shoulder abduction (primary), flexion, extension and external rotation if both branches were reinnervated	Loss of deltoid function, inability to raise the arm	Data not available

Information below are suggested guidelines. Precautions may vary according to surgeon preferences and patient factors

	Preoperative therapy	Early phase	Middle phase	Late phase
Criteria	Before surgery	0/5–1/5 MMT	2-/5 to 3/5 MMT	>3/5 MMT
Purpose of phase	Educate and establish baseline function	Understand donor and recipient relationship	Consistently activate recipient	Strengthen recipient and separate from donor activation
Precautions	Prevent glenohumeral joint stiffness	Support glenohumeral joint and minimize subluxation	Respect fatigue	Avoid resisted shoulder motion until AROM > 90° against gravity
Frequency of visits (considerations)	1–2 pre-op visits More if PROM limitations exist	1×/week until PROM is WNL and patient is independent with donor activation; then 1× monthly	1× per week to 1× per month based on patient needs and accurate, consistent demonstration of exercise program	1× every 1–2 weeks based on progress toward patient-specific goals
Orthosis considerations	NA	Full-time sling use for 4 weeks but remove for elbow ROM	Consider Kinesio® tape or Omotrain® brace to minimize glenohumeral subluxation	NA
Interventions	PROM of the shoulder in all planes	**Donor Activation:** Shoulder adduction and internal rotation (typically isometric) **Donor-Recipient Pairing**: Isometric shoulder adduction and/or internal rotation combined with passive shoulder abduction	**Active/Resisted Donor with Active Assisted Recipient:** Gravity minimized plane: isometric internal rotation into a table and simultaneously slide arm into abduction on the table Supine dowel rod exercise: bilateral pec press combined with shoulder flexion assisted by the dowel **Place and Hold**: The shoulder is supported in 90° abduction on a counter. The patient activates the pec through adduction and internal rotation. He/she slides the arm off the counter and holds it in abduction	**Resisted Donor and Recipient:** Wall push-ups or sidelying shoulder abduction/ flexion with a resistance band (isometrically contracting the pec) **Resisted Recipient:** Holding a resistance band bilaterally at his or her sides, the patient abducts both shoulders.
Additional interventions			Early anti-gravity deltoid exercises may include wall slides with a wash cloth for ease of movement	

During all phases it is essential to continue Cortical Reorganization, Psychological and Psychosocial interventions, Progress to incorporate donor/ recipient with ADLS

Pec to Axillary Nerve Transfer

Goal of Surgery: Restore the ability to raise your arm overhead

Recipient Movement = Shoulder abduction and flexion (and secondarily external rotation)

Recipient Muscle: Deltoid

Recipient Nerve: Axillary nerve

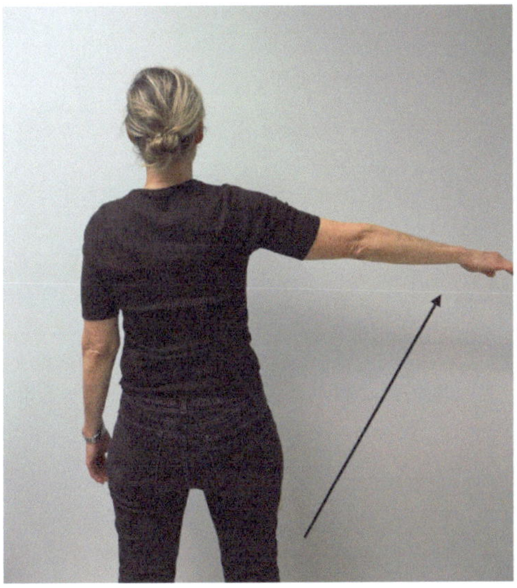

Shoulder Abduction

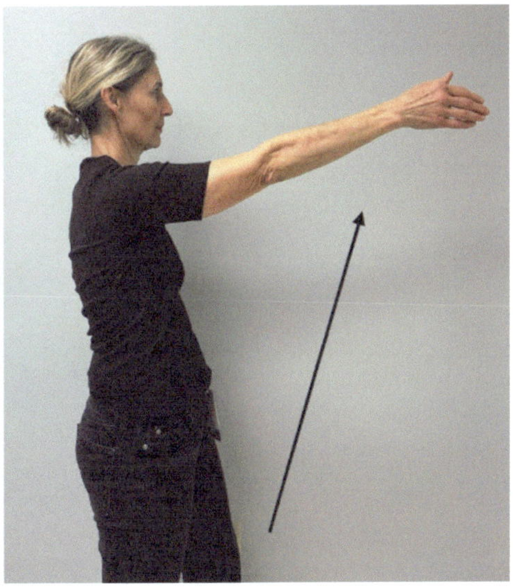

Shoulder Flexion

Donor Movement = Shoulder adduction and internal rotation
Donor Muscle: Pectoralis major
Donor Nerve: Medial pectoral nerve

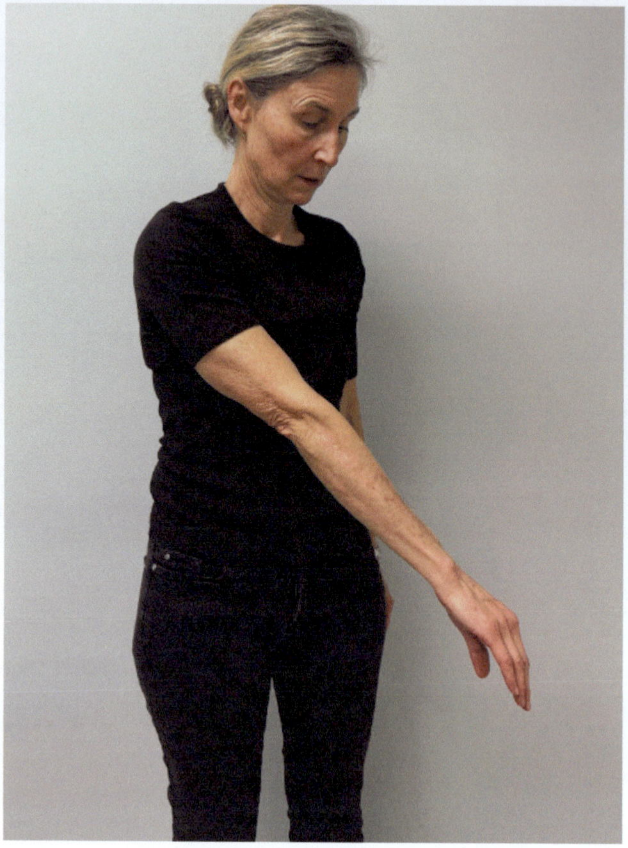

Phase 1 Pec to Axillary Nerve Transfer Exercises

☐ **Passive Range of Motion:**
Complete the below exercise 3–5 repetitions, 2–3 times per day.

- Use a pulley system anchored to a door frame. Pull the handle down with your uninjured arm, allowing your injured arm to stretch up toward the ceiling. Hold 5–10 seconds, then pull down with your injured arm and repeat.

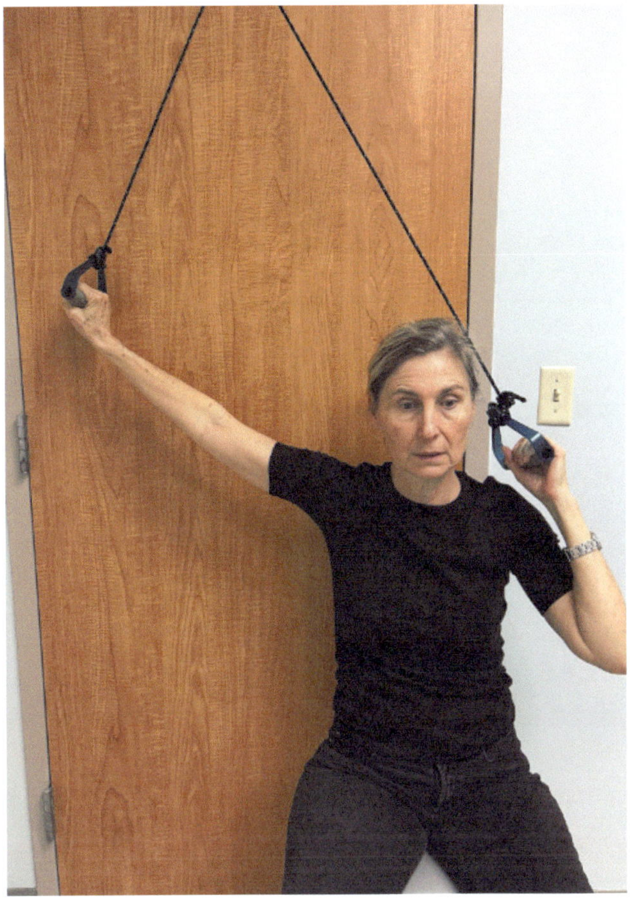

☐ **Active and Isometric Donor Movement**: **Complete 10 repetitions every hour.**

- Sit with your fingers interlocked in front of you. Press your hands together for 3–5 seconds, then relax. You may also squeeze a ball for added challenge.

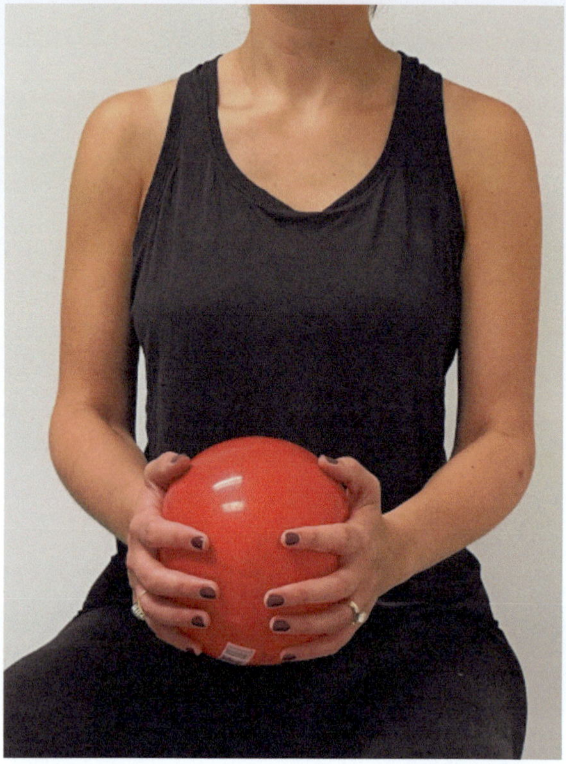

- Stand facing a doorframe with your elbow bent by your side. With a towel rolled in your hand, push the towel roll into the doorframe and hold 5–10 seconds. Relax and repeat.

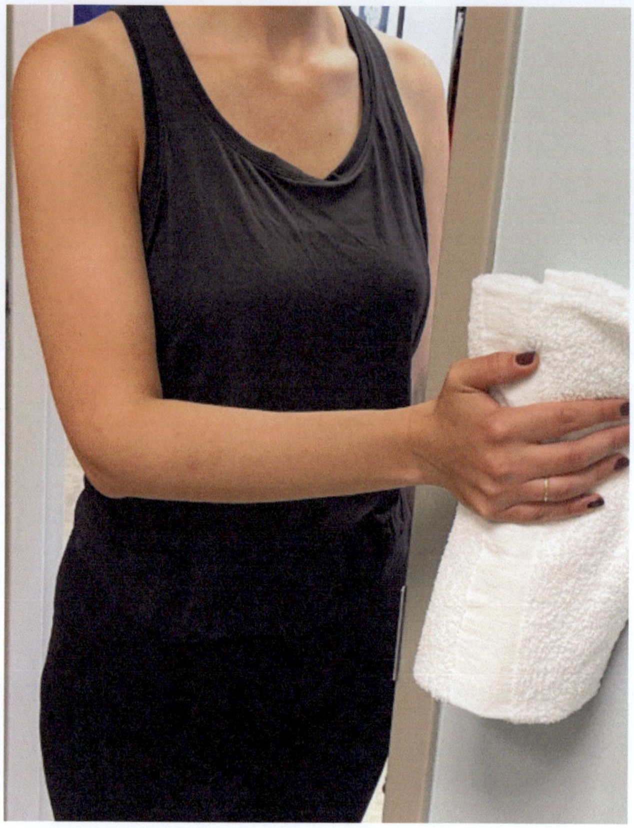

- Stand next to a wall with your uninjured arm touching the wall. Push your injured fist into the wall, moving the arm across the body. Hold 5–10 seconds, relax, and repeat.

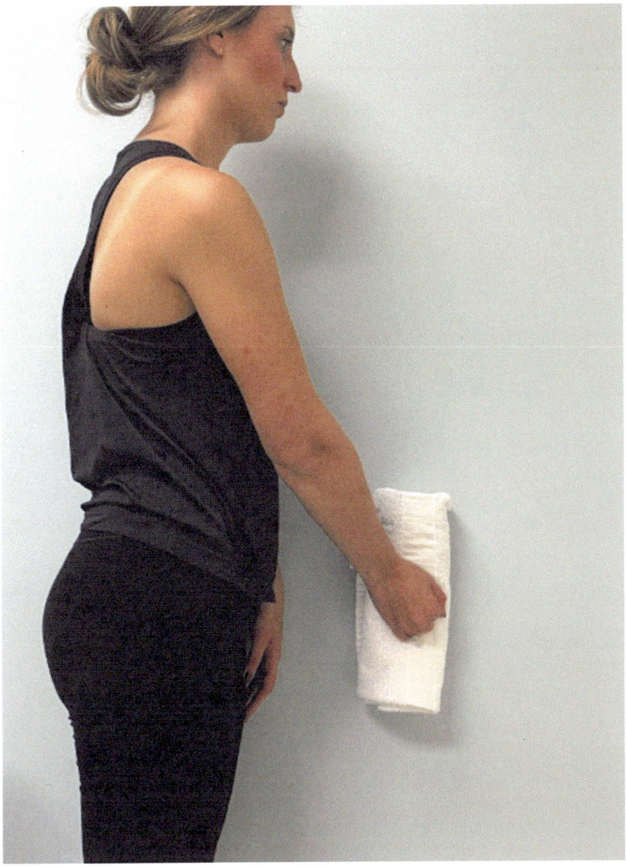

☐ **Active Donor + Passive Recipient Movement: Complete the exercise for <u>10</u> repetitions, <u>2–3</u> times per day.**

- Lie on your back holding a dowel rod or cane. Do a "chest press" by pushing your hands up toward the ceiling. Try to press your hands towards each other while raising the dowel up. Bend your elbows back down to your side and then push up again.

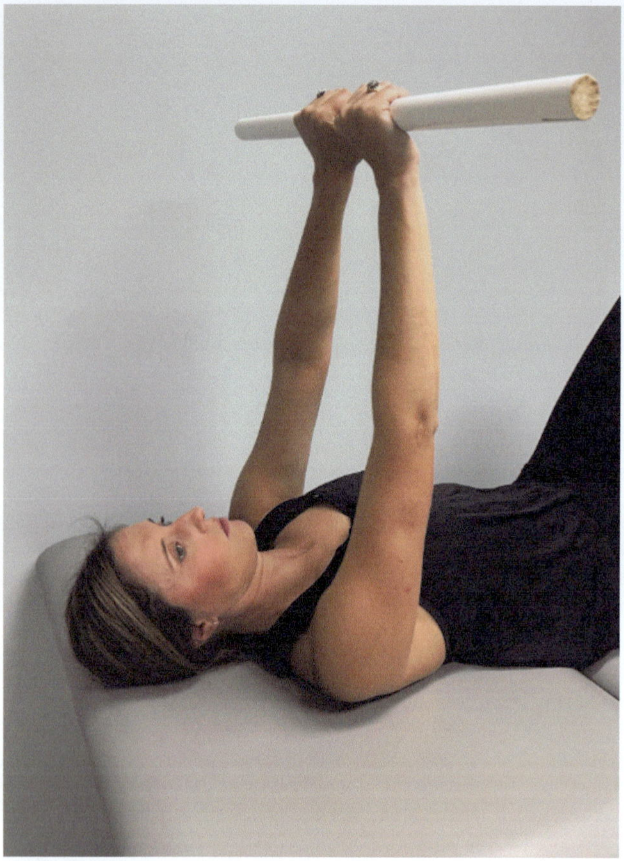

- Lie on your uninjured side with a large exercise ball in front of you. Press down on the ball while sliding the ball forward.

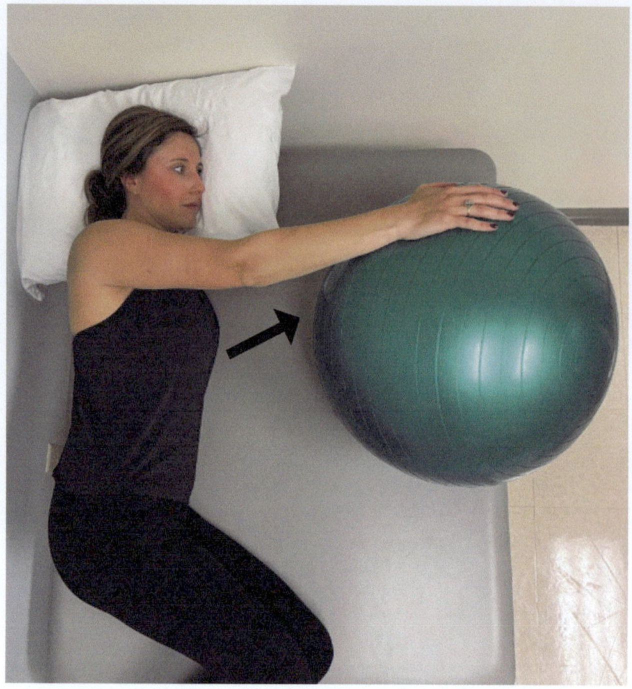

Phase 2 Pec to Axillary Nerve Transfer Exercises

☐ **Active Donor + Active-Assisted Recipient Movement: Complete these exercises <u>1–10</u> repetitions, <u>2–3</u> times per day.**

- The same "chest press" exercise outlined in Phase 1 may be continued in Phase 2. However the injured arm begins to more actively assist the dowel rod overhead (instead of the opposite arm doing all the work).
- Sit next to a table with your arm supported. Hold a dowel with the opposite hand and push the shoulder out the side. At that same time, resist the dowel rod by activating your pec muscle.

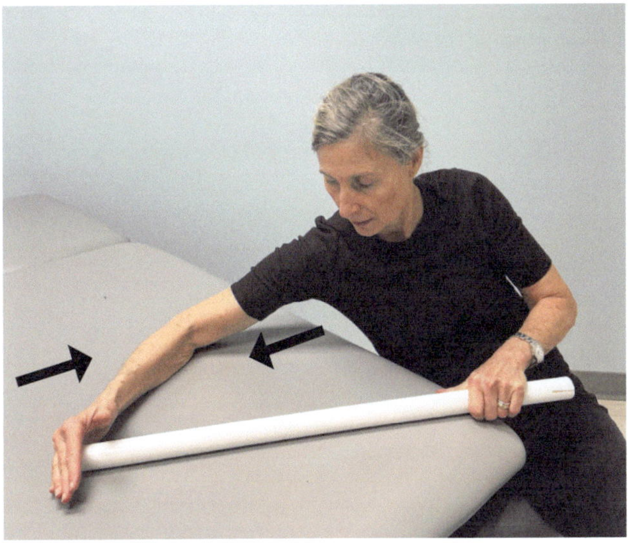

- Hold a stick or dowel rod behind your back, holding with both hands. Push both fists toward the center of the dowel and try to raise both elbows.

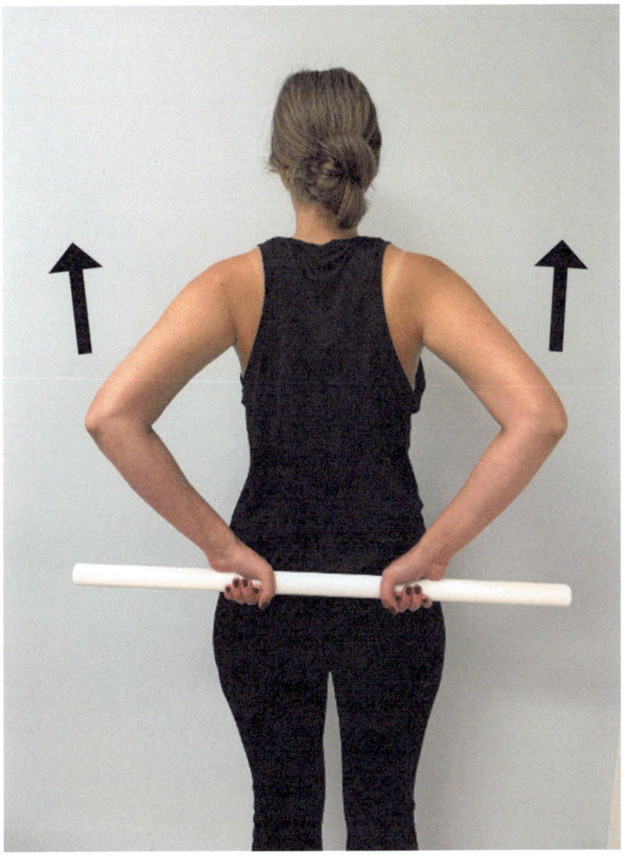

- Squeeze an inflatable ball between your hands and raise both arms above you. Hold 5 s, relax, and repeat. Try this while lying down before trying this while standing.

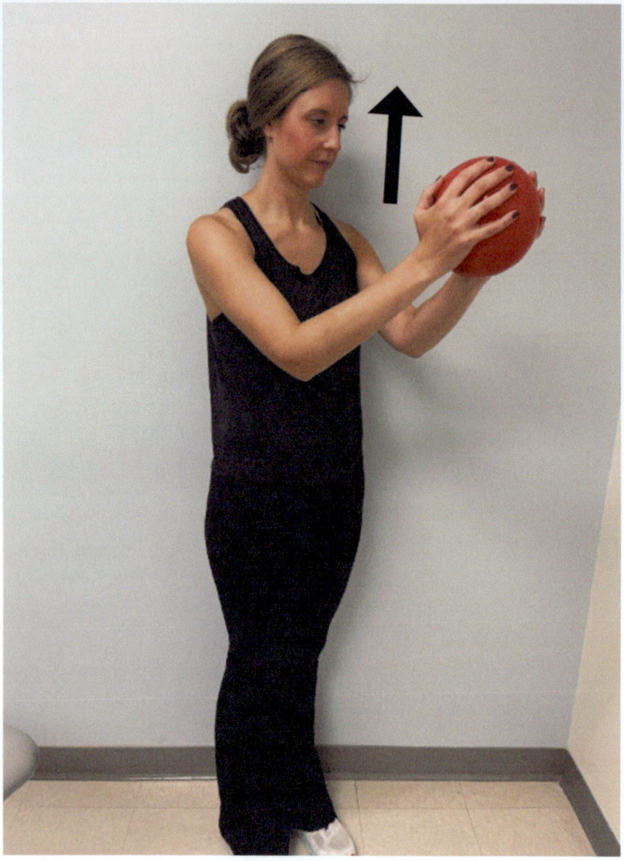

- Lie down facing a wall. Press your hand into the wall (with a washcloth between your hand and the wall). While you press into the wall, try to slide your arm up the wall.

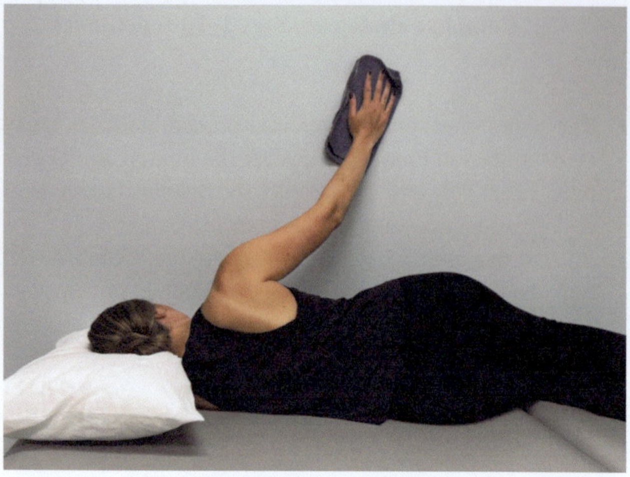

☐ **"Place and Hold"**

- Lie on a mat on your uninjured side. Use a stick or cane to push your injured arm up and out to the side. Slowly let go of the stick, and try to maintain this position for 5 seconds. Relax, then repeat.

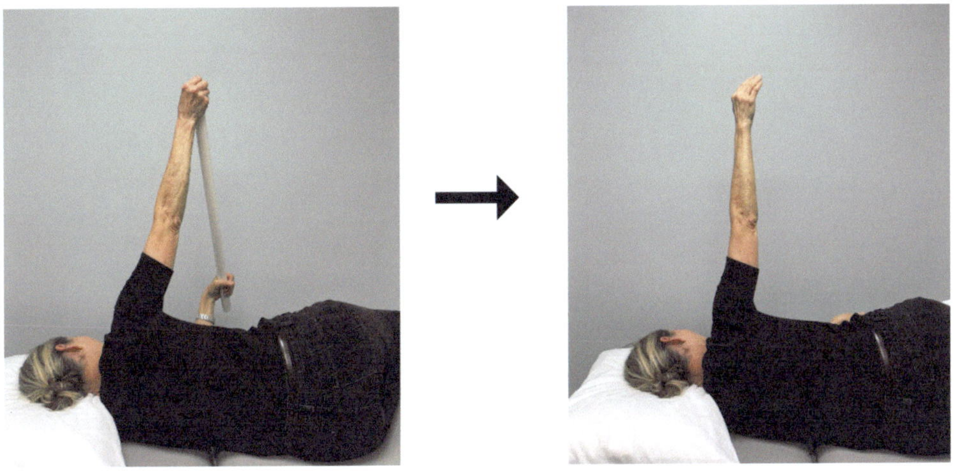

☐ **Active Donor + Active Recipient**

- Sit down with your forearm supported on a table and your elbow bent. Push your hand into the table while trying to raise the elbow toward the ceiling.

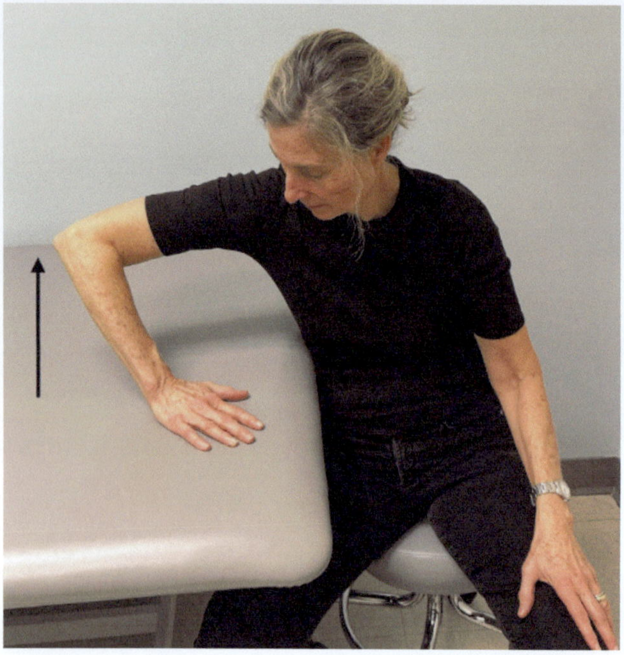

- While standing with your arms down by your side, bring both arms up *and out to the sides* like you are going to do a "snow angel" or "jumping jack."

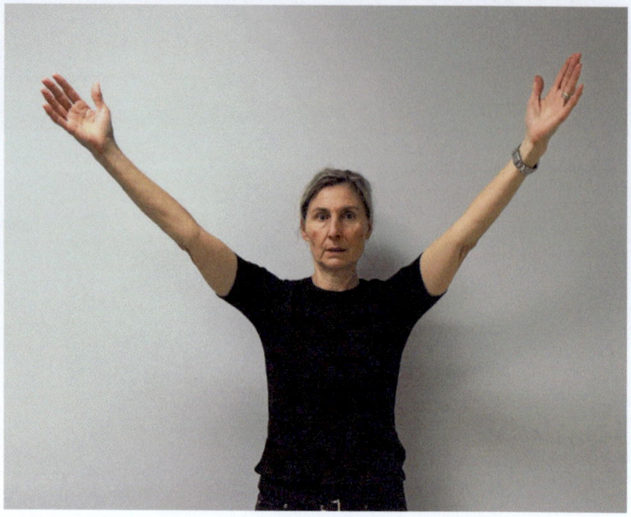

Phase 3 Pec to Axillary Nerve Transfer Exercises

Complete these exercises 1–10 repetitions, 2–3 times per day.

☐ **Resistive Donor + Resisted Recipient Movement:**

- Place both hands on a wall with your arms at shoulder height. Bend your elbows, then tighten your pecs as you straighten your elbows. Hold 5 seconds, relax, and repeat.

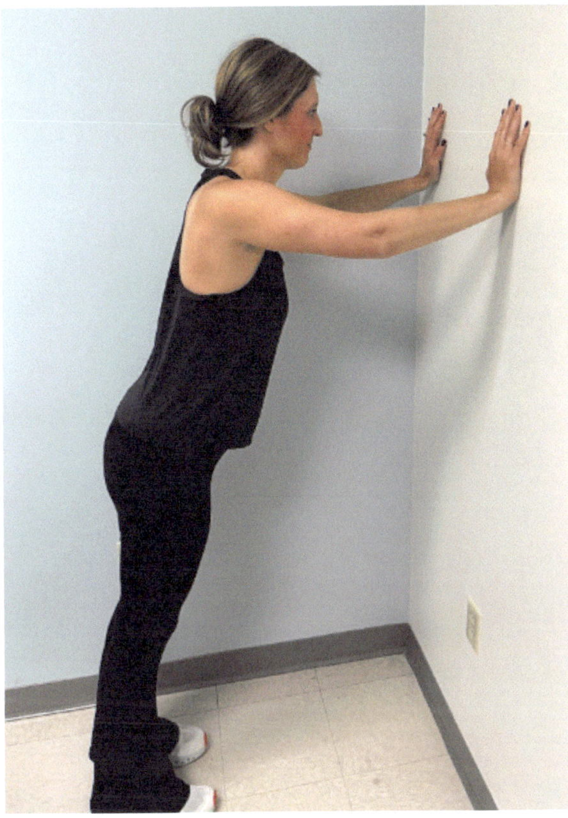

- Lie on your uninjured side with a resistance band anchored to your foot and hold the opposite end in your hand. Bring the arm out to the side and slightly in front of you. Hold 5–10 seconds, relax, and repeat.

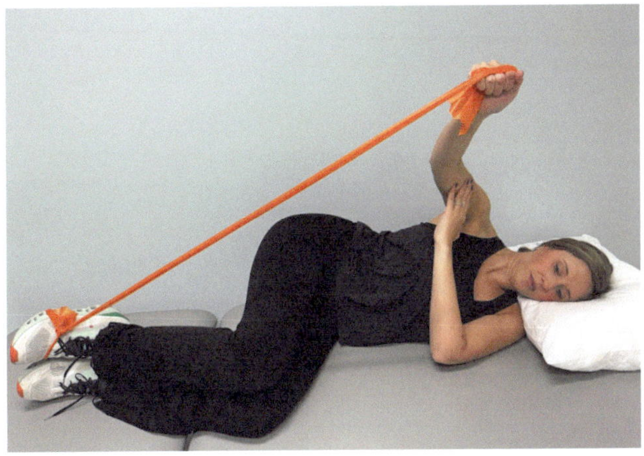

☐ **Resistive Recipient Movement**

- Lie on your back, holding the ends of a resistance band in each hand. Starting with both arms in front of you at shoulder height, spread the arms away from each other and hold 5–10 seconds. Bring the arms back toward the center, and repeat.

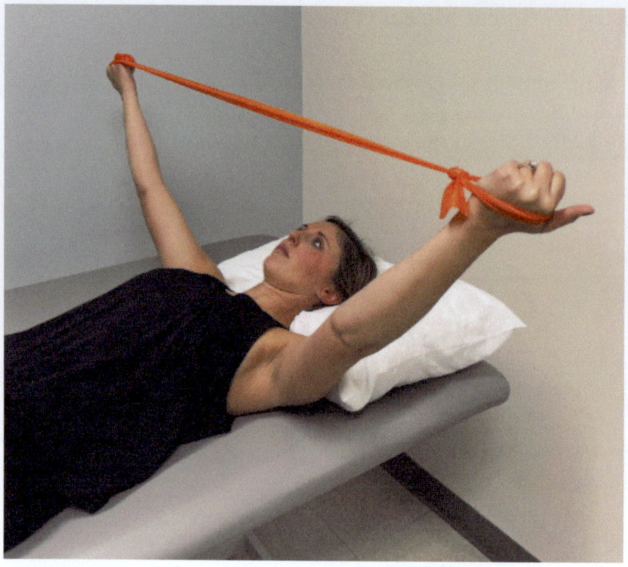

References

1. Neumann DA. Kinesiology of the musculoskeletal system-e-book: foundations for rehabilitation. Elsevier Health Sciences; 2016.
2. Hems TEJ, Mahmood F. Injuries of the terminal branches of the infraclavicular brachial plexus: patterns of injury, management and outcome. J Bone Joint Surg Br Vol. 2012;94(6):799–804.
3. Skirven TM, Osterman AL, Fedorczyk JM, Amadio PC, Feldscher SB, Shin EK. Rehabilitation of the hand and upper extremity. Elsevier; 2021. p. 644–60. (Chapter 46: Restoration of Functional After Adult Brachial Plexus Injury)
4. McCreary EK, Provance PG, Rodgers MM, Romani WA. Muscles: Testing and function with posture and pain. Lippincott Williams & Wilkins; 2005.
5. Kendall FP, McCreary EK, Provance PG, Rodgers MM, Romani WA. Muscles: testing and function with posture and pain, vol. 5. Lippincott Williams & Wilkins; 2005.
6. Koshy JC, Agrawal NA, Seruya M. Nerve transfer versus interpositional nerve graft reconstruction for posttraumatic, isolated axillary nerve injuries: a systematic review. Plast Reconstruct Surg. 2017;140(5):953–60.
7. Ray WZ, Murphy RK, Santosa K, Johnson PJ, Mackinnon SE. Medial pectoral nerve to axillary nerve neurotization following traumatic brachial plexus injuries: indications and clinical outcomes. Hand. 2012;7(1):59–65.
8. Kahn L, Moore A. Donor activation focused rehabilitation approach: maximizing outcomes after nerve transfers. Hand Clin. 2016;32(2):263–77.
9. Kahn LC, Stonner MM, Dy CJ. Key concepts for nerve transfer rehabilitation after surgical reconstruction for brachial plexus and peripheral nerve injuries. J Hand Surg. 2023;
10. Manske RC, Prohaska D. Pectoralis major tendon repair postsurgical rehabilitation. N Am J Sports Phys Therapy. 2007;2(1):22.
11. Kahn LC, Moore AM. Donor activation focused rehabilitation approach: maximizing outcomes after nerve transfers. Hand Clin. 2016;32(2):263–77. https://doi.org/10.1016/j.hcl.2015.12.014.

Spinal Accessory Nerve (SAN) to the Suprascapular Nerve (SSN) Transfer

Jennifer Q. Farrar

Background

Axonal injury to the suprascapular nerve results in denervation of the supraspinatus and infraspinatus muscles with functional loss of the rotator cuff muscles. This results in weakness of glenohumeral abduction and external rotation, two functions necessary for reaching, grooming, throwing, and many other activities of daily living (ADL). The suprascapular nerve may be damaged in isolation or as part of a complete plexus injury, but more often it occurs when the brachial plexus is injured at the upper trunk or the C5/C6 root level. A complete upper trunk injury creates a challenging situation for the individual because the primary source of arm elevation comes from a combination of supraspinatus and deltoid function. Both of these muscles are innervated by C5 and C6 of the upper trunk and are designed to work in unison to provide shoulder abduction and scaption. The most common nerve transfer to restore rotator cuff function is the spinal accessory nerve to the suprascapular nerve transfer. The spinal accessory nerve is a very practical donor due to its extraplexal nature and large number of motor fibers that are close in proximity to the target suprascapular nerve [1]. Given the varying functions of the upper, middle, and lower trapezius muscles, it is important to clarify which branch was used as a donor source. This not only will affect your donor activation function, but may also affect the stability of the scapula if a large portion is used as a donor.

Surgical Description

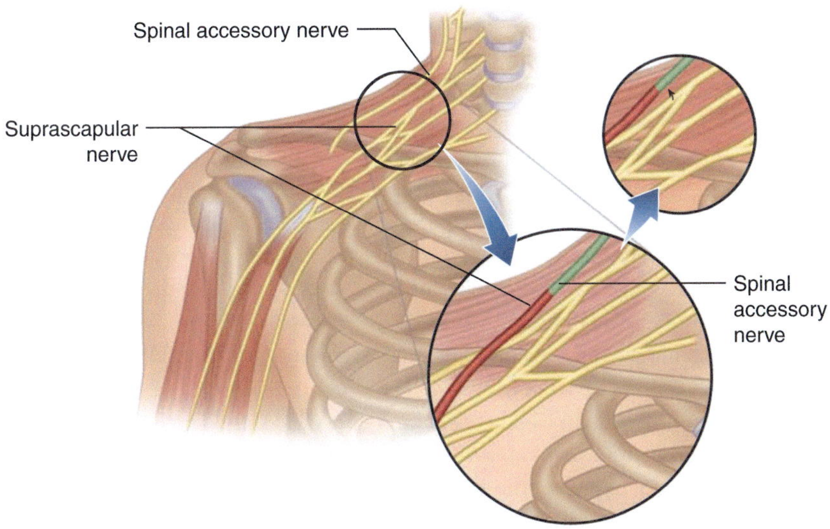

Microsurgical technique of spinal accessory nerve to axillary nerve transfer

J. Q. Farrar (✉)
Vanderbilt Health Belle Meade Clinic, Vanderbilt University Medical Center, Nashville, TN, USA
e-mail: jennifer.q.farrar@vumc.org

L. C. Kahn et al. (eds.), *Rehabilitation for Nerve Transfers of the Upper Extremity*, https://doi.org/10.1007/978-3-031-92008-0_11

Transfer of the SAN to suprascapular nerve can be done from an anterior or posterior approach, based on the particular injury pattern and concomitantly planned procedures, as well as surgeon preference and experience. Surgery from an anterior approach can be readily performed during other procedures for the brachial plexus, such as supraclavicular nerve grafting or infraclavicular nerve transfers (both intraplexal and extraplexal). Surgery from the posterior approach provides the advantage of being close to the target muscle as well as the opportunity to perform a decompression of the suprascapular notch and to inspect for additional injury to the suprascapular nerve closer to the shoulder girdle.

For an anterior approach, a transverse incision is made along the cephalad border of the clavicle. The platysma muscle is divided, and the omohyoid muscle is identified. While not necessary, it is helpful to preserve to omohyoid, as its trajectory is parallel to the course of the suprascapular nerve. The fat pad surrounding the brachial plexus is mobilized, and the upper trunk of the brachial plexus is identified. The suprascapular nerve is identified at its branching point from the upper trunk, typically lateral to the posterior and anterior divisions of the upper trunk. A nerve stimulator is used to confirm that the suprascapular nerve is not functioning, ensuring that the anesthesia team is not using any muscle paralytics. The suprascapular nerve is then neurolyzed from the upper trunk of the brachial plexus and divided proximally. The most medial aspect of the upper trapezius is released from the clavicle, allowing the surgeon to access the deep/posterior portion of the upper trapezius. After dissecting away branches to the upper trapezius, the spinal accessory nerve (supplying the middle and lower trapezius) is identified with the assistance of a handheld nerve stimulator, ensuring that the anesthesia team is not using any muscle paralytics. The spinal accessory nerve is then freed from the surrounding tissue, divided as distally as possible, and transposed to meet the suprascapular nerve. Coaptation of the spinal accessory nerve to the suprascapular nerve is performed using microsurgical technique.

For a posterior approach, the patient is positioned prone and a transverse incision is made along the cephalad border of the scapular spine. The trapezius is divided in line with its fibers, and the supraspinatus muscle is identified. Working laterally, the suprascapular notch is palpated. The surgeon then exposes the suprascapular ligament, being sure to identify and preserve the suprascapular artery. The suprascapular ligament is released, exposing the suprascapular nerve. The surgeon may choose to continue distally and release the nerve at the spinoglenoid notch. A nerve stimulator is used to confirm that the suprascapular nerve is not functioning, ensuring that the anesthesia team is not using any muscle paralytics. The surgeon then works medially, closer to the thoracic spine. Working along the medial border of the scapula, the spinal accessory nerve is identified with the assistance of a handheld nerve stimulator, ensuring that the anesthesia team is not using any muscle paralytics. The spinal accessory nerve is then freed from the surrounding tissue, divided as distally as possible, and transposed to meet the suprascapular nerve. Coaptation of the spinal accessory nerve to the suprascapular nerve is performed using microsurgical technique.

Outcomes

In a 2016 study of 22 patients, Bertelli and colleagues achieved an average of 55.55 degrees of shoulder abduction (range 40–72°) following this procedure [2]. 22.7% of patients obtained an MMT grade of 2/5; 13.6% of patients obtained an MMT grade of 3/5; and 63.6% obtained an MMT grade of 4/5. A 2019 study by Siqueira ($n = 76$) demonstrated good results for shoulder abduction, but the authors were disappointed with external rotation outcomes. In patients with upper plexus injuries, 22% of patients achieved "good" range of motion, as defined by external rotation >55° [3]. However, in those with complete plexus palsies, only 5% of patients obtained "good" range of motion. Interestingly, Suzuki found an average outcome of 32.5 degrees of external rotation if the serratus anterior was intact, but only 4 degrees of external rotation if the serratus anterior was absent, highlighting the importance of repairing the long thoracic nerve when able [1].

Phases of Rehabilitation

Phase 1

Pre-op to 1/5 MMT in the Recipient Muscle

Two weeks following surgery, patients are usually seen in the therapy clinic, often in conjunction with their first postoperative appointment with the surgeon. At that time, sutures are removed, and scar management may begin if needed. The therapist may provide a general timeline for return of shoulder external rotation and abduction. Although each patient's recovery varies, one can anticipate approximately 3–4 months for target muscle tenderness, 6–8 months for trace contraction, and 12–14 months for functional movement [4].

The shoulder should be immobilized in a sling for 3 weeks to protect the nerve coaptation. After that time, a GivMohr® or OmoTrain® brace may be used during the day to help support the weight of the affected arm and minimize glenohumeral joint subluxation (Image 1). The patient may benefit from positioning the arm in partial shoulder abduction and external rotation periodically throughout the day in order to preserve the length of the supraspinatus and infraspinatus muscles while awaiting reinnervation [5]. Following the first therapy visit, the patient should be able to identify the action of the

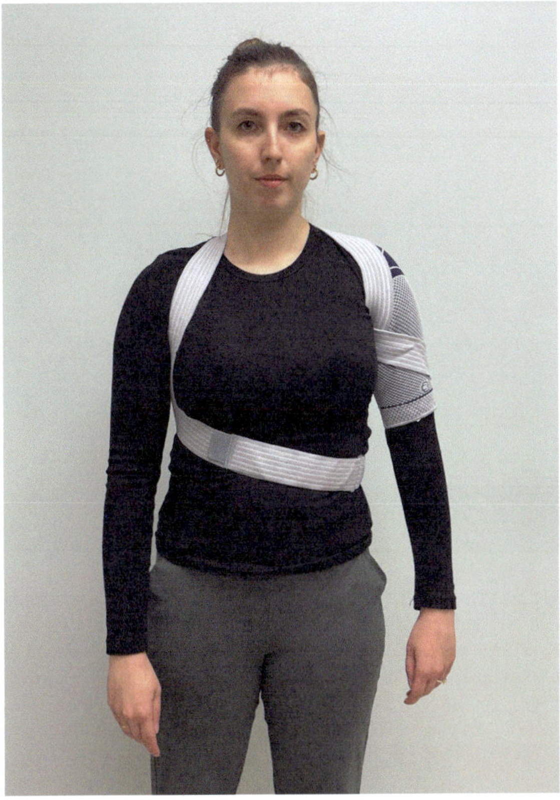

Image 1 Omotrain® brace by Bauerfeind is recommended to provide support to the shoulder and limit subluxation of the glenohumeral joint

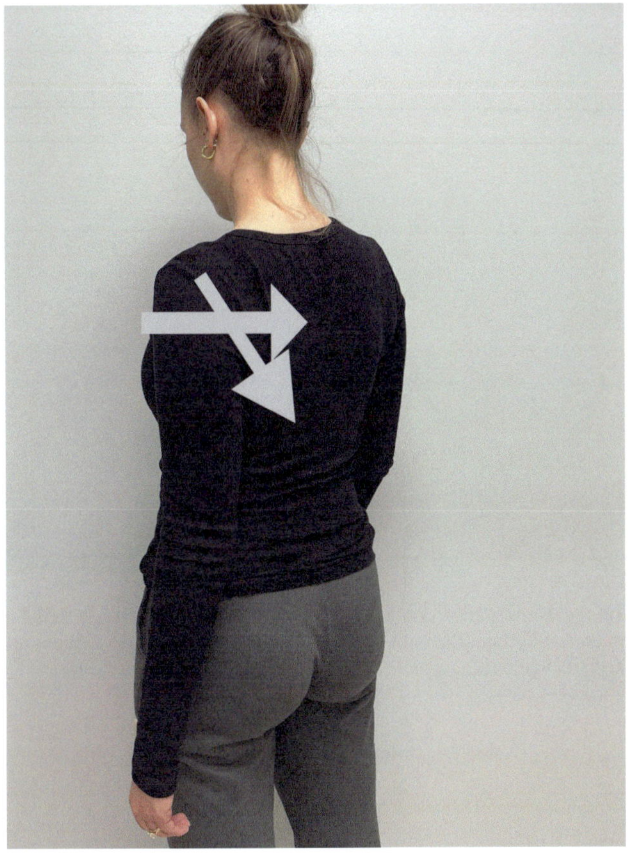

Image 2 Donor activation is demonstrated with scapular retraction and depression

donor based on information obtained from the operative note or surgeon regarding the part of the trapezius that served as a donor (scapular retraction and depression). You want the patient to develop an understanding early in the recovery that performing this movement amplifies neural messages to the target muscles (supraspinatus and infraspinatus) [5, 6].

Exercises

- ROM of Uninvolved Joints
  Patients are instructed to perform active range of motion (AROM) of uninvolved joints immediately following surgery. Exercises may include cervical flexion, rotation, extension, and side bending, along with elbow, wrist, and finger ROM.
- Donor Activation
  The concept of "flooding" the donor trapezius muscle is introduced with instruction in active scapular retraction and depression. A frequency of ten repetitions every hour is recommended (Image 2).
- Combined Donor with Passive Recipient Exercise
  At follow-up therapy visits, the patient is instructed in combined donor-recipient exercises to encourage cortical plasticity by strengthening the new motor pathway. This includes active scapular retraction/depression with passive shoulder external rotation and scaption, performed at a high frequency (ten repetitions, 4–6 times per day). The passive component of this exercise may be achieved using a dowel rod in a supine or seated position (Image 3). The same exercise may be performed with passive shoulder abduction or scaption (Image 4).

Assessment of Recovery

Infraspinatus and supraspinatus muscle function is routinely assessed monthly for early signs of reinnervation. The supraspinatus muscle is assessed in side lying or supine with the involved arm supported by the tester. As the patient performs scapular retraction, the supraspinatus is palpated to assess for tenderness or muscle tension (Image 5). Early movement would be detected in the direction of abduction, scaption, or flexion. Assessment of the infraspinatus is easier in sitting with the elbow supported on a table or by the assessor. The patient is cued to activate the donor trapezius while attempting shoulder external rotation in isolation while the examiner simultaneously palpates the infraspinous fossa for signs of tenderness or muscle tension. One will also watch for any movement of the arm into external rotation. Keep in mind that the teres minor also contributes

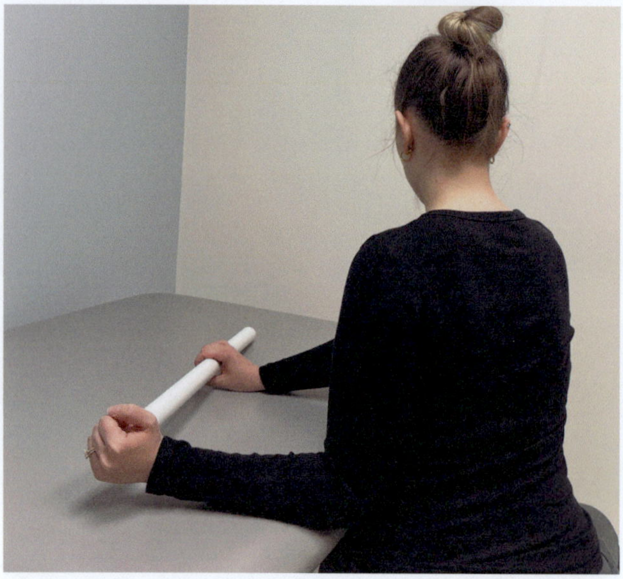

Image 3 Combined donor with passive recipient exercise is demonstrated in sitting. The individual is instructed to retract and depress the scapula while using a dowel to passively externally rotate the arm

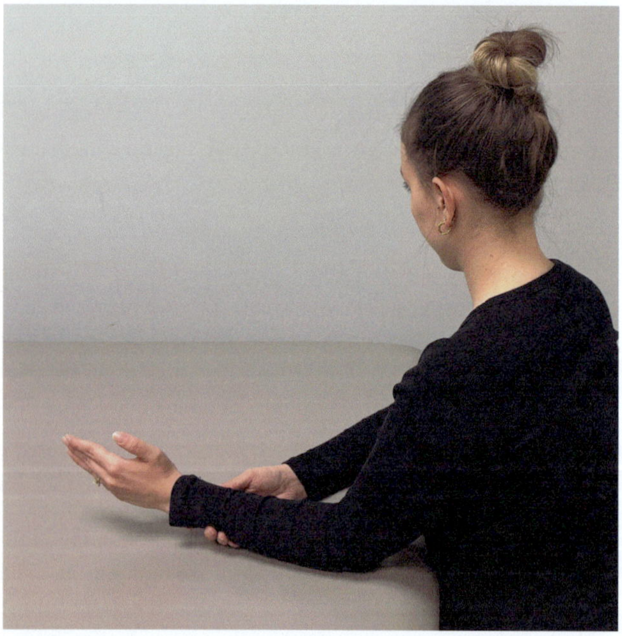

Image 4 Combined donor with passive recipient exercise is demonstrated in sitting. The supraspinatus muscle aids in initiation of arm elevation. Cues are given to retract and depress the scapula while passively sliding the arm into abduction/scaption

to this motion, and if the axillary nerve is intact, palpation of the infraspinatus is important to accurately assess the recipient, infraspinatus muscle (Image 6). When active motion is detected in these planes, the rehabilitation program is progressed to phase 2.

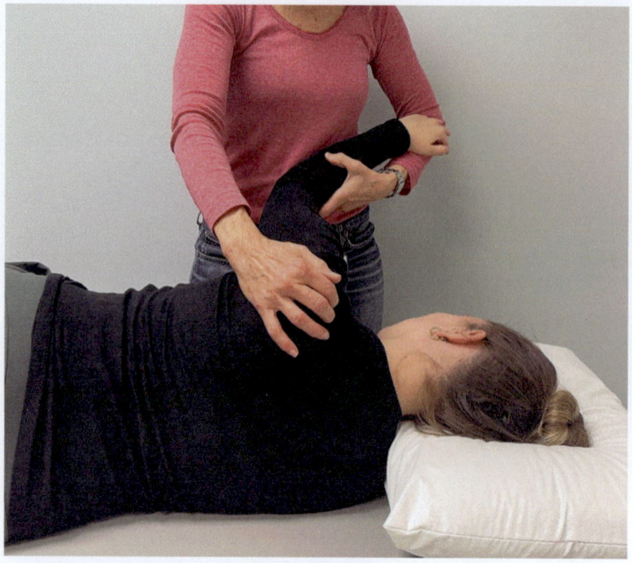

Image 5 Assessment for early signs of recovery of the supraspinatus muscle is demonstrated in side-lying. The assessor supports the involved arm and cues the individual to firmly activate the donor, trapezius, while palpating in the supraspinous fossa or at the tendon in the anterior glenohumeral joint for contraction or tension in the tissue

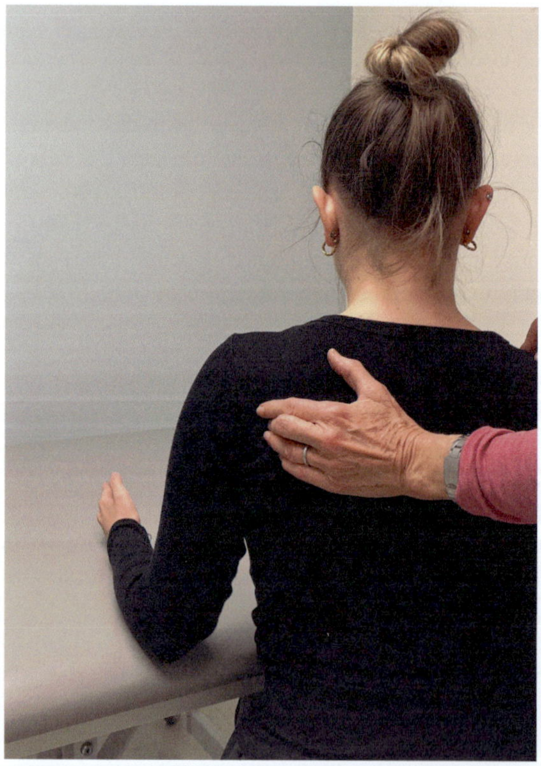

Image 6 The infraspinatus is assessed in sitting with the involved arm supported by the assessor. The individual is cued to firmly activate the donor trapezius while palpating in the infraspinous fossa and observing for any external rotation

Therapy Frequency

The patient is first seen around 2 weeks postoperatively for evaluation. After this, the patient may attend therapy once every 1–2 weeks until he or she is able to demonstrate good carryover of recommendations and transfer training techniques. Therapy frequency may vary based on the patient's needs and distance traveled to the clinic. Patients are seen several times per month if they have passive joint limitations, high pain or nerve sensitivity, excessive swelling, and/or stiffness in uninvolved joints. Otherwise, monthly visits should suffice.

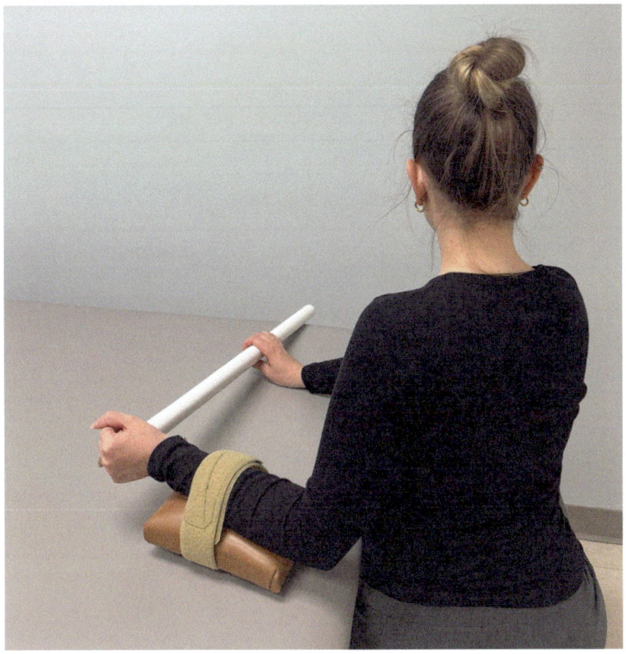

Image 7 Active-assisted external rotation is demonstrated in sitting with the forearm resting on an arm skate, supported on a table. The individual is instructed to retract the scapula while attempting external rotation. Assistance is supplied by a dowel to complete the motion

Phase 2

2−/5 to 3/5 MMT in the Recipient Muscle

Patients may progress to phase 2 of rehabilitation once they can partially abduct and externally rotate the shoulder in a gravity-minimized plane. At this point in recovery, the patient should be reliable with his or her home exercise program and demonstrate a good understanding of the donor-recipient muscle relationship. Phase 2 exercises advance from passive to active-assisted movement of the supraspinatus and infraspinatus muscles. Exercises begin in a gravity-minimized plane while demanding a strong contraction of the middle and lower trapezius. All exercises should be designed to make the movement easier for the weak shoulder/rotator cuff by adding assistance. This may be accomplished using a cane or a slick cloth under the arm and with the affected arm supported on a table. Exercises performed in a supine position may additionally facilitate movement by minimizing the effects of gravity [6].

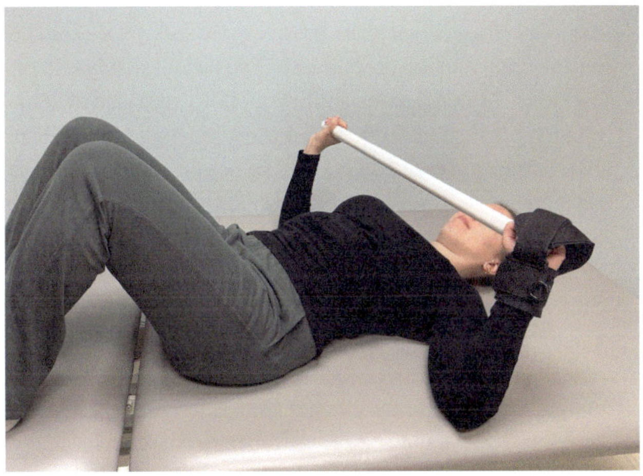

Image 8 When grip strength is insufficient to hold a dowel, a gripping aid such as the Active Hands® device may be used to complete the exercise. Here the patient is supine with both arms at 90 degrees of abduction and elbow flexion, holding a dowel rod. Gravity and the uninvolved arm assist in completing external rotation as the patient retracts the scapula

Exercises

- Active Donor with Active-Assisted Recipient
  Supraspinatus and/or Infraspinatus MMT = 2−/5 to 2/5
  The patient is positioned in a gravity-minimized plane, i.e., seated with the forearm resting on a table or mat. The arm is supported in shoulder adduction with the elbow flexed to 90°. The patient first retracts the scapula and attempts active external rotation by rotating the forearm on a skate or slick surface out and away from the chest. Holding a dowel in both hands, assistance is given to the involved arm using the uninvolved arm, to complete full-range external rotation (Image 7). A dowel may also be used for assisted external rotation in supine. With both arms abducted to 90 and the elbows flexed to 90, assistance is provided into external rotation with gravity and the help of the dowel held in both hands so the uninvolved hand may assist the involved one. For individuals who lack the ability to grasp independently, a gripping aid such as the Active Hands® device may be useful to hold the dowel (Image 8). Similarly, to achieve active-assisted supraspinatus-driven scaption, the individual is positioned in supine. Cues are given to retract the scapula while the dowel is used to assist shoulder abduction/scaption.
- "Place and Hold"
  Supraspinatus and/or Infraspinatus MMT = 2+/5
  Once the patient can actively abduct and externally rotate the shoulder through partial movement against gravity, a "place

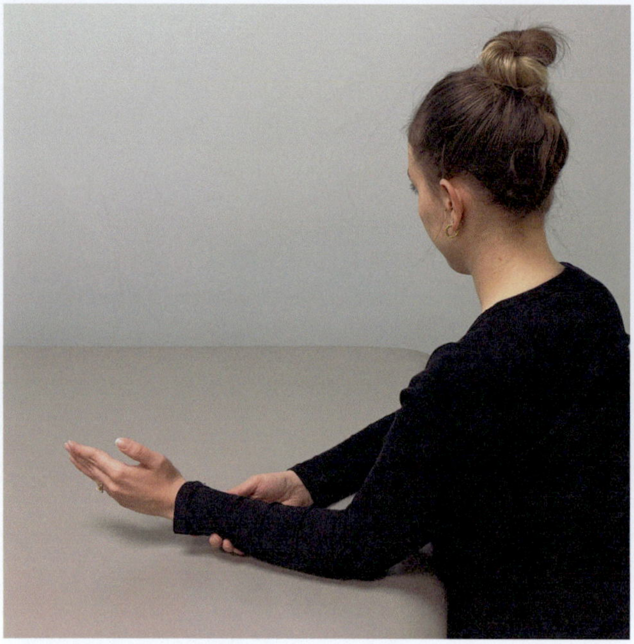

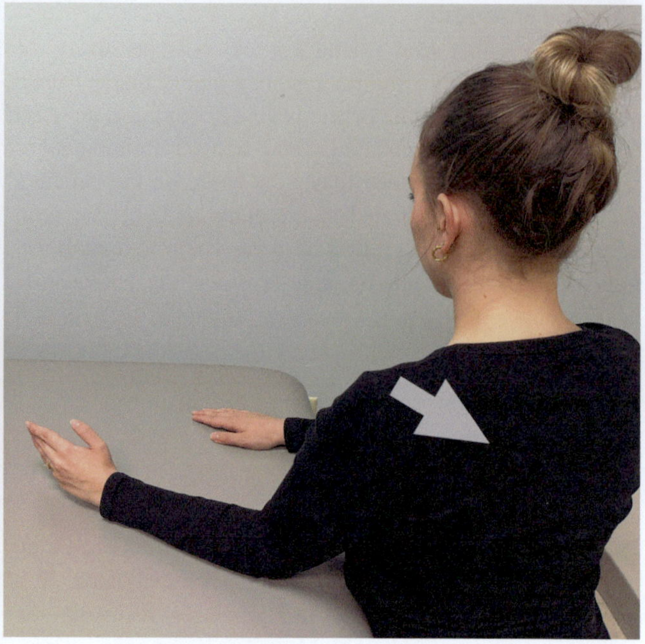

Image 9 and 10 Place and hold external rotation exercises is performed in sitting. The opposite hand or a dowel rod is used to place the involved hand into the available range of external rotation. The individual is cued to activate the trapezius donor and attempt to maintain the arm in external rotation once the assistance is removed

and hold" exercise may begin. While retracting the scapula, the patient passively assists the shoulder into external rotation or abduction. The patient slowly releases the assistive component and attempts to maintain external rotation (or flexion/abduction) against gravity (Images 9 and 10). This exercise should initially be performed with external rotation in isolation or arm elevation. Greater strength is needed to simultaneously perform both movements.

- Active Donor with Active Recipient
  Supraspinatus and Infraspinatus MMT = 3−/5 to 3/5
  Once the patient can actively demonstrate external rotation and abduction through more than 50% ROM against gravity, antigravity exercise may begin in a side-lying or standing position. The patient is instructed to perform scapular retraction/depression (donor activation) with active shoulder external rotation throughout the day with limited repetitions to avoid fatigue. Separately, active arm elevation is encouraged in limited repetitions several times throughout the day.
- Functional Activity
  Throughout phase 2, patients should try to incorporate external rotation and arm elevation movements into functional tasks. Examples of functional activities would be combing the hair, abducting the shoulder to apply deodorant, and reaching away from the body to retrieve an object from a shelf or countertop (Images 11 and 12).
- Therapy Frequency
  Therapy visits in phase 2 may occur on a weekly or biweekly basis and are dependent on the patient's needs.

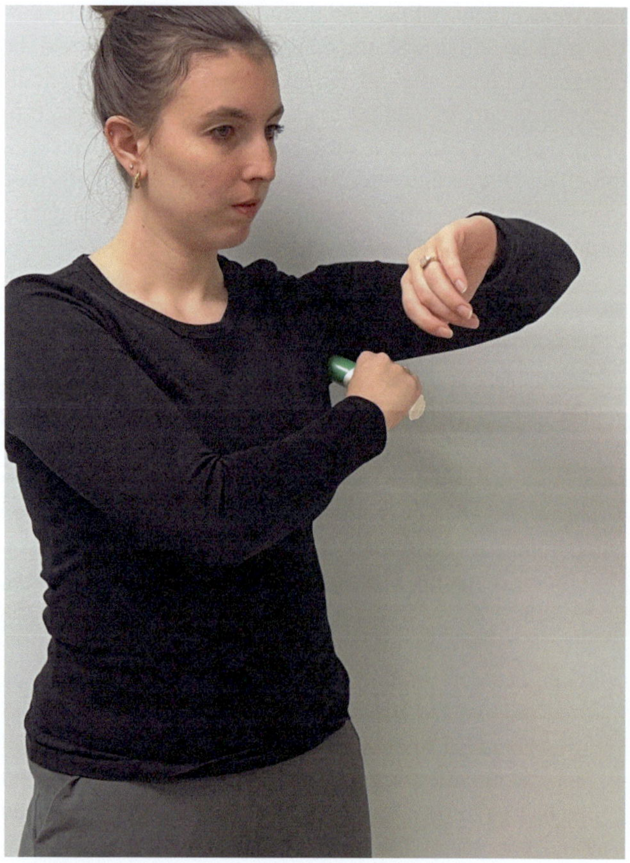

Image 11 Functional activities that incorporate active scapular retraction with arm elevation such as putting on deodorant, are encouraged

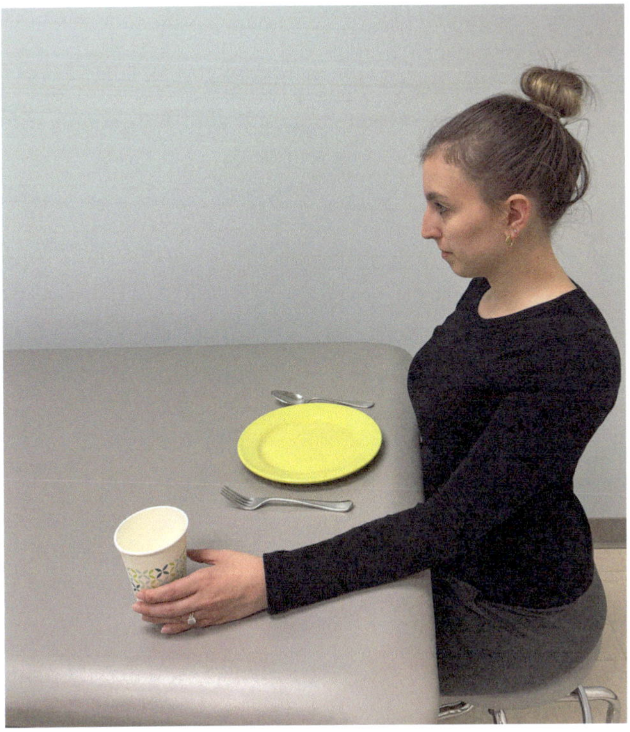

Image 12 A functional activity that combines scapular retraction with shoulder external rotation is demonstrated here with reaching for a cup out to the side

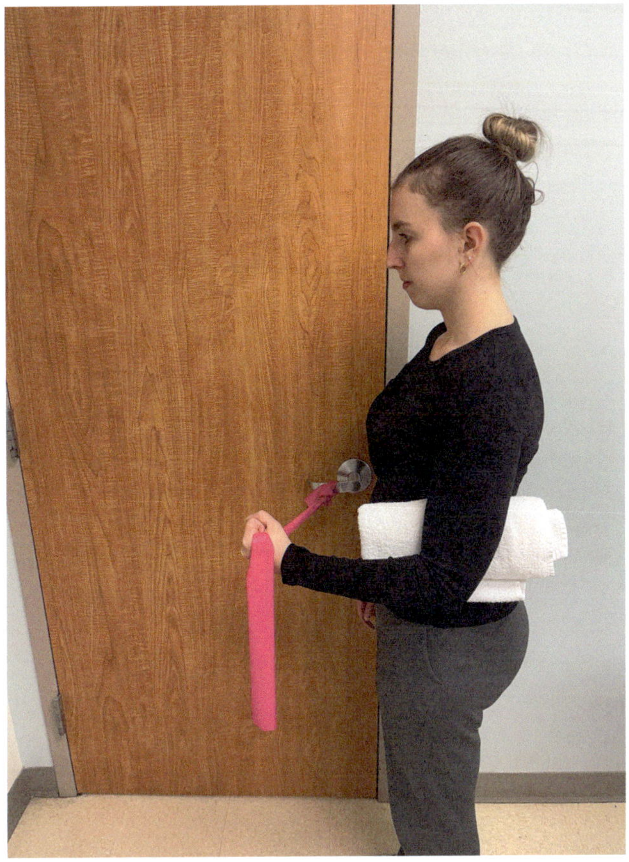

Image 13 A resistance exercise for the infraspinatus is demonstrated in standing perpendicular to a door with a resistance band attached to a doorknob. Holding the band with the elbow flexed at the side, the patient pulls the band away from their abdomen in the direction of external rotation while retracting and depressing the scapula

Phase 3

3+/5 MMT in the Recipient Muscle

Late-phase therapy begins once the infraspinatus and/or supraspinatus demonstrate full external rotation and arm elevation against gravity and can withstand light pressure. It is important that resistive exercises do not begin before 3/5 MMT strength is obtained as this often leads to fatigue, frustration, and ineffective recruitment of the target muscle. To prevent fatigue, high frequency-low resistance should remain the guiding concept during this time. It is important to note that individuals may not achieve >3/5 strength in the recipient cuff muscles. This is especially true if the deltoid was also injured.

Exercises

- Resistive Recipient Activity with Donor Contraction
  Resistive rotator cuff exercises begin with simultaneous contraction of the trapezius and infra/supraspinatus muscles. This may include holding a resistance band that is anchored in a doorframe while the patient retracts the scapula and performs either abduction in isolation or external rotation in isolation (Image 13). The patient can also be positioned in prone with the arm off the mat. The patient depresses or retracts the scapula while flexing and externally rotating the shoulder with a light weight in the hand (Image 14). Activating the donor will augment rotator cuff power, which may be functionally useful in situations when additional shoulder strength is needed.

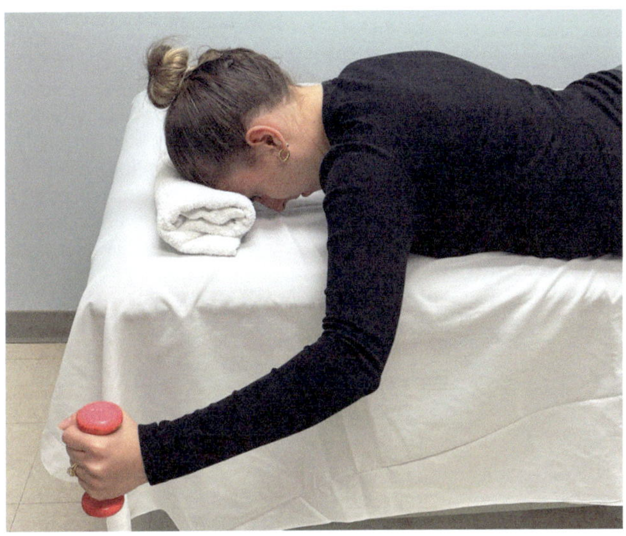

Image 14 Strengthening both the infraspinatus and supraspinatus in prone is demonstrated. Holding a light weight, the individual externally rotates and raises the arm

- Resistive Recipient Activity Without Donor Contraction
  Given the synergistic relationship between scapular stabilizer muscles like the middle and lower trapezius with the rotator cuff muscles, it is not necessary to separate donor from recipient muscle actions with this nerve transfer.
- Therapy Frequency
  Once patients achieve a 3+/5 MMT grade, therapy visits may occur once a week or every other week. Exercises are reviewed and advanced depending on the supraspinatus and infraspinatus strength and the functional needs of the patient. Duration of visits will be dependent on patient goals, insurance availability, and ability to continue to show functional gains with therapy.

Spinal accessory to Suprascapular nerve transfer

Nerve transfer overview					
Donor nerve	Donor action	Recipient nerve	Recipient action	Indications for functional restoration	Approximate months to functional movement
Spinal accessory nerve	Scapular retraction and depression	Suprascapular	Shoulder abduction and external rotation	Restore ability to reach overhead and away from the body	12–14 [2, 4, 7]

Information below are suggested guidelines. Precautions may vary according to surgeon preferences and patient factors

	Preoperative therapy	Early phase	Middle phase	Late phase
Criteria	Before surgery	0/5 to −1/5 MMT	2-/5 to 3/5 MMT	>3/5 MMT
Purpose of phase	Educate and establish baseline function	Understand donor-recipient relationship Activate donor: scapular retraction and depression	Consistently activate recipient muscles	Strengthen recipient muscles
Precautions	NA	Sling and post-operative dressings for 3 weeks after surgery	Avoid high intensity exercise Minimize fatigue and force placed on the weak recipient supra/infraspinatus	Resistive exercise should not be performed before the supra/infraspinatus demonstrates 3/5 MMT Avoid fatigue with resistance training
Frequency of visits (considerations)	1–2 visit(s); more if PROM limitations are present	1x/week until PROM is restored, and the patient is independent with the HEP Decrease to 1x/month based on progress	1× per month unless patient requires more guidance If additional nerve transfers were performed, more frequent therapy is warranted	1× per month
Orthosis considerations	Sling or Omotrain® brace for comfort if there is subluxation of the humeral head	Sling for the first 3 weeks After 3 weeks, additional shoulder support is encouraged to minimize glenohumeral subluxation: Givmohr® sling, Omotrain® brace, or Kinesio-tape®	Continue a shoulder support as needed to minimize fatigue	NA
Interventions	PROM to resolve any joint contractures	**Donor Activation:** Scapular retraction and depression 10× every hour **Donor-Recipient Pairing:** Scapular retraction and/or depression with passive shoulder abduction/external rotation 10–20 reps, 6–8× per day	**Active/Resisted Donor with Active Assist Recipient:** Scapular retraction with active-assisted shoulder abduction/external rotation is performed in a gravity minimized plane **Place and Hold:** The shoulder is supported in external rotation with the shoulder adducted. The patient retracts the scapula, removes the passive support and attempts to maintain active external rotation **Active Donor with Active Recipient**: Scapular retraction is paired with active abduction and/or external rotation against gravity	**Resisted Donor and Recipient:** Resisted shoulder abduction and external rotation while retracting the scapula. Resistance can be in the form of bands, dumbbells, or cuff weights **Resisted Recipient Without Donor Contraction:** Not recommended with this nerve transfer due to the synergistic and assistive nature of the donor trapezius muscle
Additional intervention considerations			Exercises for abduction and external rotation may occur in isolation before combined abduction/external rotation Respect fatigue	Initially focus on high frequency, low resistance exercises

During all phases it is essential to continue cortical reorganization, psychological and psychosocial interventions, and progress to incorporate donor/recipient with ADL

Spinal Accessory to Suprascapular Nerve Transfer

Goal of Surgery: Restore the ability to raise the arm and rotate it away from the body

Recipient Movements = Shoulder abduction and external rotation

Recipient Muscles: Supraspinatus and Infraspinatus

Recipient Nerve: Suprascapular nerve

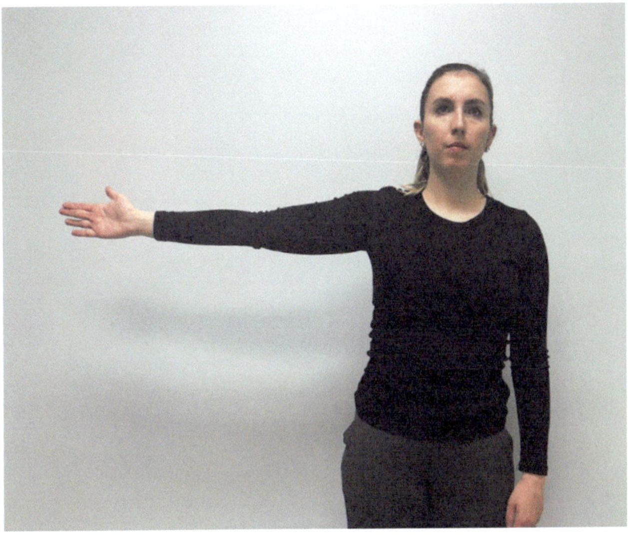

Raise arm out to the side (shoulder abduction)

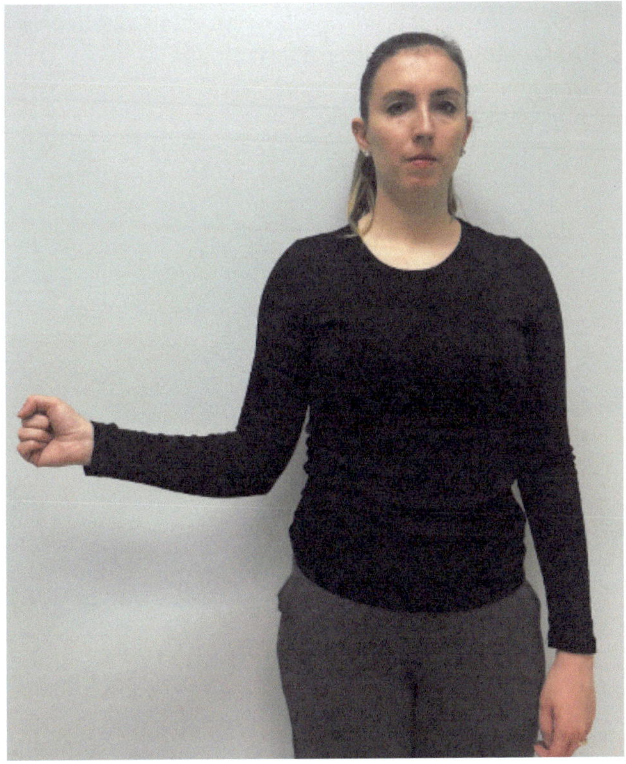

Rotate your arm away from you (shoulder external rotation)

Donor Movements = Scapular retraction and depression
Donor Muscles: Middle and lower trapezius
Donor Nerve: Spinal accessory nerve

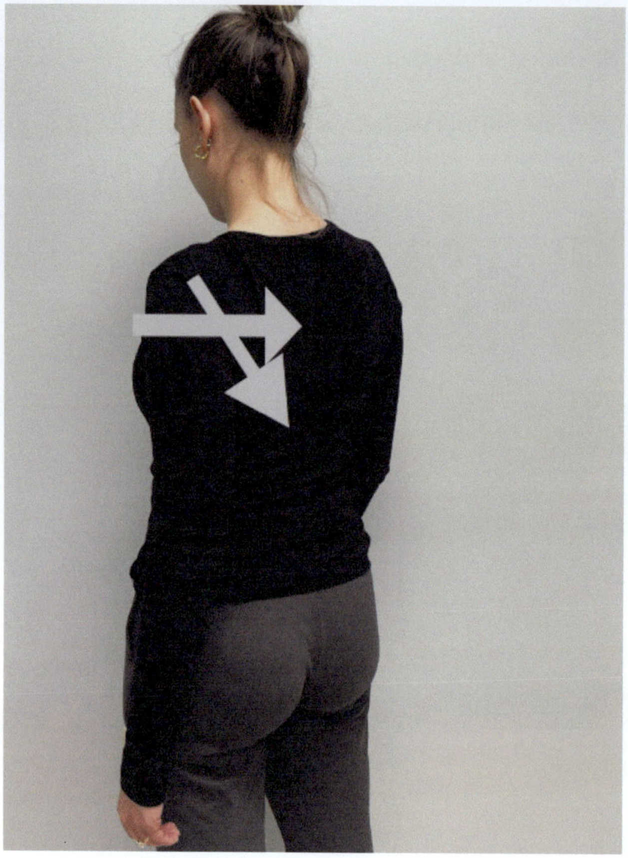

Phase 1 Spinal Accessory to Suprascapular Nerve Transfer Exercises

- **Passive Range of Motion:**

Complete the below exercises 3–5 repetitions, 2–3 times per day.

Table Slides: Sit with your arm supported on a table next to you.

- With your elbow straight, lean sideways toward the table pushing your arm away from you.

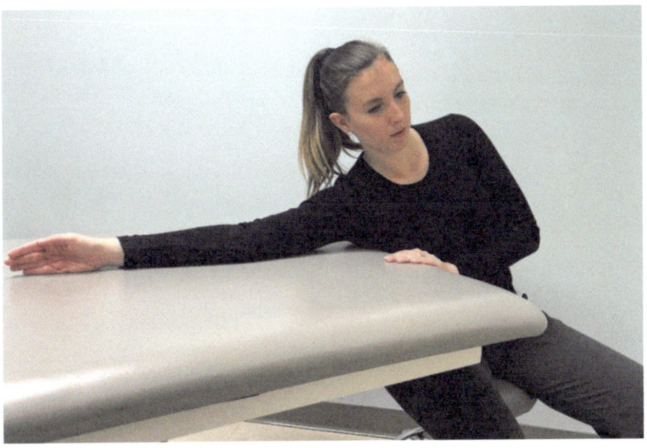

- With your arm supported on a table with the elbow bent and aligned with your knee, lean forward. Keep your elbow bent to 90° and move until you feel a stretch but not pain.

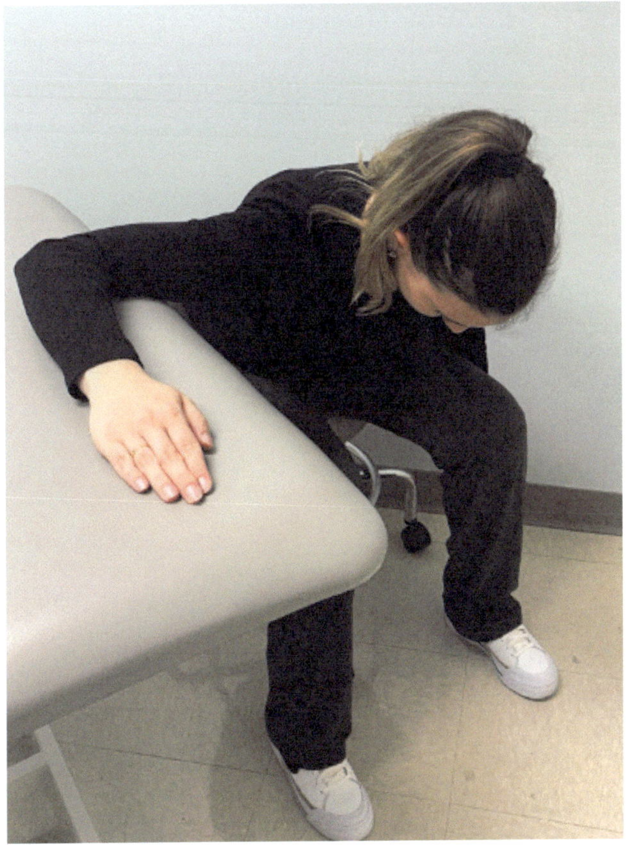

☐ **Active Donor Movement:**

- This may be performed in sitting or standing. Pull your shoulders back by pinching your shoulder blades together as you keep your shoulders down. Hold for a few seconds and release.

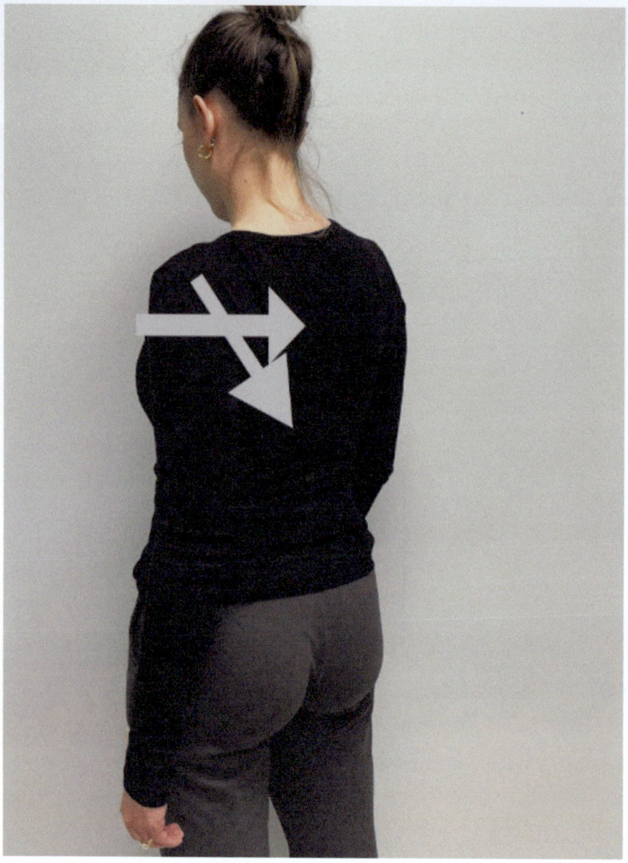

Complete 10 repetitions, every waking hour

☐ **Active Donor + Passive Recipient Movement: Complete one or both exercises <u>10</u> repetitions, <u>2–3</u> times per day**

- While lying on your back, hold one end of a dowel with your injured arm. Use your uninjured arm to push the dowel and move your injured arm out to the side while you pinch your shoulder blades together.

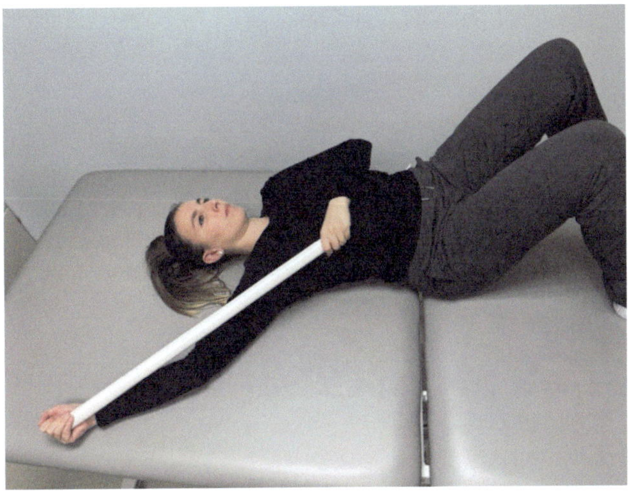

- While lying on your back, hold a dowel rod with both hands while your elbows are bent to 90°. Squeeze your shoulder blades together,and pull the dowel rod over your head to rotate the shoulders. Hold 5 seconds, relax, and repeat. If you do not have enough hand function to grasp the dowel, consider using an ActiveHand™ device as shown on the left hand.

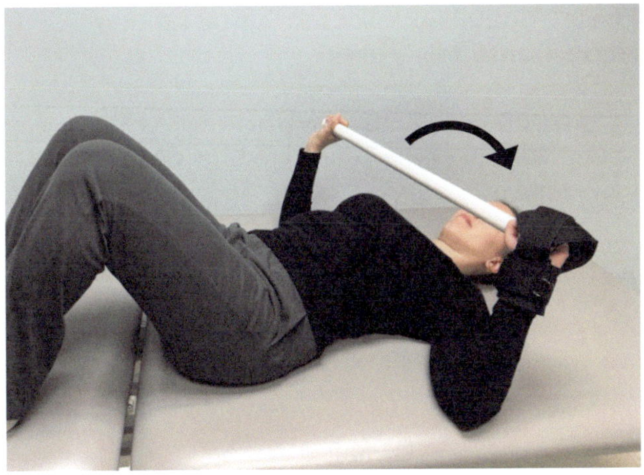

- With the involved arm supported, hold a dowel keeping the involved elbow bent and held at your side. Use your unaffected arm to push your injured hand back as you pull your shoulders back and downwards. You may use an arm skate to assist further with this motion.

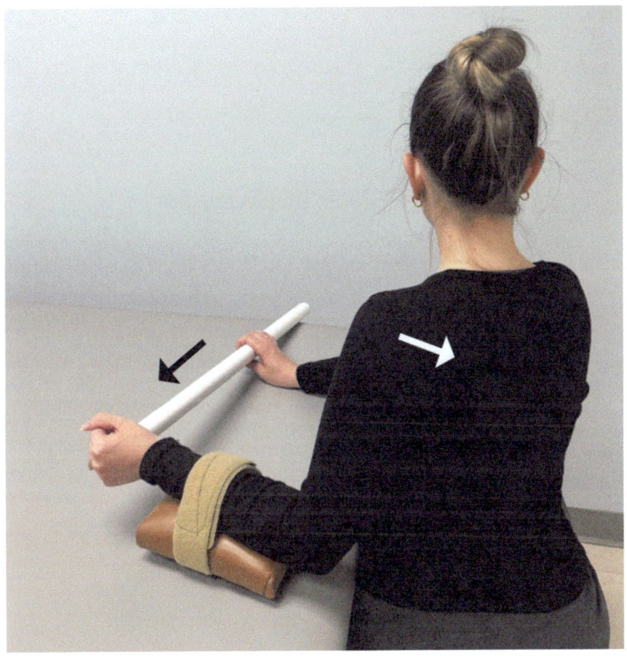

Phase 2 Spinal Accessory to Suprascapular Nerve Transfer Exercises

☐ **Active Donor + Active-Assisted Recipient Movement: Complete the below exercises 1–10 repetitions, 2–3 times per day.**

- Begin by sitting at the side of a table with your arm resting on a towel. Pinch your shoulder blades together as you slowly bend your body and arm sideways, pushing the towel across the table. Return to the starting position and repeat.

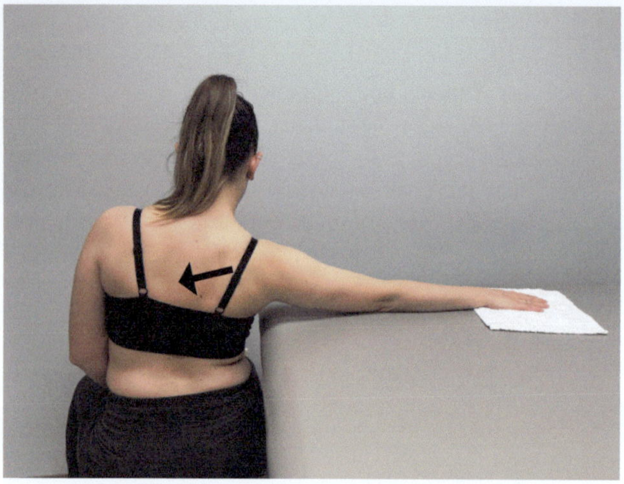

- Lie on your back and keep your elbow bent at a 90° angle by your side or in line with your shoulder (as shown). Slowly rotate your shoulder back (move the hand closer to the ground/mat) as you pinch your shoulder blades together. Bring your hand up to the starting position and repeat. Focus on slow, controlled movement.

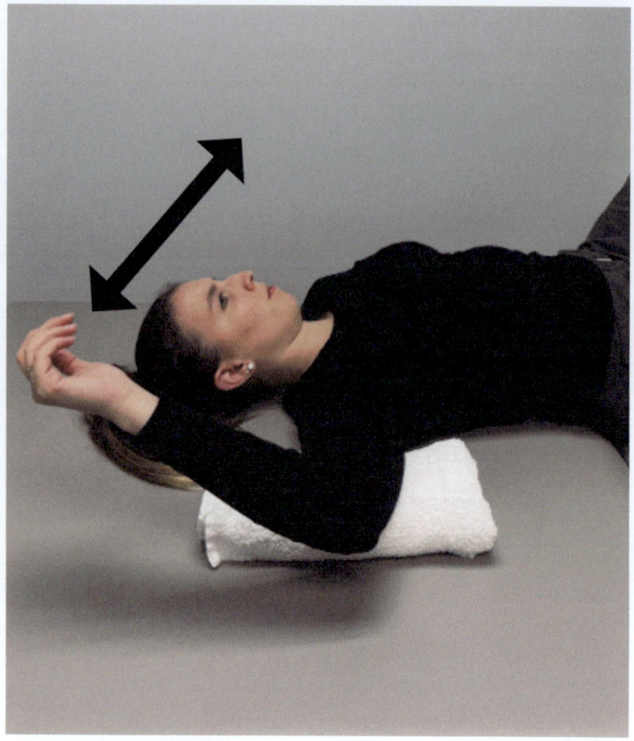

- Hold a dowel with both elbows bent and at your sides while sitting upright. Bring your shoulder blade "back and down" while you try to rotate your shoulder away from the body. Once you cannot rotate anymore, use your unaffected arm to push your injured arm further away from you. *Note- this exercise is from Phase 1 but with active initiation of external rotation before the dowel assists into end-range.*

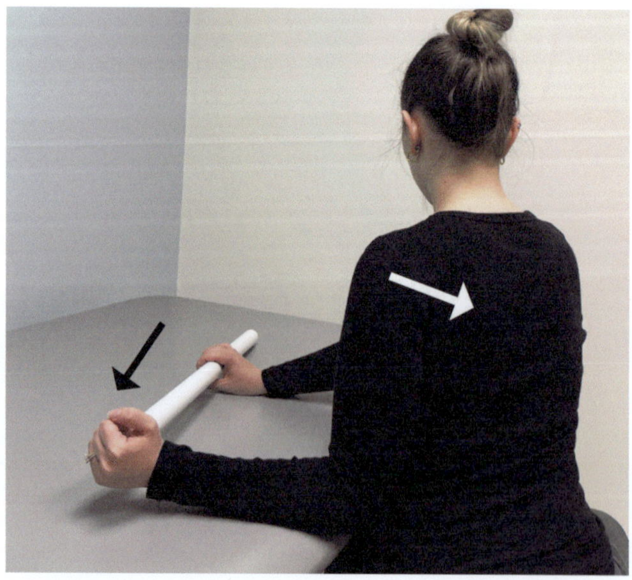

☐ **Place and Hold Exercise**

Complete the below exercises <u>1–10</u> repetitions, <u>2–3</u> times per day.

- While seated with your arm supported on a table/mat, use your unaffected hand to push and rotate the injured arm away from the body. Pull your shoulder blades "back and down," release the support of your unaffected hand, and attempt to maintain your shoulder rotated away from you for 5-10 seconds. Return to the starting position and repeat.

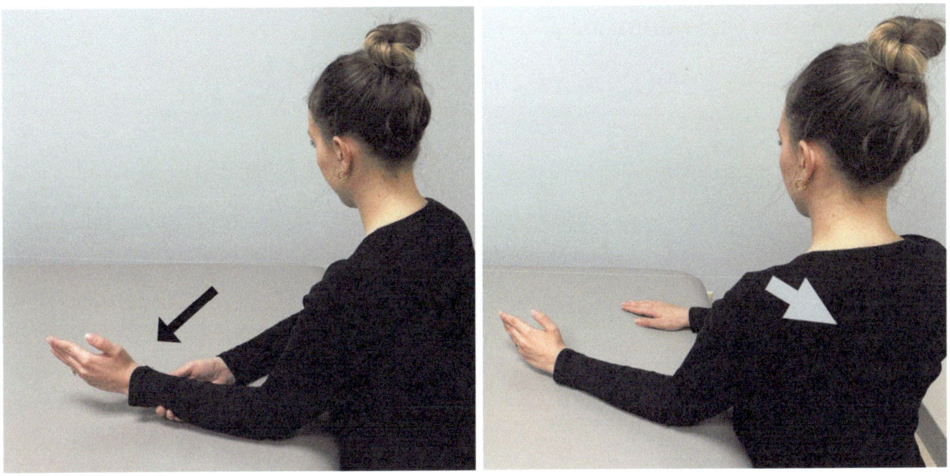

☐ **Active Donor + Active Recipient Movement:**

Complete the below exercises <u>1–10</u> repetitions, <u>2–3</u> times per day.

- Lie on your back with both arms resting by your side. Pull your shoulders back by pinching your shoulder blades together as you slide your arm out as if making a snow angel.

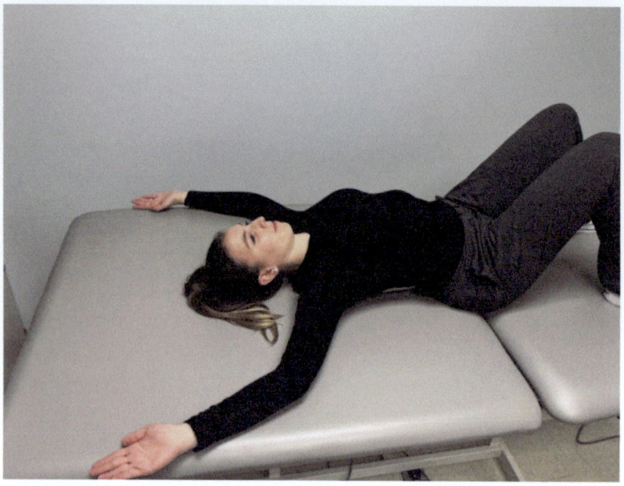

- Sit with your arm resting on a table with a washcloth underneath the forearm. Pinch your shoulder blades together as you rotate your arm away from you.

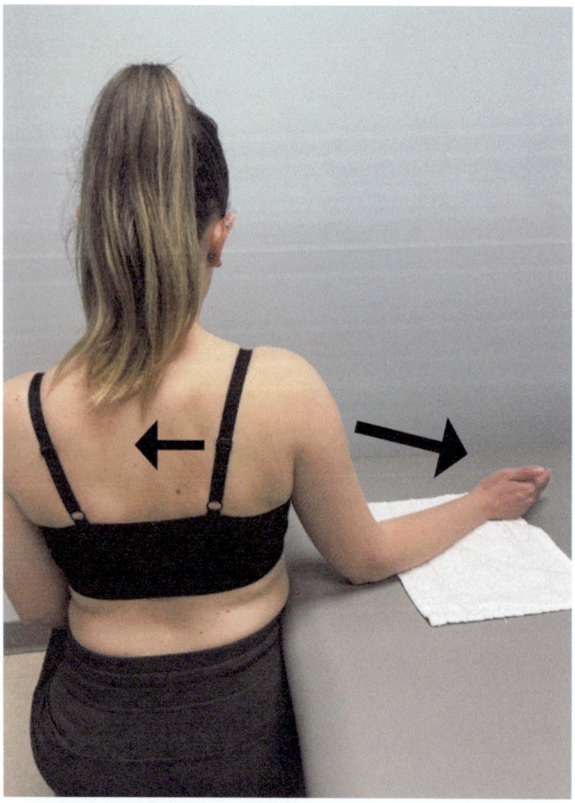

- Begin by lying on your unaffected side with your injured arm resting on your hip with the palm facing forward. Pull your shoulder back by pinching your shoulder blades together as you raise your arm upward and overhead as far as you can.

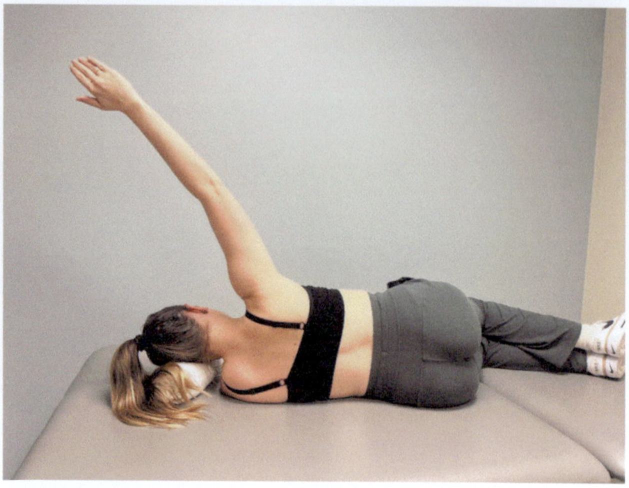

- While standing, squeeze both shoulder blades "back and down" and rotate your arms away from you. Keep your elbows at your sides. Hold 3-5 seconds, relax, and repeat.

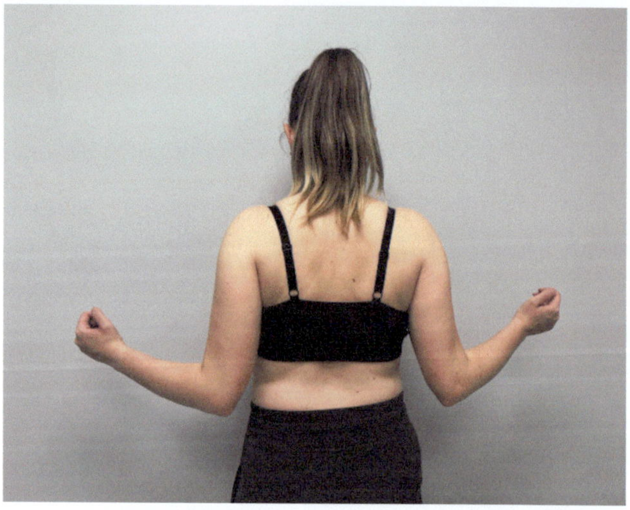

- While standing, squeeze both shoulder blades "back and down" and raise your arms up and out to the side. Hold 3-5 seconds, relax, and repeat.

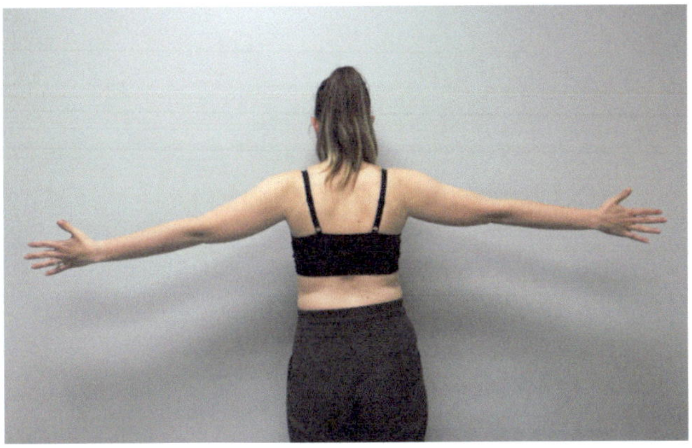

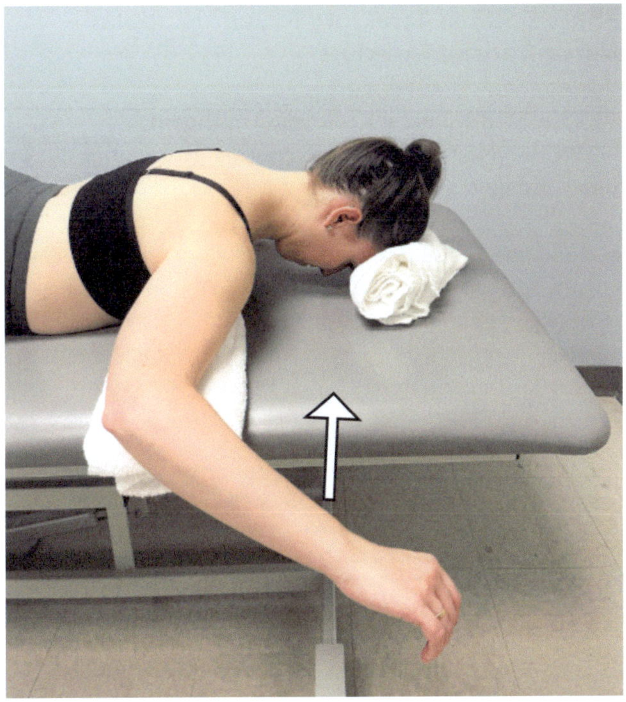

- Lie on your stomach with your injured arm hanging off the edge of the mat or bed. Squeeze your shoulder blade "back and down." Raise your arm out to the side and rotate your shoulder away from the body. Hold 3-5 seconds, relax, and repeat.

Phase 3 Spinal Accessory to Suprascapular Nerve Transfer Exercises

☐ **Resisted Donor + Recipient Movement:**

Complete the below exercises 1-10 repetitions, 2-3 times per day.

- Hold one end of a resistance band while the other end is attached to a door handle. Keep a rolled towel supported between your side and your elbow. Pinch your shoulder blade "back and down," and rotate your shoulder outward as your forearm moves out to the side. Keep your elbow bent at 90°.

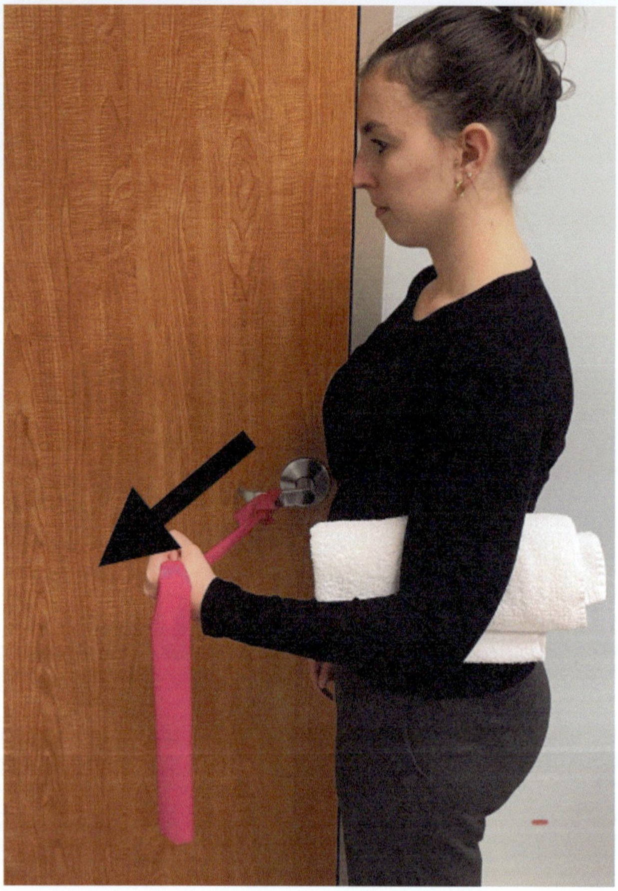

- Hold a resistance band with the opposite end anchored under your foot. Squeeze your shoulder blades together as you raise your arm up and out to the side. Hold 3-5 seconds. You can also do this same exercise holding a light dumbbell.

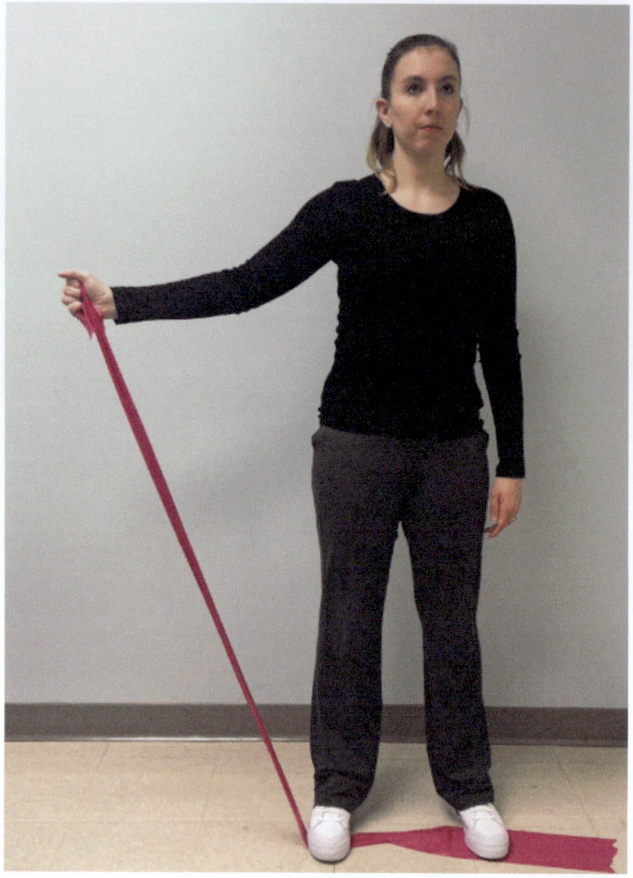

- Lie on your stomach with your arm resting off the edge of a mat/bed. With a light weight in your hand, squeeze your shoulder blade in while you raise the arm and rotate the weight up toward the ceiling. Try to keep the elbow bent to a 90-degree angle as you lift up.

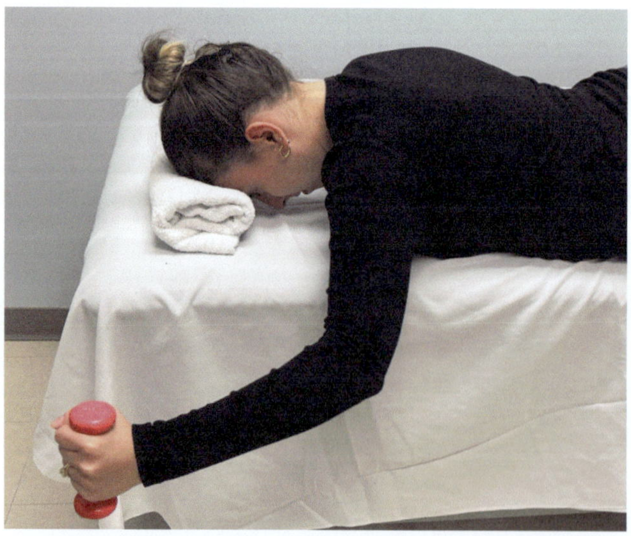

☐ **Resisted Recipient Movement:**

Strengthening the rotator cuff (recipient) without first activating the shoulder blades (donor) is NOT recommended, but the movement does not have to be as intentional once rotator cuff strength improves.

References

1. Suzuki K, Doi K, Hattori Y, Pagsaligan J. Long-term results of spinal accessory nerve transfer to the suprascapular nerve in upper-type paralysis of brachial plexus injury. J Reconstruct Microsurg. 2007;23(6):295–9.
2. Bertelli JA, Ghizoni MF. Results of spinal accessory to suprascapular nerve transfer in 110 patients with complete palsy of the brachial plexus. J Neurosurg Spine. 2016;24(6):990–5.
3. Siqueira MG, Martins RS, Solla D, Faglioni W, Foroni L, Heise CO. Functional outcome of spinal accessory nerve transfer to the suprascapular nerve to restore shoulder function: Results in upper and complete traumatic brachial plexus palsy in adults. Neurology India. 2019;67(7):77–81.
4. Hill JL, Turner LC, Jones RD, et al. The stages of rehabilitation following motor nerve transfer surgery. J Musculoskelet Surg Res. 2019;3(60)
5. Kahn L, Moore A. Donor activation focused rehabilitation approach: maximizing outcomes after nerve transfers. Hand Clin. 2016;32(2):263–77.
6. Novak CB. Rehabilitation following motor nerve transfers. Hand Clin. 2008;24(4):417–23.
7. Makel M, Sukop A, Kachlík D, Waldauf P, Whitley A, Kaiser R. Is there any difference between anterior and posterior approach for the spinal accessory to suprascapular nerve transfer? A systematic review and meta-analysis. Neurol Res. 2023;45(5):488–95.

Rehabilitation Guidelines for Specific Nerve Transfers: Elbow

Intercostal Nerves to the Biceps Branch of the Musculocutaneous Nerve Transfer

Alexandra MacKenzie

Background

Restoration of elbow flexion is vital to arm function including self-care, home management, and work. It is considered one of the most important functions to restore following paralysis due to injury of the musculocutaneous nerve [1]. Intercostal nerves (ICNs) are a reliable extraplexal donor choice to restore elbow flexion when there are no intraplexal options available because they have proximity to the infraclavicular plexus [2, 3]. ICNs are more commonly used in complete, traumatic brachial plexus avulsion or rupture injuries. Intercostal nerves have mixed motor and sensory function, and each individual ICN has a smaller axonal count than the musculocutaneous nerve (MCN). Therefore, multiple levels of intercostal nerves are often combined to boost the axonal count and improve recipient outcomes.

A. MacKenzie (✉)
Hand and Upper Extremity Therapy Center, Hospital for Special Surgery, New York, NY, USA
e-mail: mackenziea@hss.edu

L. C. Kahn et al. (eds.), *Rehabilitation for Nerve Transfers of the Upper Extremity*, https://doi.org/10.1007/978-3-031-92008-0_12

Surgery Description

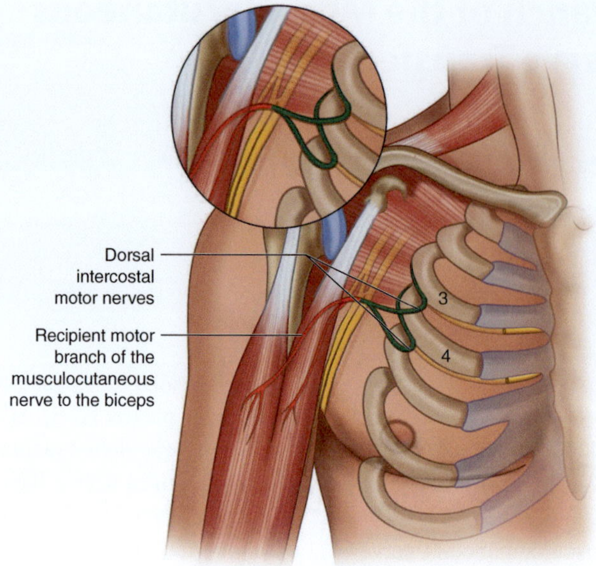

Microsurgical technique of intercostal nerves to the biceps branch of the musculocutaneous nerve transfer

A longitudinal incision is made along the midbrachial sulcus. The musculocutaneous nerve is identified deep to the biceps muscle, in the intramuscular interval between the biceps and brachialis muscles. The branch from the musculocutaneous nerve to the biceps is identified. Intraoperative stimulation is used to confirm whether the biceps branch responds. It is important to ensure that there are no long-acting paralytics being used by the anesthesia team. A separate inframammary incision is made along the chest wall. The ribs (typically the third through fifth ribs, although there is variability in which ribs are selected) and intercostal muscles are exposed. The intercostal nerve is identified, typically using a handheld nerve stimulator. The intercostal nerves are dissected free from the surrounding tissue as distal as possible (towards the sternum). Usually 2–3 intercostal nerves are used for transfer to the biceps. The donor intercostal nerves are divided distally and reflected proximally, oftentimes being passed through the slips of the serratus anterior muscle. The recipient biceps branch is neurolyzed from the musculocutaneous nerve and divided proximally. Coaptation of the intercostal nerves to the biceps branch is performed using microsurgical technique. Surgeons may also consider transferring additional intercostal nerves to the brachialis branch of the musculocutaneous nerve.

Outcomes

The ability to flex the elbow against gravity (MMT grade 3/5) is recognized as a "good" outcome following this nerve transfer. Approximately 65–72% of patients can expect to have a grade of 3/5 or greater with this transfer [4]. The variability of outcomes following the use of two, three, or four intercostal donor nerves was not considered statistically significant by Xiao's group in 2014 [5]. Elbow flexion strength outcomes in Malessey's cohort demonstrated an MMT grade of 3/5 in 8% and 4/5 in 56% [6]. He found wide outcome variability in those with two and three ICN donors and greater consistency of outcomes with those receiving four to five ICNs (two out of two patients achieved MMT 4/5 elbow flexion strength) [6]. There is some agreement that direct coaptation of the ICN to the MCN correlates with improved outcomes over nerve transfers involving indirect coaptation (nerve graft) [5]. Cho et al. explored a cohort of 15 patients undergoing two ICNs transferred to MCN with direct coaptation with a mean follow-up time of 38 months (range of 24–62 months). Sixty-six percent (66%) of patients recovered at least an MMT grade of 3/5, and 26.6% (four individuals) recovered at least MMT 4/5 biceps strength. Another 26.6% did not recover any elbow flexion [7].

Seven out of seven patients with plexus traction injuries in one report failed to recover any function [8]. Patient age has also been shown to influence outcomes of ICN-to-MCN transfers. Patients younger than 40 have better outcomes than older adults [1]. Others suggest that elbow flexion recovery is greater following ICN transfer in those younger than 30 [9, 10].

Phases of Rehabilitation

Phase 1

Preoperative to 1/5 MMT in the Recipient Muscle

The shoulder is immobilized postoperatively for 3 weeks to protect the nerve coaptation. The patient should avoid excessive end-range shoulder abduction and external rotation. Passive shoulder range of motion (ROM) is introduced and gradually increased. It is important to maintain joint flexibility because in time, a newly innervated and weak muscle will never be strong enough to produce sufficient active movement in a stiff joint. The patient should be instructed in passive elbow flexion and forearm supination. It may take anywhere from 4 to 8 months to see early signs of reinnervation [11]. A sling should be used after this nerve transfer to prevent traction on the nerve transfer and protect the length of the recovering elbow flexors. An unsupported flail elbow risks overlengthening of the biceps muscle, which may contribute to decreased force production in the elbow flexors once they reinnervate [12, 13].

Exercises

- Donor Activation
  External intercostals contribute to inspiration, while internal intercostals contribute to expiration. In addition, these muscles play a role in posture and trunk rotation. EMG studies have demonstrated that they are especially important in contralateral trunk rotation [14]. It has been demonstrated that after ICN-to-MCN transfer, there is more activity in elbow flexors with trunk flexion than with inspiration/expiration [15]. Early-phase donor activation exercises should include trunk flexion and rotation in addition to cardiovascular exercises to promote exerted inspiration and expiration.
- Combined Donor with Passive Recipient Exercise
  Trunk flexion (and rotation) exercises should simultaneously occur with passive elbow flexion and supination. It may also be helpful for the patient to mentally visualize active elbow flexion at the same time (Image 1).

Assessment of Recovery

Monthly therapy visits should include assessment of biceps motor function. This is done by having the patient forcefully flex the trunk and exhaling to activate the donor while palpating the biceps muscle and tendon for any notable change in tension (Image 2). As early as 4–5 months postoperatively, the patient may demonstrate a positive tender muscle sign. When the biceps muscly belly is squeezed, the patient may report feeling it in their chest, indicating that the donor has reached the recipient. This is typically seen before there are signs of motor activity [16] (Image 3).

A palpable proximal biceps contraction may be felt around 6–8 months postoperatively, without visible elbow motion. Patients may eventually notice that when they laugh or cough, they have a spontaneous contraction of the biceps. Active elbow flexion against gravity may appear around 12 months postoperatively [17].

Therapy Frequency

In phase 1, one therapy visit per month is usually sufficient to monitor for compliance with the home exercise program as well as to monitor for signs of biceps motor return. If the patient has very stiff joints and there is a need to work on increasing passive range of motion, then the patient may be seen more frequently. Additionally, more frequent therapy may be warranted if multiple nerve transfers were performed at the same time.

Phase 2

2−/5 to 3/5 MMT in the Recipient Muscle

Patients should continue to avoid excessive passive end-range shoulder abduction and external rotation. Exercises in this phase will primarily involve donor and recipient actions occurring together. These should be initiated at the first sign of motor return. Exercises can be performed in a gravity-minimized plane as well as "place and hold" exercises with simultaneous donor activation. Exercises should begin in a mid-range arc of motion to make the action easier for the recovering muscle to perform. Use of a slick cloth or an arm skate will reduce surface friction and allow the weak muscle to bend the elbow further [18].

Exercises

- Active Donor with Active-Assisted Recipient
  Biceps MMT = 2−/5 to 2/5

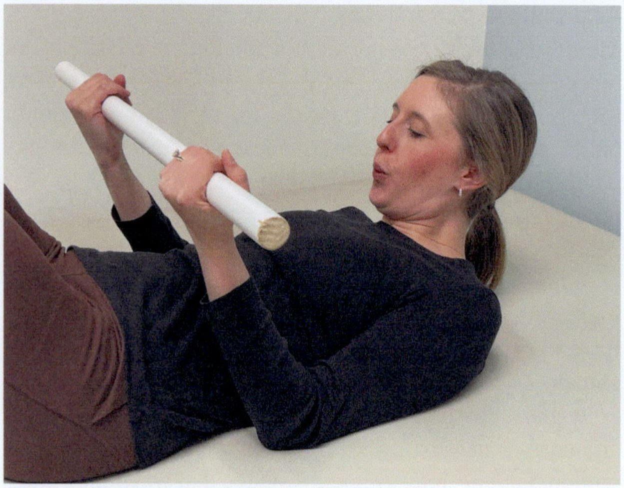

Image 1 Combined donor with passive recipient exercises are performed in supine. The individual is instructed to perform a partial sit-up with bilateral elbow flexion using a dowel to enable the uninvolved arm to passively flex the involved elbow

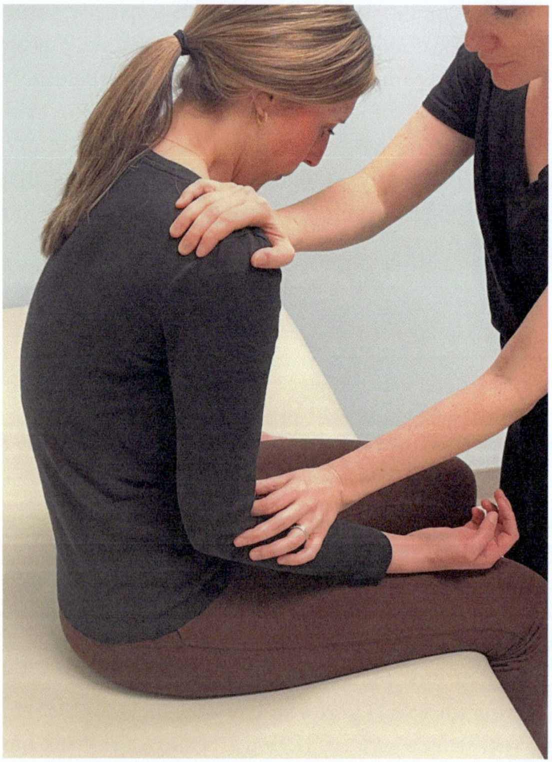

Image 2 Assessment of recovery of biceps function is performed by palpating along the biceps muscle and distal tendon while resisting trunk flexion and asking the individual to exhale. Any palpable muscle contraction with no elbow movement with donor activation is graded 1/5 on the MMT scale

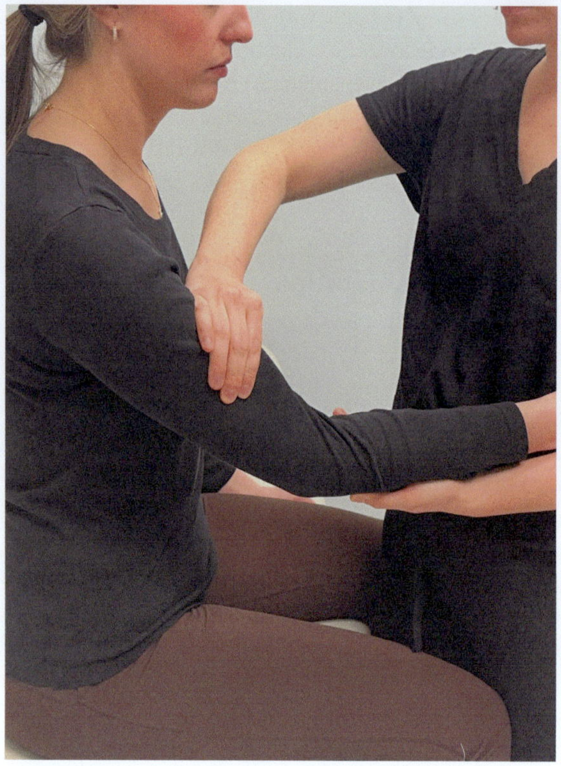

Image 3 A positive tender sign often occurs before motor function is perceived. A tender sign is performed by pinching the biceps muscle on the uninvolved side and then the involved side noting whether there is a distinct difference in tenderness in the recovering biceps

In side lying on the unaffected side, the patient flexes the trunk and exhales while attempting elbow flexion and supination with the arm supported on a table or a UE Ranger® (Image 4). An overhead pulley system can be used to hold the shoulder in flexion, allowing the elbow to flex with assistance from the contralateral hand while activating the donor intercostal muscles (Image 5).

- "Place and Hold" Exercise
  Biceps MMT = 2+/5
  The elbow is placed in 90 degrees of flexion with the forearm supinated, and the patient is asked to hold that position. Initially, this will require co-contraction of the donor. As the biceps gets stronger, the elbow can be held in varying degrees of flexion. This may be initially performed in a gravity-minimized position with the arm supported on a table (Image 6). As strength improves, this is attempted against gravity in sitting or standing (Image 7).

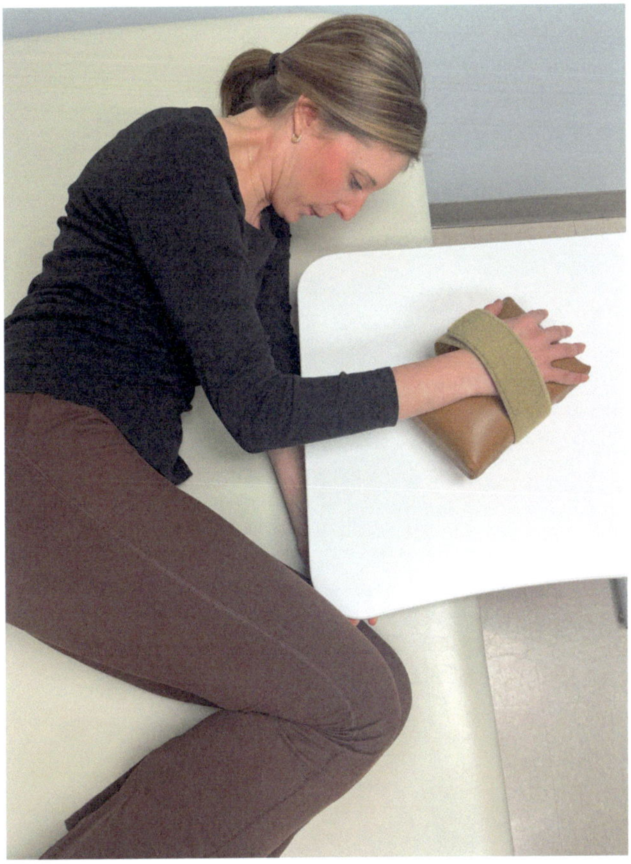

Image 4 Active donor with active-assisted recipient exercise can be performed with the patient in side-lying on the uninvolved side and the involved arm on a table with an arm skate. As the patient flexes the trunk and exhales, he or she attempts to flex the elbow from a partially flexed position

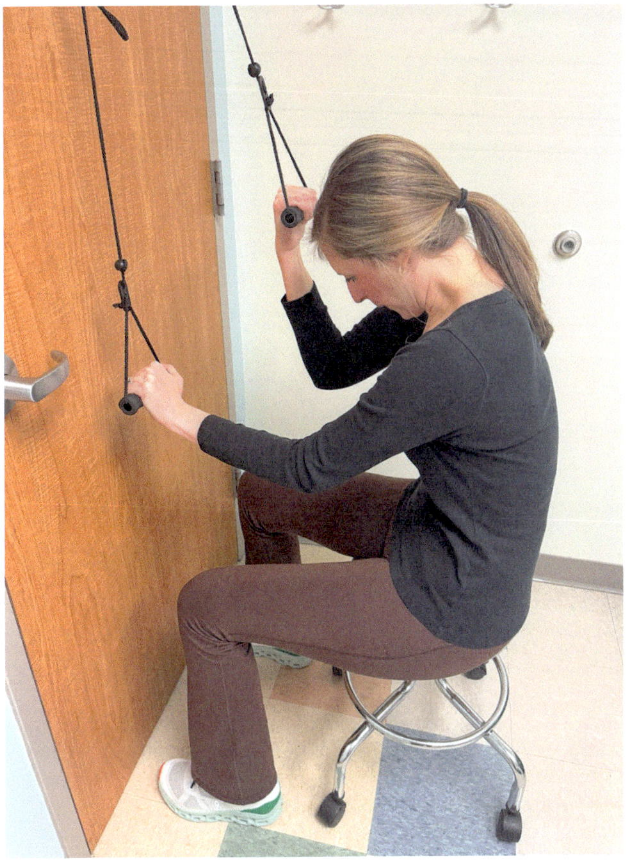

Image 5 An overhead pulley system is used perform active donor with active-assisted recipient exercise. The contralateral hand aids with elbow flexion while the patient is cued to activate the donor intercostal muscles by flexing the trunk

- Active Donor with Active Recipient
  Biceps MMT = 3−/5 to 3/5
  The patient is seated or standing while performing active elbow flexion and supination combined with forceful trunk flexion (an abdominal crunch) (Image 8).
- Functional Activity
  The patient can be taught to combine the donor and recipient actions with activities of daily living (ADLs). For example, the patient can perform active-assisted elbow flexion to bring the hand to face while eating or grooming while activating the core/trunk muscles.

Therapy Frequency

Patients may be seen once per week at this stage, with instruction in a comprehensive home exercise program. There are many factors that may warrant more or less frequent formal therapy visits.

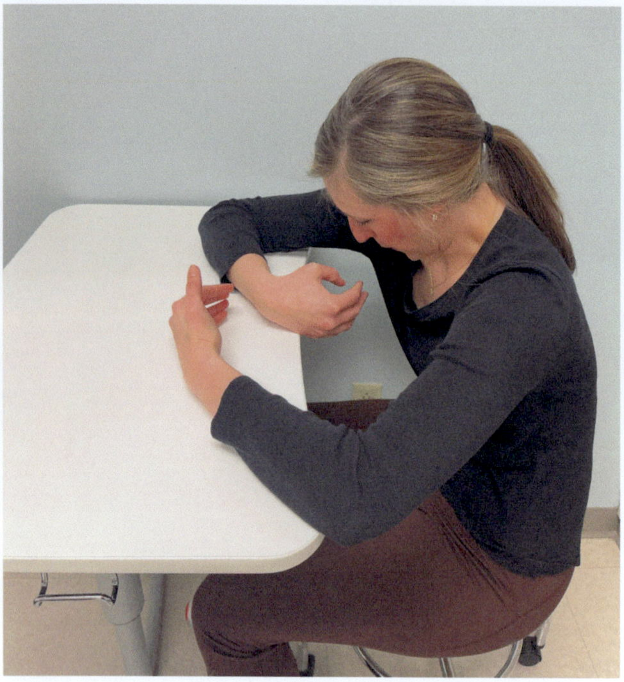

Image 6 A "place and hold" exercise is initially performed in sitting with the arm supported on a table at shoulder height. The elbow is flexed past 90 while the patient flexes the trunk, exhales, and attempts to keep the elbow in the flexed position

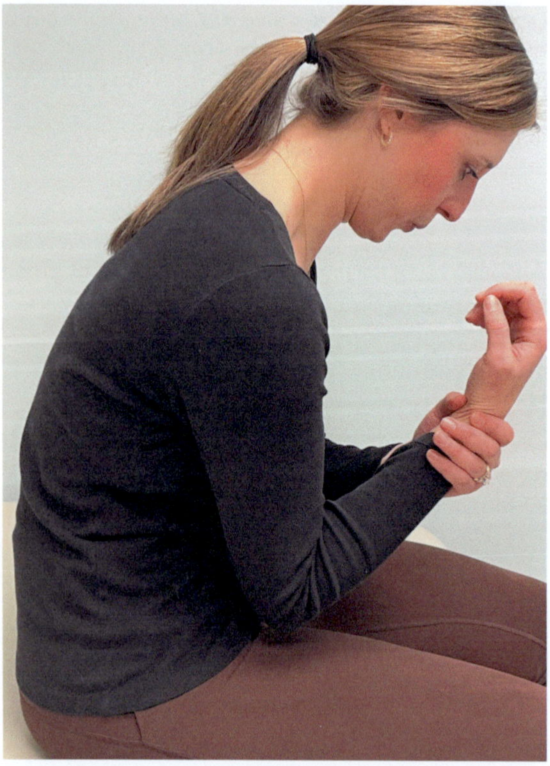

Image 7 As strength improves, "place and hold" exercises are attempted against gravity by placing the elbow in flexion while activating the donor and attempting to keep the elbow flexed

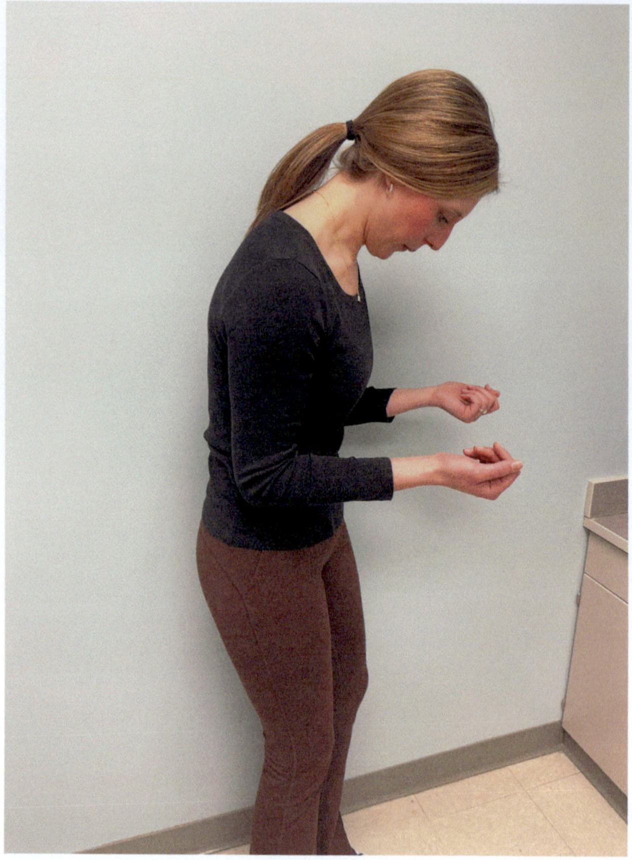

Image 8 Active donor with active recipient exercises include standing elbow flexion with trunk flexion and forceful exhalation. Performing this bilaterally enhances motor learning

Orthoses

As the patient enters phase 2 and there are signs of reinnervation, the patient can wean from the sling as the biceps get stronger. Some patients may benefit from an elbow dynamic assist orthosis [19]. This is a hinged elbow orthosis that maintains the elbow in a flexed position with the aid of elastic exercise bands (Image 9). This allows the patient to initiate elbow flexion from a more biomechanically advantageous position, promoting return of function.

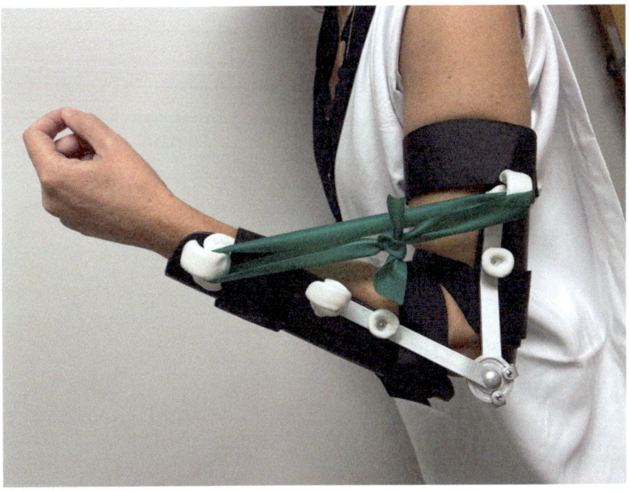

Image 9 During phase 2, the patient may benefit from a custom hinged elbow orthosis that enables him or her to flex from a more biomechanically advantageous position

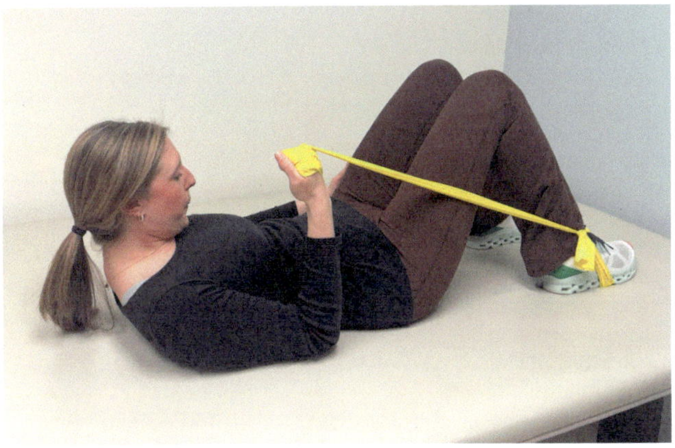

Image 10 Resistance is added to elbow flexion during phase 3. Initially, co-contraction is performed as shown here in supine with trunk flexion

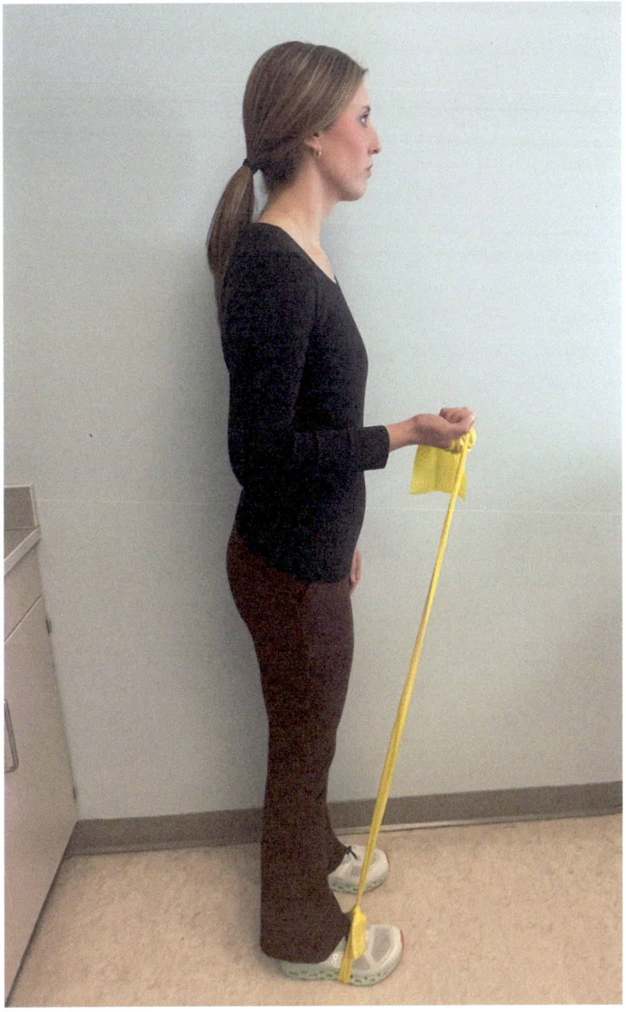

Image 11 As strength in the biceps improves, one can attempt to strengthen the biceps against gravity with resistance bands without donor input

Phase 3

3+/5 MMT in the Recipient Muscle

The goal of phase 3 is to maximize elbow flexion strength and work towards independent elbow flexion activation. Progressive resistive exercises and donor "deactivation," i.e., independent elbow flexion without core/trunk activation, are the hallmarks of this stage. This requires successful cortical remapping and may take a minimum of 2 years to reach this stage.

- Resistive Recipient Activity with Donor Contraction
- The patient can perform elbow flexion (and supination) with an elastic resistance band while simultaneously performing a crunch in supine (Image 10).
- Resistive Recipient Activity Without Donor Contraction
- The patient can perform elbow flexion (and supination) against gravity with resistance band while standing with no trunk flexion to separate the recipient function from the intercostal donor (Image 11).

Intercostal nerves to the biceps nerve transfer

Nerve transfer overview					
Donor nerve	Donor action	Recipient nerve	Recipient action	Indications for functional restoration	Approximate months to functional movement
Intercostal nerves	Trunk flexion, trunk rotation, inspiration and expiration	Musculocutaneous nerve branch to the biceps	Elbow flexion and supination	Loss of elbow flexion; complete plexus injury	12 months [17]

Information below is suggested guidelines. Precautions may vary according to surgeon preferences and patient factors

	Preoperative therapy	Early phase	Middle phase	Late phase
Criteria	Before surgery	0/5–1/5 MMT	2-/5 to 3/5 MMT	>3/5 MMT
Purpose of Phase	Educate and establish baseline function	Understand donor and recipient relationship	Consistently activate recipient	Strengthen recipient through resistance and separate from donor activation
Precautions	Prevent extension and pronation contracture of elbow	Protect elbow flexor length	Respect fatigue and prevent dominance of triceps	Avoid resisted elbow flexion until consistent 3/5 MMT is achieved. Note that not all patients achieve 3/5 strength
Frequency of visits (considerations)	1–2 pre-op visits May increase if PROM limitations exist	1×/week until PROM is WNL and patient is independent with donor activation; then 1× monthly	1× per week to 1× per month based on patient needs and accurate, consistent demonstration of exercise program	1× every 1–2 weeks based on progress toward patient-specific goals
Orthosis considerations	NA	Full-time sling and elbow support for the first 2 weeks. OK to remove for hygiene	Continue intermittent sling use to protect the length of the recovering biceps and prevent traction on the brachial plexus May consider dynamic elbow flexion orthosis	D/C as elbow flexion endurance against gravity improves
Interventions	PROM if patient lacks passive elbow flexion and forearm supination	**Donor Activation:** Primarily trunk flexion and exhalation. Others include trunk rotation and cardiovascular exercise to encourage inspiration and expiration **Donor-Recipient Pairing**: Exhalation and trunk flexion combined with passive elbow flexion in supination	**Active/Resisted Donor with Active Assisted Recipient:** Gravity minimized plane: with arm supported on table at shoulder height exhalation and trunk flexion is performed with active-assisted elbow flexion using the contralateral arm, an arm skate, or slick cloth Supine dowel rod exercise: trunk flexion and exhalation with active-*assisted* elbow flexion (in supination) **Place and Hold**: Passively place the elbow in end-range flexion and supination while flexing the trunk. Remove support from the contralateral hand and attempt to maintain this position **Active Donor with Active Recipient:** Standing trunk crunch with exhalation while independently flexing the elbow (in supination)	**Resisted Donor and Recipient:** While supine or standing and holding a resistance band, the patient performs an upper body "crunch" with elbow flexion in supination **Resisted Recipient:** While standing and holding weights or a resistance band, the patient performs elbow flexion (in supination) while keeping the trunk upright
Additional interventions			Active-assisted exercise may also include side lying with the arm supported on a large exercise ball An overhead pulley system may also be used for donor-recipient pairing	

During all phases it is essential to continue cortical reorganization, pychological and psychosocial interventions, progress to incorporate donor/recipient with ADL's

Intercostal to Biceps Nerve Transfer

Goal of Surgery: To restore elbow flexion
Recipient Movement = Elbow flexion and supination
Recipient Muscle: Biceps muscle

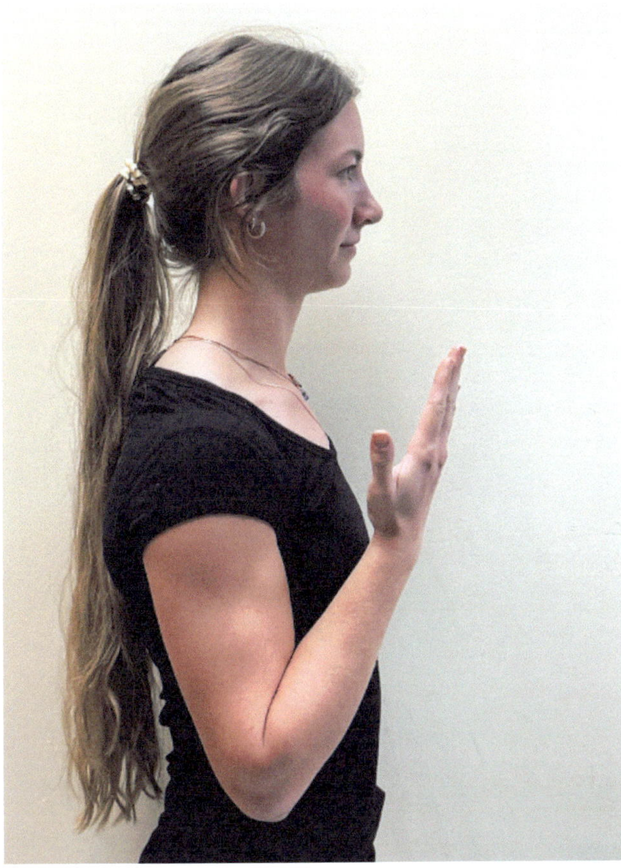

Bend elbow (palm up)

Donor Movement = Trunk flexion, exhalation, inspiration, trunk rotation

Donor Muscle: Internal and external intercostal muscles

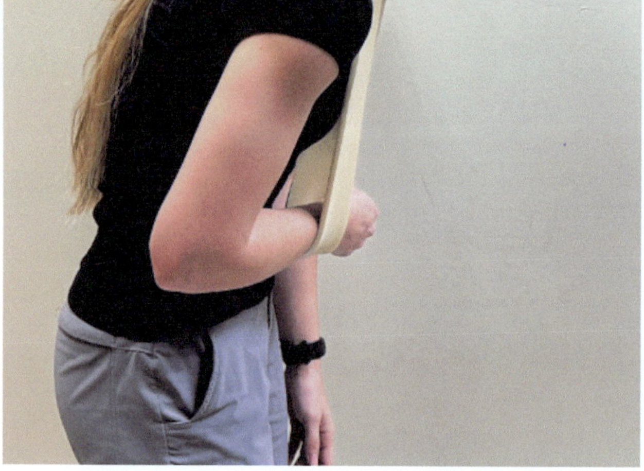

Bend trunk and exhale

Phase 1 Intercostal to Biceps Nerve Transfer Exercises

☐ **Active Donor Movement:**

- While lying on your back, exhale and do an upper body crunch, raising your shoulders off the mat. Hold 3–5 seconds and relax. You can also do this while standing or sitting.

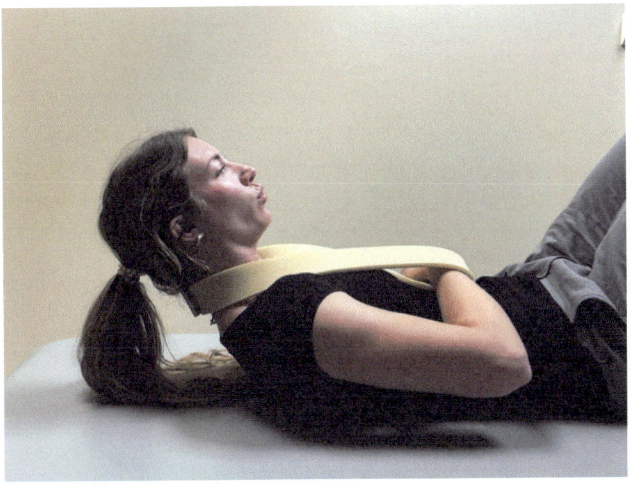

- Rotate your trunk back and forth while performing deep breathing.

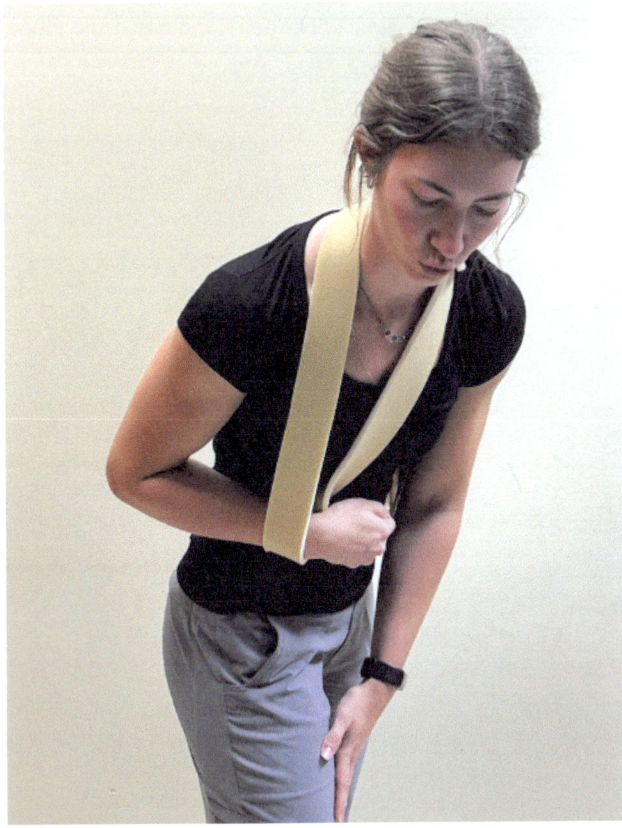

Complete 10 repetitions every hour

☐ **Combined Donor with Passive Recipient Exercise:**

- While seated or standing, take a big breath in. Forcefully breathe out, bend your upper body and assist the elbow into a bent position using your opposite hand. Try to keep the forearm in a palm-up position.

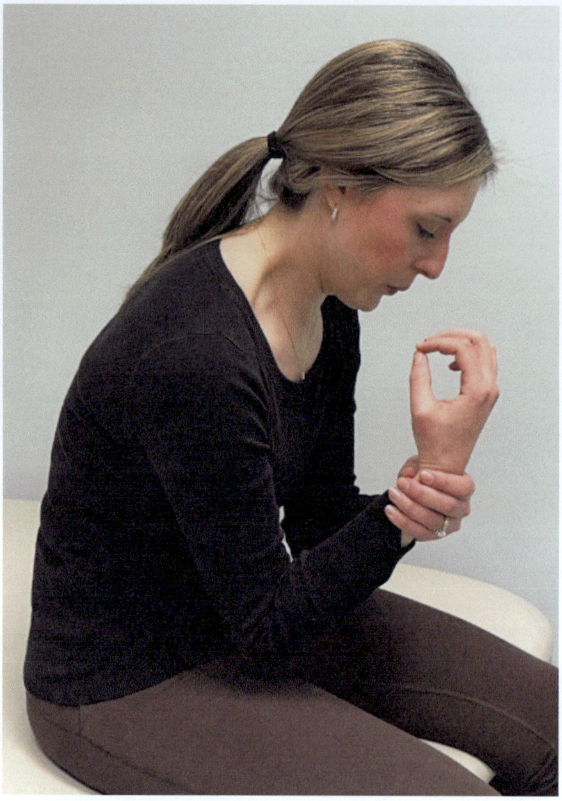

Complete 10–15 repetitions, 3–5 times per day

Phase 2 Intercostal to Biceps Nerve Transfer Exercises:

☐ **Active Donor + Active-Assisted Recipient:**

- With your arm supported on a high table, breathe out and bend your upper body. Try to slide your forearm across the table toward your chest. Once you cannot bend the elbow any further, use your opposite hand to assist the elbow into a fully bent position.
  - You may use a slick cloth under the forearm to make it easier.

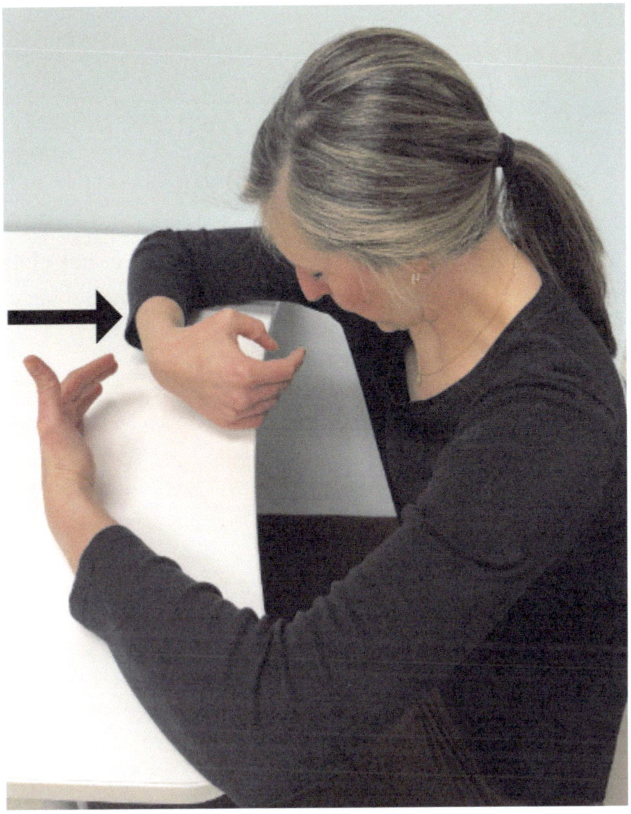

- Using an overhead pulley system, sit down facing the door and hold both handles. Make sure your injured arm holds the handle with the palm facing you. Exhale and bend your upper body while your opposite arm pulls down, allowing your injured elbow to bend.

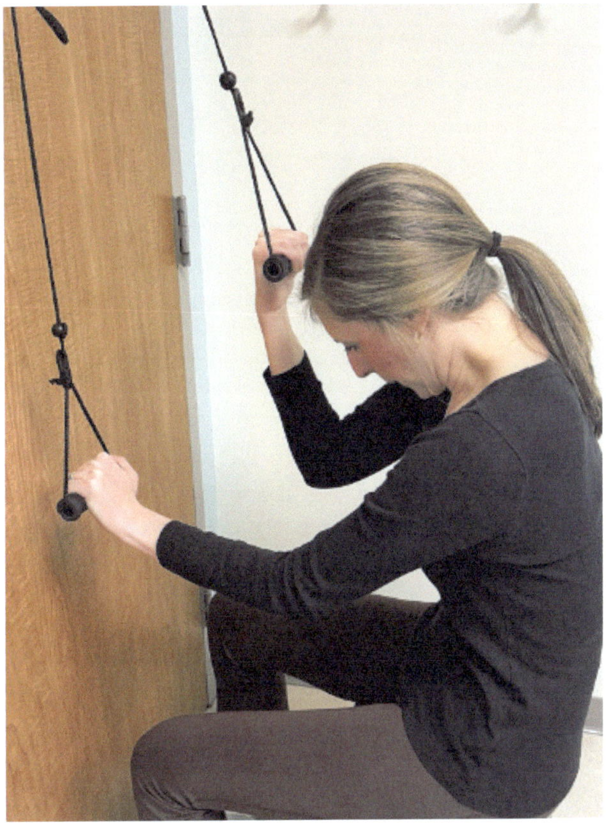

- While lying on your back, hold a dowel rod in both hands with your palms facing up. Bend your upper body, raising your shoulders off the mat and blow out. At the same time, bend both elbows so the dowel rod comes up toward your chest. Try not to rely solely on the uninjured arm.

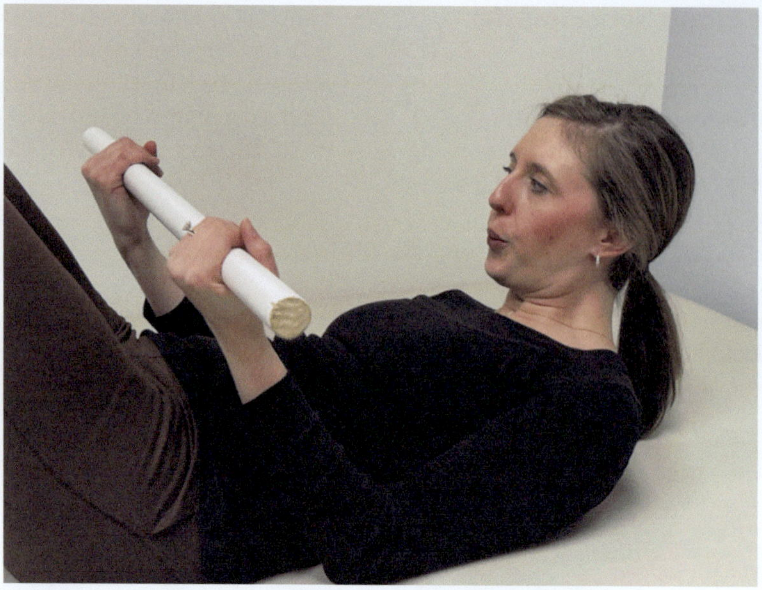

- Lie on your uninjured side. Your uninjured arm should be supported on a table in front of you. Forcefully exhale and bend your upper body forward. At the same time, try to bend your elbow on your own. You may use a a slick cloth or an arm skate to make it easier.

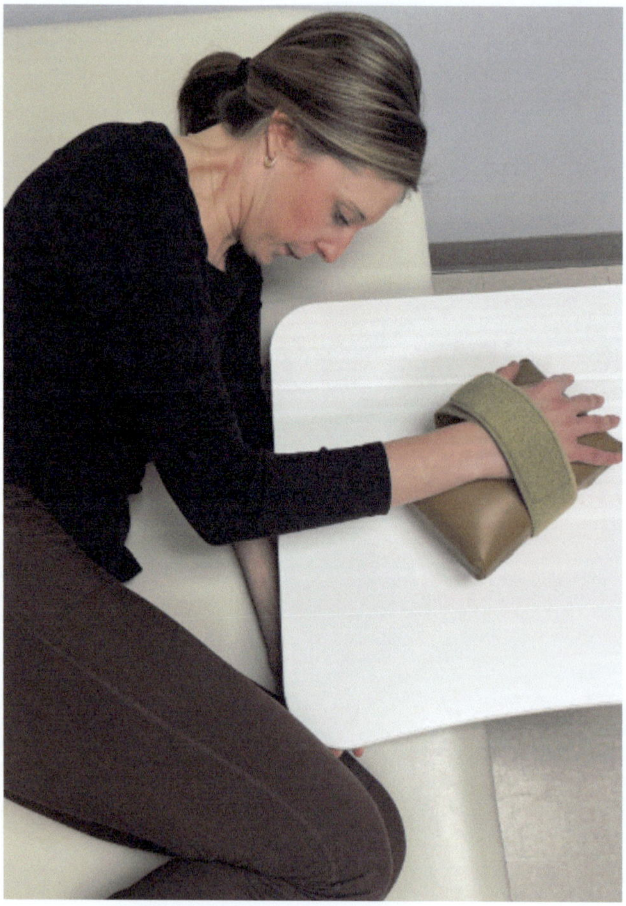

☐ **"Place and Hold"**

- While seated or standing, exhale and bend the trunk. Then use the opposite hand to bend the elbow into a fully bent (and palm-up) position. Slowly release the support of your opposite hand and try to maintain this position for a count of 5 seconds.

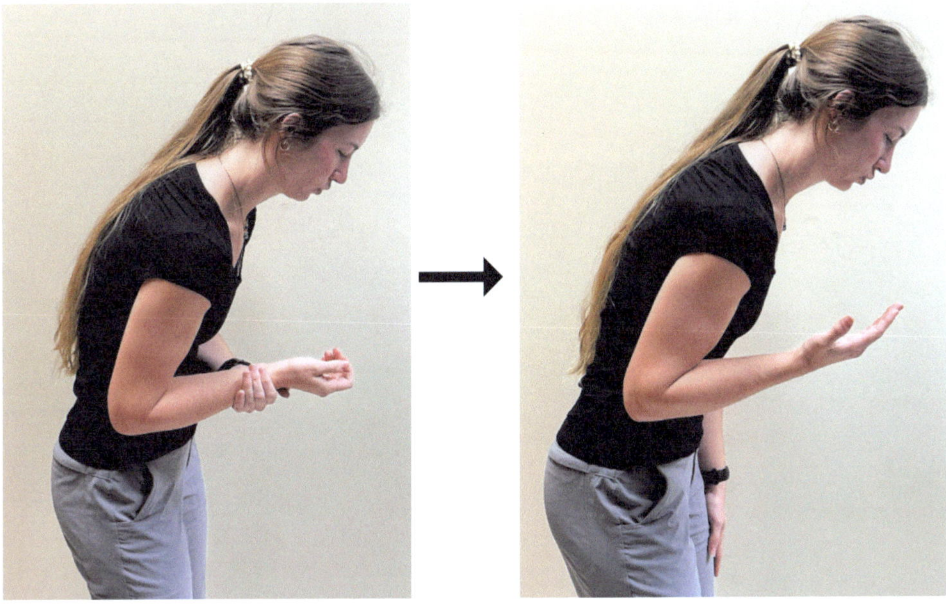

Complete 10–15 repetitions, 3–5 times per day.

☐ **Active Donor + Active Recipient Movement:**

- While seated or standing, bend the elbow (on your own) while forcefully exhaling and bending your trunk. Try to maintain a palm-up position of the forearm. Hold 3–5 seconds, relax, and repeat.
  - It may be helpful to try this exercise with both arms.

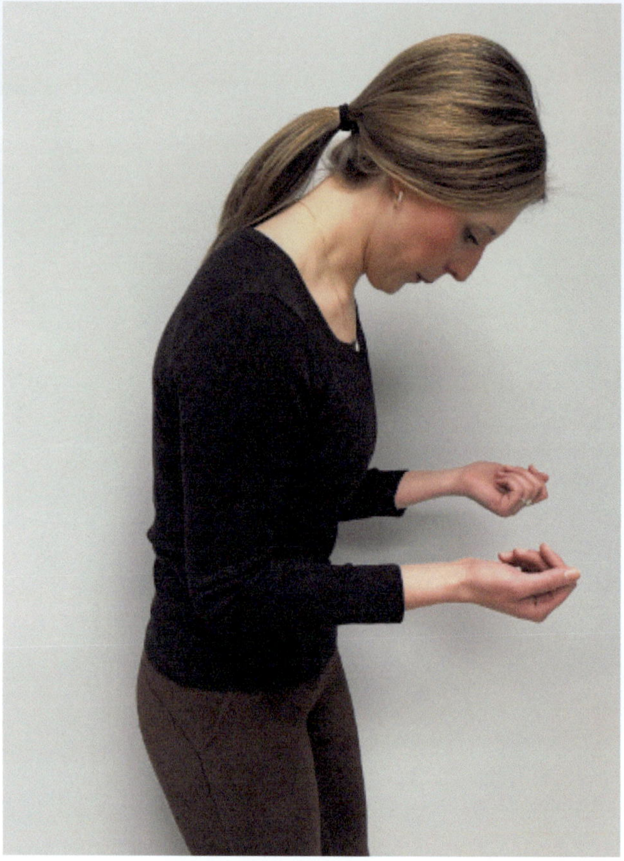

Complete 10–15 repetitions, 3–5 times per day

☐ **Functional Activities**

Complete daily activities such as washing your face in front of a sink by supporting your injured arm with the opposite arm. You can also incorporate the combined movements by holding a sandwich or fruit with both hands when eating. The key is to tighten your trunk muscles (activate your core) when doing these activities.

Phase 3 Intercostal to Biceps Nerve Transfer Exercises:

☐ **Resisted Recipient Activity with Donor Contraction:**

- Lie on your back and hold a resistance band anchored around your foot. Take a big breath out while doing an upper body crunch. At the same time, bend the elbow in a palm-up position. Hold 3 seconds, and slowly lower the arm.
  – This can also be done in a standing position holding bands or weights. If you do not have function of your fingers, arm cuffs may be used.

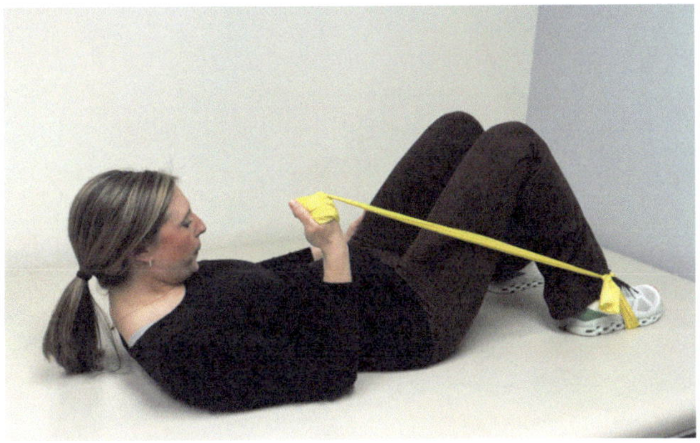

Complete 10 repetitions, 3 times per day

☐ **Resisted Recipient without Donor Contraction:**

- Hold a light weight, exercise band, or arm cuff while standing. Bend your elbow as far as you can, holding 3–5 seconds. Keep your trunk upright.

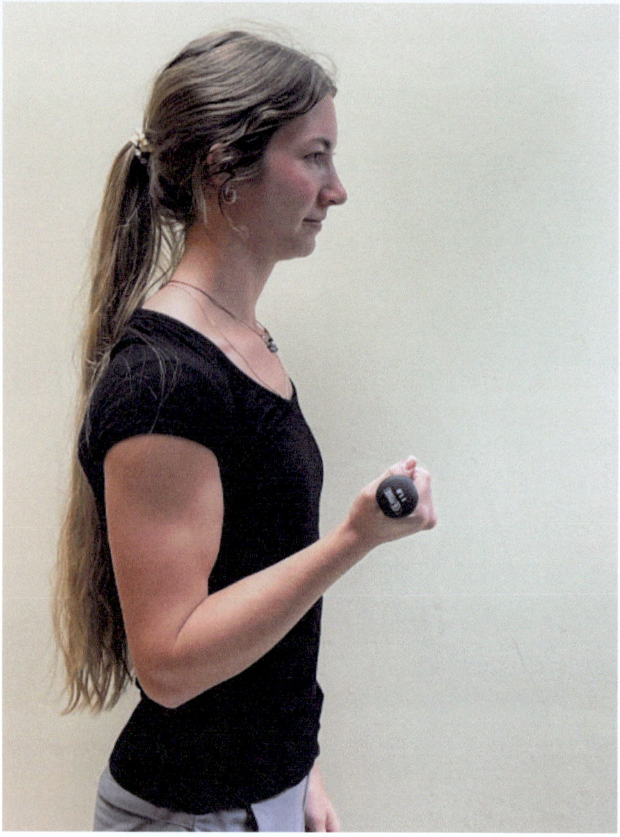

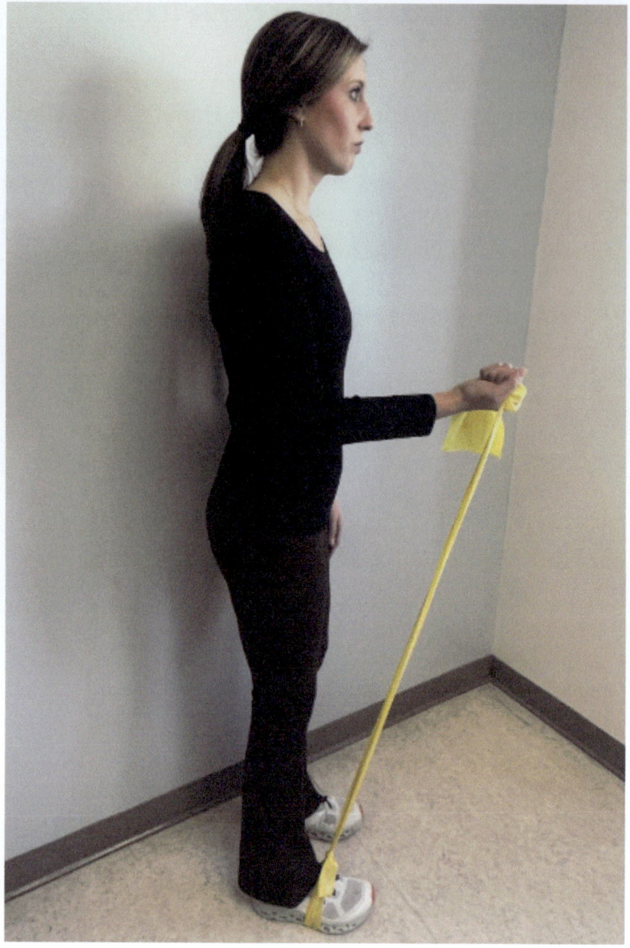

Complete 10 repetitions, 3 times per day

References

1. Allieu Y, Cenac P. Is surgical intervention justifiable for total paralysis secondary to multiple avulsion injuries of the brachial plexus? Hand Clin. 1988;4(4):609–18.
2. Azze RJ, Mattar R Jr, Ferreira MC, Starck R, Canedo AC. Extraplexal neurotization of brachial plexus. Microsurgery. 1994;15(1):28–32.
3. Shin AY, Spinner RJ, Steinmann SP, Bishop AT. Adult traumatic brachial plexus injuries. JAAOS-J Am Acad Orthop Surg. 2005;13(6):382–96.
4. Merrell GA, Barrie KA, Katz DL, Wolfe SW. Results of nerve transfer techniques for restoration of shoulder and elbow function in the context of a meta-analysis of the English literature. J Hand Surg. 2001;26(2):303–14.
5. Xiao C, Lao J, Wang T, Zhao X, Liu J, Gu Y. Intercostal nerve transfer to neurotize the musculocutaneous nerve after traumatic brachial plexus avulsion: a comparison of two, three, and four nerve transfers. J Reconstruct Microsurg. 2014;30(5):297–304.
6. Malessey MJ, Thomeer RT. Evaluation of intercostal to musculocutaneous nerve transfer in reconstructive brachial plexus surgery. J Neurosurg. 1998;88:266–71.
7. Cho AB, Iamaguchi RB, Bersani Silva G, et al. Intercostal nerve transfer to the biceps motor branch in complete traumatic brachial plexus injuries. Microsurgery. 2015;35(6):428–31.
8. Matejcik V. Analysis of the brachial plexus traumatic lesions reconstructive procedures unfavourable results. Rozhledy v Chirurgii: Mesicnik Ceskoslovenske Chirurgicke Spolecnosti. 2004;83(12):614–6.
9. Nagano A. Treatment of Brachial plexus Injury. J Orthop Sci. 1998;3:71–80.
10. Coulet B, Boretto JG, Lazerges C, Chammas M. A comparison of intercostal and partial ulnar nerve transfers in restoring elbow flexion following upper brachial plexus injury (C5-C6±C7). J Hand Surg. 2010;35(8):1297–303.
11. Chuang DCC, Yeh MC, Wei FC. Intercostal nerve transfer of the musculocutaneous nerve in avulsed brachial plexus injuries: evaluation of 66 patients. J Hand Surg. 1992;17(5)
12. Goldspink G, Tabary C, Tabary JC, Tardieu C, Tardieu G. Effect of denervation on the adaptation of sarcomere number and muscle extensibility to the functional length of the muscle. J Physiol. 1974;236(3):733–42.
13. Gossman MR, Sahrmann SA, Rose SJ. Review of length-associated changes in muscle: experimental evidence and clinical implications. Phys Ther. 1982;62(12):1799–808.
14. Whitelaw WA, Ford GT, Rimmer KP, De Troyer A. Intercostal muscles are used during rotation of the thorax in humans. J Appl Physiol. 1985;72(5):1940–4.
15. Chalidapong P, Sananpanich K, Klaphajone J. Electromyographic comparison of various exercises to improve elbow flexion following intercostal nerve transfer. J Bone Joint Surg (Br Vol). 2006;88(5):620–2.
16. Lee EY, Karjalainen TV, Sebastin SJ, Lim AY. The value of the tender muscle sign in detecting motor recovery after peripheral nerve reconstruction. J Hand Surg. 2015;40(3):433–7.
17. Hill JL, Turner LC, Jones RD, et al. The stages of rehabilitation following motor nerve transfer surgery. J Musculoskelet Surg Res. 2019;3(60)
18. Kahn L, Moore A. Donor activation focused rehabilitation approach: maximizing outcomes after nerve transfers. Hand Clin. 2016;32(2):263–77.
19. Chinchalkar SJ, Larocerie-Salgado, J., Cepek, J., & Grenier, M. L. The use of dynamic assist orthosis for muscle reeducation following brachial plexus injury and reconstruction. J Hand Microsurg 2018;10(3):172-177.

Ulnar Nerve to the Flexor Carpi Ulnaris (FCU) to the Biceps Branch of the Musculocutaneous Nerve Transfer

Macyn M. Stonner

Background

Injury to the musculocutaneous nerve (MCN) has a devastating impact on upper extremity function. The musculocutaneous nerve arises from the lateral cord with origins from C5, C6, and C7. It innervates the biceps brachii, brachialis, and coracobrachialis muscles. Loss of MCN function therefore leads to a complete loss of elbow flexion. There are few individuals who can flex the elbow with only a brachioradialis muscle. This everyday movement "brings hand to face" for eating, grooming, and majority of daily living tasks. The restoration of elbow flexion is the highest prioritized goal in the surgical management of brachial plexus injuries. The most common nerve transfer surgery to restore elbow flexion is the flexor carpi ulnaris (FCU)-to-biceps nerve transfer. This procedure is indicated in patients with C5, C6, and C7 root avulsions or injuries at the level of the upper trunk, lateral cord, or isolated musculocutaneous nerve.

The FCU-to-biceps nerve transfer was originally described by Oberlin in 1994 and has gained considerable recognition in the restoration of elbow flexion [1]. This procedure, called the "Oberlin transfer," includes the transfer of one or two fascicles of the ulnar nerve to the FCU into the MCN motor branch of the biceps brachii muscle. It has proven to be successful in part due to the close proximity of the ulnar nerve to the target musculocutaneous nerve branch of the biceps, allowing for direct coaptation with a reliable and relatively quick reinnervation of the biceps. The approximate distance from nerve coaptation to motor end plate is 8 cm.

M. M. Stonner (✉)
Milliken Hand Rehabilitation Center, WashU Medicine, St. Louis, MO, USA
e-mail: macyn.stonner@wustl.edu

Surgical Description

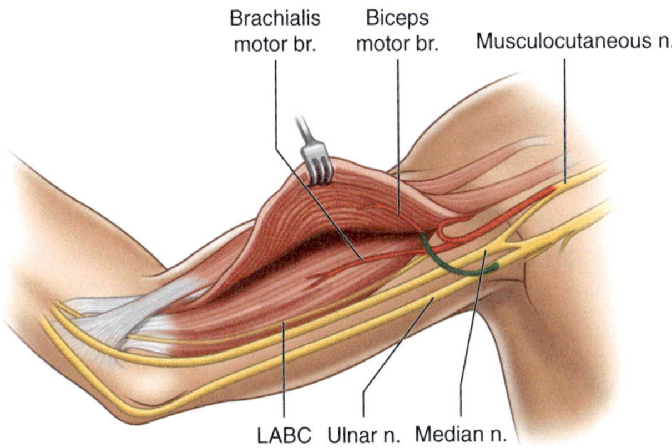

Microsurgical technique of Ulnar nerve to the flexor carpi ulnaris (fcu) to the biceps branch of the musculocutaneous nerve transfer

A longitudinal incision is made along the midbrachial sulcus. The musculocutaneous nerve is identified deep in the biceps muscle, in the intramuscular interval between the biceps and brachialis. The branch from the musculocutaneous nerve to the biceps is identified. Intraoperative stimulation is used to confirm whether the biceps branch responds. It is important to ensure that there are no muscle paralytics being used by the anesthesia team. The ulnar nerve is then identified near the intermuscular septum, just anterior to the triceps muscle. Intraoperative stimulation is used to confirm the identity of the ulnar nerve, and an internal neurolysis is performed to select a portion of the ulnar nerve that matches the caliber of the recipient biceps branch. When selecting the donor fascicle, it is important to ensure that stimulation of the donor fascicle is predominantly resulting in wrist flexion (and not intrinsic muscle firing). The donor fascicle is neurolyzed from the remainder of the ulnar nerve and divided distally. The recipient biceps branch is neurolyzed from the musculocutaneous nerve and divided proximally. Coaptation of the FCU branch of the ulnar nerve to the biceps branch is performed using microsurgical technique. Surgeons may

L. C. Kahn et al. (eds.), *Rehabilitation for Nerve Transfers of the Upper Extremity*,
https://doi.org/10.1007/978-3-031-92008-0_13

also consider transferring a portion of the median nerve to the brachialis branch of the musculocutaneous nerve.

Outcomes

Oberlin's original surgical description included a cohort of four patients and also a cadaver study. Of these four patients, three obtained elbow flexion manual muscle testing (MMT) strength of 4/5, and one achieved 3/5 MMT strength [1]. A clinical series of 18 patients subsequently followed this in 1997, in which 11 patients recovered elbow flexion after nerve transfer [2]. Five patients in this study required additional Steindler flexorplasty, yet these patients underwent nerve transfer more than 1 year following their injury. More recent outcomes by Sedain et al. (2011) demonstrate elbow flexion strength ≥3/5 MMT in 77.8% of patients with an average of 12.2 months from injury to surgery [3]. In 2005, Mackinnon and colleagues described a refined technique to restore elbow flexion with the addition of transferring median nerve fascicles into the MCN motor branch of the brachialis muscle. The original study led to excellent results in six patients (mean MMT grade 4+/5) and is now widely used and recognized as the "double fascicular transfer" (DFT) [4].

A 2020 systematic review showed that DFT outcomes are superior to the single Oberlin transfer, demonstrating elbow flexion MMT ≥ 4/5 in 83% of subjects versus 63% of subjects [5]. This chapter highlights the single FCU-to-biceps nerve transfer.

Phases of Rehabilitation

Phase 1

Pre-op to 1/5 MMT in the Recipient Muscle

Both the surgeon and therapist should provide thorough yet simple education about the anatomy involved in the nerve transfer, with specific rationale for precautions and therapy/timeline expectations. The patient should be educated on the importance of protecting the length of the target biceps muscle by positioning the elbow in 90 degrees of flexion and supination preoperatively and in the early postoperative phase. Proper positioning is first achieved in the operating room using a postoperative dressing, which later transitions to a sling after 1–2 weeks. The patient is referred to an initial therapy visit around this time, often in conjunction with the first postoperative appointment with the surgeon.

Between 10 days and 3 weeks (pending wound healing and surgeon preference), sutures are removed. Scar management may begin once the wound is fully healed. Instrument-assisted soft tissue mobilization (IASTM) is not recommended after nerve surgery. The therapist may provide a general timeline about the anticipated timeframe for functional return of elbow flexion. Although each patient's recovery varies, one can anticipate approximately 3–4 months for target muscle tenderness, 4–5 months for trace contraction, and 12+ months for functional movement [6]. By the first therapy visit, the patient should be able to verbalize the action of the donor (wrist flexion) and that performing this movement amplifies neural messages to the biceps [7, 8].

Exercises

- ROM of Uninvolved Joints
  Patients are instructed to perform active range of motion (AROM) of uninvolved joints immediately following surgery. Exercises may include scapular retraction, shoulder flexion and abduction, and finger flexion and extension. This may help minimize swelling and joint stiffness. If joint limitations occur, passive range of motion (PROM) should be initiated.
- Donor Activation
  As early as 2 weeks from surgery, patients are seen for their first therapy visit. They should be instructed in the concept of "flooding the donor." Donor activation is performed with active (or isometric) wrist flexion exercises at a recommended frequency of ten repetitions every hour. During subsequent visits, resistive wrist flexion with weights or isometrics (Image 1) can be added to increase effort.
- Combined Donor with Passive Recipient Exercise
  At follow-up therapy visits, the patient is instructed in combined donor-recipient exercises to strengthen the new motor pathway. This would include active wrist flexion with passive or "assisted" elbow flexion in supination,

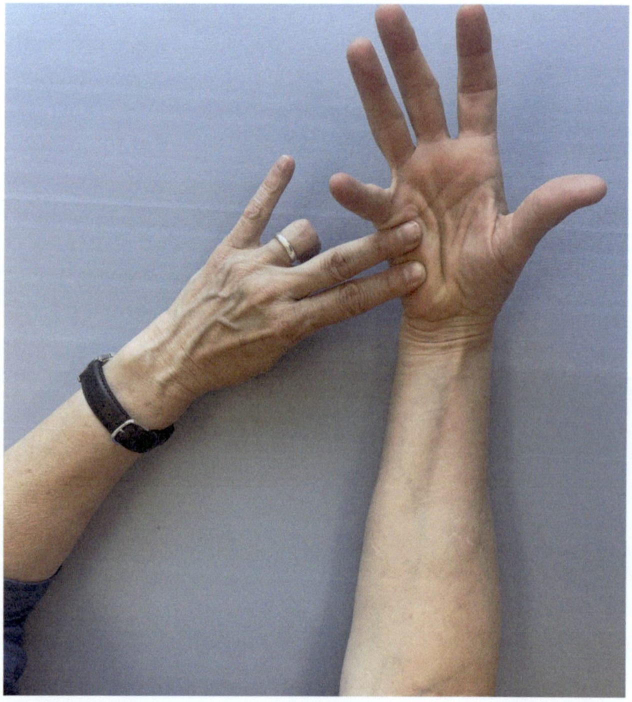

Image 1 Donor activation is performed by flexing the wrist in slight ulnar deviation at a frequency of 10×/hour. Resistance may be added, as shown

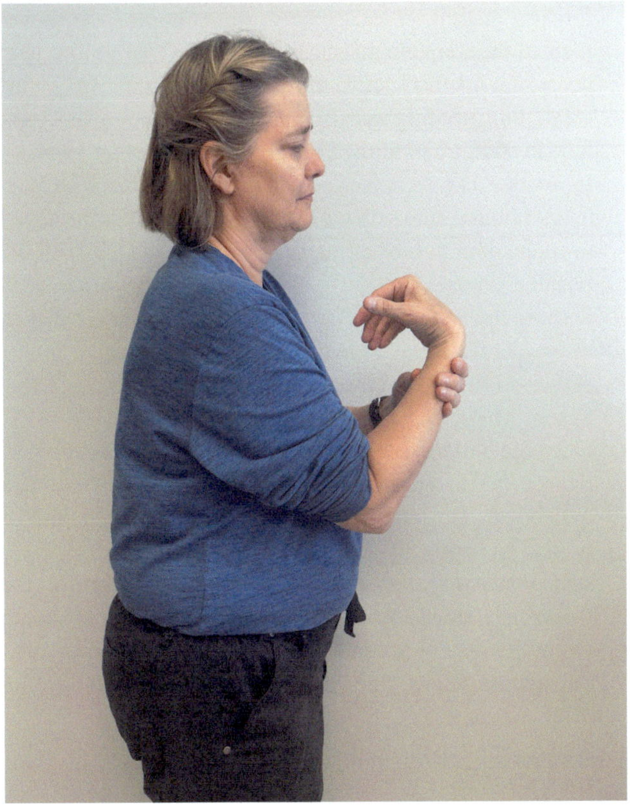

Image 2 An example of combined donor with passive recipient exercise is demonstrated. The individual is instructed to flex the wrist while the uninvolved hand passively flexes the elbow in supinated position

performed at a high frequency (10–20 repetitions, 6–8 times per day) with no resistance (Image 2).

Assessment of Recovery

Once therapy visits occur on a monthly basis (see below section on therapy frequency), biceps function is routinely reassessed. Reinnervation of the muscle is assessed as the patient performs active or resisted wrist flexion while supported in forearm supination and in varying degrees of elbow flexion. The examiner simultaneously palpates the biceps muscle or tendon to evaluate for contraction (Image 3). Once patients can partially flex the elbow in a gravity-minimized plane, they may progress to phase 2 of rehabilitation.

Therapy Frequency

Patients may attend their first therapy visit around 2 weeks postoperatively. In the first 6 weeks, they may be seen approximately 4–6 total visits depending on their physical recovery, distance to travel, and insurance coverage. Patients are seen more frequently (as needed 2–3 times per week) if they have passive joint limitations, high pain or nerve sensitivity, excessive swelling, and/or stiffness in uninvolved joints. Patients often need more therapy sessions if they undergo multiple nerve transfers at the same time.

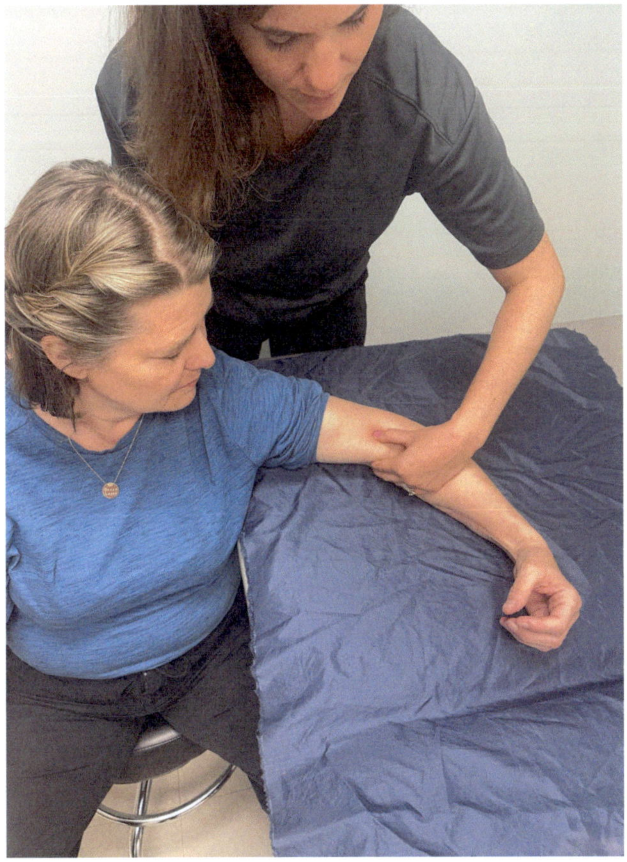

Image 3 Assessment of recovery of biceps function is performed with the arm supported in supination and partial elbow flexion in a gravity lessened plane. The examiner resists wrist flexion while palpating along the biceps muscle and tendon for a change in tension or movement

Phase 2

2−/5 to 3/5 MMT in the Recipient Muscle

Patients may progress to phase 2 of rehabilitation once they can partially flex the elbow in a gravity-minimized plane. At this point in recovery, the patient should be reliable with his or her home exercise program and demonstrate a good understanding of the donor-recipient muscle relationship. Phase 2 exercises advance from passive to active movement of the biceps. Exercises are performed in a gravity-minimized or *assisted* plane while demanding a strong contraction of the FCU. All exercises should be designed to make the movement easier for the biceps. This may be accomplished using a slick cloth under the forearm, an arm skate, and/or gravity-minimized positions of the extremity [7]. The patient should continue intermittent use of the elbow sling in phase 2 to minimize fatigue and prevent overstretching of the biceps muscle [9, 10]. The patient may remove the sling for light activity, rest, and therapy exercises.

Exercises

- Active Donor with Active-Assisted Recipient
  Biceps MMT = 2−/5 to 2/5

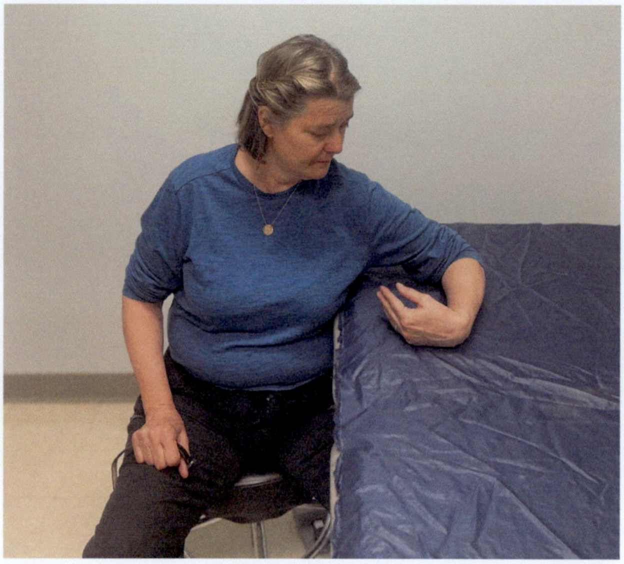

Image 4 Active donor with assisted recipient muscle exercise is demonstrated in sitting. The arm is abducted on a raised surface to reduce the effect of gravity. The individual is instructed to flex the wrist while attempting to flex the elbow with assistance of the opposite hand with friction reduced by the slick fabric to make it easier for the weak arm to move

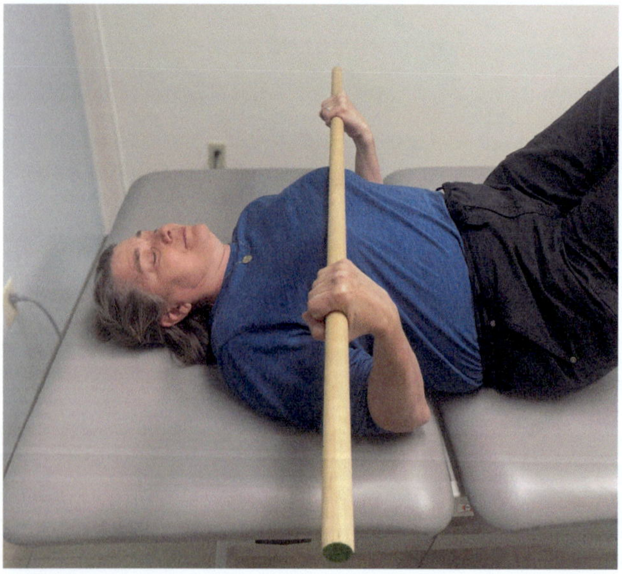

Image 5 Active donor with assisted recipient muscle exercise can also be performed in supine. Using a dowel in both supinated hands, the uninvolved arm assists with bilateral elbow flexion as the individual is instructed to flex the wrists

In the first exercise of phase 2, the patient is positioned in a gravity-minimized plane. He or she may be seated with the arm resting on a table or mat. The arm is supported in shoulder abduction (approximately 60–90°) and the forearm in neutral rotation. The patient first flexes the wrist and attempts active elbow flexion, sliding the forearm along the table (Image 4). To make the movement easier for the biceps, the forearm may rest on a slick cloth or an arm skate. The patient may also try this in a pool, with the forearm resting on a kickboard, for example. The movement of the recipient muscle is considered "active assisted" because it involves active movement, but the biceps is still weak, thus needing assistance from gravity or a slick surface in addition to limited support from the other hand.
In another exercise, the patient may be supine with both hands holding onto a dowel rod. The patient holds the dowel in supination, flexes both wrists, and simultaneously flexes bilateral elbows (Image 5). This movement is "assisted" because the contralateral arm assists the movement, which also occurs in a gravity-minimized plane (supine).

- "Place and Hold" Exercise
  Biceps MMT = 2+/5
  Once the patient can actively flex the biceps through partial movement against gravity, a "place and hold" exercise may begin. The patient may be seated or standing, and he or she passively places the elbow in full flexion while strongly flexing the wrist (Image 6a). The support to the forearm is slowly released from the contralateral hand, while the patient attempts to maintain active elbow flexion against gravity (Image 6b) while maintaining a strong FCU contraction.
- Active Donor with Active Recipient
  Biceps MMT= 3−/5 to 3/5
  Anti-gravity exercise may begin once the patient can actively flex the elbow more than 50% range of motion (approximately 65°). The patient may perform a few repetitions of active elbow flexion routinely throughout the day, slowly and with cues to avoid fatigue. The patient should continue to first demand a strong contraction of the FCU prior to anti-gravity elbow flexion (Image 7). Patients should be cued to supinate the forearm while flexing the elbow, as this is the primary action of the biceps and is argued to be more functionally useful compared to elbow flexion in pronation.
- Functional Activity
  Once patients can perform active elbow flexion against gravity, they should try to incorporate this movement into functional tasks throughout the day. Elbow flexion is crucial for eating and grooming. Examples of functional activities would be bringing a fork to the mouth, washing the face, and bringing a brush to the hair (Image 8). Each of these tasks becomes more challenging as the end target is anatomically more superior compared to the preceding one. If the patient lacks hand function, the goal of an FCU-to-biceps transfer is to support items in the forearm as the elbow is flexed to 90°. An example of a functional activity in this scenario may be holding a fork and bring it to their mouth with their elbow supported in a gravity lessened plane.
- Therapy Frequency
  Therapy visits in phase 2 may occur on a weekly basis (or two times per month depending on the patient's needs), which is increased in frequency compared to phase 1.

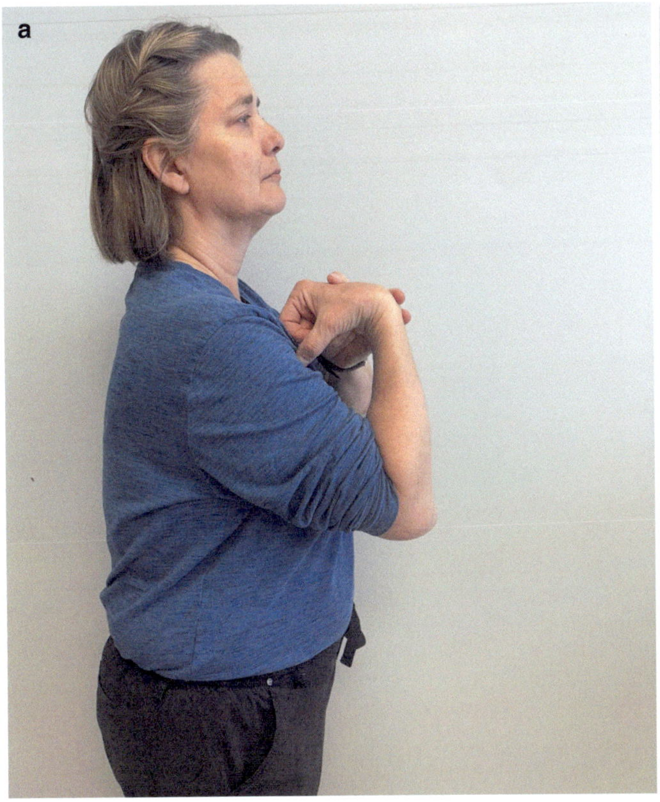

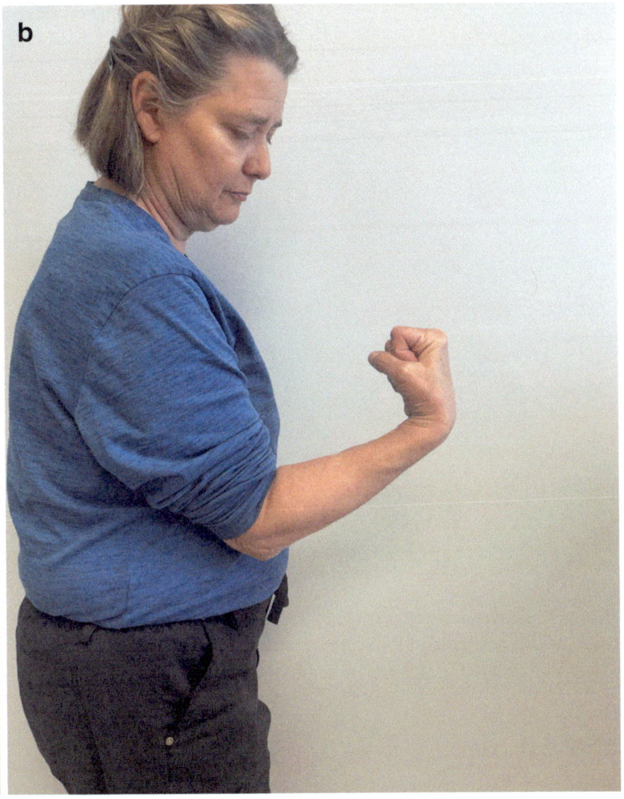

Image 6 (**a**) "Place and hold" elbow flexion is performed by placing the elbow in end range elbow flexion and supination with firm activation of the donor FCU (wrist flexion towards the small finger side). (**b**) "Place and hold" is completed as the support from the uninvolved hand is removed as the individual is cued to attempt to maintain wrist flexion and elbow flexion

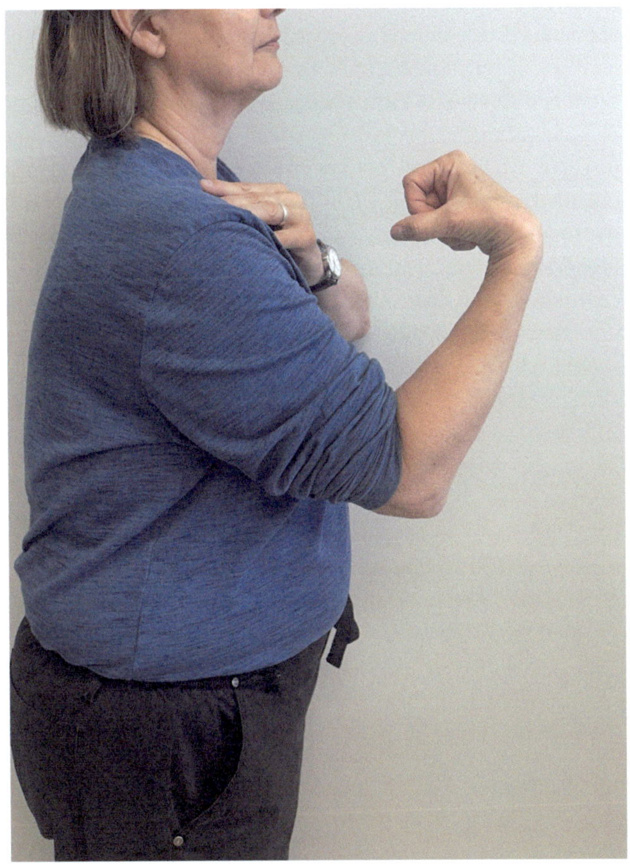

Image 7 An active donor with active recipient exercise is demonstrated in an anti-gravity position. The individual is instructed to flex the wrist to the ulnar side as she attempts to flex the elbow

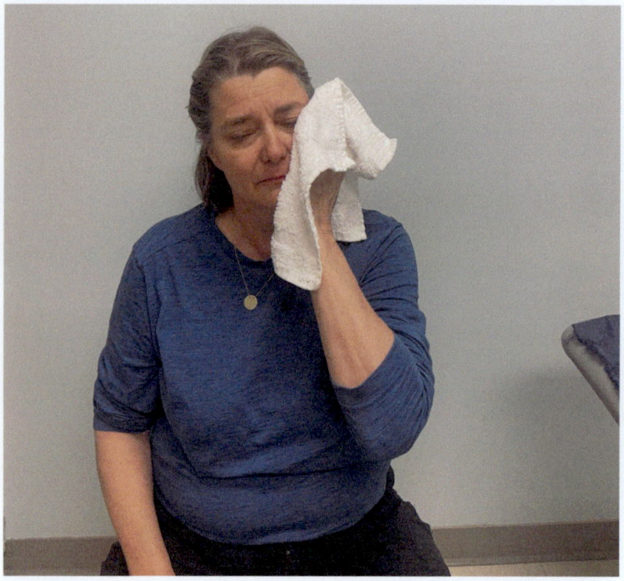

Image 8 Functional activities are encouraged as elbow flexion strength returns. One example of anti-gravity elbow flexion is teaching the individual to wash his or her face with the involved hand

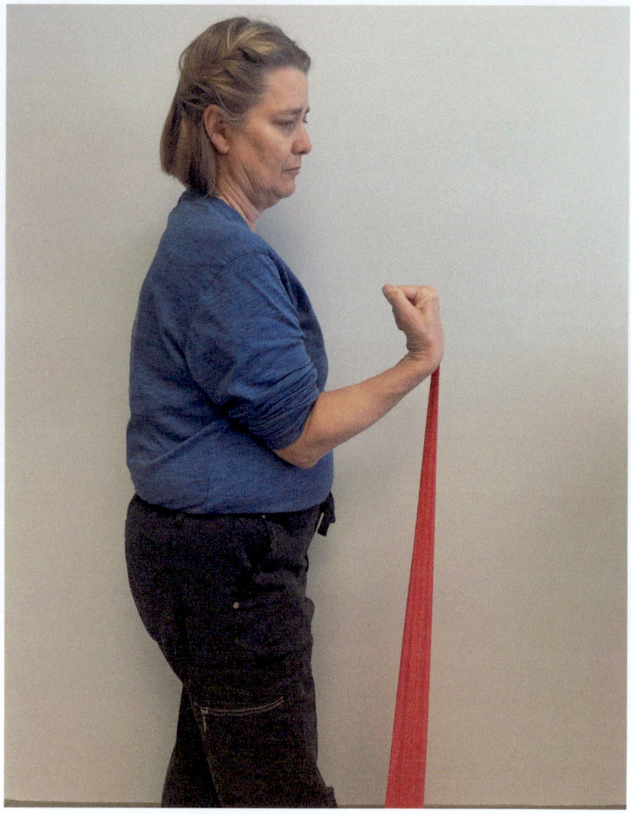

Image 9 Strengthening with resistance to the biceps occurs in phase 3. Early in this phase co-contraction of the FCU is often needed to develop adequate strength to flex the elbow against a resistance band

Phase 3

3+/5 MMT in the Recipient Muscle

Late-phase therapy begins once the biceps muscle demonstrates the ability to flex the elbow through full motion against gravity and withstand slight pressure. The use of an elbow sling is no longer necessary on a full-time basis. Patients should be encouraged to continue to wear it intermittently until fatigue and loss of function are no longer an issue. The presence of a dominant antagonist triceps will also affect this decision. Phase 3 is characterized by resistive exercise. It is imperative that resistive exercise does not begin before 3/5 MMT strength is obtained as this often leads to fatigue, frustration, and ineffective recruitment of the target muscle. In order to prevent fatigue, high frequency/low resistance should remain an important concept during this time. As biceps strength increases, exercises may slowly exclude the assistive action of the FCU. Therapists should educate patients on realistic outcomes such that final strength grades vary among patients. Additionally, it may take 2–3 years to obtain maximal strength, and pre-injury elbow flexion (5/5 MMT) is rarely achieved [11].

Exercises

- Resistive Recipient Activity with Donor Contraction
  Resistive elbow flexion begins with simultaneous contraction of the FCU. This may involve holding a resistance band and flexing the elbow in supination while the wrist maintains a flexed position (Image 9). Maintaining wrist flexion will augment biceps power, which may be functionally useful when additional elbow flexion strength is needed.
- Resistive Recipient Activity Without Donor Contraction
  Once patients demonstrate consistent, synergistic elbow flexion with wrist flexion, they may learn to separate the two functions. For example, patients may work on resistive elbow flexion with the wrist in neutral extension in order to have sufficient biceps strength during ADLs that require varying wrist positions (Image 10).
- Therapy Frequency
  Once patients achieve a 3+/5 MMT grade, therapy visits occur once a week or every other week. Exercises are reviewed and advanced depending on biceps strength and functional needs of the patient.

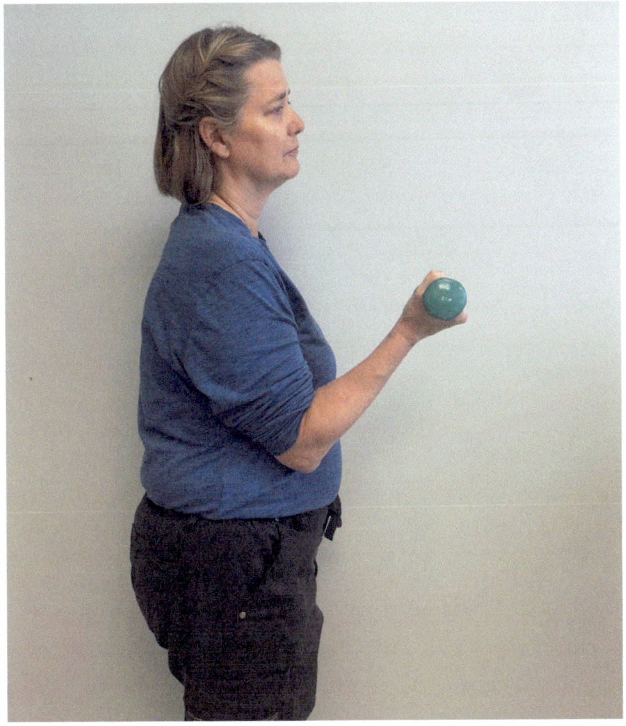

Image 10 Separation of donor from recipient is addressed once there is adequate biceps strength. The individual is instructed to maintain the wrist in varying degrees of wrist extension while attempting to flex the elbow with resistance

FCU to Biceps nerve transfer

Nerve transfer overview					
Donor nerve	Donor action	Recipient nerve	Recipient action	Indications for functional restoration	Approximate months to functional movement
Ulnar nerve branch to the flexor carpi ulnaris	Wrist flexion with ulnar deviation	Musculocutaneous nerve branch to the biceps	Elbow flexion with supination	Loss of elbow flexion	12 months [3, 6]

Information below are suggested guidelines. Precautions may vary according to surgeon preferences and patient factors

	Preoperative therapy	Early phase	Middle phase	Late phase
Criteria	Before surgery	0/5–1/5 MMT	2-/5 to 3/5 MMT	>3/5 MMT
Purpose of Phase	Educate and establish baseline function	Understand donor and recipient relationship	Consistently activate recipient	Strengthen recipient and separate from donor activation
Precautions	Prevent pronation and extension contractures of the forearm and elbow	Protect elbow flexor length	Respect fatigue and prevent dominance of triceps	Avoid resisted elbow flexion until consistent 3/5 MMT is achieved
Frequency of visits (considerations)	1–2 pre-op visits May increase if PROM limitations exist	1×/week until PROM is within-normal-limits and patient is independent with donor activation; then 1× monthly	1× per week to 1× per month based on patient needs and accurate, consistent demonstration of exercise program	1× every 1–2 weeks based on progress toward patient-specific goals
Orthosis considerations	NA	Full-time sling for the first 3 weeks. OK to remove for hygiene. Replace with other elbow support as needed after 3 weeks	Continue intermittent sling use to protect the length of the recovering biceps muscle	NA unless fatigue remains an issue
Interventions	PROM if patient lacks passive supination and elbow flexion	**Donor Activation:** Wrist flexion with ulnar deviation **Donor-Recipient Pairing**: Active wrist flexion with passive elbow flexion in supination	**Active/Resisted Donor with Active Assisted Recipient:** Supine dowel rod exercise: bilateral wrist flexion in supination with active-*assisted* elbow flexion Gravity minimized plane: Arm supported on table at shoulder height: wrist flexion with active elbow flexion using towel or arm skate **Place and Hold**: Passively place the elbow in end-range flexion and supination (while flexing wrist). Remove support from the contralateral hand and attempt to maintain this position	**Resisted Donor and Recipient:** Holding weights or resistance bands, the patient performs an elbow curl while the forearm is in supination and the wrist is flexed **Resisted Recipient:** Holding weights or resistance bands, the patient flexes the elbow with the forearm supinated and the wrist is in neutral or extension
Additional interventions			Active-assisted elbow flexion precedes active elbow flexion Gravity minimized recipient movement precedes anti-gravity recipient movement	

During all phases it is essential to continue cortical reorganization, psychological and psychosocial interventions, and progress to incorporate donor/recipient with ADLs

FCU to Biceps Nerve Transfer

Goal of Surgery: Restore the ability to bend the elbow and bring the hand to the face.

Recipient Movement = Bend Elbow and Turn Palm Up (Elbow Flexion and Forearm Supination)

Recipient Muscle: Biceps

Recipient Nerve: Musculocutaneous Nerve

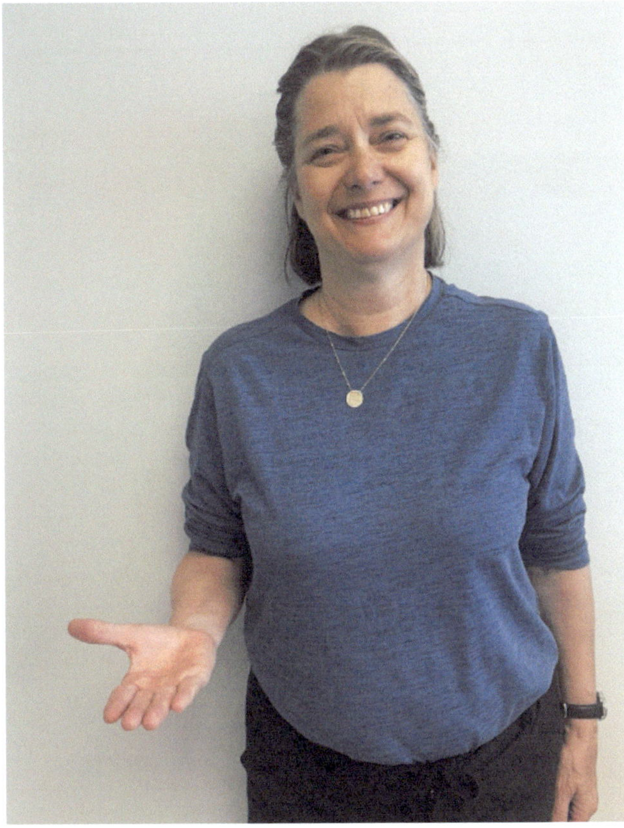

Donor Movement = Bend Wrist Forward (Wrist Flexion)
Donor Muscle: Flexor Carpi Ulnaris (FCU)
Donor Nerve: Ulnar Nerve

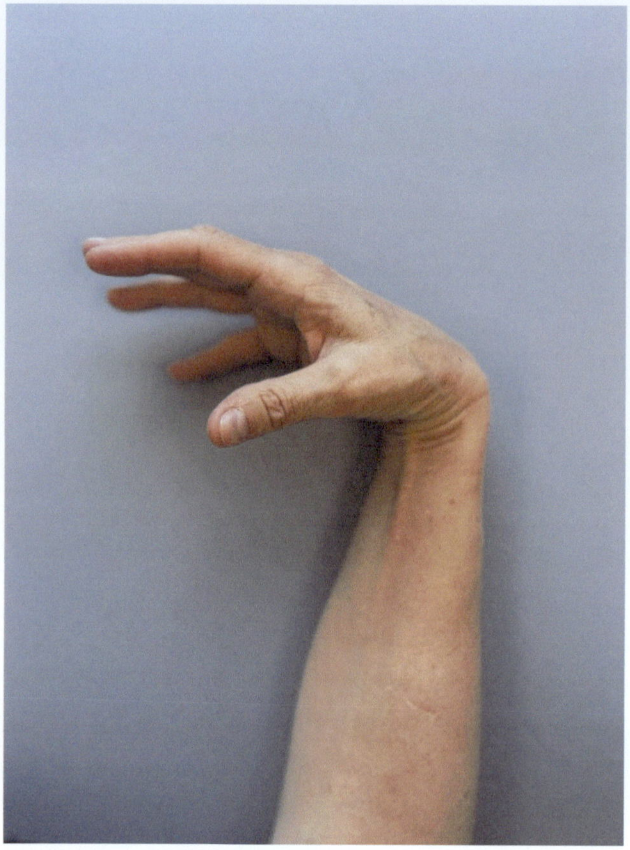

Phase 1 FCU to Biceps Nerve Transfer Exercises

Use a sling to keep your elbow bent and your forearm resting with your palm up to protect your transfer during the day.

☐ **Active or Resisted Donor Movement:**

Complete one of the below exercises 10 repetitions, every waking hour.

1. Sit with your elbow bent and your forearm resting on a table. With your palm facing up, bend your wrist forward. Return to the start position and repeat.

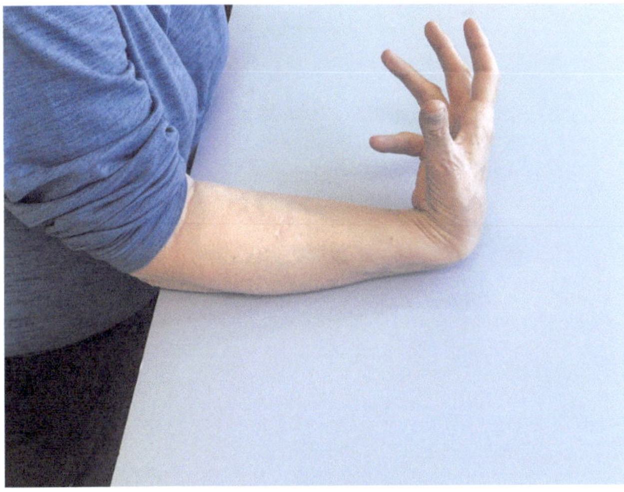

2. Sit with your elbow bent and your forearm resting on a table. With your palm facing up, slowly bend your wrist forward. Using your other hand, apply gentle resistance to the small finger side of your palm as you bend your wrist forward. You may complete the motion with your opposite hand. Return to the start position and repeat.

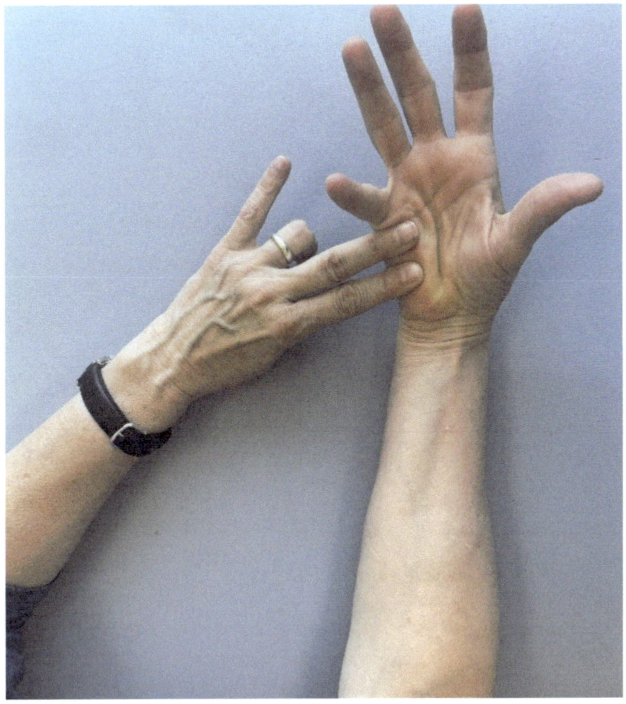

☐ **Active Donor + Passive Recipient Movement:**

Sit or stand with your arm by your side. Using your other hand, support your forearm with the palm up and elbow bent. Bend your wrist forward. Using your other hand, bend your elbow to bring your hand toward your shoulder.

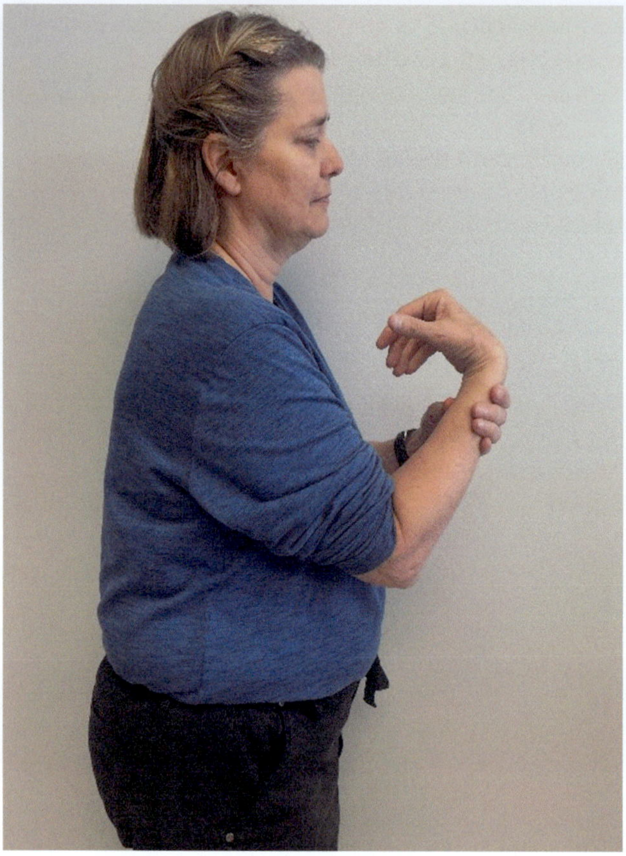

Complete 10 repetitions, 3 times per day

Phase 2 FCU to Biceps Nerve Transfer Exercises

Wear your sling throughout the day. Remove for light activity, rest, and during therapy exercises.

☐ **Active Donor + Active-Assisted Recipient Movement:**

Complete one of the below exercises 10 repetitions, 3 times per day.

1. While seated, begin with your arm supported on a table out to your side with your elbow bent and the thumb side of your hand facing the ceiling. Rest your forearm on a slick cloth such as a pillowcase or piece of nylon (pictured). Bend your wrist forward as you try to bend your elbow, sliding your forearm toward you. You may complete the motion with your opposite hand. Return to the start position and repeat.

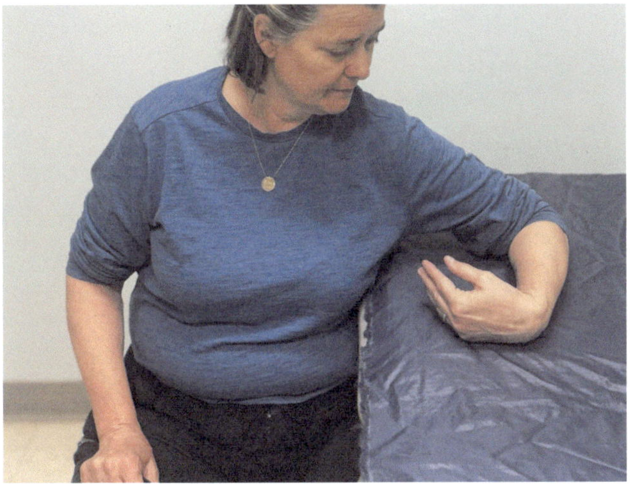

2. Lying on your back, hold a dowel, broomstick, or cane with both hands in a palm-up position. Begin with your arms down by your side and elbows straight. First, curl both wrists forward as you bend your elbows and bring the dowel toward your chest. Return to the start position and repeat.

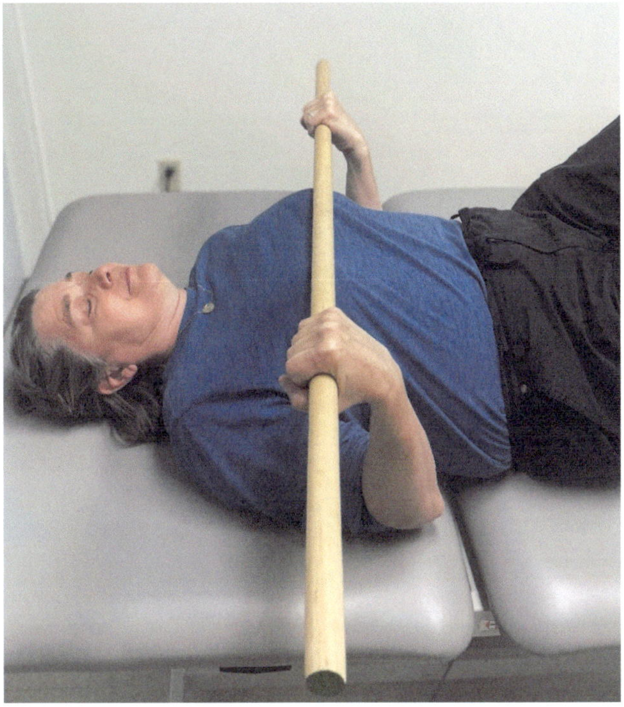

☐ **"Place and Hold" Exercise**

Begin sitting or standing with the arm by your side. Firmly bend your wrist forward. Using your other hand to support the forearm, bend your elbow. Keep your wrist bent and SLOWLY let go of your forearm as you try to keep the elbow bent without the help of your other hand.

Hold 3–5 seconds. Return to the start position and repeat.

- Start by only bending your elbow halfway.
- As strength improves, bend your elbow as far as it will comfortably go.
- Try to maintain a palm-up position during this exercise.

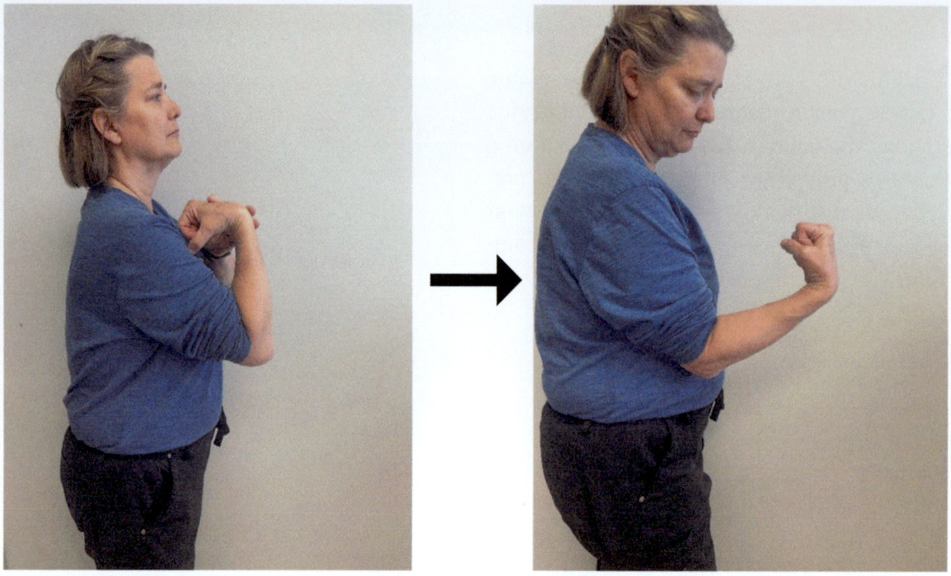

Complete 1–10 repetitions, 2–3 times per day

☐ **Active Donor + Active Recipient Movement:**

Begin sitting or standing with the arm by your side. Firmly bend your wrist forward as you bend your elbow on your own (no assistance from your other hand). Reach your hand toward your shoulder. If this is too difficult, begin the exercise with your elbow supported in a partially bent position.

Complete 5–10 repetitions, 3 times per day

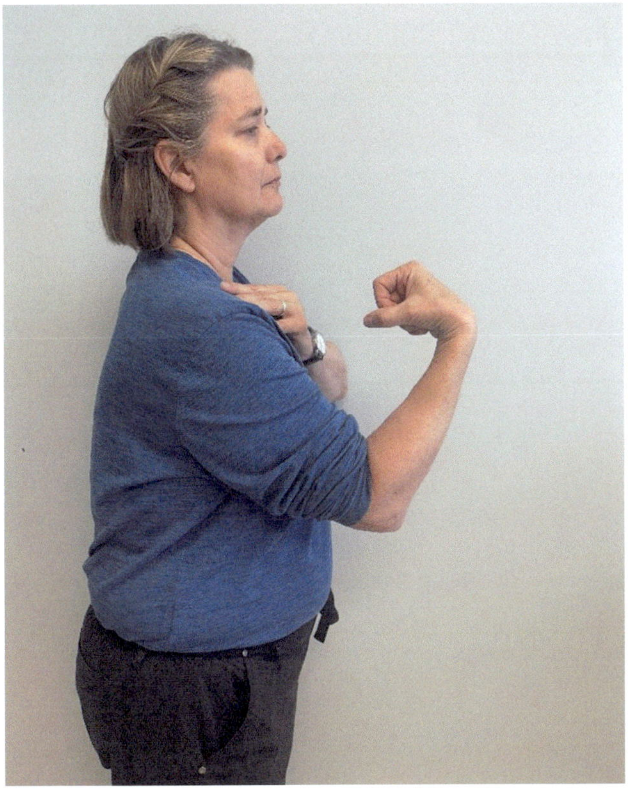

Phase 3 FCU to Biceps Nerve Transfer Exercises

☐ **Resisted Donor + Resisted Recipient Movement:**

In sitting, hold a resistance band in your hand with your palm up and arm by your side. Pull the resistance band by strongly bending your wrist forward. Then, bend your elbow, pulling the band toward your shoulder. Return to the start position and repeat.

Complete 5–10 repetitions, 2–3 times per day.

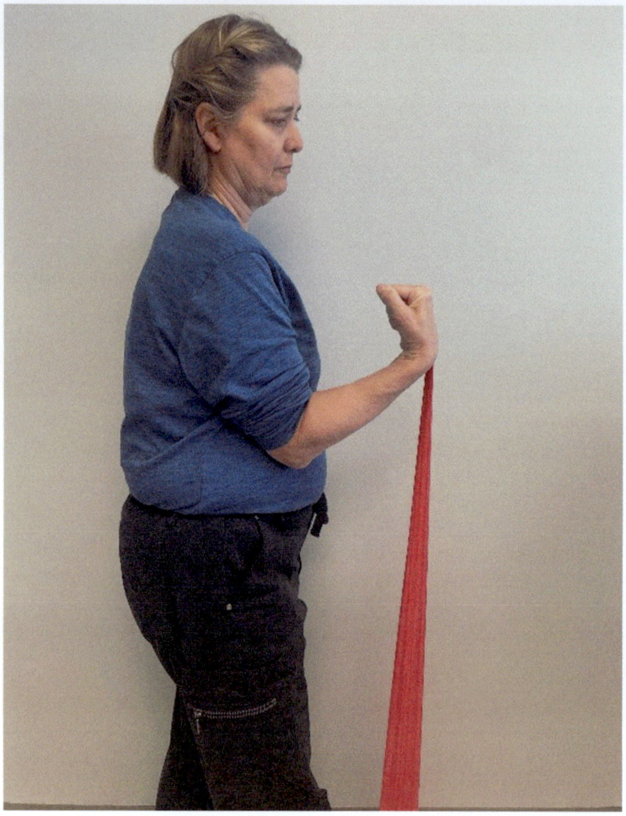

☐ **Resisted Recipient Movement without donor co-contraction:**

Complete one of the below exercises 5–10 repetitions, 2–3 times per day.

Complete the following exercises while standing, if able. *Try to avoid bending your wrist forward or bending your body forward.*

1. Use a __________ pound weight. Hold the weight with your palm up and arm by your side. Bend your elbow to bring the weight toward your shoulder. Then, slowly lower the weight back down to the start position. Repeat.

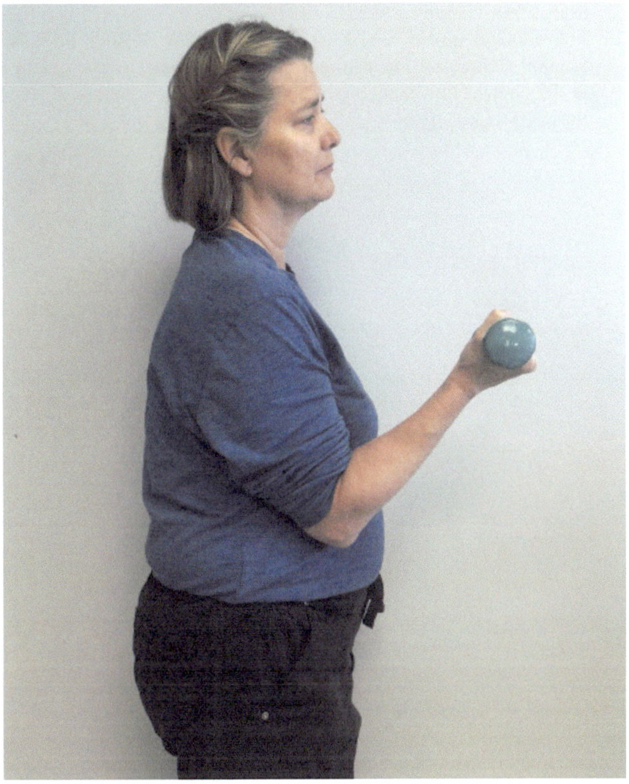

2. Hold a resistance band in your hand with your palm up and arm by your side. Bend your elbow, pulling the band toward your shoulder. Then, slowly straighten your elbow back to the start position and repeat.

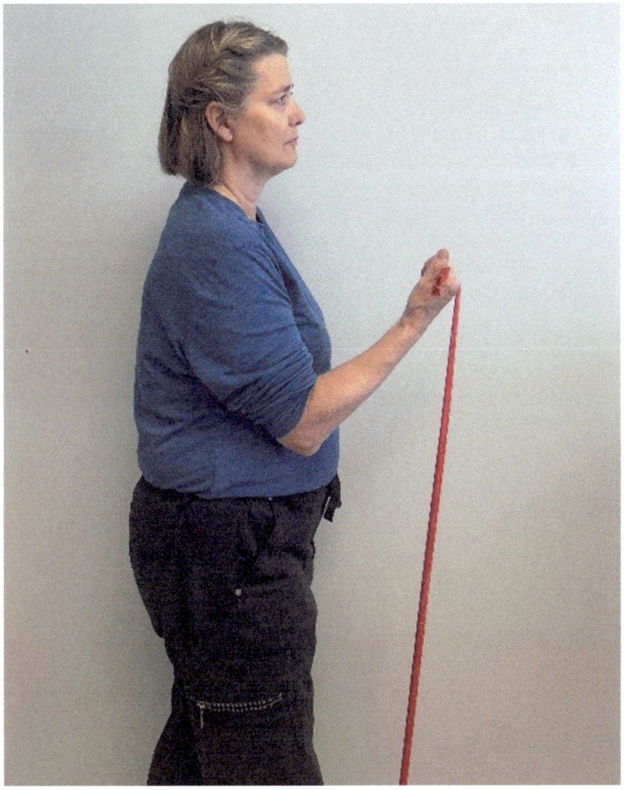

References

1. Oberlin C, Beal D, Leechavengvongs S, Salon A, Dauge MC, Sarcy JJ. Nerve transfer to biceps muscle using a part of ulnar nerve for C5–C6 avulsion of the brachial plexus: anatomical study and report of four cases. J Hand Surg. 1994;19(2):232–7.
2. Loy S, Bhatia A, Asfazadourian H, Oberlin C. Ulnar nerve fascicle transfer onto to the biceps muscle nerve in C5-C6 or C5-C6-C7 avulsions of the brachial plexus. Eighteen cases. Ann Hand Upper Limb Surg. 1997;16(4):275–84.
3. Sedain G, Sharma M, Sharma B, Mahapatra A. Outcome after delayed Oberlin transfer in brachial plexus injury. Neurosurgery. 2011;69(4):822–7.
4. Mackinnon SE, Novak CB, Myckatyn TM, Tung TH. Results of reinnervation of the biceps and brachialis muscles with a double fascicular transfer for elbow flexion. J Hand Surg. 2005;30(5):978–85.
5. Donnelly MR, Rezzadeh KT, Vieira D, Daar D, Hacquebord J. Is one nerve transfer enough? A systematic review and pooled analysis comparing ulnar fascicular nerve transfer and double ulnar and median fascicular nerve transfer for restoration of elbow flexion after traumatic brachial plexus injury. Microsurgery. 2020;40(3):361–9.
6. Hill JL, Turner LC, Jones RD, et al. The stages of rehabilitation following motor nerve transfer surgery. J Musculoskelet Surg Res. 2019;3(60)
7. Kahn L, Moore A. Donor activation focused rehabilitation approach: maximizing outcomes after nerve transfers. Hand Clin. 2016;32(2):263–77.
8. Novak CB. Rehabilitation following motor nerve transfers. Hand Clin. 2008;24(4):417–23.
9. Goldspink G, Tabary C, Tabary JC, Tardieu C, Tardieu G. Effect of denervation on the adaptation of sarcomere number and muscle extensibility to the functional length of the muscle. J Physiol. 1974;236(3):733–42.
10. Gossman MR, Sahrmann SA, Rose SJ. Review of length-associated changes in muscle: experimental evidence and clinical implications. Phys Therapy. 1982;62(12):1799–808.
11. Merrell GA, Barrie KA, Katz DL, Wolfe SW. Results of nerve transfer techniques for restoration of shoulder and elbow function in the context of a meta-analysis of the English literature. J Hand Surg. 2001;26(2):303–14.

FCR/FDS Branch of the Median Nerve to Brachialis Branch of the Musculocutaneous Nerve Transfer

Elizabeth Westland

Background

The brachialis muscle is the prime mover of elbow flexion [1–4]. It sits deep to the biceps with the greatest muscle volume of the three elbow flexors and contributes to elbow flexion regardless of forearm position [1, 2]. The brachialis is innervated by the musculocutaneous nerve (MCN) and works in synergy with the biceps and the radial-innervated brachioradialis muscle.

The musculocutaneous nerve arises from the spinal roots C5, C6, and C7 and branches from the lateral cord of the brachial plexus [2, 3]. The nerve crosses the anterior shoulder to innervate the primary elbow flexors of the upper arm, the biceps and brachialis muscles, as well as the coracobrachialis which aids in shoulder flexion [3]. It innervates the elbow joint and terminates as the lateral antebrachial cutaneous nerve, which provides sensation to the radial side of the forearm [2, 3]. Injury to this nerve may result in loss of elbow flexion and forearm supination strength as well as loss of sensation to the radial forearm. A lack of elbow flexion is a devastating functional loss as this contributes to the daily motion of "bringing hand to face" for eating and grooming along with lifting and stabilization of objects. For patients with pan-plexus injuries, the restoration of elbow flexion is the most prioritized reconstructive goal among surgeons.

There are a variety of mechanisms in which the musculocutaneous nerve can be injured, most notably in motorcycle, car, and snowmobile accidents [4–7]. Isolated injuries to the musculocutaneous nerve are rare; however, etiology may include blunt trauma to the head or shoulder, penetrating injuries, and throwing injuries [3, 7].

Following injury to the musculocutaneous nerve, surgery may be recommended if there is no recovery of elbow flexion and no indication of potential recovery from electrodiagnostic testing at 3–6 months post-injury. There are a variety of surgical options available to restore elbow flexion. These include nerve transfers using donors from the ulnar nerve, thoracodorsal nerve, medial pectoral nerve, or median nerve [4–6]. The most cited of these options is the Oberlin procedure where the flexor carpi ulnaris (FCU) branch of the ulnar nerve is transferred to biceps. Given the fact that the biceps is a primary supinator and secondary elbow flexor, this surgery does not consistently generate sufficient strength or endurance to adequately provide functional elbow flexion. Outcomes following the single Oberlin procedure vary widely from excellent to poor results [5, 6, 8]. A double fascicular nerve transfer (DFT), which aims to reinnervate the brachialis muscle as well as the biceps, has been shown to improve outcomes allowing for stronger elbow flexion ability [6, 7]. The donor nerve for the brachialis is typically the median nerve branch to the flexor carpi radialis (FCR) and/or flexor digitorum superficialis (FDS). There is limited evidence available for outcomes of the isolated FCR/FDS-to-brachialis nerve transfer as the literature primarily describes it in the context of the DFT.

The median nerve is a viable option for this transfer due to the number of expendable fascicles available and close anatomic relationship to the brachialis branch of the MCN [5]. The median nerve arises from the spinal roots of C5, C6, C7, C8, and T1 and branches from the lateral and medial cords [2, 3]. It innervates the muscles of the radial forearm including

E. Westland (✉)
Athletico Physical Therapy/ Hand Therapy, Saint Louis, MO, USA

L. C. Kahn et al. (eds.), *Rehabilitation for Nerve Transfers of the Upper Extremity*, https://doi.org/10.1007/978-3-031-92008-0_14

pronator teres (PT), flexor carpi radialis (FCR), flexor digitorum superficialis (FDS), and palmaris longus (PL). The source of fascicles used for this nerve transfer to restore elbow flexion via the brachialis is typically the FCR and/or FDS. The FCR is responsible for wrist flexion and radial deviation. It may also assist with pronation of the forearm and flexion of the elbow. The FDS flexes the proximal interphalangeal joints of the second, third, fourth, and fifth digits. It also assists with flexion of the metacarpophalangeal joints and with flexion of the wrist.

Surgical Description

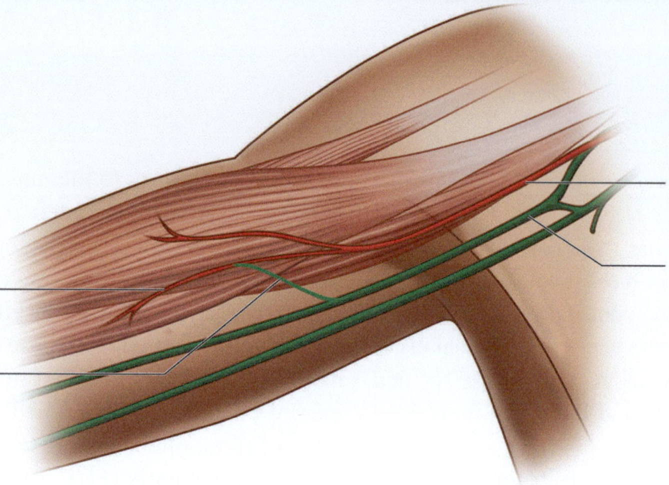

Microsurgical technique of FCR/FDS branch of the median nerve to brachialis branch of the musculocutaneous nerve transfer

A longitudinal incision is made along the mid-brachial sulcus. The musculocutaneous nerve is identified deep to the biceps muscle, in the intramuscular interval between the biceps and brachialis. The branch from the musculocutaneous nerve to the brachialis muscle is identified. Intraoperative stimulation is used to confirm whether the brachialis branch responds. It is important to ensure that there are no muscle paralytics being used by the anesthesia team. The median nerve is then identified adjacent to the brachial artery. Intraoperative stimulation is used to confirm the identity of the median nerve, and an internal neurolysis is performed to select a portion of the median nerve that matches the caliber of the recipient brachialis branch. When selecting the donor fascicle, it is important to ensure that stimulation of the donor fascicle is predominantly resulting in wrist flexion and PIP flexion (and not thenar function, finger DIP flexion, or thumb IP flexion). The donor fascicle is neurolyzed from the remainder of the ulnar nerve and divided distally. The recipient biceps branch is neurolyzed from the musculocutaneous nerve and divided proximally. Coaptation of the FCR/FDS branch of the median nerve to the brachialis branch is performed using microsurgical technique. Surgeons may also consider transferring a portion of the ulnar nerve to the biceps branch of the musculocutaneous nerve.

Outcomes

There is limited research available on outcomes for this surgery in isolation. Available data refers to outcomes following the FCU to biceps (Oberlin 1) and FCR/FDS to brachialis (Oberlin 2) together, the double fascicular nerve transfer (DFT), as coined by Mackinnon. When performed as a part of a DFT, the ability to regain elbow flexion function is greater than with the FCU-to-biceps nerve transfer alone [4–8]. The average length of time for the first sign of reinnervation for elbow flexion has been documented to occur between 5.3 and 5.5 months from surgery [4, 6, 7]. Long-term outcomes when a double fascicular nerve transfer is performed yield excellent to good recovery of elbow flexion with most patients regaining a muscle strength of 4/5 MMT or greater [4–6, 8].

Phases of Rehabilitation

Phase 1

Preoperative to 1/5 MMT in the recipient muscle

Preoperative

Preoperative therapy includes baseline motor function assessment and clarification of expectations for postoperative therapy. Evaluation measurements should include active (AROM) and passive (PROM) range of motion of the shoulder, elbow, forearm, wrist, and digits. It is important to determine the extent of the nerve injury, as damage to the entirety of the musculocutaneous nerve will have implications for the shoulder as well as the elbow. In the setting of an upper trunk injury, complete assessment of the shoulder is warranted as this injury would severely affect shoulder function in addition to elbow flexion. Communication with the referring physician is important to confirm the extent of nerve injury and to ensure that there are no precautions regarding ROM at the shoulder. If there are no shoulder precautions but deficits are present, ROM is initiated in all planes. Patients should maintain full passive flexion of the elbow prior to surgery. Therapists may educate patients to protect the recipient elbow flexor length, especially in the setting of absent musculocutaneous nerve function [9]. A sling (or other device) that maintains the elbow in flexion is recommended. Baseline sensation measurements of the involved limb, especially the lateral forearm, are also included in the preoperative evaluation.

Postoperative Management

Following surgery, the patient is placed in a surgical dressing and a sling. If a drain is used at the surgical site, it is typically removed 2–3 days postoperatively. Caution should be taken to limit shoulder abduction and elbow extension. Sling use will continue at least until the postoperative dressing is removed, between post-op days 10 and 14. At that time, therapy may begin or resume. ROM restrictions of the shoulder or elbow are rare following the postoperative rest period. If continued precautions exist, it is likely because other surgical procedures were simultaneously performed. Closure of the surgical site in the medial arm is performed with sutures, glue, or staples. Wound care preferences will be physician specific, and it is important to be in contact with the surgeon regarding these preferences to appropriately educate patients.

During the first postoperative visit, instruction is given in edema management and wound care. Exercise instruction will include "donor flooding" (wrist and finger flexion) as well as AROM of uninvolved joints. Passive elbow flexion is encouraged to optimize joint mobility. Passive elbow extension is generally unnecessary due to the unopposed active of the triceps muscle. During this early postoperative period, it is important to educate patients on expectations, healing timelines, expected outcomes, postoperative precautions, and donor activation.

Precautions

For the first 10–14 days after surgery, full-time sling use and restricted shoulder and elbow motion are required. Following that time, a sling or other form of elbow flexion support is strongly encouraged when the person is standing or walking, to avoid overlengthening the elbow flexor muscles [9–12].

Exercises

- ROM of Uninvolved Joints
  Maintenance of shoulder and hand mobility is important for activities of daily living and is needed to ensure that no secondary complications (i.e., joint stiffness) occur. Exercises may include table slides into shoulder flexion, pendulum exercises, or dowel exercises. Postural exercises are encouraged to counteract sling use and sustained arm positioning. If needed, scapular retraction, chin tucks, and/or side-lying scapular clocks may be added to the home exercise program.
- Donor Activation
  If flexor carpi radialis (FCR) was used at the donor, active or isometric wrist flexion should be performed.
  If flexor digitorum superficialis (FDS) was used as the donor, the following exercises may be included in the home exercise program: active straight fist, tendon gliding exercises (Image 1), and/or putty gripping into a full fist or straight fist.
- Combined Donor with Passive Recipient Exercise
  The patient activates the donor muscle (straight fist for FDS and/or wrist flexion for FCR) while passively flexing the elbow in a gravity-lessened plane, such as on a table with a nylon material to reduce friction [12] (Image 2). Brachialis function is biased when the forearm is positioned in pronation. This puts the biceps and brachioradialis at some disadvantage to increase isolation of the brachialis muscle. Because the recipient movement (elbow flexion) is purely passive in this stage, active-donor with passive-recipient exercise could also be against gravity.

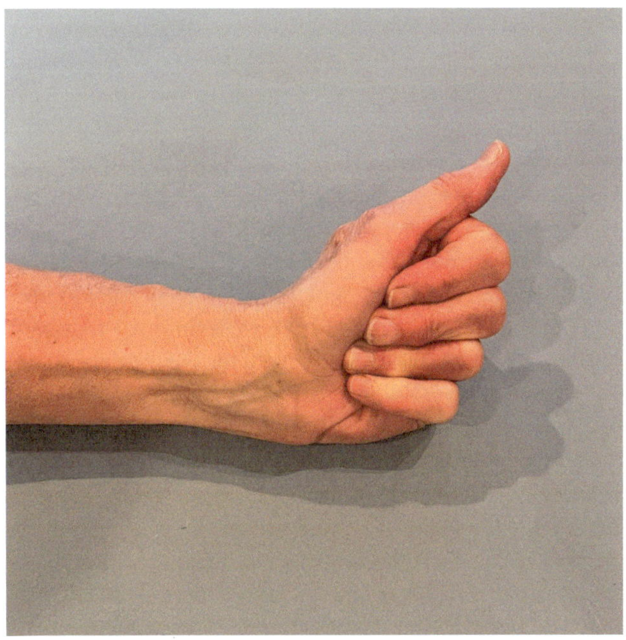

Image 1 If a median branch to the flexor digitorum superficialis (FDS) is included in the donor nerves early activation exercises should include straight or flat fist. With the DIP joints in extension, flexing the MP and PIP joints favors the FDS muscle

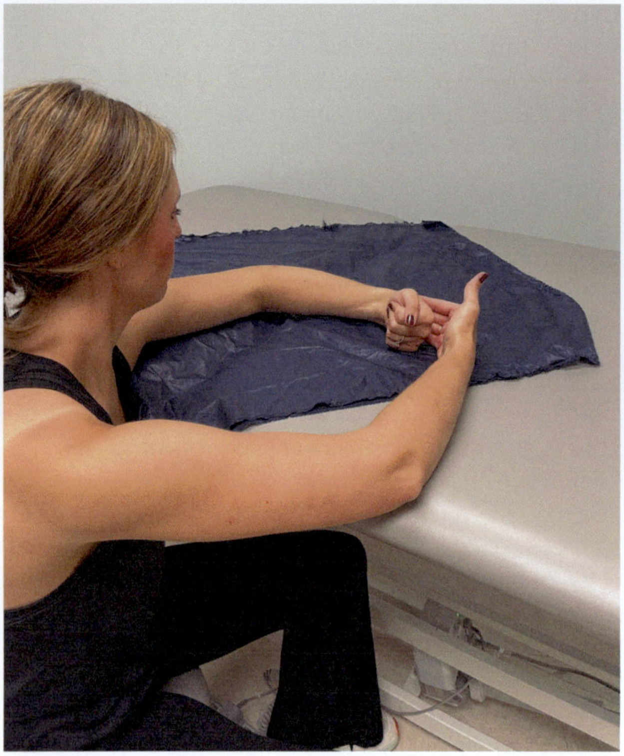

Image 2 Combined donor with passive recipient exercises are achieved by flexing the fingers and/or wrist while passively flexing the elbow in a gravity lessened plane

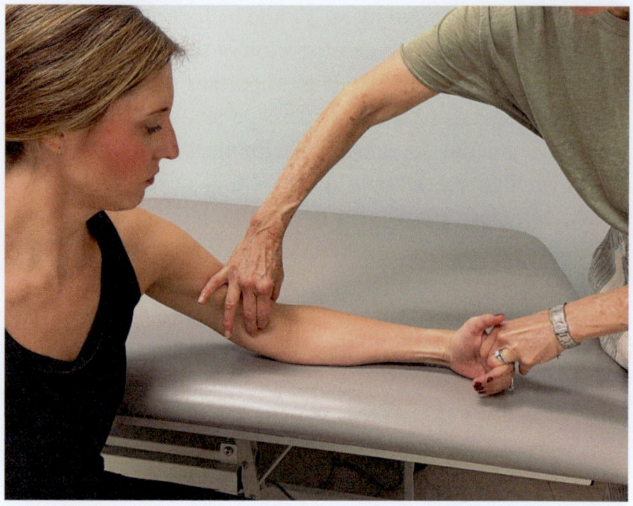

Image 3 To assess for early recovery of the brachialis muscle position the arm on a table and resist finger and /or wrist flexion while palpating for the brachialis on either side of the biceps tendon where tension in the muscle can be more easily perceived

Assessment of Recovery

To evaluate for recipient brachialis reinnervation, resistance is applied to the donor (wrist flexion/FCR or finger flexion/FDS) as the patient attempts active elbow flexion from a partially flexed position (Image 3). The examiner palpates the brachialis muscle for signs of contraction. The lateral edge of the brachialis can be palpated from the deltoid tuberosity distally down the lateral side of the upper arm; however, it is easiest to identify the muscle distally on the humerus by palpating medial and lateral to the biceps tendon where the flat wide distal portion of the brachialis is exposed. If there is a twitch in the brachialis muscle, the patient should then attempt independent active elbow flexion in a gravity-minimized position, i.e., seated with the arm abducted on a table/mat around 70–90 degrees of shoulder abduction.

Therapy Frequency

Frequency of visits in this phase will vary greatly depending on the needs of the individual patient. Factors to consider when establishing frequency of visits should include patient anxiety, understanding of precautions, understanding of basic donor-recipient exercise concepts, and insurance limitations. If patients have limitations in passive ROM, difficulty understanding donor/recipient concepts, or issues with wound closure or hypersensitivity, they should be seen once a week for a few weeks. If patients have near-full PROM, no pain, normal wound healing, and a basic understanding of motor reeducation concepts, they could be seen once or twice per month.

Phase 2

2−/5 to 3/5 MMT in the Recipient Muscle

Once the patient can partially flex the elbow in a gravity-lessened plane, phase 2 of therapy is initiated. During this time, regaining elbow flexion will be the most feasible in gravity-lessened positions while the brachialis is slowly gaining strength. These include supine, side lying, and seated with the shoulder abducted to 70–90°. During this phase, there is an increased focus on pairing the donor and recipient muscle actions. Activities should be performed to the level of fatigue but not beyond it. This will be patient specific and will vary over time limiting the sets and repetitions that one is able to perform. Phase 1 exercises can be performed as a warm-up and are not necessarily discontinued. Use of a sling or hip support for the arm (Image 4) is encouraged to maintain the recipient brachialis in a shortened position. This may minimize the risk of the recipient muscle overlengthening, which limits the muscle's ability to generate sufficient force once it is reinnervated [9–12].

Exercises

- Active Donor with Active-Assistive Recipient Brachialis MMT = 2−/5 to 2/5
  The patient is seated with the shoulder abducted 70–90°, supported on a table or mat. The elbow should be positioned in partial flexion on slick material to reduce fric-

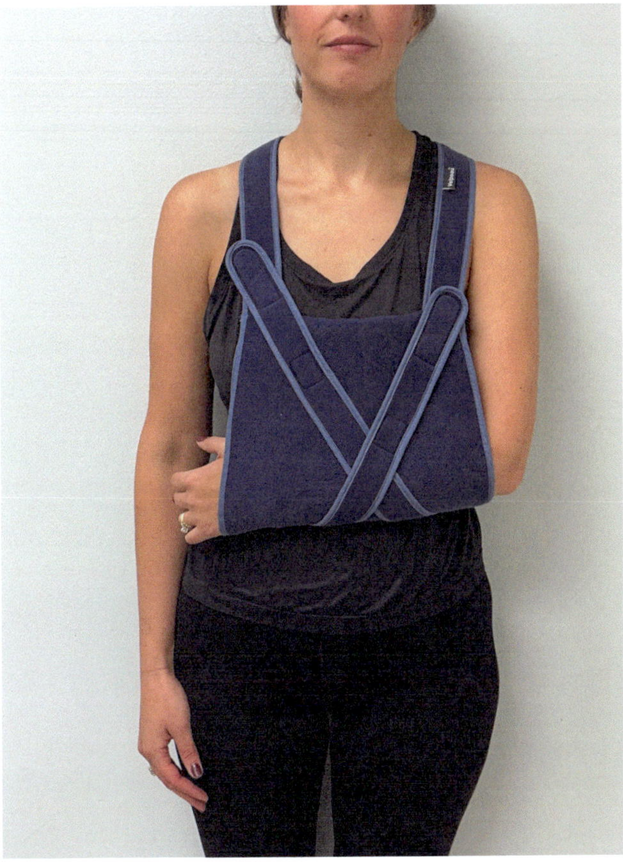

Image 4 Use of a sling or other support is encouraged to maintain the elbow in flexion and prevent overlengthening of the recipient muscle

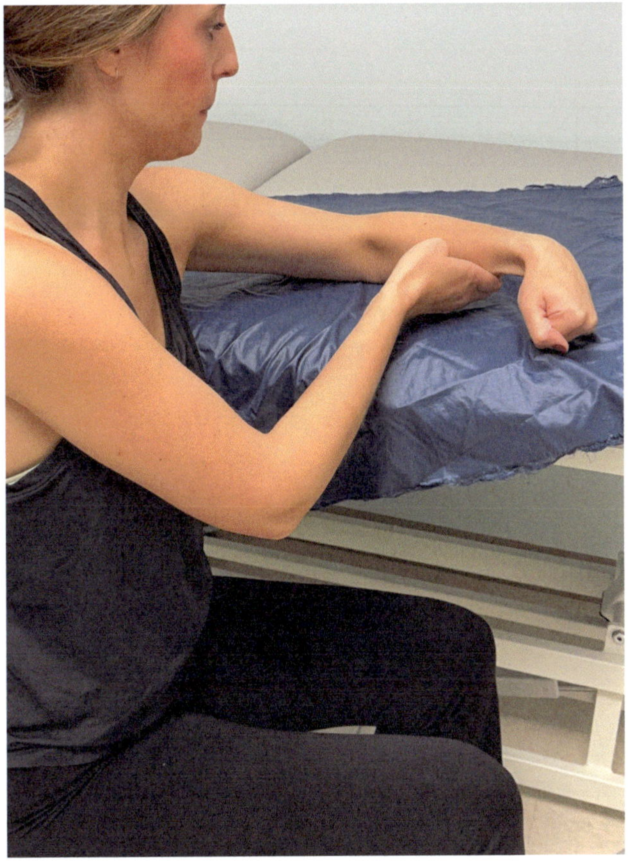

Image 5 In phase 2, pairing the donor and recipient muscles is performed in a gravity-lessened plane with assistance from the opposite hand

tion and thus facilitate movement. The patient first performs donor activation (straight fist for FDS and/or wrist flexion for FCR) and simultaneously attempting active elbow flexion. Once the patient cannot flex the elbow further, he or she assists the elbow into end-range flexion with the contralateral hand (Image 5). The forearm should be positioned in either neutral or pronation to better isolate brachialis function.

Dowel Exercise: The patient may also perform elbow flexion holding a dowel in both hands (while pronated). The patient first flexes the wrist and then assists into elbow flexion using support from the dowel and contralateral hand (Image 6). As the brachialis strengthens in time, the unaffected hand will provide less assistance.

- "Place and Hold"
  Brachialis MMT=2+/5
  The patient passively flexes the elbow using the contralateral hand. He or she activates the donor by flexing the wrist and/or fingers and slowly releases the support of the contralateral hand while attempting to maintain independent elbow flexion. This exercise should be done against gravity (seated or standing) and can also be done at varying degrees of elbow flexion, as needed, to isolate motion throughout the range.

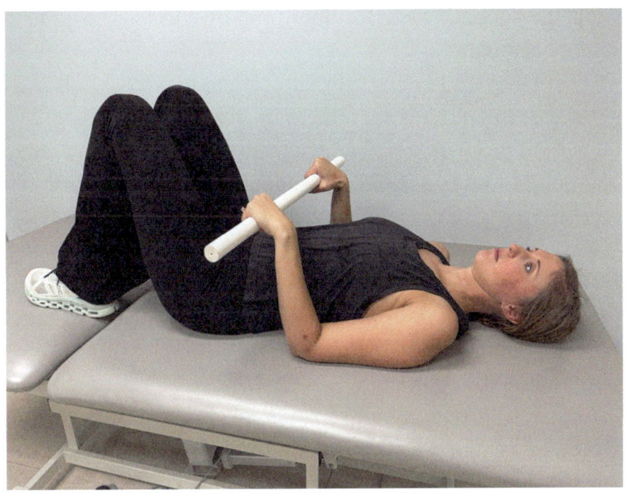

Image 6 Active-assisted elbow flexion may also be performed in supine with both hands holding a dowel in wrist flexion and the uninvolved arm assisting elbow flexion of the involved arm

- Active Donor with Active Recipient
  Brachialis MMT = 3−/5
  In an antigravity position (seated or standing), the patient performs wrist flexion and/or finger flexion while actively flexing the elbow from varying degrees of partial elbow flexion (Image 7).

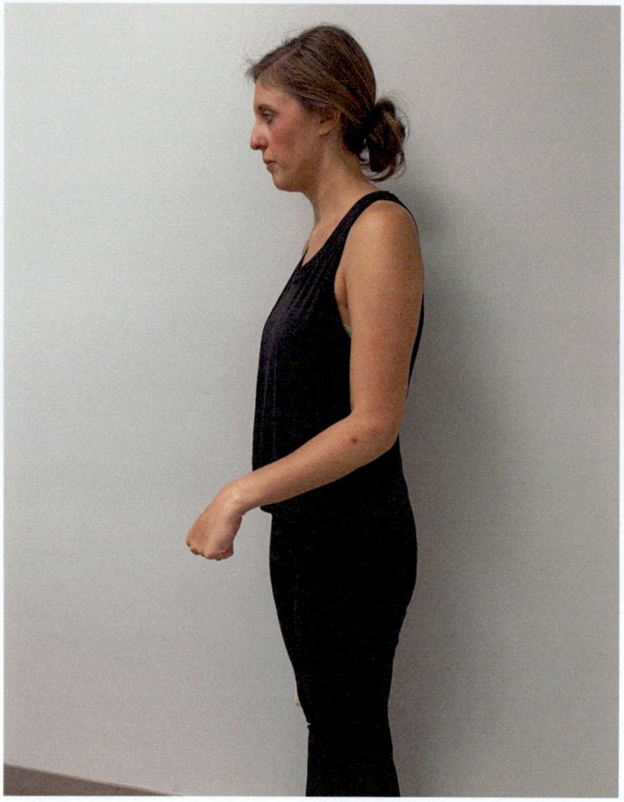

Image 7 Independently flexing the elbow is gradually attained in anti-gravity positions with forceful co-contraction of the wrist and finger flexors

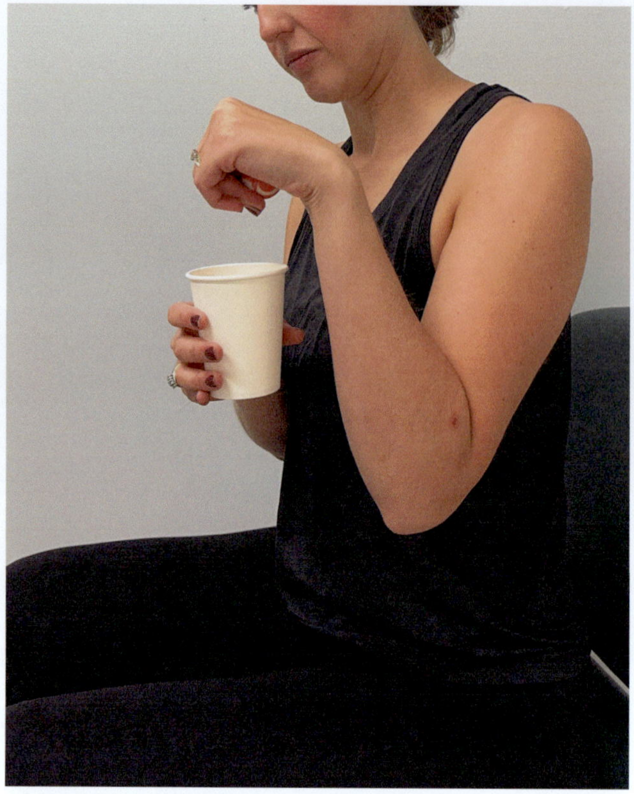

Image 8 An example of an activity that involves active elbow flexion with finger and wrist flexion includes picking up small objects like marbles and placing then in a cup held close to the shoulder

Cone Activity: While holding a cone in hand, cues are given to activate the donor muscles (wrist/finger flexion) as the patient flexes the elbow and tries to tap the cone to each shoulder.

Ball Drop into High Cup: The patient is seated with marbles or small balls on a table in front of him or her. The patient picks up a ball and actively flexes the elbow in an attempt to place it in a cup being held near the shoulder (Image 8).

Functional Activity

Once patients can perform active elbow flexion against gravity, they should try to incorporate this movement into functional tasks throughout the day. Elbow flexion is crucial for eating and grooming. Examples of functional activities would be bringing a cup to the mouth, applying deodorant, and brushing teeth.

Assessment of Recovery

To evaluate for brachialis reinnervation, the examiner applies resistance to the donor(s) (wrist flexion/FCR or finger flexion/FDS) as the patient attempts active elbow flexion. The examiner simultaneously palpates the brachialis muscle for signs of contraction. Demonstrating any progress is highly motivating to the patient. Using a goniometer, the therapist should assess the actual degrees of elbow flexion achieved in a gravity-minimized plane each visit (Image 9).

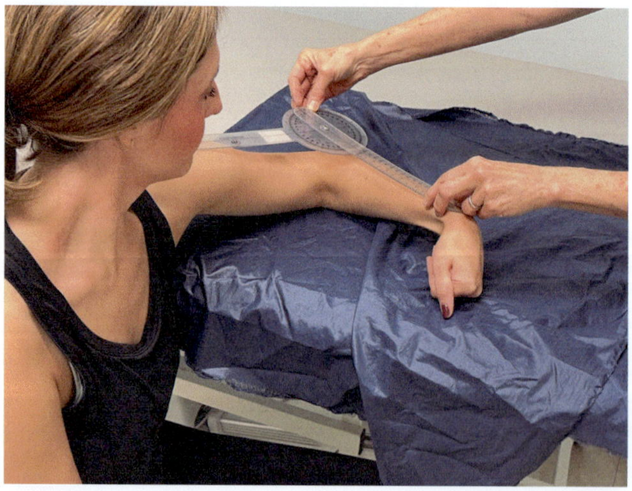

Image 9 As brachialis function improves monthly assessments include goniometrivc measures of elbow flexion in a gravity lessened plane

Therapy Frequency

The recommended therapy frequency depends on the patient's needs. For most patients, once a week or every other week is appropriate. At this time, the patient should have a strong understanding of the donor-recipient relationship, donor flooding activities, and use of donor activation with elbow flexion exercises.

Phase 3

3+/5 MMT or Greater in the Recipient Muscle

Once the patient can fully flex the elbow against gravity and can withstand slight resistance, phase 3 of therapy begins. This phase is characterized by the addition of strengthening for the recipient muscle. There are no surgical precautions in phase 3; however, excessive fatigue should continue to be avoided with all activities. Given the limited endurance of the recovering brachialis, repetitions for each activity may be fewer than what the patient may expect from this phase. It is important to set reasonable expectations with the patient and make sure that he or she can recognize signs of fatigue. These may include muscle fasciculations, cramping, soreness, and inability to perform repetitions as well as they previously could. Endurance limitations can take a year or more to improve. Therefore, patients should understand that strengthening activities should be balanced with rest, which will continue far past their last therapy session.

Exercises

- Resistive Recipient Activity with Donor Contraction
  The patient flexes the elbow while holding a resistance band with the wrist in partial flexion and the fingers flexed. Donor activation will still augment elbow flexion power early in this phase. If the FDS was the only donor, the patient focuses on finger flexion around the band to provide stronger recipient response (Image 10). Elbow flexion exercises are performed with the forearm either pronated or in neutral, and it is eventually advanced to a supinated position.
  Elbow flexion may be performed with free weights during phase 3. Patients should start with a very light weight, such as a cell phone. Additionally, exercises may begin with eccentric elbow flexion, which is easier and functionally important. Starting with the elbow flexed to end range (and the donor simultaneously activated), the patient slowly lowers the arm into elbow extension. Once the patient can hold the weight easily, he or she should begin concentric elbow flexion starting from a partially flexed range to full flexion (Image 11). This can be advanced by having the patient start from a more elbow extended position.
- Resistive Recipient Activity Without Donor Contraction
  All of the abovementioned phase 3 exercises can be performed with less (or no) demand of the donor muscle. If the FCR was the donor, resistive elbow flexion may be attempted in wrist extension or neutral. If FDS was the donor, the patient may wrap a resistance band around the palm (without finger flexion involved) to eliminate the assistive action of the FDS.

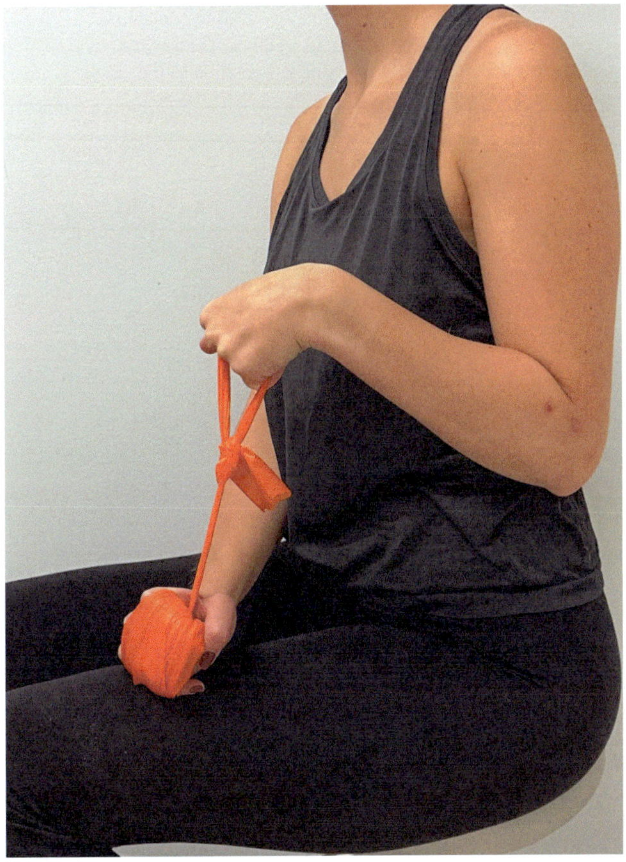

Image 10 In phase 3, resistance to the brachialis is initially performed with strong donor wrist and finger flexion as shown

Therapy Frequency

Therapy frequency continues to be patient dependent. Patients who are very independent and motivated may benefit from once a month, while other patients may choose to maintain their weekly or bimonthly therapy sessions to ensure adequate performance and progression. During the strengthening phase, it is important that activities are geared toward patient goals and promoting independence with functional activities.

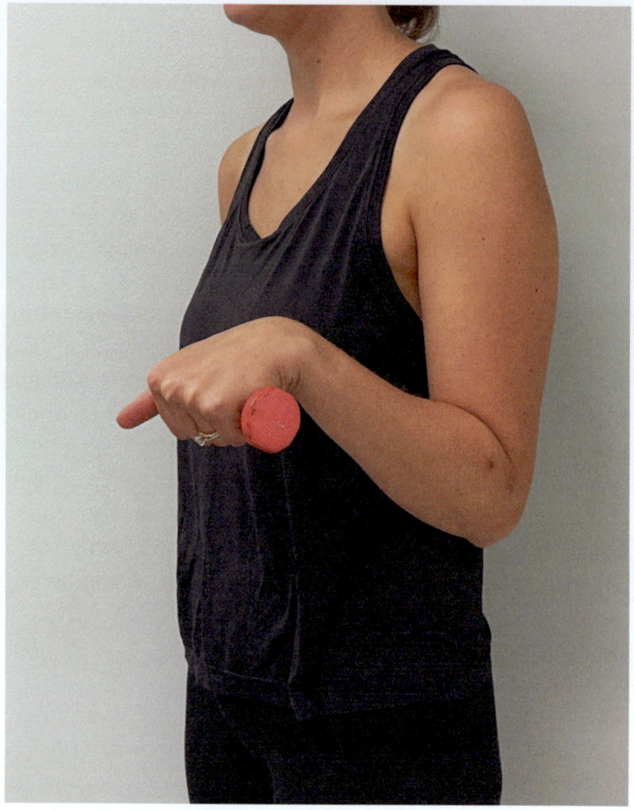

Image 11 Light weights are gradually added to concentric elbow flexion, starting in 90 degrees of elbow flexion and gradually starting from a more extended position of the elbow

Median (FCR, FDS) to brachialis nerve transfer

Nerve transfer overview					
Donor nerve	Donor action	Recipient nerve	Recipient action	Indications for functional restoration	Approximate months to functional movement
Median nerve branch to the flexor carpi radialis and/or flexor digitorum superficialis	Wrist flexion with radial deviation and/ or finger flexion	Musculocutaneous nerve branch to the brachialis	Elbow flexion (regardless of forearm position)	Loss of elbow flexion	12 months [13]

Information below is suggested guidelines. Precautions may vary according to surgeon preferences and patient factors

	Preoperative therapy	Early phase	Middle phase	Late phase
Criteria	Before surgery	0/5–1/5 MMT	2-/5 to 3/5 MMT	>3/5 MMT
Purpose of Phase	Educate and establish baseline function	Understand donor and recipient relationship	Consistently activate recipient	Strengthen recipient and separate from donor activation
Precautions	Prevent extension contracture of elbow, maintain elbow ROM	Protect elbow flexor length	Respect fatigue and prevent dominance of triceps	Avoid resisted elbow flexion until consistent 3/5 MMT is achieved
Frequency of visits (considerations)	1-2 pre-op visits May increase if PROM limitations exist	1×/week until PROM is WNL and patient is independent with donor activation; then 1× monthly	1x per week to 1x per month based on patient needs and accurate, consistent demonstration of exercise program	1× every 1-2 weeks based on progress toward patient-specific goals
Orthosis considerations	NA	Full-time sling and elbow support for the first 2 weeks. OK to remove for hygiene Replace with other elbow support as needed after 2 weeks	Continue intermittent sling use to protect the length of the recovering brachialis muscle	NA
Interventions	PROM if patient lacks passive elbow flexion and forearm rotation	**Donor Activation:** Wrist flexion with radial deviation and/or finger flexion **Donor-Recipient Pairing**: Active wrist flexion and/or finger flexion with passive elbow flexion in pronation	**Active/Resisted Donor with Active Assisted Recipient:** Gravity minimized plane: Arm supported on table at shoulder height: wrist and finger flexion with active elbow flexion using towel or arm skate Supine dowel rod exercise: bilateral wrist flexion (and finger flexion around dowel) in pronation with active-*assisted* elbow flexion **Place and Hold**: Passively place the elbow in end-range flexion and pronation (while flexing wrist and fingers). Remove support from the contralateral hand and attempt to maintain this position	**Resisted Donor and Recipient:** Holding weights or a resistance band, the patient performs an elbow curl while the forearm is in pronation and the wrist/fingers are flexed **Resisted Recipient:** Holding weights or a resistance band, the patient performs an elbow curl while the forearm is in pronation and the wrist/fingers are extended
Additional Interventions			Exercises should first prioritize elbow flexion in pronation prior to forearm-neutral or supination	

During all phases it is essential to continue cortical reorganization, psychological and psychosocial interventions

Median to Brachialis Nerve Transfer

Goal of Surgery: To restore elbow flexion

Recipient Muscle Movement = Elbow flexion (regardless of forearm position)

Recipient Muscle: Brachialis muscle

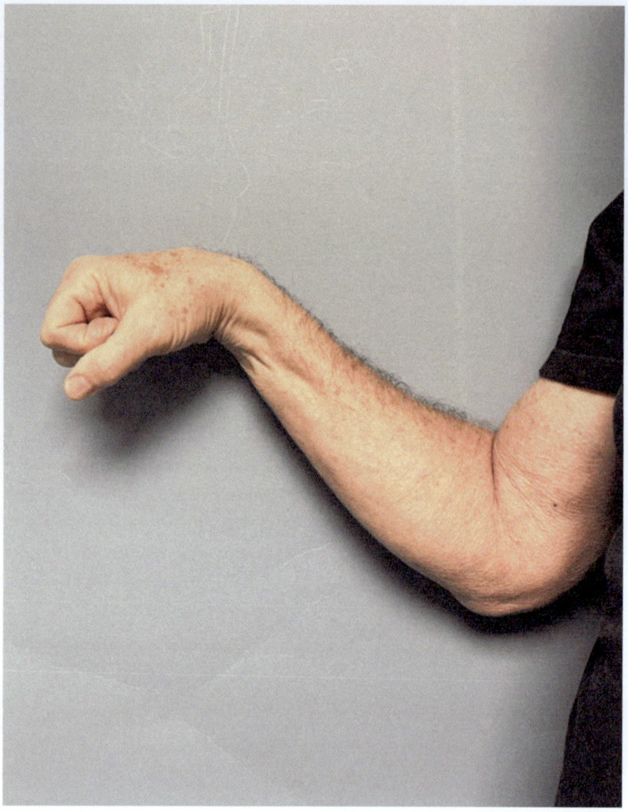

Bend elbow (flexion)

Donor Movements =

Wrist flexion and radial deviation: flexor carpi radialis, FCR

Finger flexion (primarily PIP joints): flexor digitorum superficialis, FDS

Donor Muscles: Flexor carpi radialis (FCR) and/or flexor digitorum superficialis (FDS)

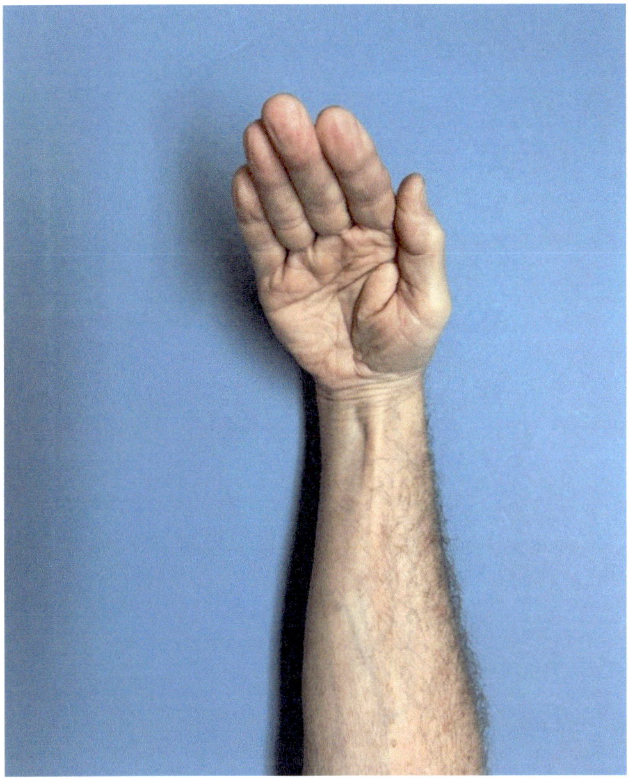

Bend wrist (flexion)

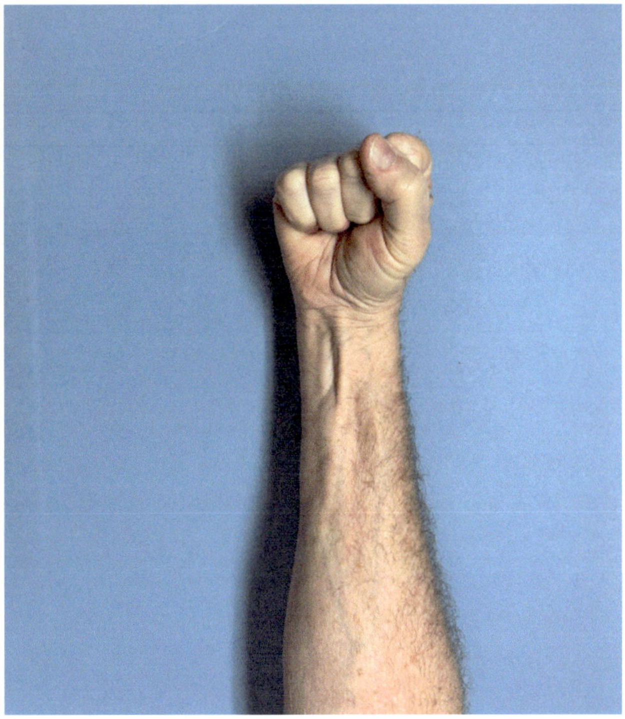

Bend fingers (flexion)

Phase 1 Median to Brachialis Nerve Transfer Exercises

☐ **Active or Resisted Donor Movement:**

- Bend the wrist forward and hold 3–5 seconds. Relax the wrist and repeat.

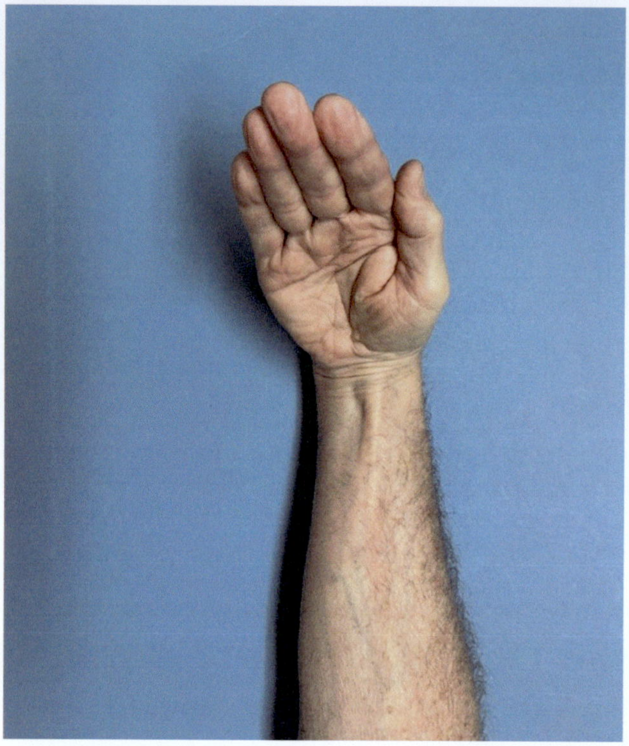

- Bend the fingers into a fist or a "straight" fist. Open the fingers and repeat.

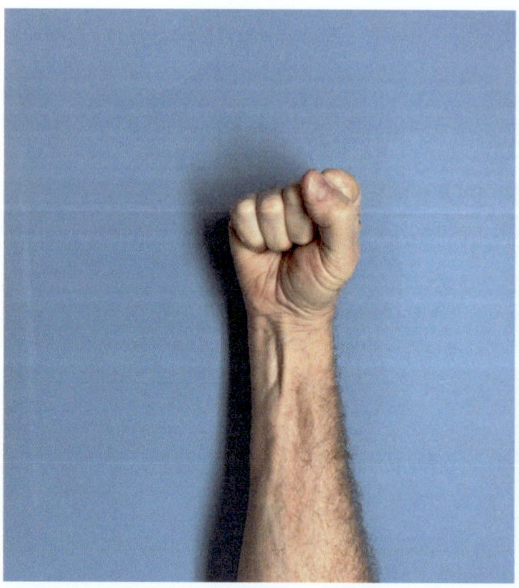

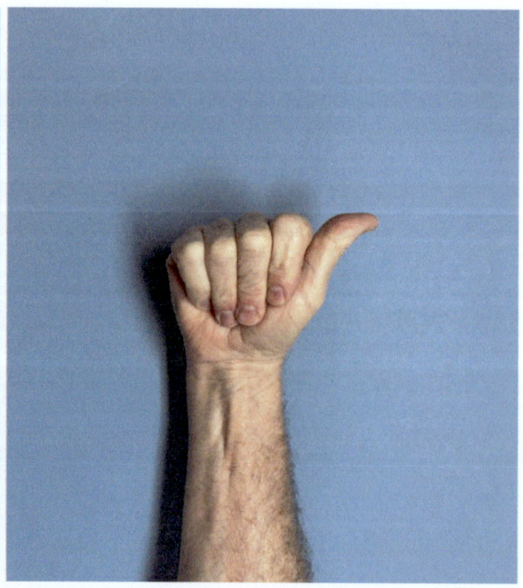

Complete 10 repetitions every hour

- Bend the wrist forward. Use your opposite hand to apply resistance to the palm while your injured wrist resists this pressure.

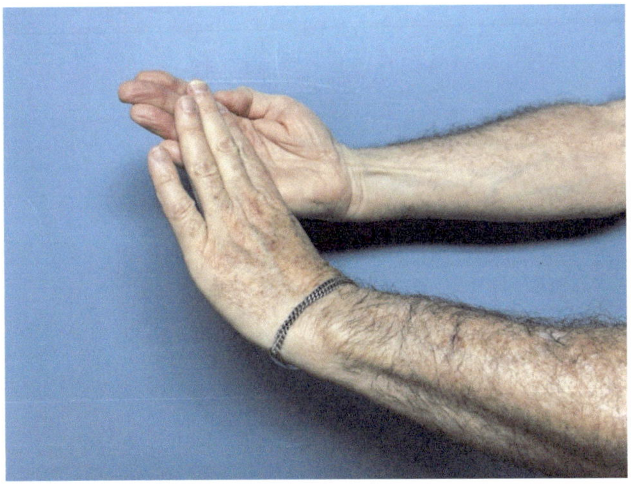

- Squeeze light therapy putty or a gripper tool.

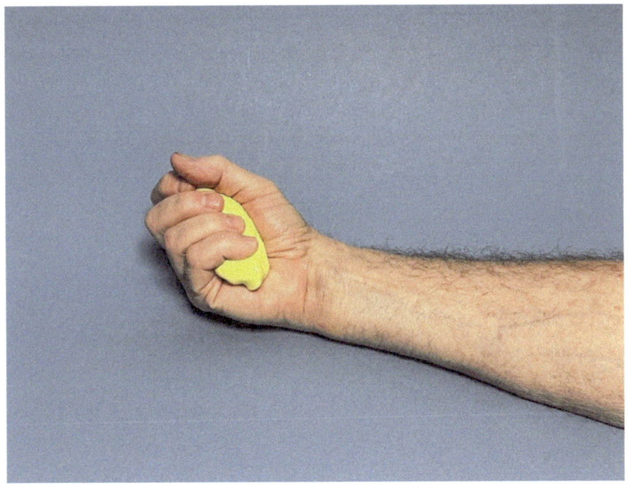

☐ **Combined Donor with Passive Recipient Exercise:**

- Bend the wrist and/or fingers forward and use your opposite hand to bend the elbow at the same time. Try to make sure your forearm is facing palm down. Hold 5 seconds, then relax and repeat.

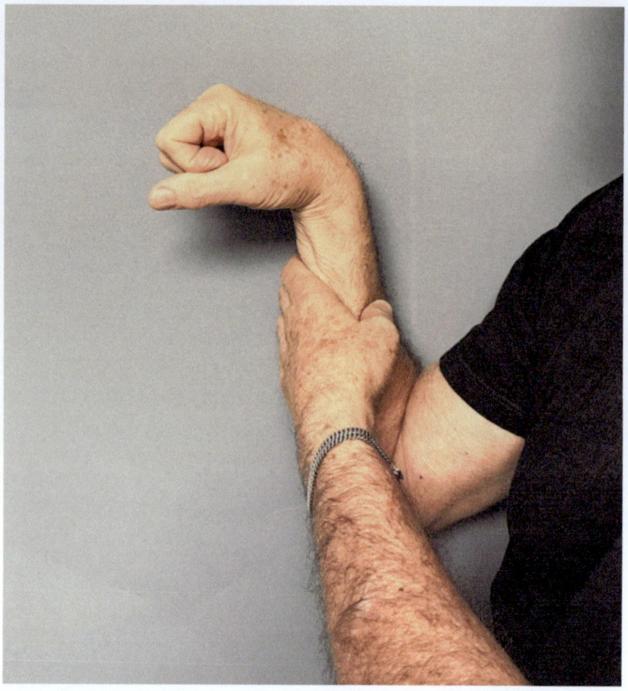

Complete 10-15 repetitions, 3-5 times per day

Phase 2 Median to Brachialis Nerve Transfer Exercises:

☐ **Active Donor + Active-Assisted Recipient:**

- Sit next to a table or mat with your arm out to the side. Bend your wrist and/or fingers while trying to independently bend the elbow across the table. Once you cannot bend the elbow any further, use your opposite hand to assist the elbow into a fully bent position.
  - You may use a slick cloth under the forearm to make it easier.

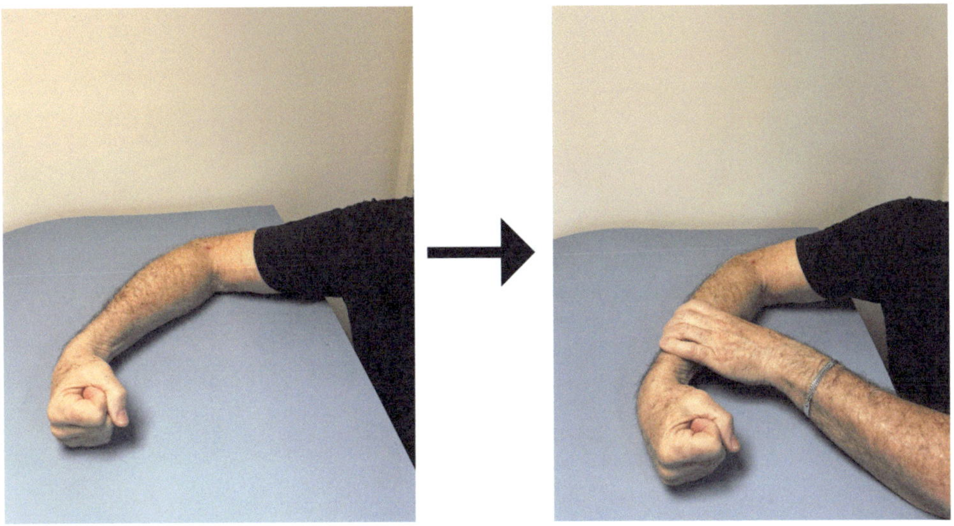

- While lying on your back, hold a dowel rod in both hands with your forearms facing palm-down. First squeeze your fingers and bend your wrists. At the same time, bend both elbows so the dowel rod comes up toward your chest. Try not to rely solely on the uninjured arm.

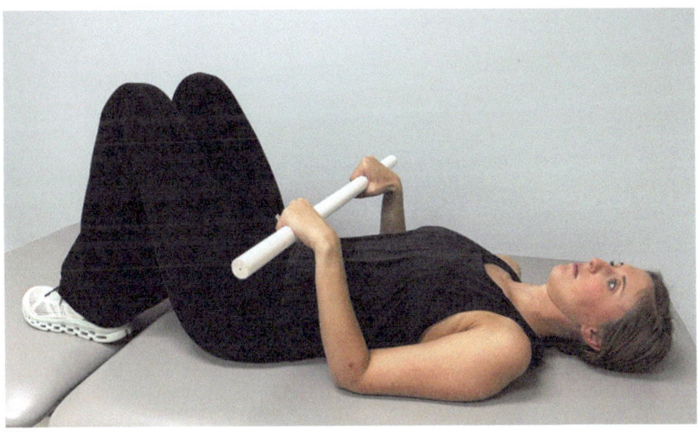

☐ **"Place and Hold"**

- While seated or standing, bend the fingers and wrist. Then use the opposite hand to bend the elbow into a fully bent position. Slowly release the support of your opposite hand and try to maintain this position for a count of 5 seconds.

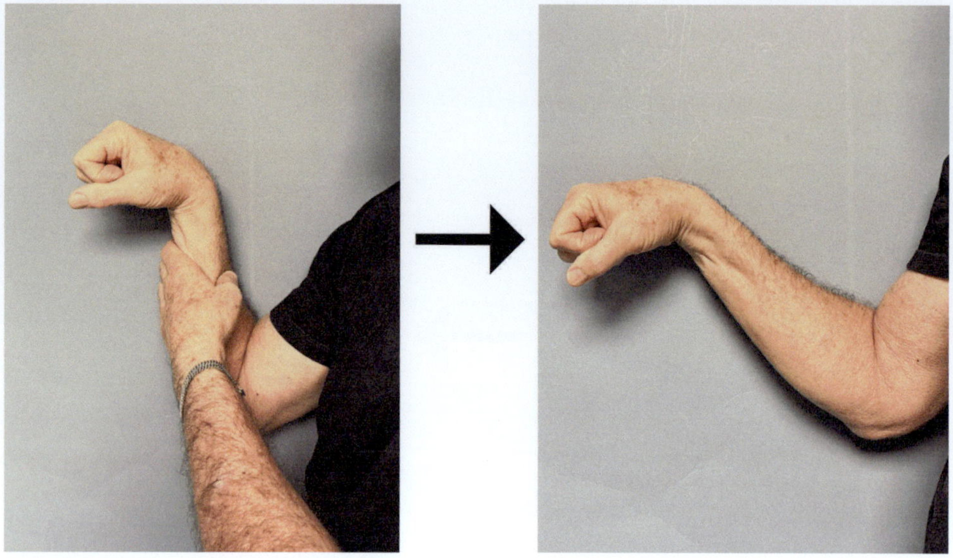

Complete 10-15 repetitions, 3-5 times per day

☐ **Active Donor + Active Recipient Movement:**

- While seated or standing, bend the fingers and wrist. Then independently bend the elbow as much as you can. Try to maintain a palm-down position of the forearm. Hold 3-5 seconds, relax, and repeat.

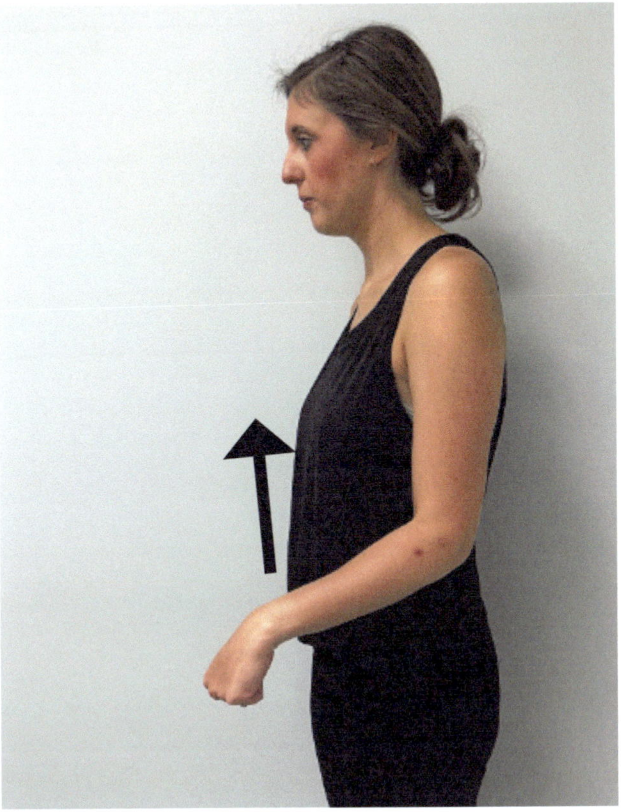

- Hold a cone or lightweight cylindrical object that is resting on a surface. Bend the wrist forward and try to touch the object to the shoulder.

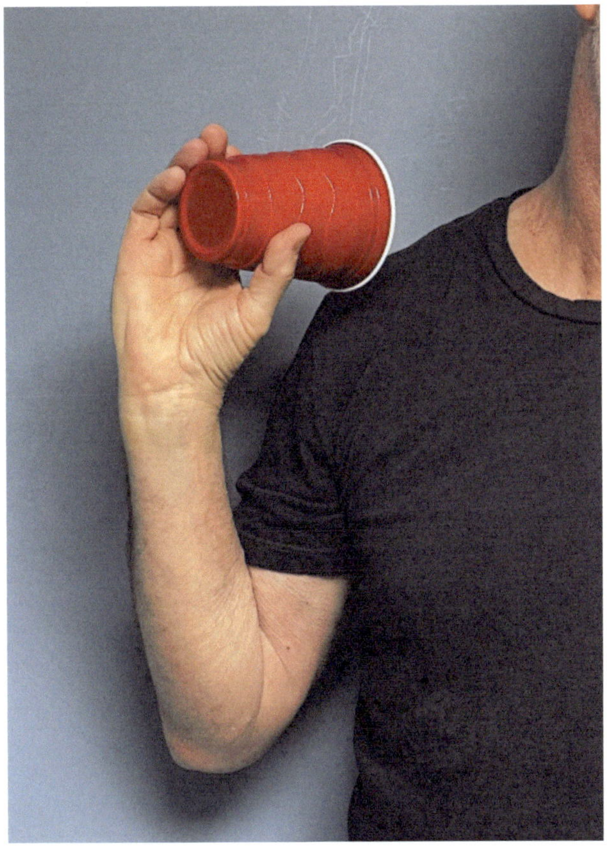

Complete 10-15 repetitions, 3-5 times per day

Phase 3 Median to Brachialis Nerve Transfer Exercises:

☐ **Resisted Recipient Activity with Donor Contraction:**

- Hold a resistance band with the opposite end held by your other hand. Bend the wrist and fingers while bending the elbow. Hold 3-5 seconds.

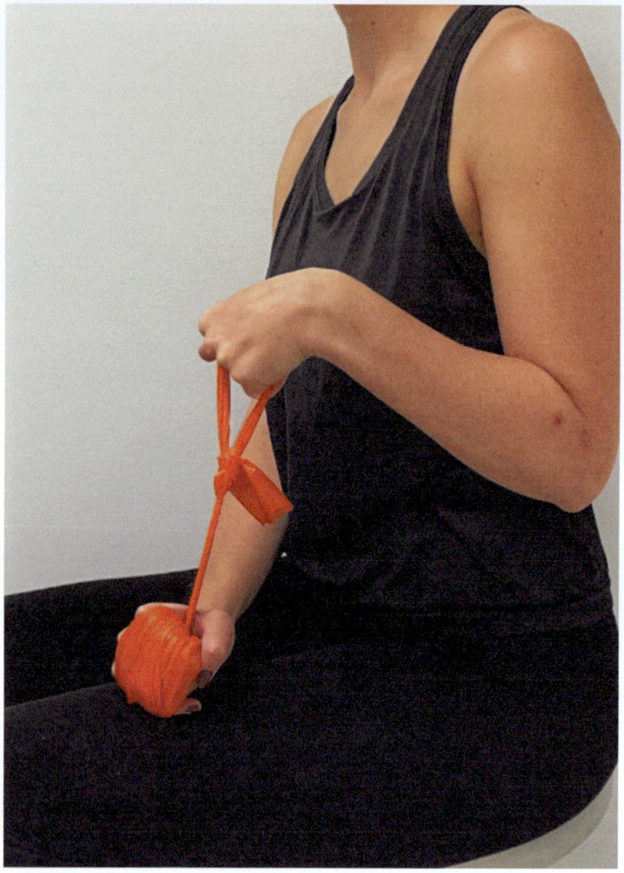

- Hold a light weight, bend the wrist, and bend the elbow at the same time. Hold 3-5 seconds.

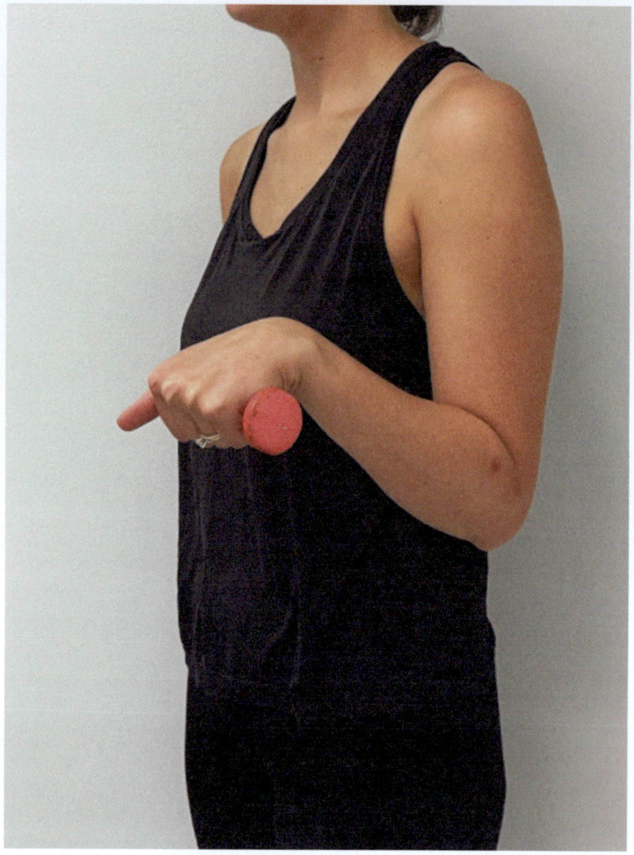

Complete 10 repetitions, 3 times per day

Try to master these exercises first with the forearm in a palm-down position, then with the forearm neutral/sideways, and finally in a palm-up position.

☐ **Resisted Recipient without Donor Contraction:**

- Hold a light weight with the wrist pulled backward into extension. At the same time, bend the elbow and hold 3–5 seconds.

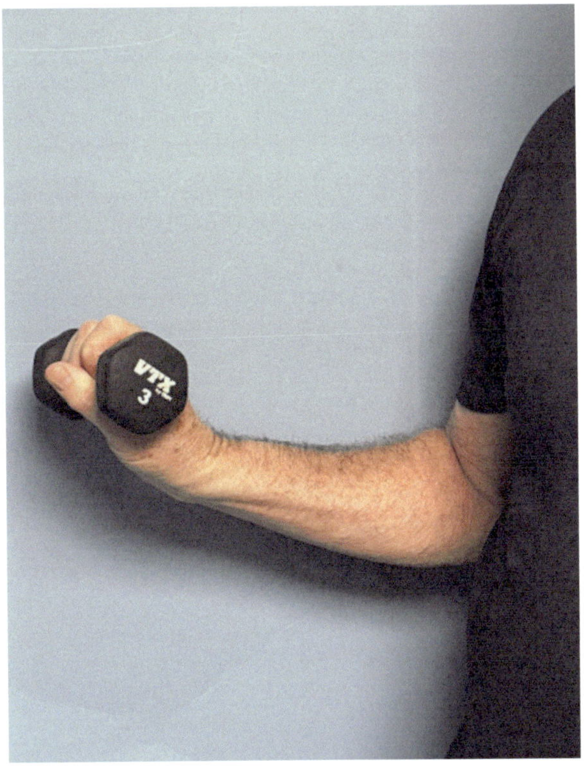

- Place a resistance band around your palm, holding the with the opposite end of the band with your unjured hand (or anchored under your foot). Keep you injured arm in a palm-up position with your fingers open while you bend the elbow. Hold 3-5 seconds and repeat.

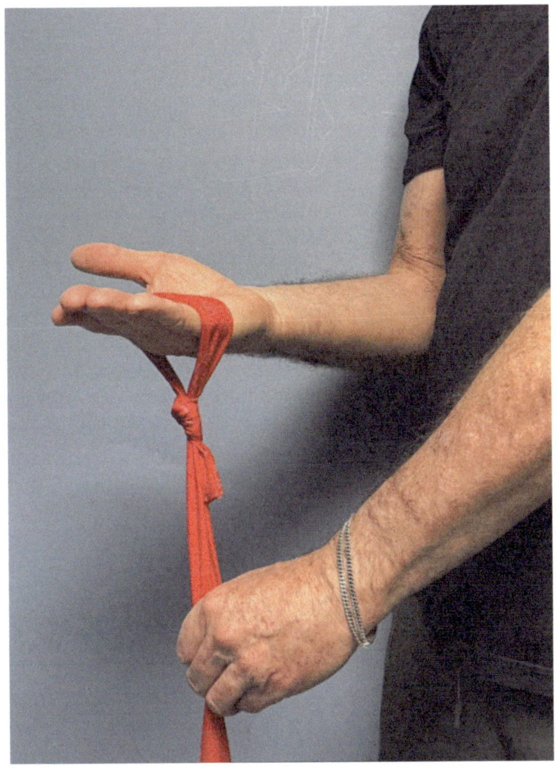

Complete 10 repetitions, 3 times per day

References

1. McCreary EK, Provance PG, Rodgers MM, Romani WA. Muscles: testing and function with posture and pain. Lippincott Williams & Wilkins; 2005.
2. Neumann DA. Kinesiology of the musculoskeletal system-e-book: foundations for rehabilitation. Elsevier Health Sciences; 2016.
3. Mackin E, Pierrie SN, Loeffler BJ. Common nerve injuries about the shoulder. Rehabilitation of the hand and upper extremity, vol. 7. St. Louis: Mosby; 2002. p. 661–76.
4. Mackinnon SE, Novak CB, Myckatyn TM, Tung TH. Results of reinnervation of the biceps and brachialis muscles with a double fascicular transfer for elbow flexion. J Hand Surg. 2005;30(5):978–85.
5. Kokkalis ZT, Bavelou A, Papanikos E, Konofaos P, Efstathopoulos DG, Soucacos PN. Reconstruction of elbow flexion with a modified Oberlin procedure: a comparative study. Injury. 2019;50:S71–6.
6. Ray WZ, Pet MA, Yee A, Mackinnon SE. Double fascicular nerve transfer to the biceps and brachialis muscles after brachial plexus injury: clinical outcomes in a series of 29 cases. J Neurosurg. 2011;114(6):1520–8.
7. Tung TH, Novak CB, Mackinnon SE. Nerve transfers to the biceps and brachialis branches to improve elbow flexion strength after brachial plexus injuries. J Neurosurg. 2003;98(2):313–8.
8. Nath RK, Lyons AB, Bietz G. Physiological and clinical advantages of median nerve fascicle transfer to the musculocutaneous nerve following brachial plexus root avulsion injury. J Neurosurg. 2006;105(6):830–4.
9. Kahn LC, Stonner MM, Dy CJ. Key concepts for nerve transfer rehabilitation after surgical reconstruction for brachial plexus and peripheral nerve injuries. J Hand Surg. 2023;
10. Gossman MR, Sahrmann SA, Rose SJ. Review of length-associated changes in muscle: experimental evidence and clinical implications. Phys Ther. 1982;62(12):1799–808.
11. Goldspink G, Tabary C, Tabary JC, Tardieu C, Tardieu G. Effect of denervation on the adaptation of sarcomere number and muscle extensibility to the functional length of the muscle. J Physiol. 1974;236(3):733–42.
12. Kahn L, Moore A. Donor activation focused rehabilitation approach: maximizing outcomes after nerve transfers. Hand Clin. 2016;32(2):263–77.
13. Hill JL, Turner LC, Jones RD, et al. The stages of rehabilitation following motor nerve transfer surgery. J Musculoskelet Surg Res. 2019;3(60)

Intercostal Nerves to Triceps Branch of the Radial Nerve Transfer

Alexandra MacKenzie

Background

Restoring triceps function following brachial plexus injury is not often a top priority. Elbow flexion and shoulder abduction vie for valuable available nerve donors before the triceps in a partial or complete plexus injury. However, loss of elbow extension should not be minimized. Triceps function is important for many daily activities where power beyond just the weight of the arm is required. Triceps function can be important in activities requiring stabilization of an object on a table, such as holding a paper while writing on it and holding a plate while cutting food. It also plays a role in functional mobility, such as pushing oneself up from sit to stand or using an assistive mobility device (such as a walker). It is important for overhead reaching activities, including dressing or reaching for an object while the arm is stabilized on a table [1]. In addition, having triceps function can improve the function of the biceps as an antagonist and stabilizer.

Triceps function can be restored with a nerve transfer of the intercostal nerves (ICNs) from thoracic roots 3–5 to the triceps branch of the radial nerve, provided that the ICN has not already been used as a donor for the biceps. Reports vary in the literature, but generally two to three intercostal nerves are required for this transfer [2]. Gao and colleagues describe using this transfer in combination with a phrenic nerve transfer to the biceps [2]. Use of the intercostal nerves as donors for nerve transfers generally does not create respiratory deficits [2].

Surgery Description

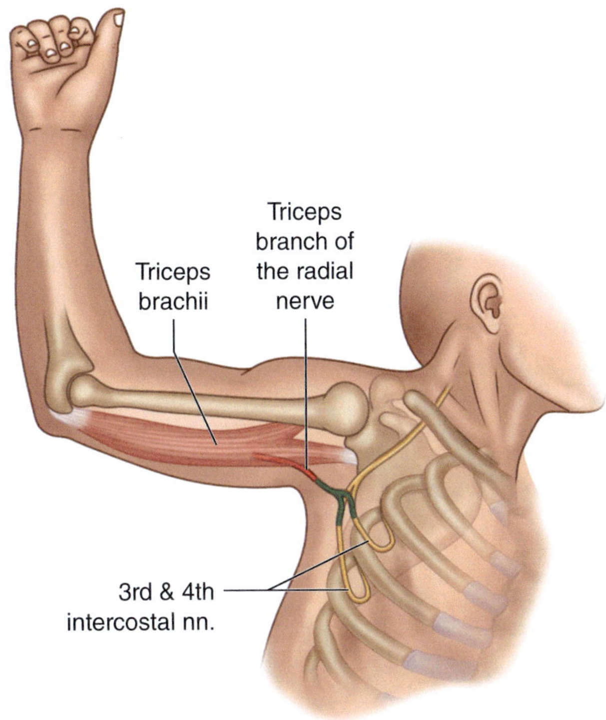

Straighten the elbow against gravity

An incision is made in the deltopectoral interval. The pectoralis major insertion is detached from the humerus, ensuring that it can be reattached at conclusion of the procedure. The pectoralis major muscle is elevated, taking care to preserve the nerve branches entering its undersurface (deep aspect). The posterior cord is then identified adjacent to the anterior aspect of the glenohumeral joint. The radial nerve is identified at the anterior aspect of the triangular interval, and triceps branches (typically to the lateral head) can be identified at this level. Intraoperative stimulation is used to confirm that the

A. MacKenzie (✉)
Hand and Upper Extremity Therapy Center, Hospital for Special Surgery, New York, NY, USA
e-mail: mackenziea@hss.edu

L. C. Kahn et al. (eds.), *Rehabilitation for Nerve Transfers of the Upper Extremity*, https://doi.org/10.1007/978-3-031-92008-0_15

triceps branch is not functioning, and the triceps branch is then neurolyzed from the radial nerve and divided proximally. A separate inframammary incision is made along the chest wall. The ribs (typically the third through fifth ribs, although there is variability in which ribs are selected) and intercostal muscles are exposed. The intercostal nerve is identified, typically facilitated by using a handheld nerve stimulator. The intercostal nerves are dissected free from the surrounding tissue as distal as possible (towards the sternum). Usually 2–3 intercostal nerves are used for the transfer to the triceps. The donor intercostal nerves are divided distally and reflected proximally, oftentimes being passed through the slips of the serratus anterior muscle. Coaptation of the intercostal nerves to a triceps branch of the radial nerve is performed using microsurgical technique.

Outcomes

Studies have demonstrated that the ICN-to-triceps nerve transfer is reliable and effective; 57–72% of patients can expect to have good results (manual muscle score of a 3 or greater) [1–4]. Positive factors that influence recovery include normal body mass index (BMI), shorter time from injury to surgery, as well as if the surgery was performed on the dominant limb [1]. The average time to see trace muscle contraction is 7 months (with a range from 5 to 11 months), and the average time to recover extension against resistance is 15 months (with a range of 13–20 months) [1–4].

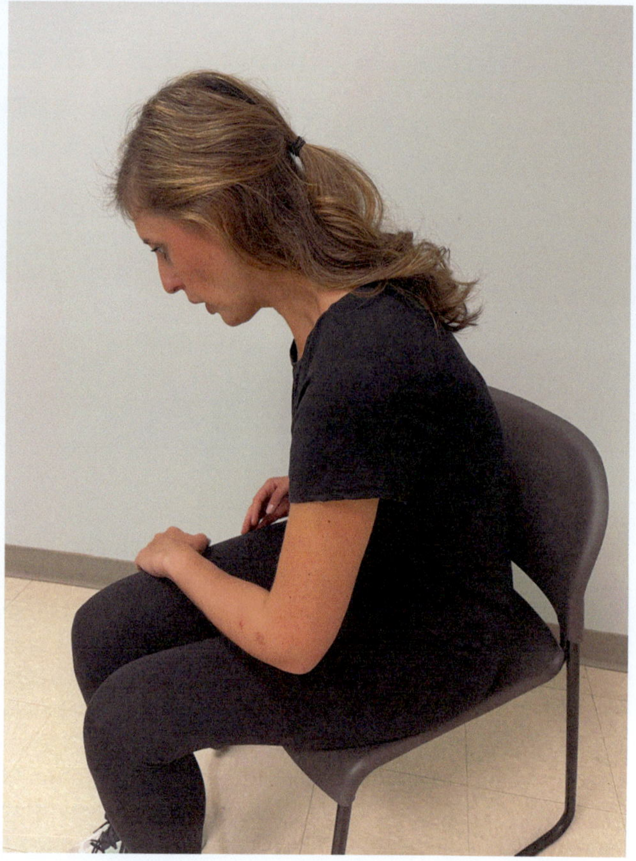

Image 1 Intercostal donor activation is demonstrated with active trunk flexion and rotation in sitting

Phases of Rehabilitation

Phase 1

Pre-op to 1/5 MMT in the Recipient Muscle

After surgery, patients are immobilized in a sling or shoulder immobilizer for 3–4 weeks [3]. Maintaining shoulder internal rotation at the side for 4 weeks is required for those individuals whose surgery involved detachment and subsequent repair of the pectoralis major tendon. This also prevents traction on the nerve transfer and limits seroma formation. During this period, patients are advised to avoid active or passive shoulder abduction and external rotation beyond 45° with ADLs such as hygiene. Passive shoulder range of motion (ROM) is introduced in the second month and is gradually increased. It is important to restore and maintain shoulder and elbow joint flexibility because in time, the newly reinnervated, weak triceps muscle will struggle to produce sufficient force to move a stiff joint. The patient should be instructed in passive elbow extension to prevent flexion contracture from prolonged sling positioning, especially when the elbow flexors are intact and unopposed.

The general concepts of motor reeducation are outlined early in phase 1. The names and actions of the donors and recipient muscles are introduced, and donor activation is encouraged [5]. Realistic expectations should be set and timelines for recovery discussed. Following this nerve transfer, it will take anywhere from 5 to 11 months to see early signs of reinnervation [1–4].

Exercises

- Donor Activation

  The intercostal nerves innervate the intercostal muscles. External intercostals contribute to inspiration, while internal intercostals contribute to expiration. In addition, these muscles play a role in posture and trunk rotation. EMG studies have demonstrated that they are especially important in contralateral trunk rotation [6]. It has been demonstrated that after ICN-to-musculocutaneous nerve (MCN) transfer, there is more activity in elbow flexors with co-contraction of the donor that focused on trunk flexion than with inspiration/expiration [7]. While the literature for ICN-to-triceps transfer is scant, it can be postulated that the same would be true when the ICNs are the donor, no matter the recipient. Early-phase donor activation exercises should include trunk flexion and rotation (Image 1). This can be performed in sitting or supine. Additionally, cardiovascular exercises are encouraged to promote exerted inspiration and expiration.

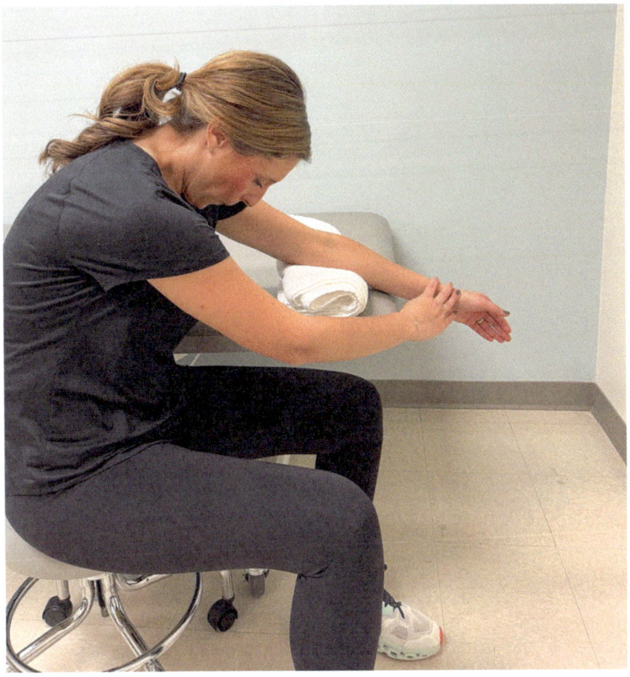

Image 2 In sitting, active donor with passive recipient exercise is demonstrated. The individual is instructed to perform an abdominal "crunch" as he or she flexes the trunk while the uninvolved hand assists in elbow extension

- Combined Donor with Passive Recipient Exercise
  The long head of the triceps extends the elbow. Due to its origin on the infraglenoid tubercle of the scapula, it also contributes to shoulder adduction and extension [8]. Trunk flexion and rotation exercises should be performed with passive extension of the elbow. These exercises can be done in supine, side lying, or sitting. It may be helpful to cue the patient to visualize active elbow extension while the combined donor and recipient actions are being performed. In sitting, the patient performs partial trunk flexion while the elbow is passively extended with the uninvolved hand (Image 2). In supine, passive elbow extension can be achieved by the therapist or family member or with the assistance of gravity.

Clinical Pearl
The patient is supine with an inflatable elbow sleeve (or an orthosis) maintaining the affected elbow in extension. A partial sit-up with exhalation (for donor activation) is performed as the patient slides the arm into shoulder abduction along the mat (Image 3). Performing this bilaterally will promote cortical plasticity and aid in learning the new pattern of trunk flexion while maintaining the elbow in extension. This can also be performed in sitting with arms resting on a table.

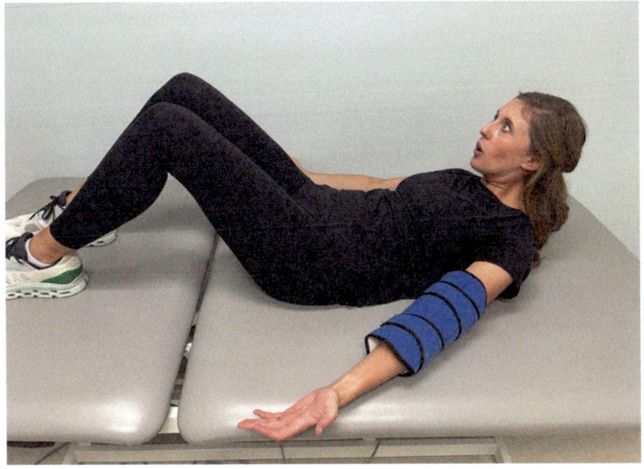

Image 3 Independent pairing of active intercostal donors with passive triceps is demonstrated in supine with a splint holding the elbow in extension. As the individual performs trunk flexion, he or she is cued to abduct the shoulder along the mat while thinking about extending the elbow

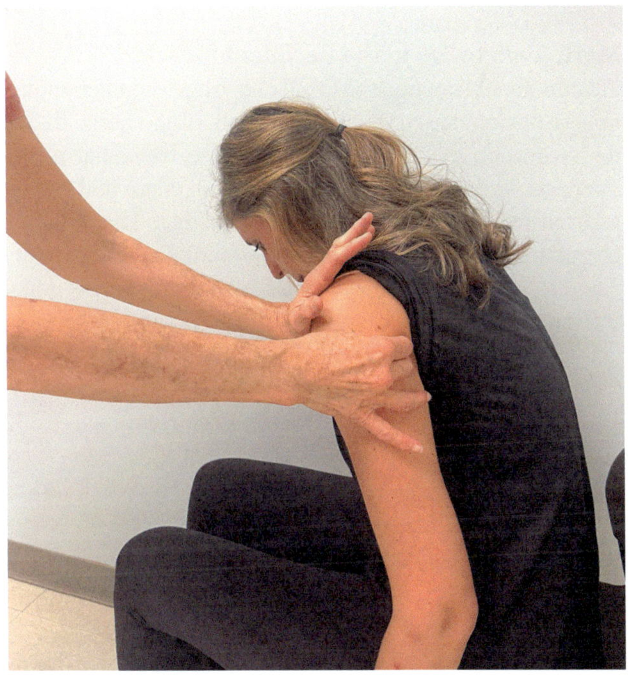

Image 4 Assessment of triceps reinnervation is performed monthly. The individual performs active trunk flexion with or without resistance from the examiner while palpating along the long head of the triceps

Assessment of Recovery

Monthly visits should include assessment of potential recovery of triceps motor function. This is done by having the patient perform donor activation of trunk flexion with forceful exhalation while simultaneously having them attempt elbow extension. The therapist palpates along the long head of the triceps, looking for a notable change in tension (Image 4). As early as 4–5 months post-op, the patient may demonstrate a tender muscle sign [9]. When the triceps muscle belly is squeezed, the patient may report feeling it in their chest or in the triceps muscle, indicating that the donor has reached the recipient. This is typically seen before signs of motor activity [9]. Active elbow extension against gravity may appear around 13–20 months postoperatively [1–4].

Therapy Frequency

In phase 1, one therapy visit per month is usually sufficient to monitor for compliance with the home exercise program as well as to monitor for signs of triceps muscle recovery. If the patient has very stiff joints and there is a need to work on increasing passive joint range of motion, then the patient may be seen more frequently. Additionally, if multiple nerve transfers were performed at the same time, additional visits may be needed to ensure adequate performance of motor reeducation.

Phase 2

MMT: 2−/5 to 3/5 in the Recipient Muscle

Patients should continue to avoid end-range shoulder abduction or flexion due to the limited length of the nerve due to the coaptation of the intercostal nerve to the radial nerve. Exercises in this phase will involve active donor and active-assisted recipient actions occurring together. These should be initiated at the first signs of motor return. Exercises should begin in a gravity-minimized plane with simultaneous donor activation.

Exercises

- Active Donor with Active-Assisted Recipient Triceps MMT: 2−/5 to 2+/5

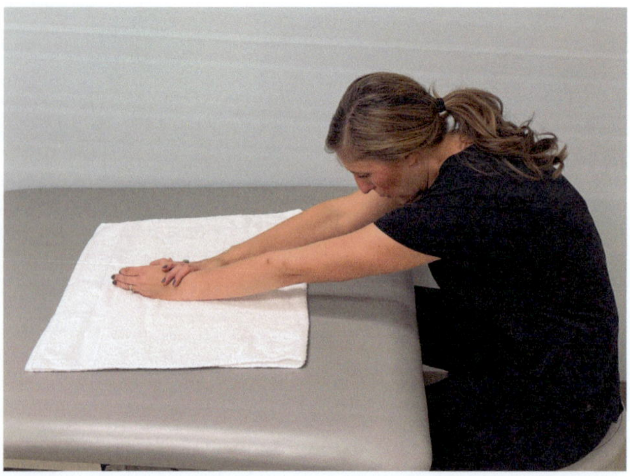

Image 5 Combined active donor with assisted triceps motion is performed in sitting with arms supported on a table. As the individual forcefully flexes the trunk, the arms slide forward, and end-range elbow extension is achieved with the assistance of the uninvolved hand

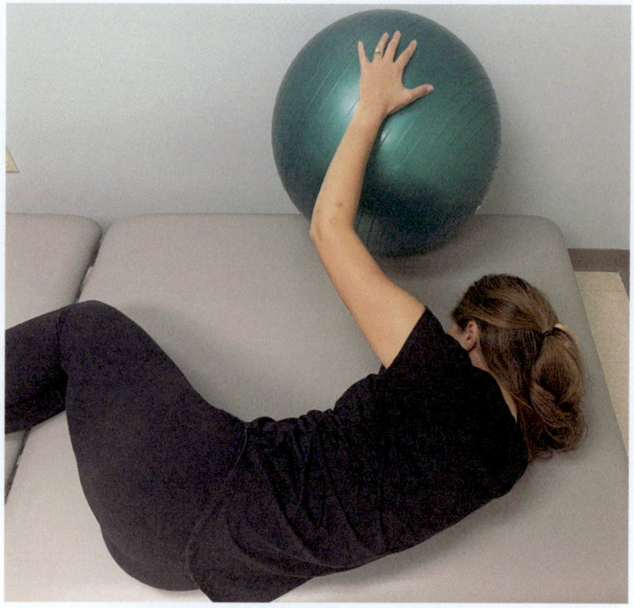

Image 6 Active donor with assisted elbow extension is achieved in side-lying with the involved arm on a large exercise ball. The individual is instructed to flex the trunk, sliding the arm forward, which allows gravity to assist with elbow extension

The patient is seated with both arms on a table in front of him or her with elbows bent and hands clasped. Forceful trunk flexion or a forward "crunch" motion is performed as the patient slides the arms forward, straightening the elbows with assistance from the uninvolved hand (Image 5). A slick cloth under the arm may facilitate ease of triceps activation [5, 10].

A physio ball or UE Ranger® is helpful in achieving active-assisted motion in the recipient muscle. In side lying on the unaffected arm, the injured arm is positioned in 90° of shoulder flexion and is supported by the ball or glider. The patient attempts independent, active elbow extension while performing trunk flexion, or a "crunch" motion (Image 6). As the ball rolls forward, it assists in elbow extension. The therapist should monitor for compensatory motions to ensure that the patient is not just adducting or externally rotating the shoulder or moving the ball into the mat/floor, but rather eliciting a true triceps contraction while pushing.

An overhead pulley system, when available, can be used to hold the shoulder in flexion, allowing the elbow to extend in a gravity-eliminated plane.

Gravity is also used to assist in elbow extension in supine. With the hands on the thighs or abdomen, the patient is instructed to partially flex the trunk and exhale while attempting to extend the elbow as he or she slides the hands off the thighs onto the mat (Image 7).

- Active Donor with Active Recipient Triceps MMT: 3−/5 to 3/5

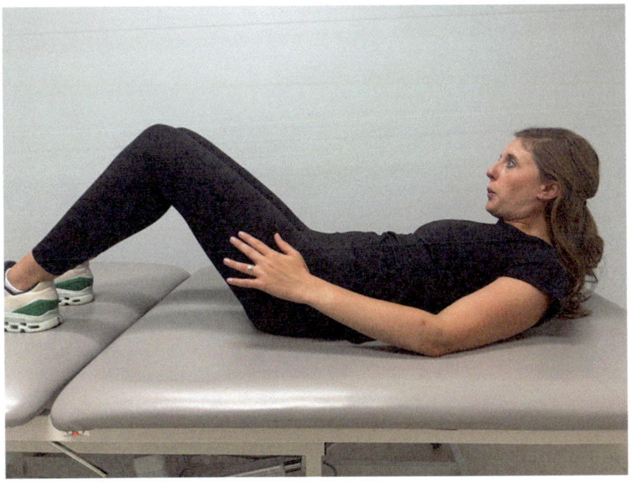

Image 7 The individual is positioned in supine for active donor with assisted triceps exercise. Gravity assists the elbow to complete extension during trunk flexion as the arms slide off the thighs on to the mat

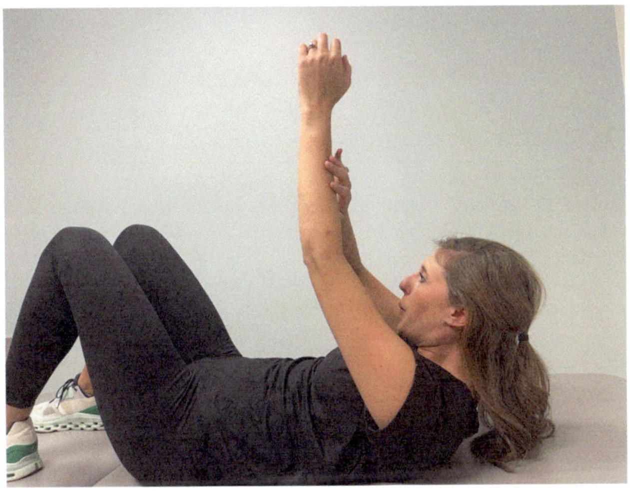

Image 8 As active elbow extension strength improves, "place-and-hold" elbow extension is performed. Here, the individual is supine, activating the donor with trunk flexion and the shoulder flexed to 90°. The uninvolved hand assists the elbow to end-range extension and releases it while attempting to maintain end-range elbow extension

In supine with the shoulder flexed to 90°, the patient performs the trunk "crunch" motion while attempting to maintain the elbow in full extension with varying amounts of manual support (from the therapist or the patient's opposite hand) (Image 8). In the same position, the patient could also do a triceps concentric contraction while simultaneously performing a sit-up.

- Functional Activity
  At this stage, the patient should be encouraged to combine the donor and recipient actions with activities of daily living (ADLs). For example, they can combine short-arc trunk flexion with reaching the arm into a sleeve using elbow extension.

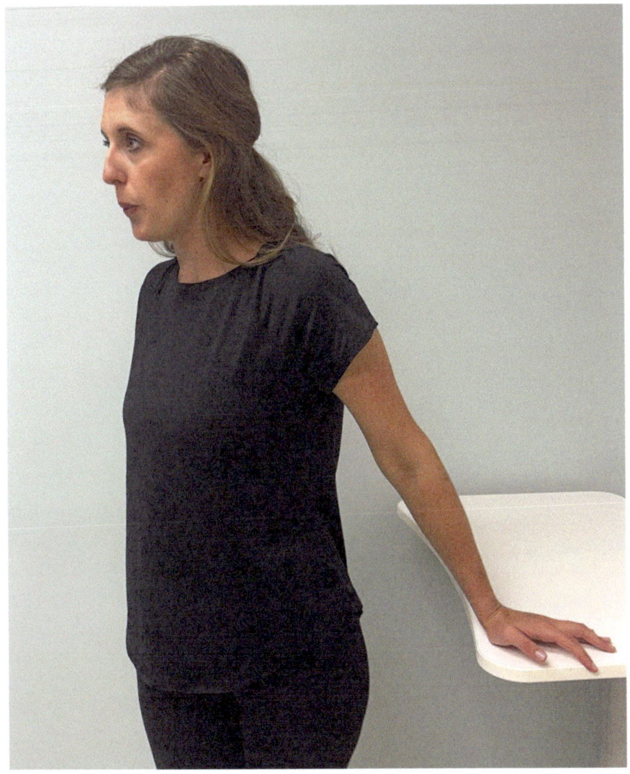

Image 9 With the hand resting on a table, the patient attempts to actively contract the triceps, extending the elbow while rotating the trunk and exhaling

Therapy Frequency

Patients may be seen once or twice per week in addition to a comprehensive home exercise program. Certain patients may do well with once per month as motor reinnervation is slow, especially if the patient is compliant, has full PROM, and demonstrates a good understanding of the donor-recipient relationship.

Phase 3

3+/5 MMT in the Recipient Muscle

The goal of phase 3 is to maximize elbow extension strength and work towards independent triceps activation without having to activate the donor. Progressive resistive triceps exercises and donor "deactivation" (independent elbow extension without trunk/core/forced respiratory activation) are the hallmarks of this stage. This requires successful cortical remapping and may take 2–4 years to achieve [1].

- Resistive Recipient Activity with Donor Contraction
  While standing, the patient is instructed to rotate the trunk to the contralateral side while simultaneously actively extending the elbow, pressing the palm into a countertop to achieve isometric triceps strength (Image 9). End-range extension assist may be provided by the uninvolved hand.

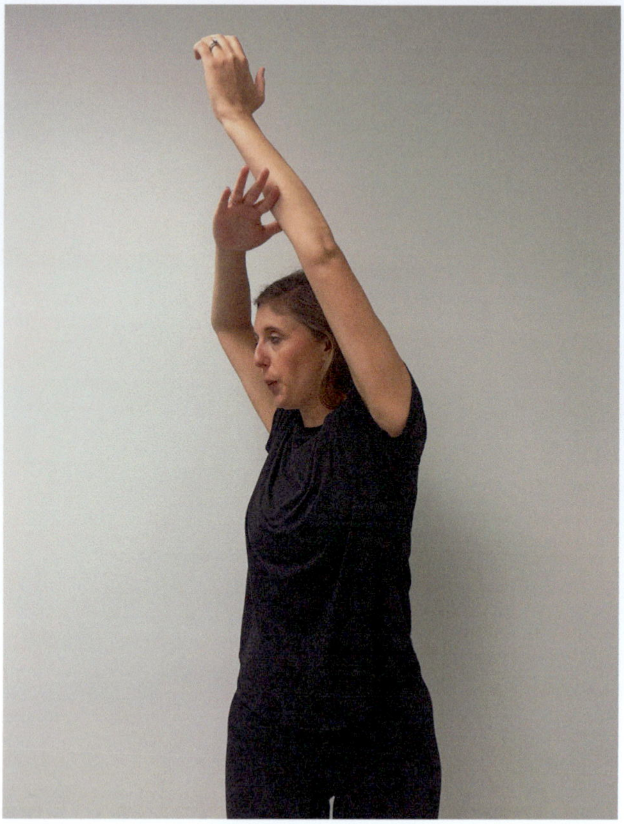

Image 10 Resisted elbow extension is demonstrated against gravity while standing with the shoulder fully flexed. The patient is instructed to rotate the trunk and exhale while attempting full elbow extension

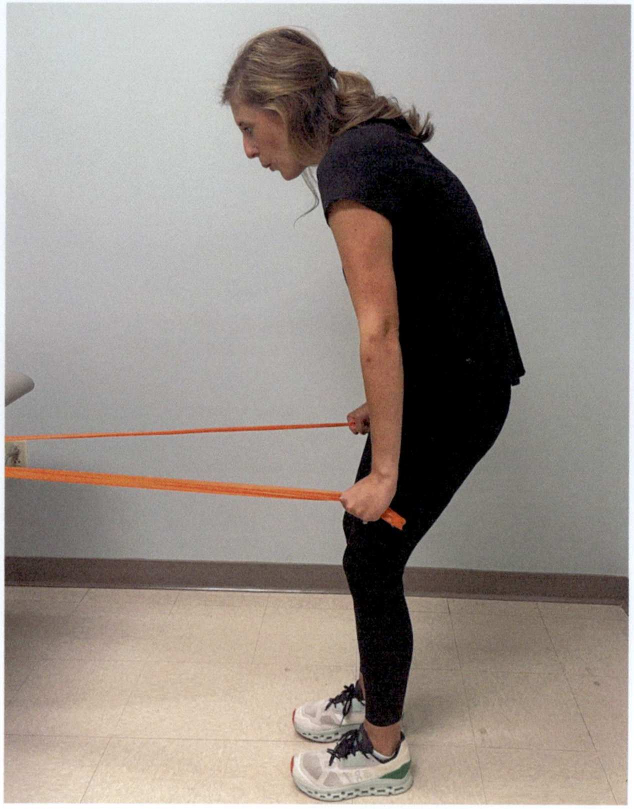

Image 11 Resisted triceps exercises are demonstrated with a light resistance band. Simultaneous trunk flexion provides co-contraction of the donor intercostal muscles

Also, while standing, gravity will provide resistance to the triceps when the shoulder is fully flexed. Trunk rotation is performed to activate the donor while extending the elbow against gravity (Image 10).

A light resistive exercise band may be introduced for resisted triceps/elbow extension with simultaneous contralateral trunk rotation OR with short abdominal crunch (Image 11). Manual resistance to the donor by resisting the trunk motion may enhance the recipient response.

- Resistive Recipient Activity Without Donor Contraction

  Strengthening exercises performed in prone will target the long head of the triceps while de-emphasizing donor action. Both elbow and shoulder extension are achieved in this position. Once full elbow extension against gravity is reached, a dumbbell, cuff weight, or resistive exercise band may be added (Image 12).

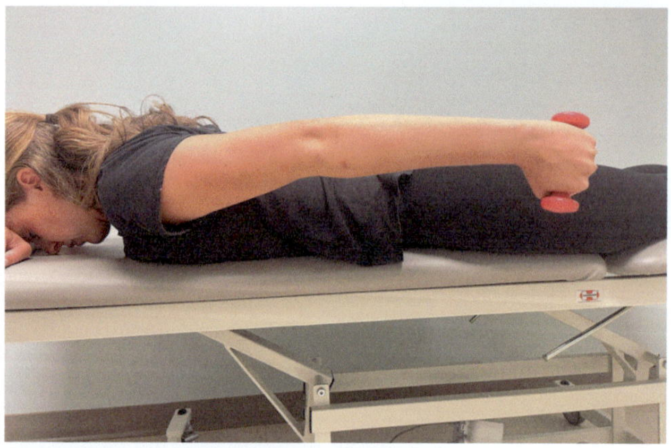

Image 12 Triceps curls with light weights are performed in prone to discourage and disassociate the recipient intercostal muscles from the donor action

Orthosis/Positioning Considerations: This transfer is rarely done in isolation, so it is presumed that the patient may already be wearing a sling to protect an injured biceps. As triceps strength returns, if it is unopposed by intact elbow flexors, intermittent sling use is recommended to prevent shortening of the triceps and/or elbow extension contracture.

Intercostal-to-triceps nerve transfer

Nerve transfer overview					
Donor nerve	Donor action	Recipient nerve	Recipient action	Indications for functional restoration	Approximate months to functional movement
Intercostal nerves	Inspiration, expiration, trunk flexion, and trunk rotation	Triceps branch of the radial nerve	Elbow extension	Regain the ability to reach, stabilize objects, propel a wheelchair, perform transfers, and perform pressure relief in a wheelchair	13–20 [1–4]

	Preoperative therapy	Early phase	Middle phase	Late phase
Criteria	Before surgery	0/5 to 1/5 MMT	2−/5 to 3/5 MMT	>3/5 MMT
Purpose of phase	Educate and establish baseline function	Understand donor and recipient relationship Begin pairing donor and recipient muscles to aid in cortical plasticity	Consistently activate recipient in gravity-lessened planes	Strengthen recipient through resistance, and gradually separate from donor activation Use triceps during functional tasks
Precautions	NA	Sling immobilization × 3–4 weeks	Respect fatigue	NA
Frequency of visits (considerations)	1–2 pre-op visits May increase if PROM limitations are present	Once every 1–2 weeks until able to demonstrate supple joint mobility and accurate donor activation and then monthly to monitor for signs of motor return	1×/week to 1×/month based on patient needs and accurate, consistent demonstration of exercise program	1× every 1–2 weeks based on progress toward patient-specific goals
Orthosis considerations	NA	Sling immobilization × 3–4 weeks	NA	NA
Interventions		**Donor activation**: Trunk flexion, trunk rotation, inspiration, and expiration **Donor-recipient pairing**: Expiration + trunk flexion with passive elbow extension	**Active/resisted donor with active assist recipient**: While seated, the patient exhales, flexes, and/or rotates the trunk while he or she tries to extend the elbow. Then, the contralateral hand assists the elbow into end-range extension **Active donor with active recipient**: While supine or seated, the patient flexes the trunk while reaching to lift the arms and straighten the elbows	**Resisted donor and recipient**: While standing and holding a resistance band, the patient exhales and flexes the trunk while extending the elbows and shoulders **Isolated resisted recipient**: In prone, the patient holds a weight and extends the shoulder and elbow
Additional interventions		Exercises can be performed bilaterally to improve motor learning. The patient is instructed to visualize the motion *before and during* the actual movement	Elbow extension should be initiated from a midrange position rather than from full elbow flexion until strength improves Triceps exercises should be performed in supine or sitting prior to prone	

During all phases, it is essential to continue cortical reorganization and psychological and psychosocial interventions and progress to incorporate donor/recipient with ADLs

Intercostal-to-Triceps Nerve Transfer

Goal of Surgery: Restore the ability to straighten the elbow.

Recipient Movement = Straighten the elbow (elbow extension)

Recipient Muscle: Long head of triceps

Recipient Nerve: Radial nerve branch to long head of triceps

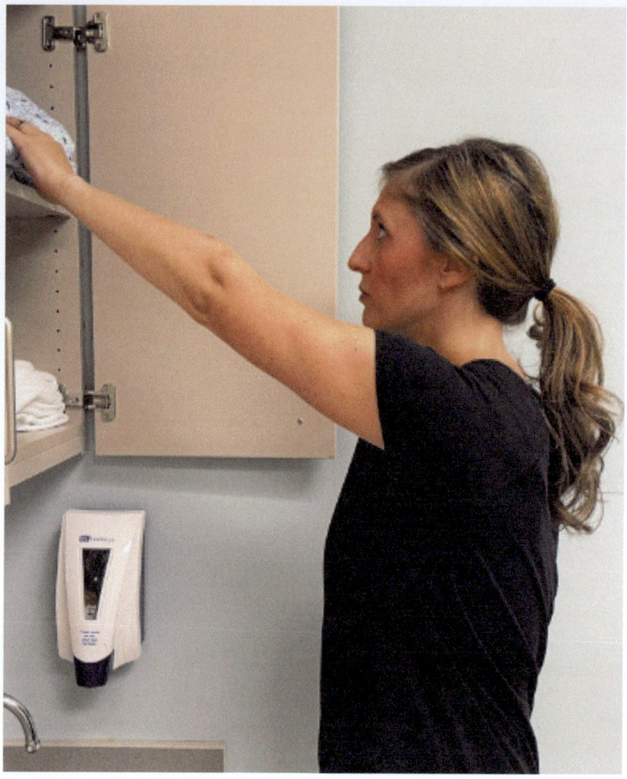

Straighten the elbow against gravity

Donor Movement = Bend trunk forward and rotate trunk, breathe in and out (spinal flexion/rotation and inspiration/expiration)

Donor Muscle: Intercostal muscles

Donor Nerve: Intercostal nerves (third, fourth, and fifth)

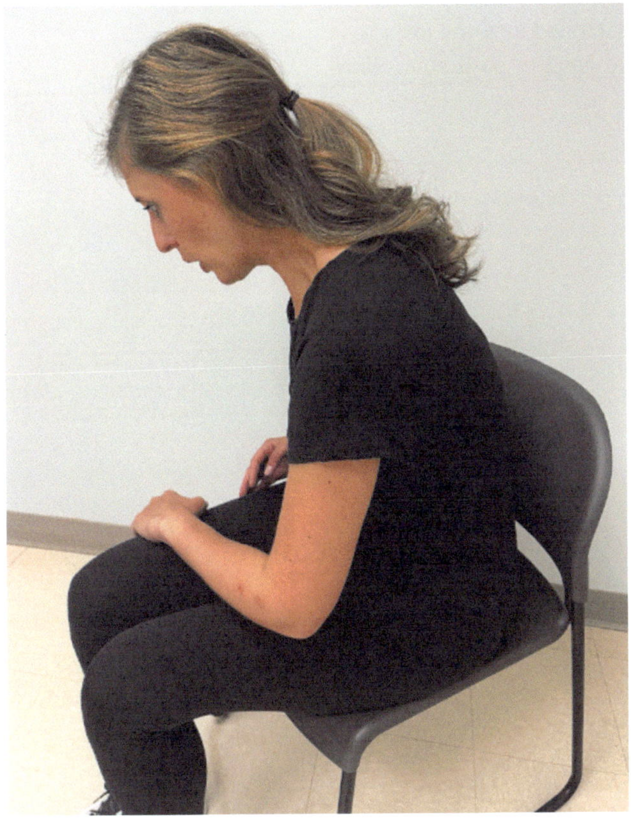

Breathe out while flexing and rotating the trunk

Phase 1 Intercostal-to-Triceps Nerve Transfer Exercises

☐ **Passive Range of Motion**:

- Rest your arm on a table with a rolled-up towel just above the elbow. Use your opposite hand to push your elbow into a straight position.

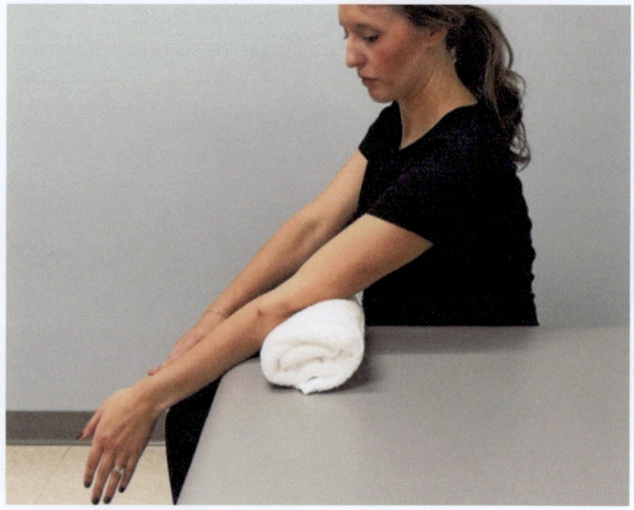

Complete 3–5 repetitions, 2–3 times per day

☐ **Active Donor Movement**:

- While seated, take a big breath and bend your trunk forward as you forcefully breathe out. Rest in between repetitions to prevent yourself from getting lightheaded.

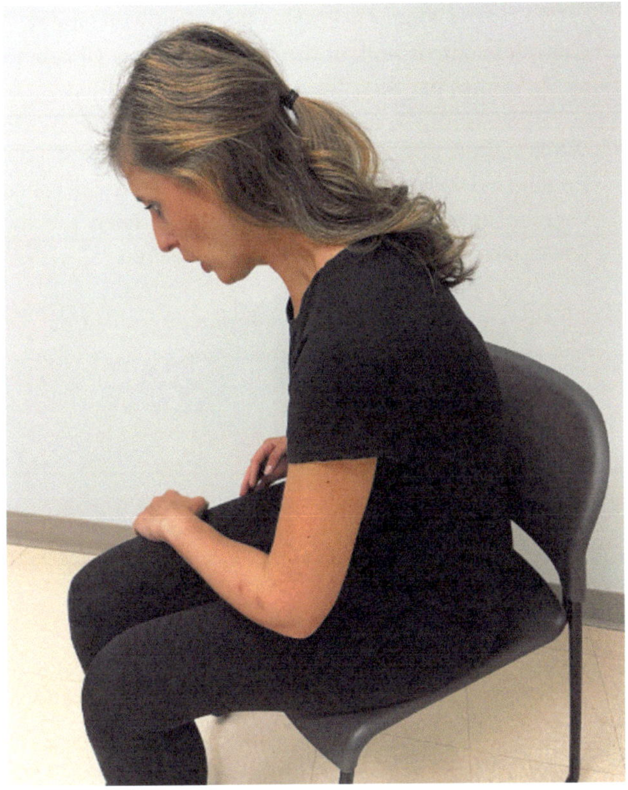

Complete 10 repetitions every waking hour

☐ **Active Donor + Passive Recipient Movement: Complete one or both of the below exercises 10 repetitions, 2–3 times per day.**

- While seated, rest your arm on a table in front of you. Breathe in while sitting upright. Breathe out as you round your upper body forward (upper body "crunch") while you stretch your elbow into a straight position.

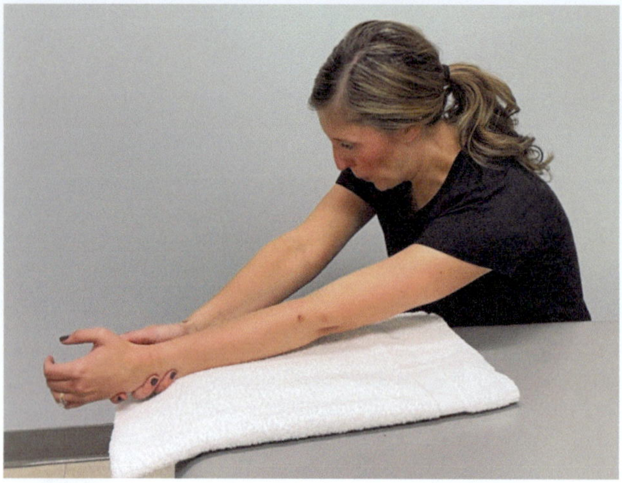

- While standing, hold a dowel rod in both hands. Exhale and bend your trunk forward while pushing your arm out to the side to straighten the elbow.

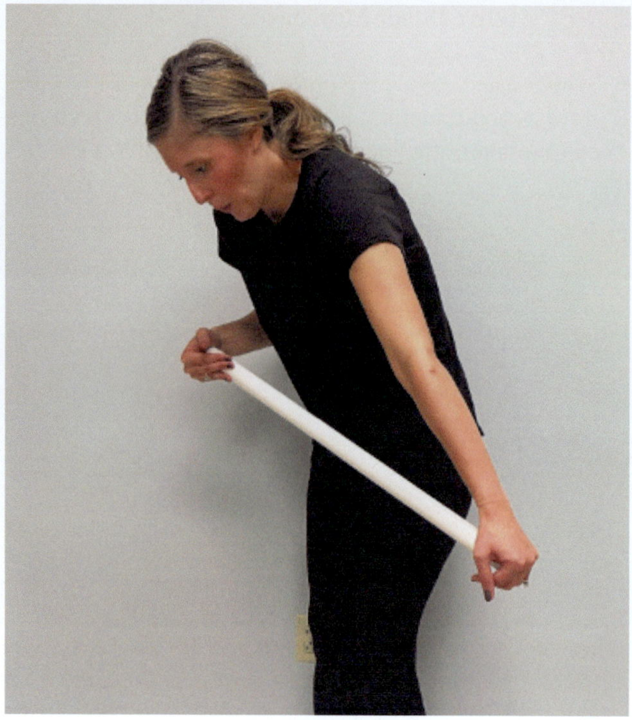

Phase 2 Intercostal-to-Triceps Nerve Transfer Exercises

☐ **Active Donor + Active-Assisted Recipient Movement**:

Complete one or more of the below exercises 1–10 repetitions, 2–3 times per day.

1. While seated, rest both arms on the table out in front of you with a towel under your forearms. Breathe in while sitting upright. Forcefully breathe out as you round your upper body forward as you straighten your elbows, allowing the arms to slide forward on the table.

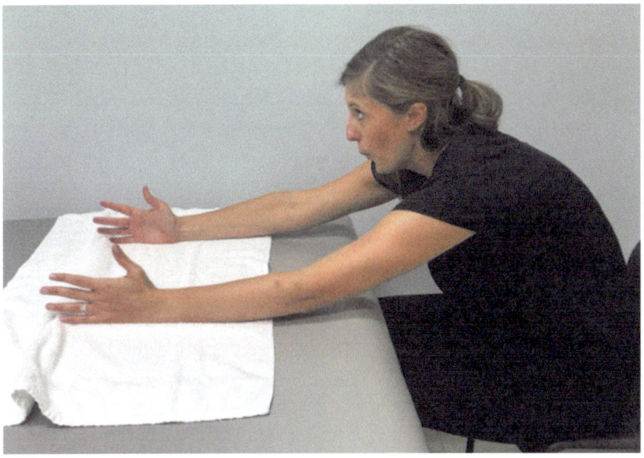

2. Lay on your uninvolved side with your surgical arm resting on an exercise ball. Curl your trunk forward as you forcefully breathe out and roll the ball forward while attempting to straighten your elbow.

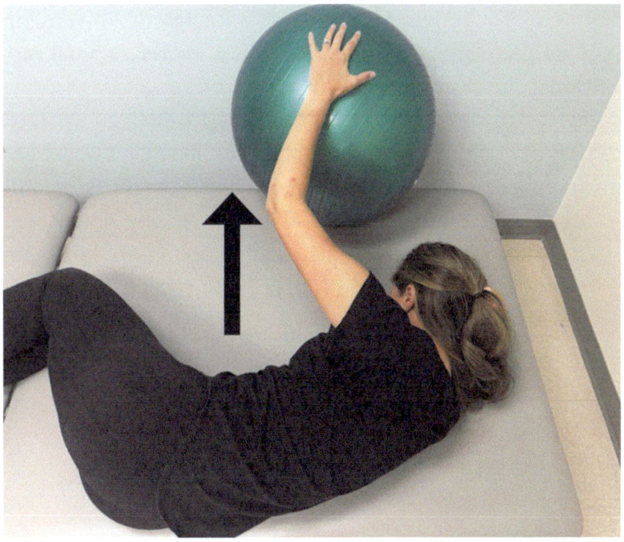

3. Begin lying on your back with your knees bent and feet flat. Rest both hands on your belly or thighs. Breath in before you move. Breathe out as you round your upper body forward and gently slide your hands off your thighs, down to the mat, allowing the elbows to straighten.

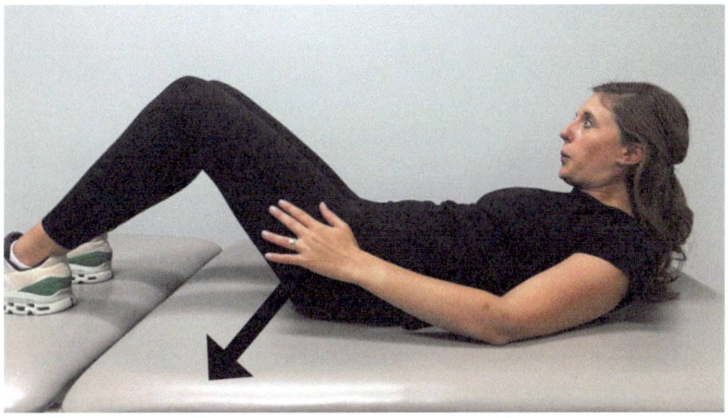

☐ **Active Donor + Active Recipient Movement**: **Complete one or more of the below exercises 5–10 repetitions, 2–3 times per day.**

1. Begin lying on your back with knees and elbows bent and feet flat. Breathe in before you move. Forcefully breathe out as you straighten your elbows, reaching your hands forward. At the same time, round your upper body forward toward the ceiling (upper body crunch). Return to the start position, and repeat.

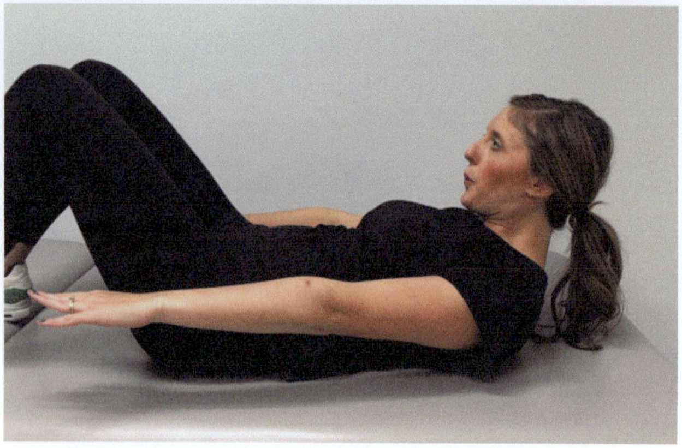

2. While standing, reach your arms overhead while you rotate your trunk from one side to the other.

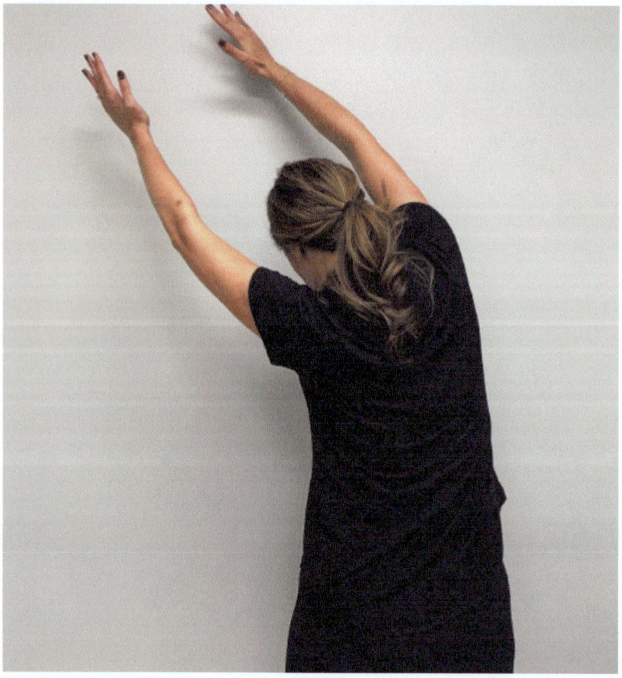

- This may also be done holding a ball between your hands and reaching overhead. At the same time, rotate your trunk side to side.

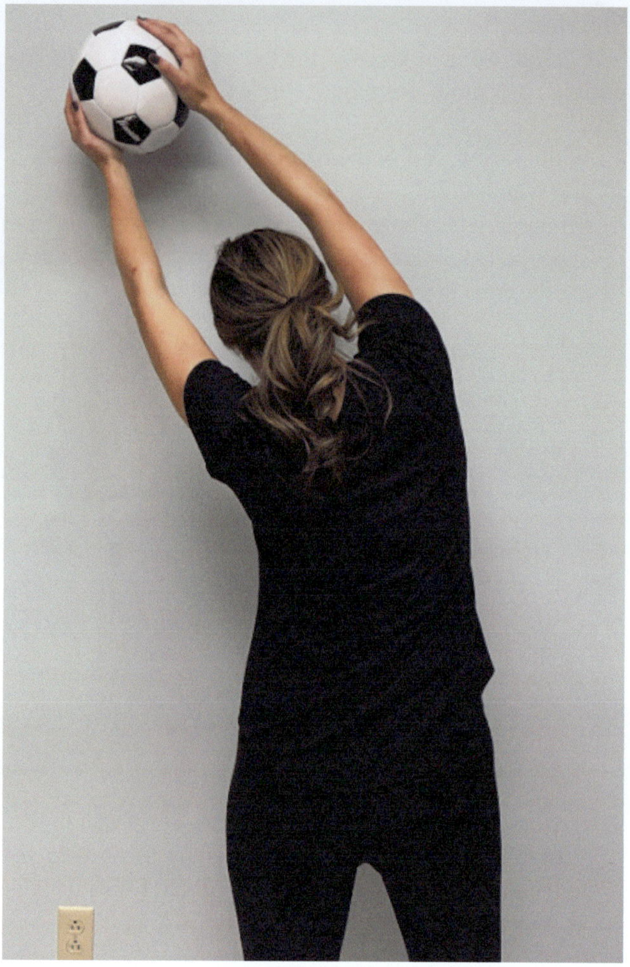

Phase 3 Intercostal-to-Triceps Nerve Transfer Exercises

☐ **Resisted Donor + Active Recipient Movement**: **Complete one or more of the below exercises 1–10 repetitions, 2–3 times per day.**

1. While standing, hold the ends of a resistance band secured in front of you. Keeping your elbows straight, pull your arms back as you round your upper body slightly forward (short abdominal crunch).

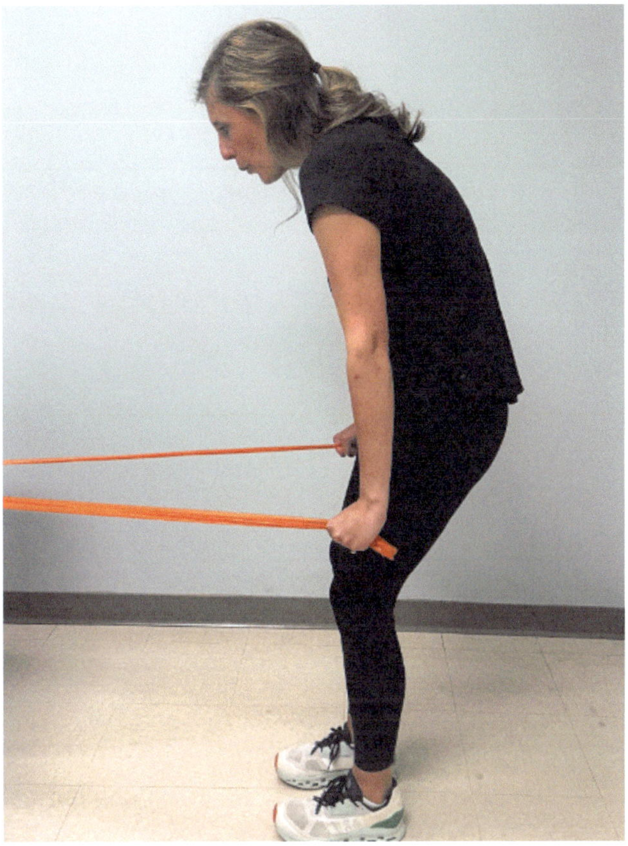

2. Stand with your hand firmly planted on a countertop and your elbow straight. Press your hand into the countertop to create resistance as you rotate your trunk away from that arm. Hold for 3–5 s. Return to the start position, and repeat.

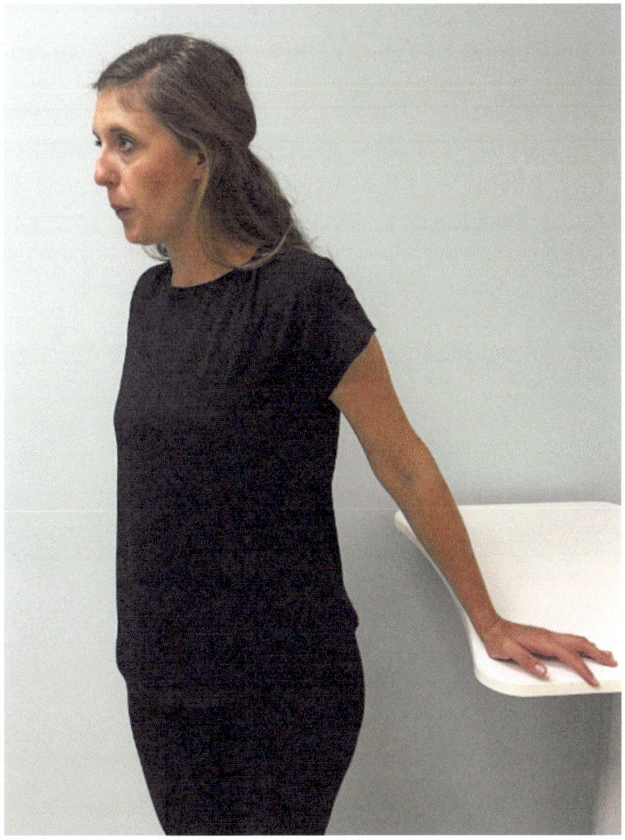

☐ **Resisted Recipient Movement**:

Complete one or more of the below exercises 5–10 repetitions, 2–3 times per day.

1. Begin lying on your back with your knees bent and feet flat. Hold a _____ pound weight in your hand. Begin with your elbow bent and your hand resting by your ear. Straighten your elbow, bringing the weight toward the ceiling. Return to the starting position, and repeat.

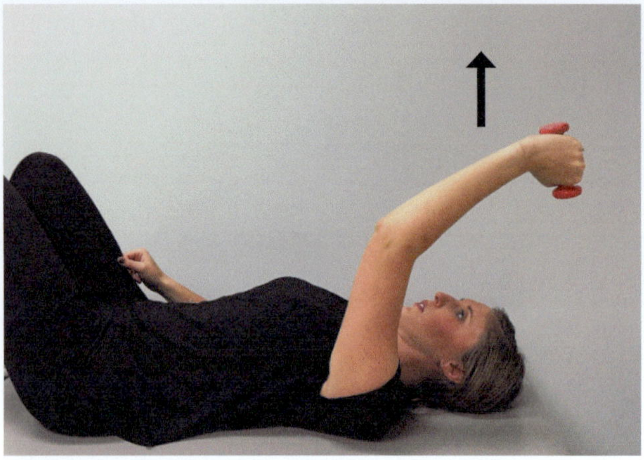

2. Lay on your belly with your arm down by your side. Hold a ___ lb weight in your hand. Lift your hand up toward the ceiling while keeping your elbow fully straight. Return to the starting position, and repeat.

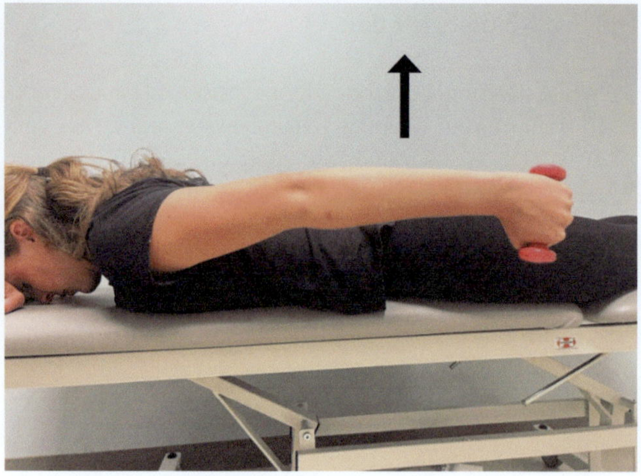

References

1. Kittithamvongs P, Leechavengvongs S, Malungpaishrope K, Pongpinyopap W, Anantavorasakul N, Uerpairojkit C. The intercostal nerves transfer to the radial nerve branch to the long head of the triceps muscle: influencing factor and outcome of 55 cases. J Hand Surg. 2023;48(7):733–e1.
2. Gao KM, Lao J, Zhao X, Gu YD. Outcome after transfer of intercostal nerves to the nerve of triceps long head in 25 adult patients with total brachial plexus root avulsion injury. J Neurosurg. 2013;118:606–10.
3. Goubier JN, Teboul F. Transfer of intercostal nerves to the nerve of the long head of the triceps to recover elbow extension in brachial plexus palsy. Tech Hand Up Extrem Surg. 2007;11(2):139–41.
4. Goubier JN, Teboul F, Khalifa H. Reanimation of elbow extension with intercostal nerves transfers in total brachial plexus palsies. Microsurgery. 2011;31:7–11.
5. Kahn L, Moore A. Donor activation focused rehabilitation approach: maximizing outcomes after nerve transfers. Hand Clin. 2016;32(2):263–77.
6. Whitelaw WA, Ford GT, Rimmer KP, De Troyer A. Intercostal muscles are used during rotation of the thorax in humans. J Appl Physiol. 1985;72(5):1940–4.
7. Chalidapong P, Sananpanich K, Klaphajone J. Electromyographic comparison of various exercises to improve elbow flexion following intercostal nerve transfer. J Bone Joint Surgery. 2006;88(5):620–2.
8. Neumann DA. Kinesiology of the musculoskeletal system-e-book: foundations for rehabilitation. Elsevier Health Sciences; 2016.
9. Lee EY, Karjalainen TV, Sebastin SJ, Lim AY. The value of the tender muscle sign in detecting motor recovery after peripheral nerve reconstruction. J Hand Surg Am. 2015;40(3):433–7.
10. Kahn LC, Stonner MM, Dy CJ. Key concepts for nerve transfer rehabilitation after surgical reconstruction for brachial plexus and peripheral nerve injuries. J Hand Surg Am. 2023;49:160.

Posterior Branch of the Axillary Nerve to the Triceps Branch of the Radial Nerve Transfer

Alexandra MacKenzie

Axillary-to-Triceps Nerve Transfer

Background

The axillary-to-triceps nerve transfer is useful in restoring triceps function both in patients with lower plexus injuries (C7 and below) as well as for patients with mid-level cervical spinal cord injuries (SCIs). The need for elbow extension is often underestimated. Triceps function is important for many daily activities where some extension power is required (more than just the weight of the arm), such as stabilization of an object on a table (holding a paper while writing on it, holding a plate while cutting food). It is important in reaching for an object [1], and for those who can reach, it improves the ability to grasp [2] as well as reach from a supine position so that the arm does not fall and hit them in the face [3]. In addition, a working triceps can improve the function of the biceps as an antagonist and stabilizer. In the SCI population, triceps function is helpful in weight shifting for pressure relief as well as during transfers and propelling a wheelchair.

The function of the triceps can be restored with a nerve transfer from the posterior motor branch of the axillary nerve to the long head of the triceps branch of the radial nerve. Nerve root function from C5 to C6 needs to be intact for this transfer to work because the axillary nerve derives from this upper trunk contribution to the posterior cord. The axillary nerve innervates the deltoid and teres minor muscles. The teres minor contributes external rotation force to the rotator cuff, along with the infraspinatus muscle. Together, the deltoid and teres minor contribute to arm elevation in anterior, posterior, and lateral directions. The teres minor branch can be used alone as a donor if preservation of the posterior deltoid is desired [4]. This may be a reasonable synergistic relationship as external rotation has been demonstrated to aid in elbow extension through altered kinematics of the glenohumeral and scapulothoracic joints in the spinal cord population [5]. When the teres minor is used alone, the posterior deltoid is left as a potential donor for a tendon transfer at a later time [6]. However, when branches to both teres minor and posterior deltoid are combined to coapt to the long head branch of the radial nerve, there may be a better nerve fiber count match [7]. It is important to discuss with the referring surgeon what branches of the axillary nerve were used because this will determine the appropriate motor reeducation program.

In the SCI population, timing of nerve transfers depends on the level of upper motor neuron (UMN) involvement, which will be determined with electrodiagnostic studies [8]. There is not the same level of urgency to perform nerve transfers within 6 months of injury if there is only UMN involvement, as the muscle does not become denervated. However, if there is both upper and lower motor neuron (LMN) involvement, timing becomes crucial [6]. In looking at electrodiagnostic studies, Fox and colleagues found that up to 92% of quadriplegics experiencing triceps loss have LMN involvement [8]. In their study, no patients who presented greater than 1 year post-injury were eligible for axillary-to-triceps transfer, so early electrodiagnostic studies and timing for this transfer are important in this population [8].

A. MacKenzie (✉)
Hand and Upper Extremity Therapy Center, Hospital for Special Surgery, New York, NY, USA
e-mail: mackenziea@hss.edu

L. C. Kahn et al. (eds.), *Rehabilitation for Nerve Transfers of the Upper Extremity*,
https://doi.org/10.1007/978-3-031-92008-0_16

Surgery Description

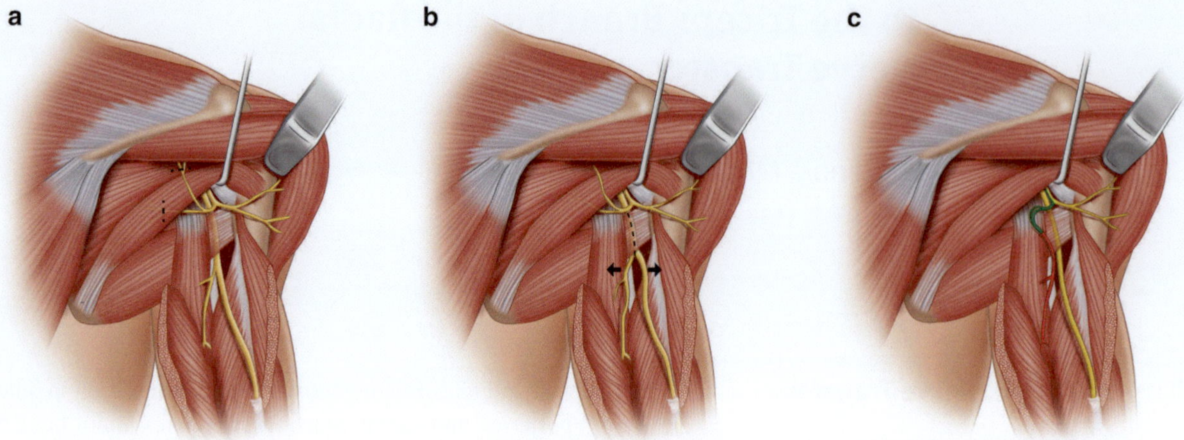

Axillary to triceps

A longitudinal incision is made along the posterior brachium, beginning just cephalad to the posterolateral corner of the acromion and continuing to the mid-brachium. The interval between the posterior deltoid and triceps is identified. It can be helpful, but not necessary, to identify the posterior cutaneous branch from the axillary nerve, which can be used as a guide to the axillary nerve proper. Retracting the posterior head of the deltoid, the quadrangular space is exposed. Being sure to preserve the circumflex humeral artery and its branches, the anterior and posterior branches of the axillary nerve are identified. The posterior branch of the axillary nerve is isolated and neurolyzed from the axillary nerve. A nerve stimulator is used to confirm that the remaining anterior branch of the axillary nerve provides robust shoulder abduction, therefore confirming that the posterior branch is expendable as a donor nerve.

If these criteria are met, the posterior cutaneous nerve is dissected free from the motor portion of the posterior branch of the axillary nerve so as to maximize motor neurons in the donor nerve. The surgeon then exposes the radial nerve in the triangular interval, identifying branches from the radial nerve to the triceps. The selection of a recipient nerve to the lateral, long, or middle heads of the triceps (or multiple branches) is based on surgeon preference. A nerve stimulator is used to confirm absence of triceps function when stimulating the recipient nerve, ensuring that the anesthesia team is not using muscle paralytics. The donor posterior branch of the axillary nerve is then divided distally and transposed to meet the recipient triceps branches, which have been neurolyzed from the radial nerve proper. Coaptation of the posterior branch of the axillary nerve to the triceps branches of the radial nerve is performed using microsurgical technique.

Outcomes

Few studies have evaluated outcomes following this transfer, but evidence shows that trace muscle contraction appears around 5–6 months, and elbow extension against resistance occurs around 12–14 months from surgery [6, 7]. In a small study of two patients who underwent axillary-to-triceps nerve transfer, one patient regained fair (3/5 manual muscle testing/MMT) strength, and the other patient regained good (4/5 MMT grade) strength [9].

Phases of Rehabilitation

Phase 1

Pre-op to 1/5 MMT in the Recipient Muscle

After surgery, patients are immobilized in a sling or shoulder immobilizer for 10 days to 3 weeks [4, 7]. Once the rest period is over, patients may resume normal activities but should avoid excessive end-range shoulder abduction and external rotation for a month. Passive shoulder range of motion (PROM) is introduced and gradually increased within a symptom-free range. It is important to maintain shoulder and elbow joint flexibility because during recovery, the reinnervating weak triceps muscle will struggle to produce sufficient force to actively move a stiff joint. Passive elbow extension should be addressed, if needed, to prevent stiffness or contracture from prolonged sling use. Motor reeducation begins in the first month to familiarize the patient with the donor and recipient muscle action, donor activation exercises, and timelines for recovery.

Exercises

- Donor Activation
  After reviewing the operative note to identify the specific donor muscle, the patient should be instructed in frequent activation of shoulder extension, with abduction (if posterior deltoid branch was used as a donor) (Image 1) and/or external rotation (if teres minor branch is included). Shoulder extension with abduction can also be performed with a light resistance band for added challenge to the donor (Image 2).
- Combined Donor with Passive Recipient Exercise
  In standing or sitting, the patient performs active shoulder extension/abduction (with or without external rotation) with the elbow resting in extension *or* holding a dowel to maintain extension with the help of the uninvolved hand (Image 3). Donor activation with the elbows in extension can also be performed bilaterally to reinforce the new motor pathway. In supine, gravity will provide the passive component of elbow extension. The patient is instructed to visualize extending the elbow during this movement.

Assessment of Recovery

Monthly visits should include assessment of triceps motor function. This can be done by having the patient activate the donor (shoulder extension with abduction with or without external rotation) against manual resistance while the therapist simultaneously palpates whichever head of the triceps was chosen for the nerve transfer, looking for a notable change in tension (Image 4). This can be performed in sev-

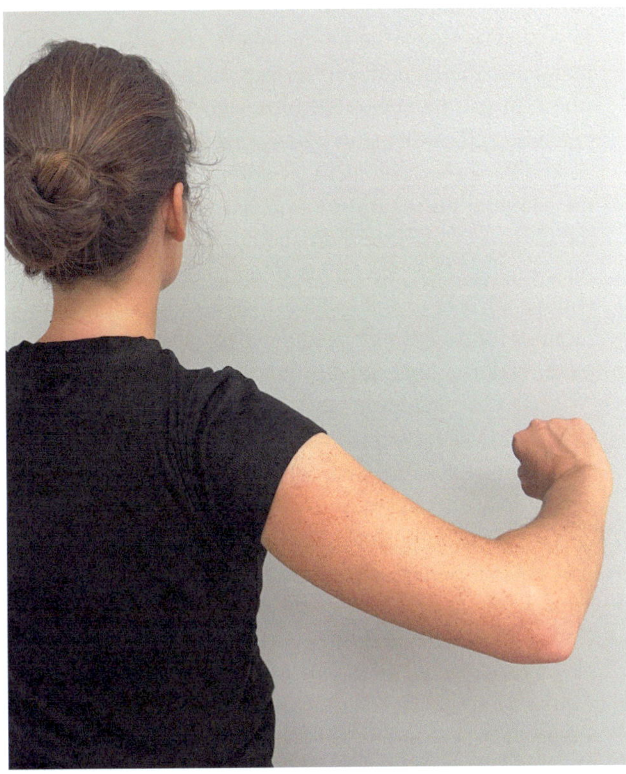

Image 1 Donor activation of the posterior head of the deltoid includes active shoulder abduction with extension

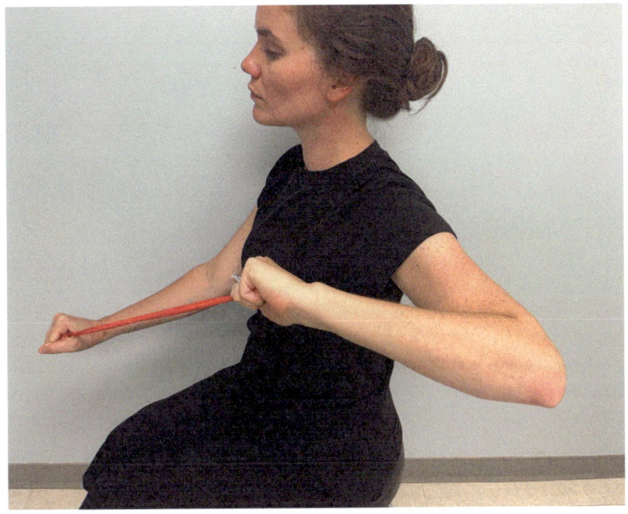

Image 2 Resisted axillary donor activation is demonstrated with a resistance band in the direction of shoulder abduction with extension and external rotation

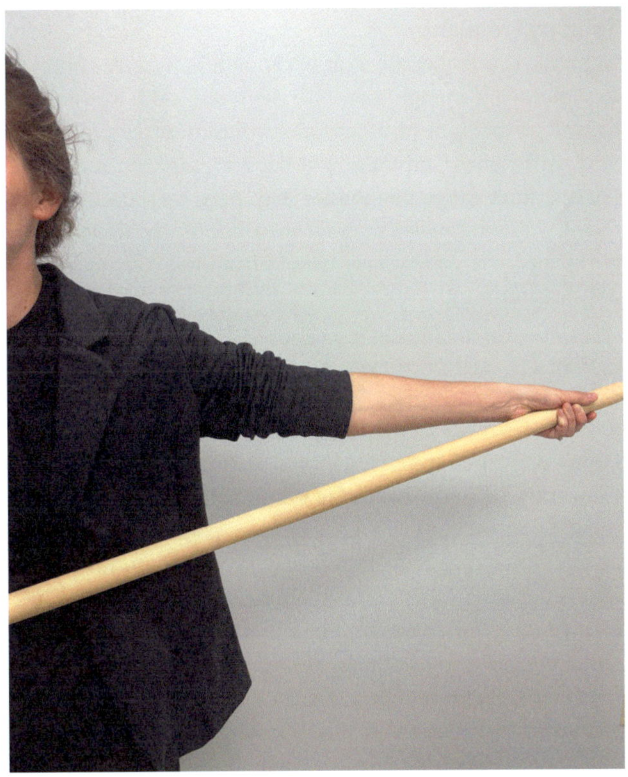

Image 3 Combined donor with passive recipient exercises are performed in phase 1. The individual is instructed to actively extend and abduct the shoulder, with or without external rotation, holding a dowel to maintain elbow extension with the help of the uninvolved hand

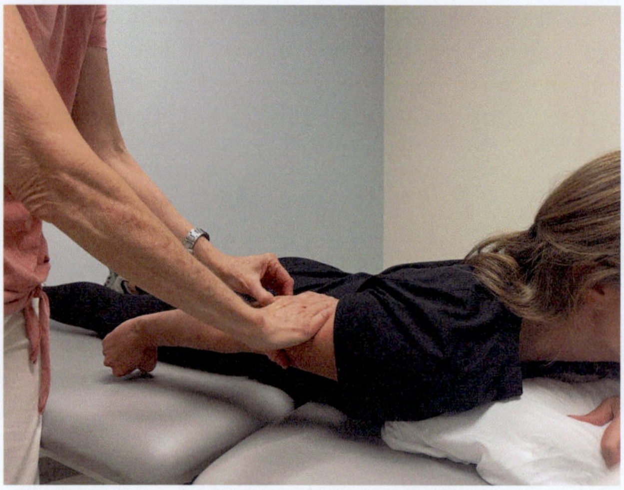

Image 4 Assessment of recovery of the triceps is demonstrated in prone. Resistance is applied to the donor/posterior deltoid while palpating the tendons or heads of the triceps muscle for any sign of tone or tension

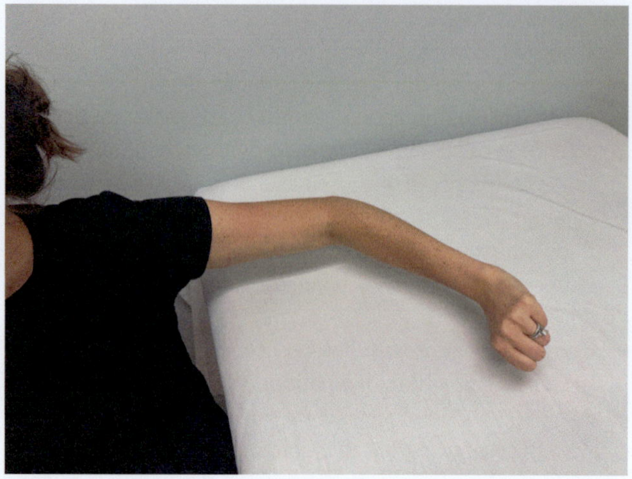

Image 5 The triceps muscle works best when in approximately 80 degrees of elbow flexion. Early in phase 2 of therapy, this position is recommended to aid the recovering triceps in producing force while activating the donor deltoid

eral positions, but they may get a greater response in prone where the donor will have to work harder. It will take anywhere from 5 to 11 months to see early signs of reinnervation. Active elbow extension strength against gravity may appear around 12–14 months postoperatively [6, 7].

Therapy Frequency

In phase 1, one therapy visit per month is usually sufficient to monitor for compliance with the home exercise program as well as for signs of triceps motor return. If the patient has very stiff joints, and there is a need to work on increasing passive joint range of motion, they may be seen more frequently. Additionally, if more than one nerve transfer was performed, the patient may benefit from more frequent therapy sessions.

Phase 2

2−/5 to 3/5 MMT in the Recipient Muscle

Donor activation exercises should continue to be performed frequently in phase 2. Pairing donor activation with passive recipient movement will advance to *active-assisted* recipient action with donor activation. These should be initiated at the first signs of triceps reinnervation. Exercises can be performed in a gravity-minimized plane for the triceps with simultaneous active (or resisted) donor activation. While the long head of the triceps can maintain a relatively constant force across a wide range of elbow angles, volitional triceps contraction forces are greatest when the elbow is in about 80 degrees of flexion [10], so it may be beneficial to initiate elbow extension from this angle, rather than from a position of maximum flexion (Image 5).

Exercises

- Active Donor with Active-Assisted Recipient
  Triceps MMT: 2−/5 to 2/5
  While sitting next to a table with a cloth under the hand, the patient abducts (and extends) the shoulder while independently extending the elbow, as able. The contralateral hand then assists the elbow into end-range extension (Image 6a, b).
  In supine or side lying on the unaffected side, the patient maintains the shoulder in an externally rotated position (the arm can be supported on a stack of pillows) while extending elbow in a gravity-assisted position. The patient should be actively abducting (with or without extending) the shoulder during this motion. The therapist should cue the patient to squeeze their shoulder blades together and raise the hand off the pillow to enhance donor activation (Image 7). The patient should be instructed on how to monitor for triceps fatigue and maladaptive compensatory patterns during this stage.
- "Place and Hold" Exercise
  Triceps MMT = 2+/5
  While sitting next to a table with a cloth under the hand, the patient abducts (and extends) the shoulder while using the opposite hand to push the elbow into end-range extension. The patient is instructed to maintain this fully extended position once the contralateral hand releases the support. Once this becomes easy, the patient may then lift the arm off the table while attempting to hold the elbow in extension.
- Active Donor with Active Recipient
  Triceps MMT = 3−/5
  The patient may be standing (Image 8) or prone to partial side lying (Image 9) while he or she externally rotates and

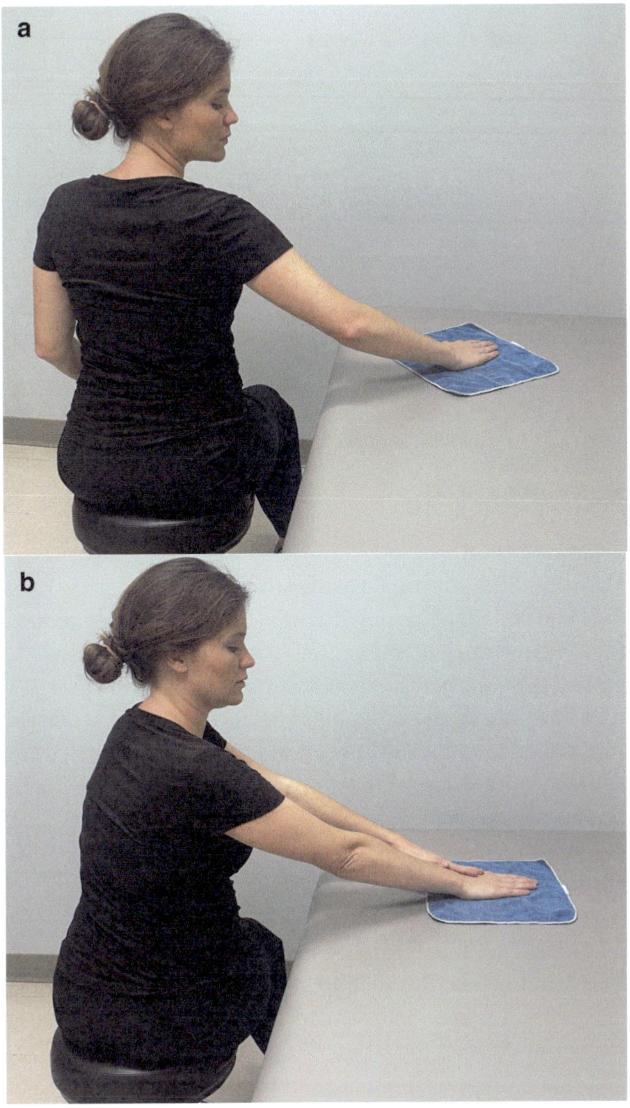

Image 6 (**a**, **b**) Active donor (deltoid and teres minor) with active-assisted recipient (triceps) is demonstrated with active shoulder posterior abduction with simultaneous active elbow extension across the table. Once the triceps cannot extend further, the contralateral hand assists the arm into end-range elbow extension

extends the shoulder while attempting to maintain elbow extension.

- Functional Activity
  The patient can be taught to combine the donor and recipient actions with activities of daily living (ADLs). For example, the patient can externally rotate and posteriorly abduct the shoulder while extending the elbow and reaching into a sleeve for triceps activation (Image 10).

Assessment of Recovery

Triceps reinnervation should continue to be assessed during monthly therapy visits. The patient performs shoulder extension (and/or external rotation), while the therapist palpates the long head of the triceps evaluating for active movement—first in a gravity-minimized plane. The best target muscle response will be in prone where the donor will have to work harder.

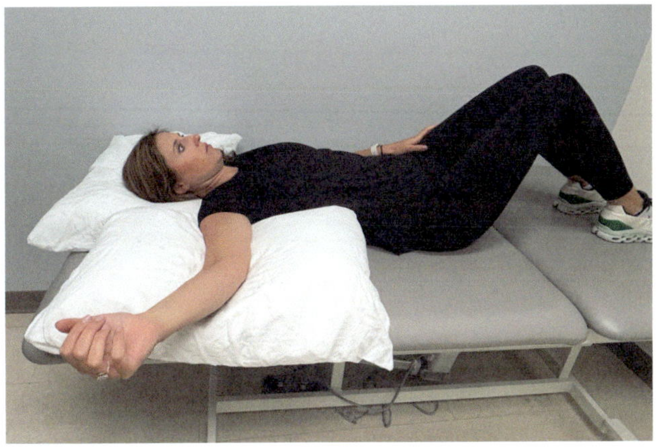

Image 7 Active donor (deltoid and teres minor) with active-assisted recipient/triceps is demonstrated in supine. The involved arm is positioned in shoulder abduction and external rotation on a pillow. Cues are given to raise the arm into shoulder abduction (and external rotation) as the elbow slides into extension with the assistance of gravity

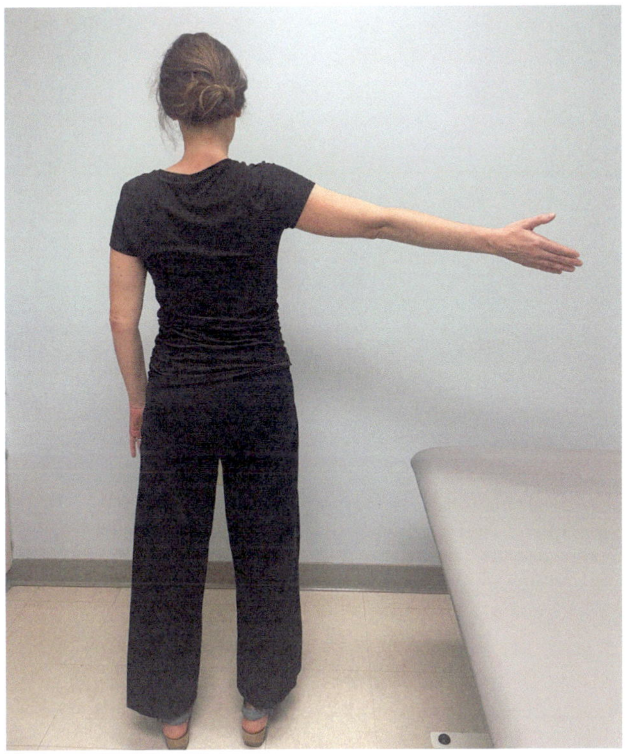

Image 8 While standing, the individual is instructed to posteriorly abduct (with external rotation) while simultaneously extending the elbow

Therapy Frequency

Patients can be seen once per week at this stage with instruction in a comprehensive home exercise program.

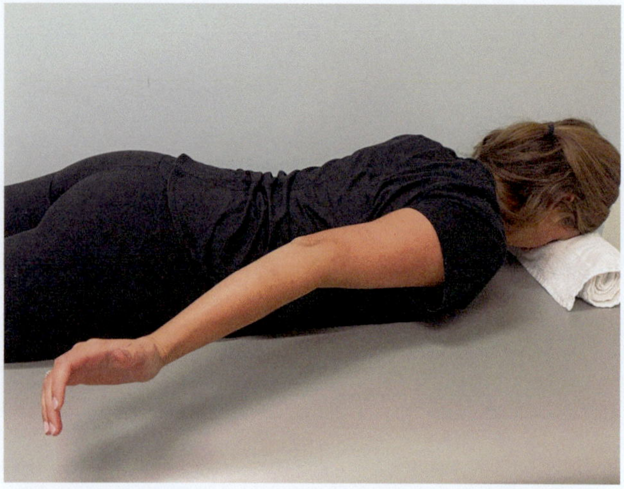

Image 9 Lying prone or partial side lying, the individual is instructed to externally rotate and extend the shoulder while maintaining elbow extension

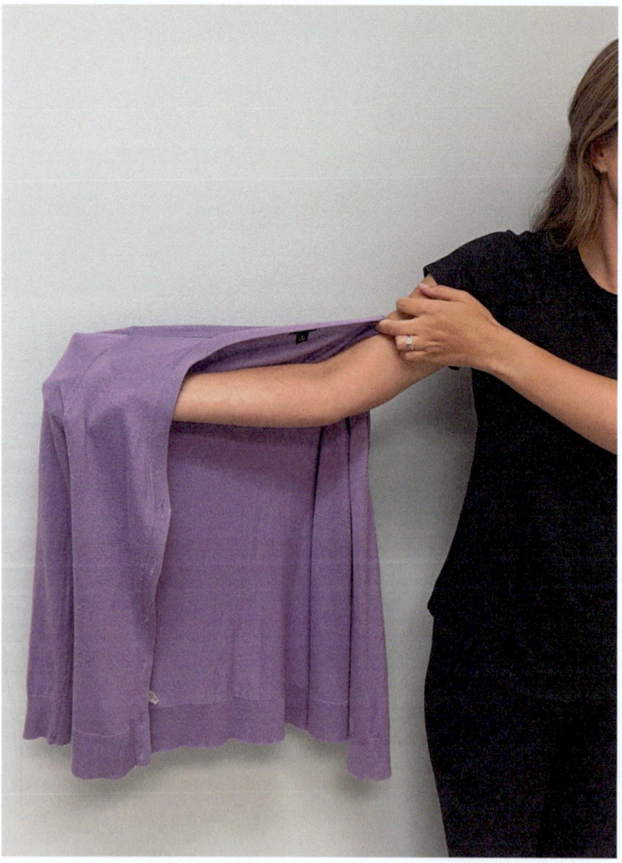

Image 10 Incorporate combined donor and recipient activation for ADL activities such as dressing. The patient is instructed to abduct the shoulder and attempt to extend the elbow while placing it in a shirtsleeve

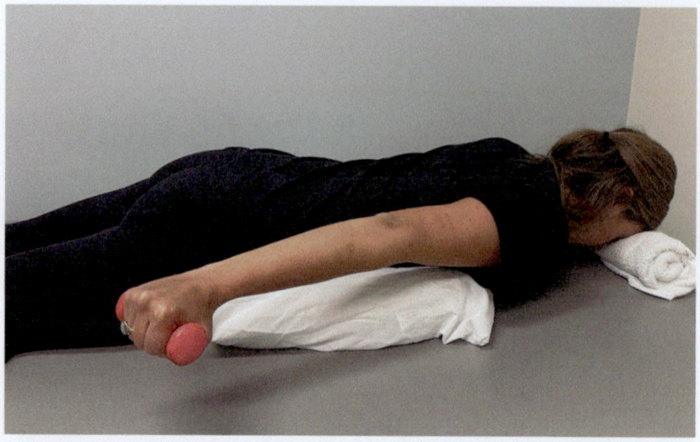

Image 11 Resistance is added in phase 3. With the individual in prone, elbow and shoulder extension is performed while holding a lightweight dumbbell

Orthosis/Positioning Considerations

No sling or splint is required at this stage. As strength returns, intermittent sling can be used for patient comfort if the patient lacks sufficient elbow flexion strength. However, it is important not to let the shoulder get too stiff from prolonged immobilization. Patients undergoing this nerve transfer presumably have shoulder function, and there is less concern for traction on the nerve repair after postoperative week 3.

Phase 3

3+/5 MMT or Greater in the Recipient Muscle

The goal of phase 3 is to maximize elbow extension strength and work towards independent triceps activation without having to activate the donor. Progressive resistive exercises and donor "deactivation," i.e., independent elbow extension without donor activation, are the hallmarks of this stage. Highest maximum force of the triceps occurs with the shoulder in 80 degrees of flexion and 60–80 degrees of elbow flexion [10, 11], so incorporating this positioning into the rehabilitation program may be useful for some patients as they advance the strengthening program.

- Resistive Recipient Activity with Donor Contraction
  To target the long head of the triceps, the patient can perform triceps and shoulder extension from a prone position with a dumbbell, cuff weight, or resistive exercise band (Image 11).
  Low rows: While sitting and holding a resistance band, the patient can perform bilateral resisted shoulder extension (with the elbows flexed) followed by resistive elbow extension (Image 12).

Wall slides: While standing with a resistance band looped around the wrists, the patient is instructed to pull the wrists apart (external rotation) while sliding up the wall into elbow extension (Image 13).

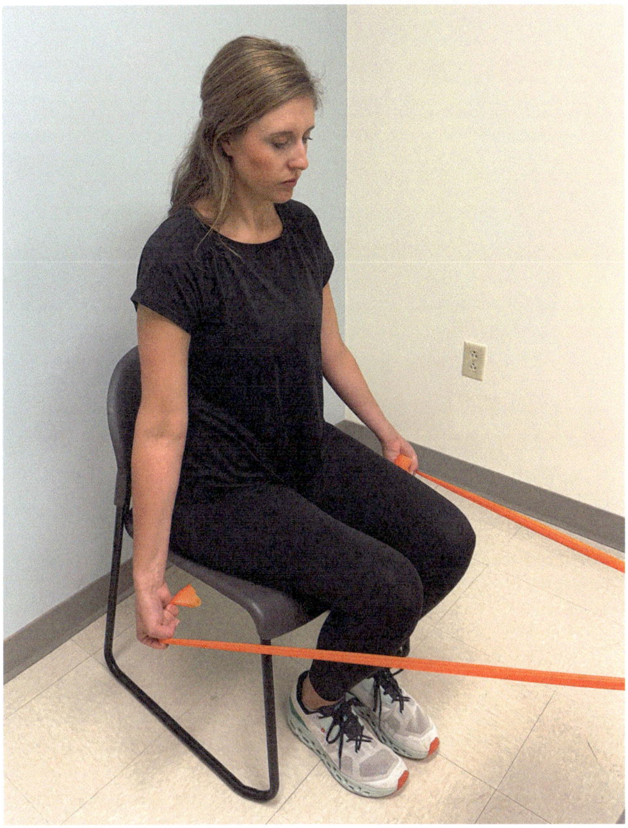

Image 12 Low rows performed in sitting with a resistance band are demonstrated for combined resisted donor and recipient muscle exercise. The individual extends the shoulder (with the elbows flexed) and then attempts resisted elbow extension. Patients may do this bilaterally for added plasticity training

- Resistive Recipient Activity Without Donor Contraction
Once the patient demonstrates reliable triceps strength, the patient may deactivate the donor by working on triceps resistance without the assistive component of shoulder extension/external rotation. The patient can be supine with the shoulder flexed at 90° while performing triceps extension with a light weight. The weight can be advanced in time per patient tolerance. A functional activity that may achieve donor deactivation would be pushing a weighted object across a table while extending the elbows.

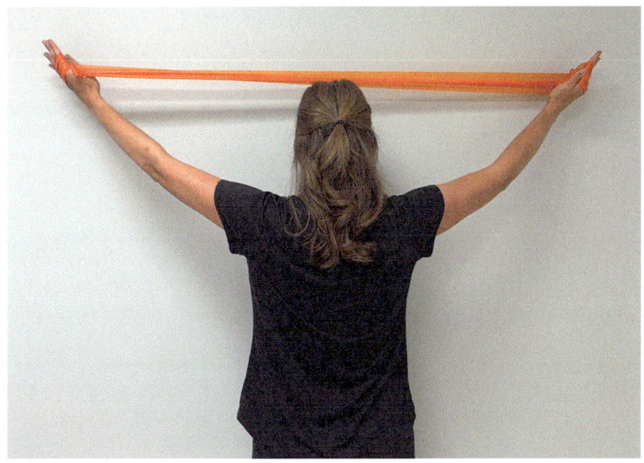

Image 13 In standing, resisted elbow extension with resisted donor is achieved with wall slides. A resistance band provides resistance as the individual pulls the arms apart and slides up the wall into shoulder abduction (and external rotation) with elbow extension

Axillary-to-triceps nerve transfer

Nerve transfer overview					
Donor nerve	Donor action	Recipient nerve	Recipient action	Indications for functional restoration	Approximate months to functional movement
Posterior branch of the axillary nerve	Shoulder extension with abduction and sometimes external rotation if teres minor branch was used	Radial nerve	Elbow extension	Regain the ability to reach, stabilize objects, propel a wheelchair, perform transfers, and perform pressure relief in a wheelchair	12–14 [6, 7]

	Preoperative therapy	Early phase	Middle phase	Late phase
Criteria	Before surgery	0/5 to 1/5 MMT	2−/5 to 3/5 MMT	>3/5 MMT
Purpose of phase	Educate and establish baseline function	Understand donor and recipient relationship Begin pairing donor and recipient muscles to aid in cortical plasticity	Consistently activate recipient in gravity-lessened planes	Strengthen recipient through resistance and gradually separate from donor activation Use triceps during functional tasks
Precautions	NA	Sling immobilization × 10 days to 3 weeks Avoid end-range passive shoulder abduction/external rotation for 1 month	Respect fatigue	NA
Frequency of visits (considerations)	1–2 pre-op visits May increase if PROM limitations are present	Once every 1–2 weeks until ability to demonstrate supple joint mobility and accurate donor activation and then monthly to monitor for signs of motor return	1×/week to 1×/month based on patient needs and accurate, consistent demonstration of exercise program	1× every 1–2 weeks based on progress toward patient-specific goals
Orthosis considerations	NA	Sling immobilization × 10 days to 3 weeks	NA	NA
Interventions		**Donor activation**: Shoulder extension with abduction (with or without external rotation) Can add resistance/bands for added challenge to donor **Donor-recipient pairing**: Active shoulder abduction and extension with passive support to maintain the elbow in extension Resisted shoulder external rotation +/− shoulder extension/abduction performed with elbow straight at patient's side	**Active/resisted donor with active assist recipient**: With the shoulder in extension and 90 degrees of abduction on a table, the patient attempts independent elbow extension. The contralateral hand then assists the elbow into end-range extension **Place and hold**: The arm is supported in elbow extension with the shoulder abducted/extended. Elbow support is removed as the patient attempts to maintain elbow extension	**Resisted donor and recipient**: Resisted shoulder abduction/extension with resisted elbow extension Bands, dumbbell, or cuff weights can be used **Isolated resisted recipient**: Resisted elbow extension with the arm at side, in 0 abduction
Additional interventions		Exercises can be performed bilaterally to improve motor learning. The patient is instructed to visualize the motion *before and during* the actual movement	Elbow extension should be initiated from a midrange position rather than from full elbow flexion until strength improves Triceps exercises should be performed in supine or sitting prior to prone	

During all phases, it is essential to continue cortical reorganization and psychological and psychosocial interventions and progress to incorporate donor/recipient with ADLs

Axillary-to-Triceps Nerve Transfer

Goal of Surgery: Restore the ability to straighten out the elbow against gravity

Recipient Movement = Straighten the elbow
Recipient Muscle: Triceps brachii
Recipient Nerve: Radial nerve branch to the triceps

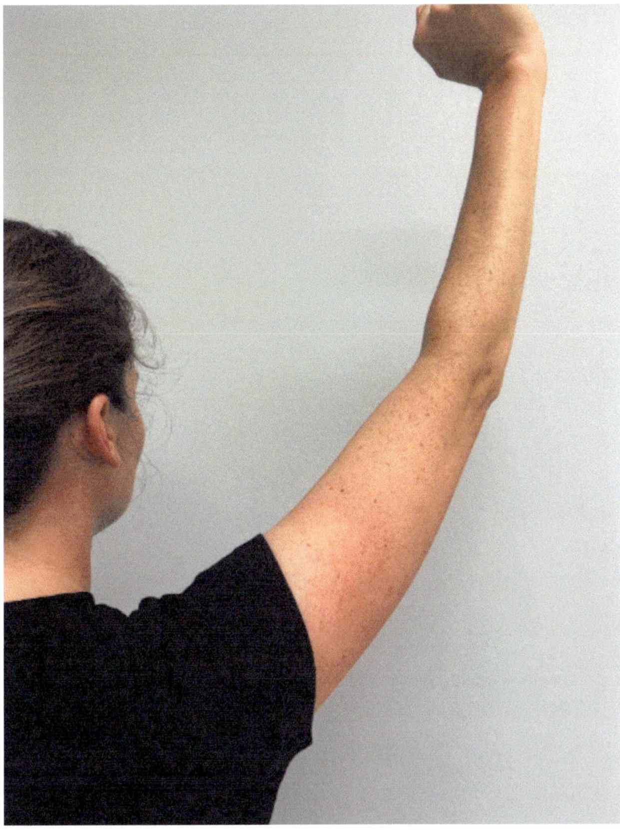

Donor Movement = Rotate the shoulder out and bring the shoulder back

Donor Muscle: Posterior deltoid and teres minor

Donor Nerve: Posterior branch of the axillary nerve

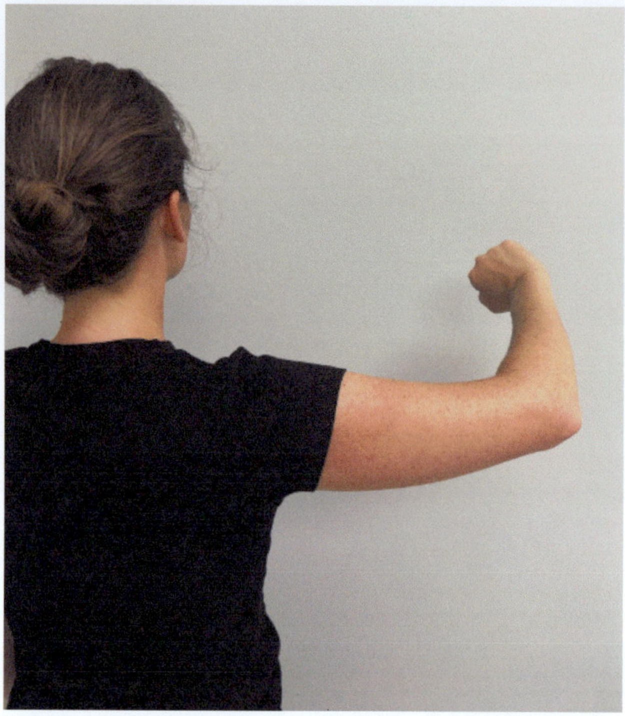

Phase 1 Axillary-to-Triceps Nerve Transfer Exercises

☐ **Passive Range of Motion**:

Complete the below exercise 3–5 repetitions, 2–3 times per day.

- Rest your arm on a table with a rolled-up towel just above the elbow. Use your opposite hand to push your elbow into a straight position.

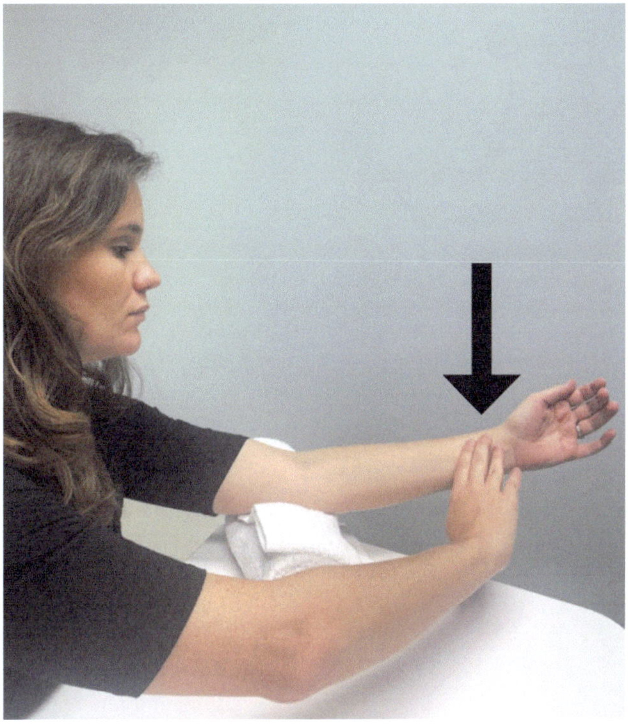

☐ **Active Donor Movement**:
Complete <u>10</u> repetitions every hour.
Shoulder Abduction with Extension

- While standing, lift your shoulder out to the side and slightly behind you. Pretend like you are going to "elbow" someone behind you. Keep your elbow relaxed, and bring your upper arm backward as comfortably as possible. Return to the starting position, and repeat.

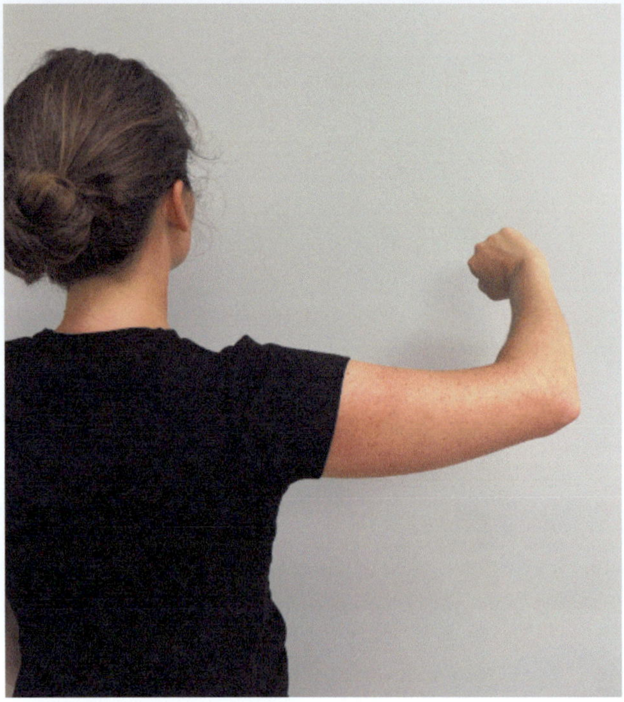

- You may hold a resistance band with both hands. Keep your opposite arm in front of you in a straight position. With the injured side, pull the shoulder backwards and away from you.

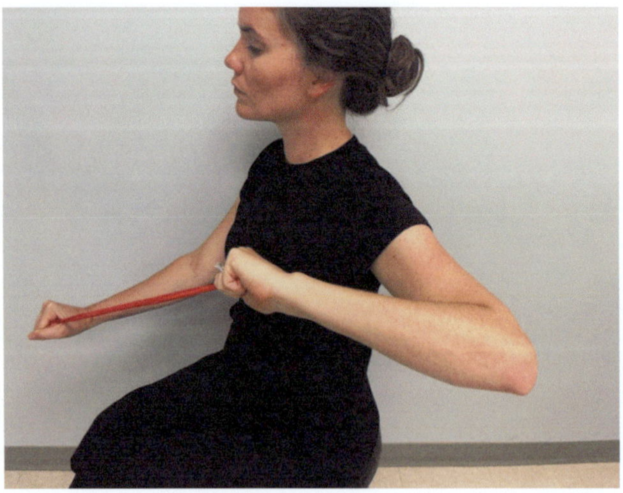

External Rotation

- Lie on your uninjured side. Put a rolled towel between your arm and side with your elbow bent. Starting with your hand against your belly, slowly raise it, rotating your forearm away from your body. Hold the position for a count of three, return to the starting position, and repeat.

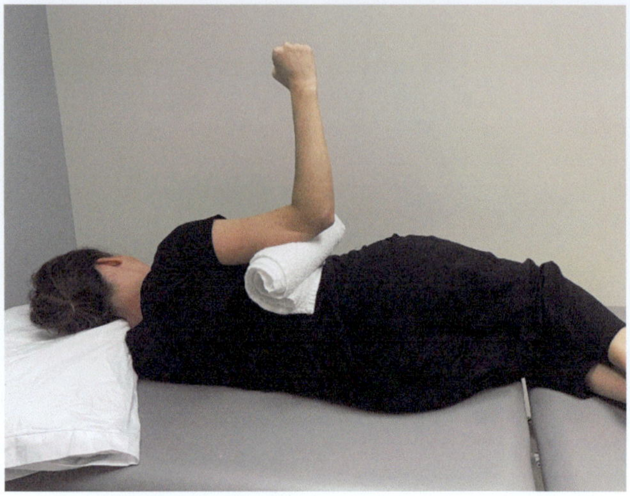

  – If advised by your therapist, you may do the same exercise with a light weight.
- Hold the ends of a resistance band with both hands, with your uninjured arm staying down by your side. With your injured arm, bring your shoulder out to the side, rotating your forearm away from you. Relax back to the starting position, and repeat.

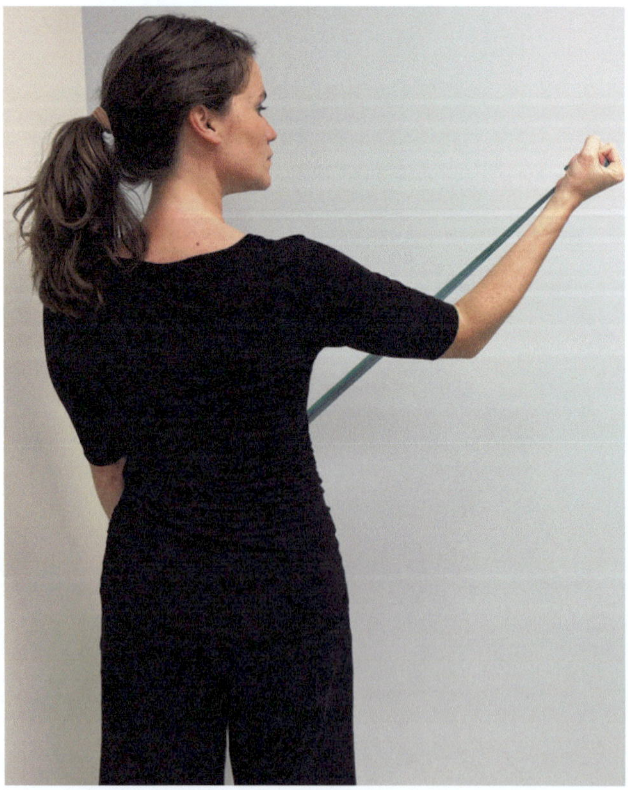

☐ **Active Donor + Passive Recipient Movement: Complete the exercise for <u>10</u> repetitions, <u>2–3</u> times per day.**

- While standing, use both hands to grasp a lightweight dowel or broomstick. Raise your injured shoulder out the side and slight behind you. Maintain the elbow in a straight position using assistance from the dowel rod.

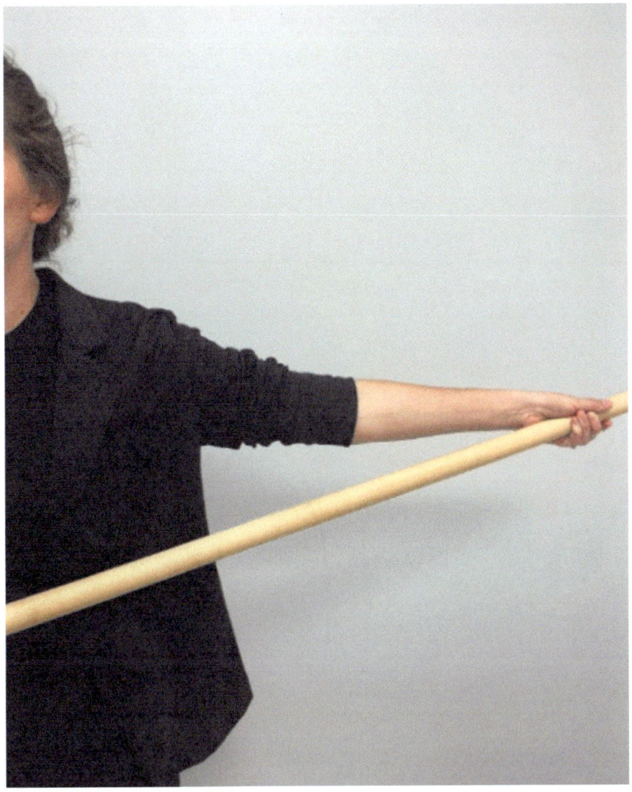

- Begin by lying on your back with your arm supported on a pillow or towel. Rotate your forearms so that your palms face the ceiling. Then, slide your shoulder/arm out to the side, and allow your elbow to straighten. Return to the starting position, and repeat.

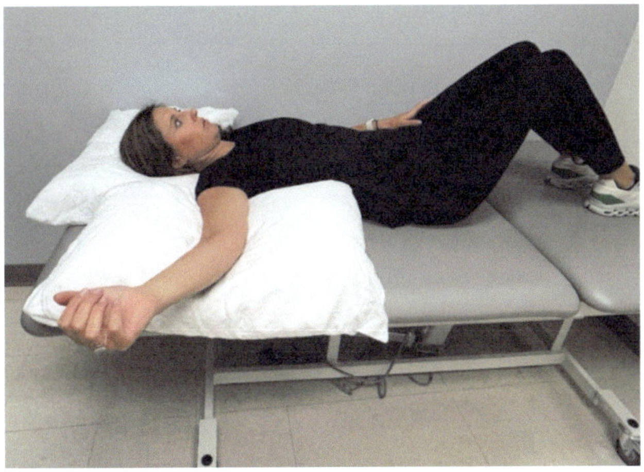

Phase 2 Axillary-to-Triceps Nerve Transfer Exercises

☐ **Active Donor + Active-Assisted Recipient Movement**:

Complete these exercises <u>1–10</u> repetitions, <u>2–3</u> times per day.

- Sit at a table with your hand resting on a towel. Straighten your arm out the side as far as you can, sliding your forearm across the table. Once you cannot straighten the elbow anymore, use your opposite hand to assist it further into a straight position.

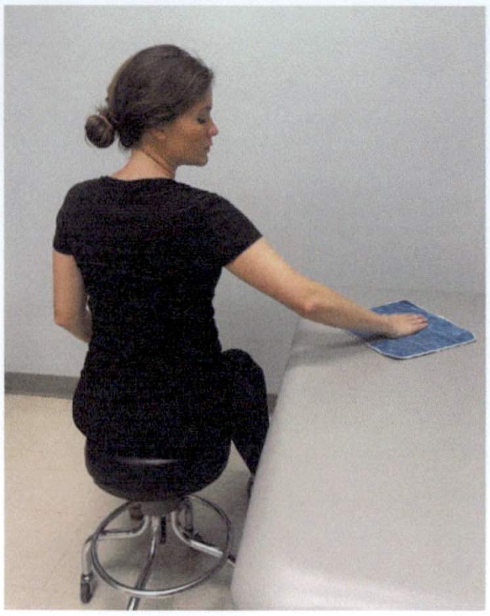

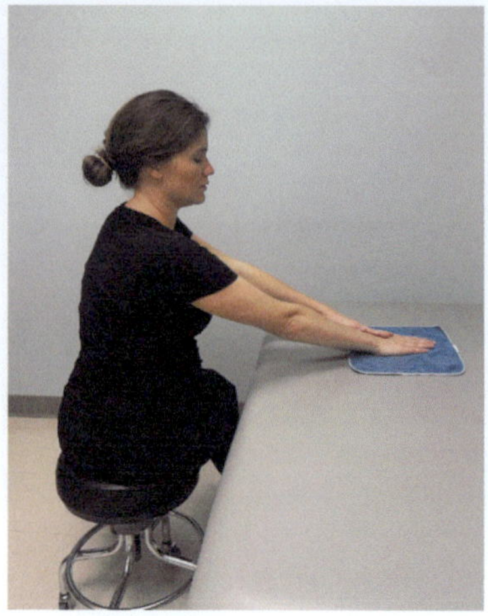

☐ **"Place and Hold"**

- Sit at a table with your hand resting on a towel. Use your opposite hand to place your elbow into a straight position with your shoulder out to the side. Let go with the opposite hand, and try to maintain your elbow into "end-range" extension or as straight as it will go.

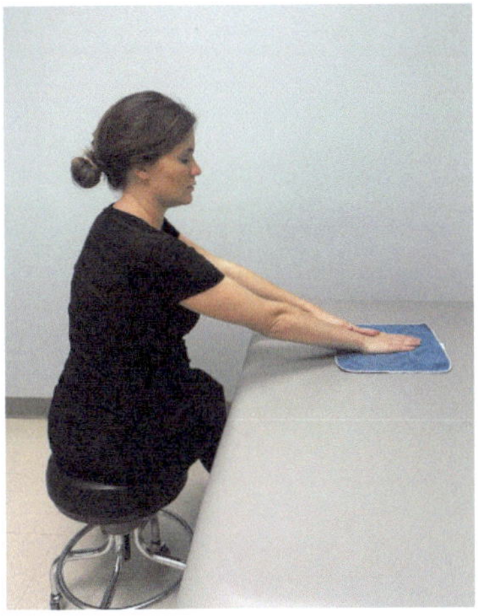

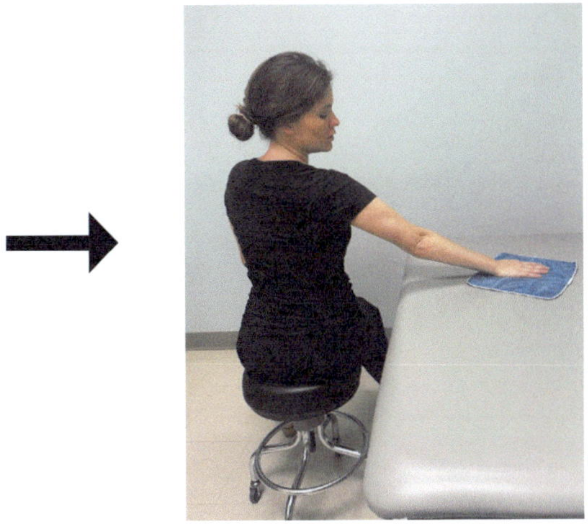

- Once you can achieve this fully extended position, raise your arm completely off the table with the shoulder out the side and elbow fully straight, and hold this position for a count of 5 s.

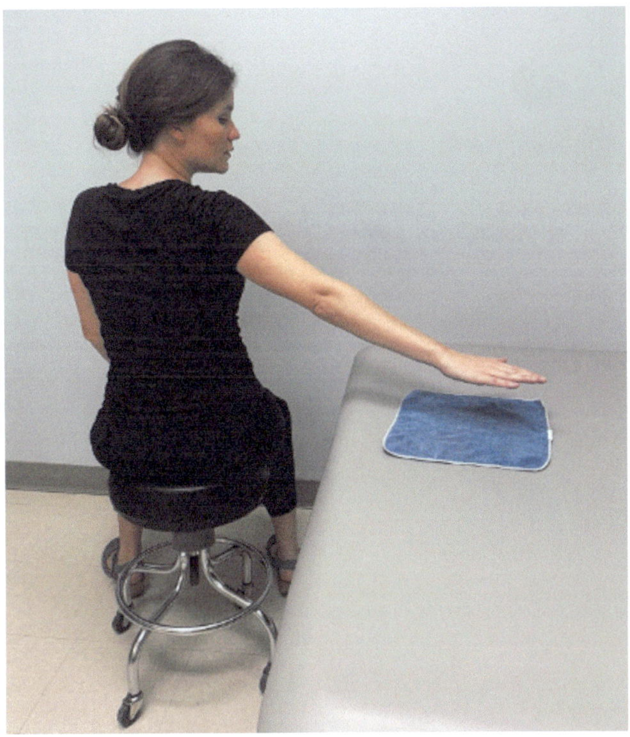

☐ **Active Donor + Active Recipient**

- Lie on your belly (prone) with your forehead supported on a rolled towel. Rotate your shoulder so that your thumb is facing away from you. Lift your shoulder up while straightening your elbow at the same time. Relax to the starting position and repeat.

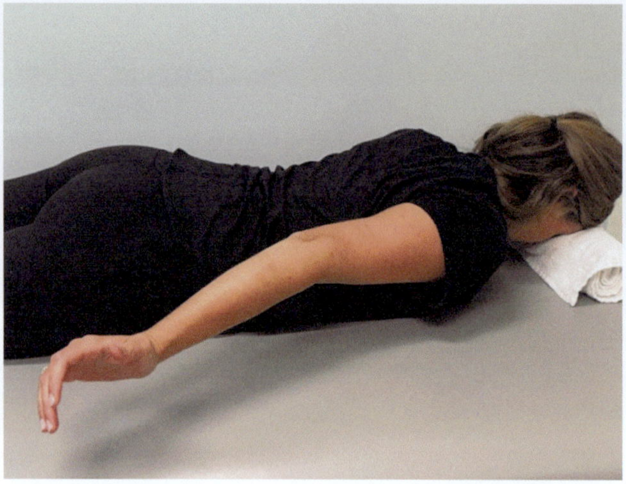

- While standing, lift your arm out to side and slightly behind you while keeping your elbow firmly in a straight position.

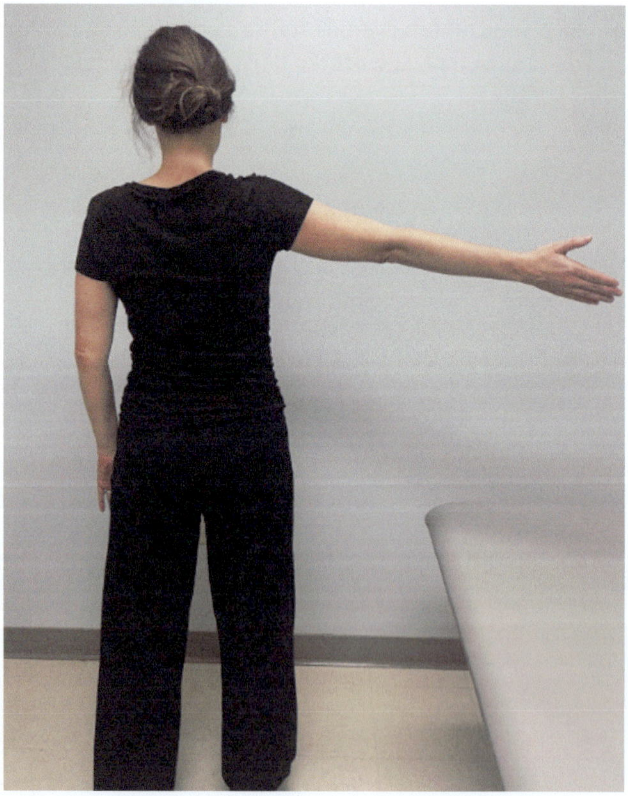

Phase 3 Axillary-to-Triceps Nerve Transfer Exercises

Complete these exercises 1–10 repetitions, 2–3 times per day.

☐ **Resistive Donor + Active Recipient Movement**:

1. Shoulder and Elbow Extension Pulls with External Rotation

   Either while standing or seated, hold the ends of a resistance band secured in front of you. Keep your elbows straight as you pull your arms back while rotating your arms to turn the thumbs out.

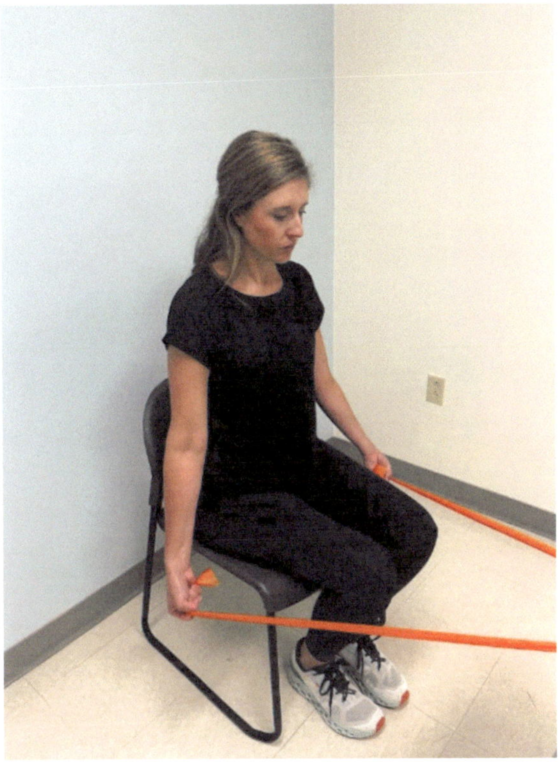

2. Wall Slides

   Stand in front of a wall with a resistance band looped around your wrists. Place both hands on the wall to the same level of your face. Pull the resistance band apart as you slide both hands up the wall and straighten your elbows. Slide down to the starting position, and repeat.

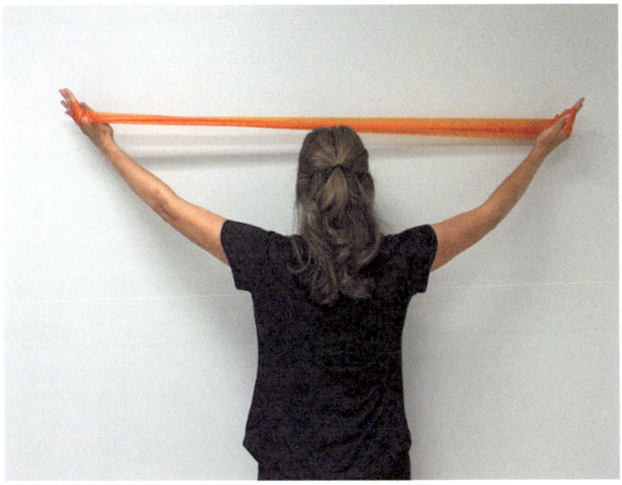

☐ **Resistive Recipient Movement**

1. Supine with Elbow Extension

   On your back, hold a ___ lb weight in your hand. Support your shoulder in front of you, and straighten your elbow up toward the ceiling. Relax the elbow into a bent position, and then repeat.

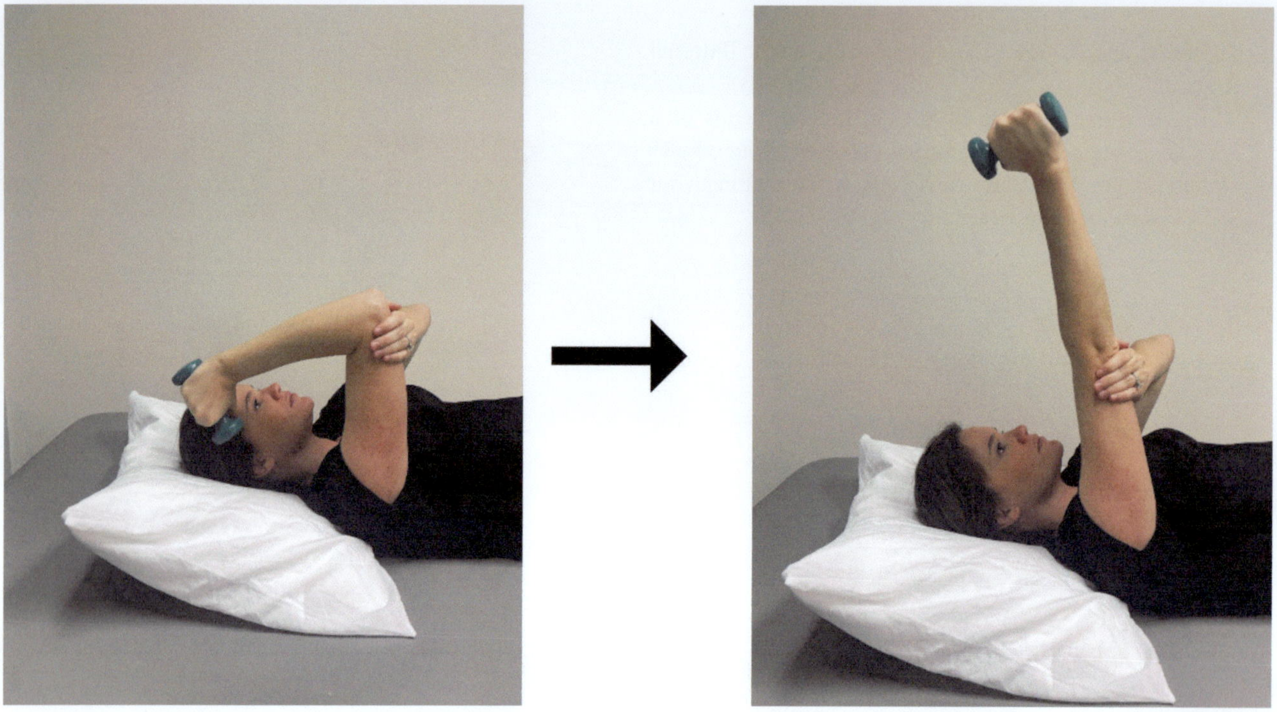

2. Standing Triceps Curl

   While standing, lean forward slightly with your elbow bent and held against your side. Hold a weight in your hand, and straighten the elbow fully. Hold for 3–5 seconds.

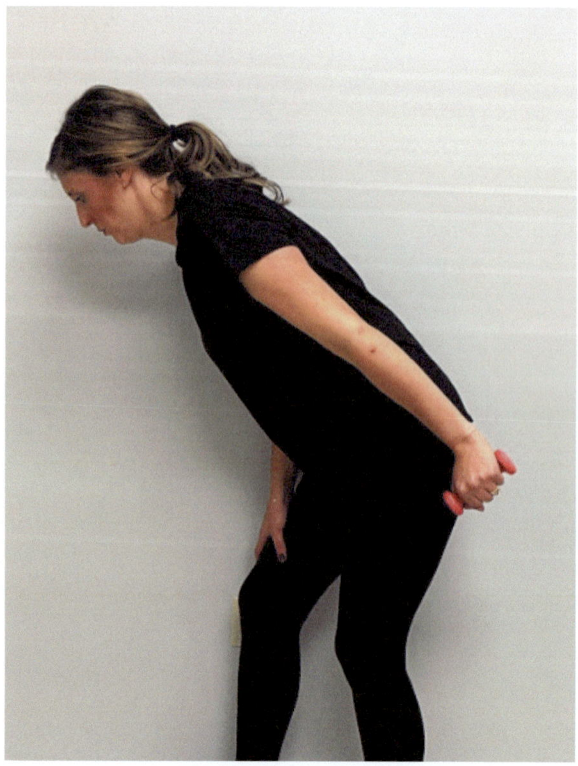

References

1. Kittithamvongs P, et al. The intercostal nerves transfer to the radial nerve branch to the long head of the triceps muscle: influencing factor and outcome of 55 cases. J Hand Surg Am. 2023;48(7):733.e1–7.
2. Bertelli JA, Tacca CP, Winkelmann Duarte EC, Ghizoni MF, Duarte H. Transfer of axillary nerve branches to reconstruct elbow extension in tetraplegics: a laboratory investigation of surgical feasibility. Microsurgery. 2011;31(5):376–81.
3. Bazarek S, et al. Axillary to radial nerve transfer for recovery of elbow extension after spinal cord injury. Op Neurosurg. 2023;25(6):e324–9.
4. Bertelli JA, Ghizoni MF, Tacca CP. Transfer of teres minor motor branch for triceps reinnervation in tetraplegia: case report. J Neurosurg. 2011;114:1157–460.
5. Mateo S, Roby-Brami A, Reilly KT, Rossetti Y, Collet C, Rode G. Upper limb kinematics after cervical spinal cord injury: a review. J Neuroeng Rehabil. 2015;12:9. https://doi.org/10.1186/1743-0003-12-9.
6. Zlotolow DA, Kripke LA, Kozin SH. Current concepts in elbow extension reconstruction for the tetraplegic patient. J Am Acad Orthop Surg. 2023;32:221–8.
7. Klika BJ, Spinner RJ, Bishop AT, Kircher AF, Shin AY. Posterior branch of the axillary nerve transfer to lateral triceps branch for restoration of elbow extension: case report. J Hand Surg. 2013;38A:1145–9.
8. Fox IK, Novak CB, et al. The use of nerve transfers to restore upper extremity function in cervical spinal cord injury. Plast Reconstr Surg. 2018;10:1173–84.
9. Alolabi N, Lovy AJ, Kircher MF, Spinner RJ, Bishop AT, Shin AY. Distal nerve transfers to the triceps brachii muscle: surgical technique and clinical outcomes. J Hand Surg Am. 2020;45(2):155.e1–8.
10. Landin D, Thompson M, Jackson M. Functions of the triceps brachii in humans: a review. J Clin Med Res. 2018;10(4):290–3.
11. Neumann DA. Chapter 6: Elbow and forearm. In: Kinesiology of the musculoskeletal system: foundations for rehabilitation. 3rd ed. Elsevier; 2017. p. 175–214.

Rehabilitation Guidelines for Specific Nerve Transfers: Wrist

Flexor Digitorum Superficialis Branch of the Median Nerve to the Extensor Carpi Radialis Brevis Branch of the Radial Nerve Transfer

Amy M. Young

FDS-to-ECRB Nerve Transfer

Background

Of the three major nerves in the upper extremity, the radial nerve is the largest and most often compromised by injury. It arises from the posterior cord of the brachial plexus with origins from C5, C6, C7, C8, and T1 nerve roots. Radial nerve injuries lead to insufficient elbow, wrist, finger, and thumb extension. A high radial nerve injury affects the muscles innervated by the radial nerve and posterior interosseous nerve (PIN). The radial nerve innervates the triceps brachii, anconeus, brachioradialis, extensor carpi radialis longus (ECRL), supinator, and extensor carpi radialis brevis (ECRB). The PIN innervates extensor carpi ulnaris (ECU), extensor digitorum communis (EDC), extensor digiti minimi (EDM), abductor pollicis longus (APL), extensor pollicis longus (EPL), extensor pollicis brevis (EPB), and extensor indicis proprius (EIP). A common nerve transfer to restore wrist extension is the FDS (median nerve) to the ECRB nerve transfer. The goal of this surgery is to restore the ability to extend the wrist to place the hand in a position of grasp and to provide stabilization of the wrist while gripping.

The FDS-to-ECRB nerve transfer is often performed in conjunction with the FCR-to-PIN nerve transfer, which provides finger and thumb extension. This pair of nerve transfer is also frequently combined with pronator teres (PT)-to-ECRB tendon transfer to provide more immediate internal wrist stability [1]. Unlike radial nerve tendon transfers where wrist and finger extension can only occur in isolation, a benefit of this nerve transfer duo is the potential ability to simultaneously extend the wrist and fingers together [2]. An additional benefit is gaining individual finger extension in comparison with tendon transfer outcomes.

A. M. Young (✉)
Northwestern Medicine Center for Surgery of the Hand, Chicago, IL, USA
e-mail: Amy.Young@nm.org

Surgical Graphic

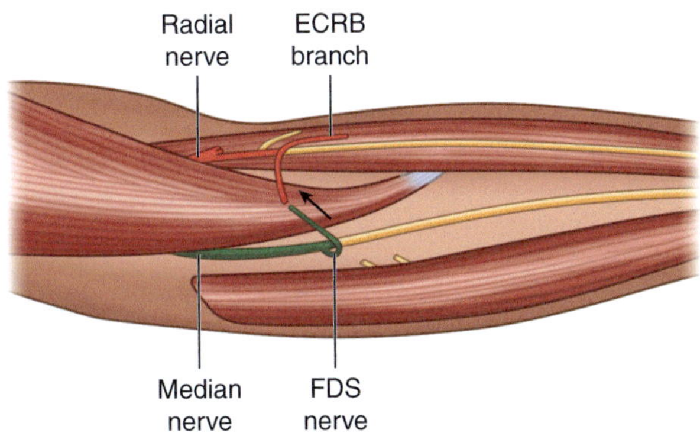

Microsurgical technique of flexor digitorum superficialis branch of the median nerve to the extensor carpi radialis brevis branch of the radial nerve transfer

A curvilinear incision is made along the volar aspect of the proximal two-thirds of the forearm. The brachioradialis muscle is identified, and the superficial radial nerve is dissected on the undersurface of the brachioradialis muscle. The superficial radial nerve is used as a guide to dissect retrograde (distal to proximal) to identify the posterior interosseous nerve and the radial nerve proper. There is typically a branch to the ECRB identified close to the point where the PIN and SRN branch from the radial nerve proper. Intraoperative stimulation is used to confirm whether the ECRB branches (which are visually confirmed to reach the ECRB muscle) respond. It is important to stimulate these branches within 30 min of the tourniquet being inflated (if one is being used) and to ensure that the anesthesia team is not using any muscle paralytics. After doing so, the lacertus fibrosus is identified, and after releasing the lacertus fibrosus, the median nerve is identified deep to the lacertus fibrosus and along the inner surface of the flexor pronator mass. After decompressing the median nerve, the branching pattern of the median

L. C. Kahn et al. (eds.), *Rehabilitation for Nerve Transfers of the Upper Extremity*,
https://doi.org/10.1007/978-3-031-92008-0_17

nerve is identified. It is helpful to decompress the FDS arch and subsequently identify the anterior interosseous nerve (AIN) coming off the median nerve proper, being sure to protect the AIN. A handheld nerve stimulator is used to identify the branches of the median nerve to the FDS, again ensuring that this is done within 30 min of the tourniquet being inflated (if one is being used) and that there are no muscle paralytics being used by the anesthesia team. After doing so, the FDS branch of the median nerve is dissected as distally as possible, being sure to identify any additional branch of the median nerve that innervates the FDS. The donor nerve is divided distally, and the recipient nerve is divided proximally after dissecting the ECRB branch as proximally as possible. Coaptation of the FDS branch of the median nerve to the ECRB branch of the radial nerve is performed using microsurgical technique.

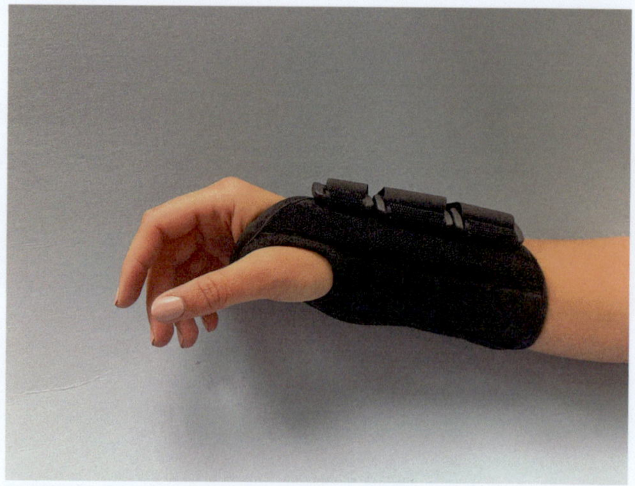

Image 1 Individuals with wrist drop should wear a wrist extension orthosis to support the hand in a position for functional grasp and prevent wrist flexor shortening. A prefabricated orthosis is acceptable if it provides adequate wrist extension support

Outcomes

FDS-to-ECRB nerve transfer was first described in 2002 from a report of two cases. Both patients obtained between 40 and 45 degrees of active wrist extension against gravity within 14 months from surgery [4]. Another early-outcome study described two cases following C5, C6, and C7 avulsion injury; one patient achieved 40 degrees of wrist extension and the other 70°. Both were able to withstand moderate resistance against gravity [5]. Ray and Mackinnon described their outcomes following median-to-radial nerve transfers in 2011. Out of 13 patients who underwent FDS-to-ECRB nerve transfer, 12 of them (92.3%) achieved a 4/5 manual muscle testing (MMT) score for wrist extension [6]. The authors suggest this transfer be performed within 9 months of injury. Bertelli and Ghizoni later published a study of three patients with C5–C8 injuries, in which all subjects gained active wrist extension from full flexion to neutral. Yet none achieved antigravity wrist extension past neutral [7]. Nerve transfers to restore wrist extension have gained momentum in the last decade, and although more studies with higher sample sizes are warranted, the FDS-to-ECRB nerve transfer is an intuitive, synergistic transfer with promising results in the brachial plexus population.

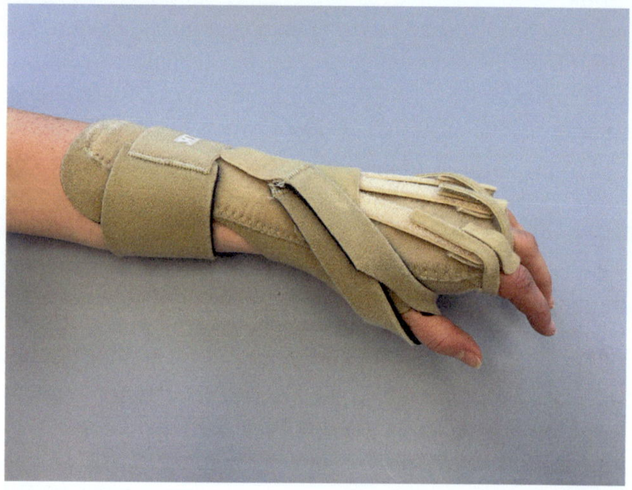

Image 2 Finger and thumb extension may also be affected when wrist drop is present. A forearm-based prefab orthosis like the Benik W-711 is recommended to support the length of the denervated muscles and improve hand function during the day

Phases of Rehabilitation

Phase 1

Pre-op to 1/5 MMT in the Recipient Muscle

Precautions

Avoid prolonged positioning in wrist flexion, which can contribute to both flexor shortening and overlengthening of the weak, reinnervating ECRB. If the FCR-to-PIN transfer was simultaneously performed, patients should avoid prolonged composite digit flexion to prevent flexor shortening and overlengthening of the finger and thumb extensors. According to the length-tension relationship of muscle, overlengthening may contribute to biomechanical failure of the muscle to produce desired movement and strength once reinnervation of the recipient muscle occurs. A general rule to follow is to preserve recipient muscle length whenever possible.

Orthoses

Therapy may be initiated preoperatively to address potential joint contractures by initiating passive wrist extension exercises. The patient is fit with an orthosis to support the wrist in extension. This can be a custom volar wrist orthosis or a prefabricated style (Image 1). The posterior interosseous nerve is typically injured as well. In this situation, the patient is fit with a forearm-based orthosis that supports wrist, thumb, and finger MCP extension, such as the prefabricated BENIK™ (Image 2) or a similar custom orthosis. Donor activation may begin with finger interphalangeal (IP) joint flexion exercises within the confines of the orthosis. MMT strength and range-of-motion measurements of the recipient muscle, donor muscle, and other affected muscles and joints will be helpful to track progress following surgery. Grip strength measurements are useful preoperatively as wrist stability is inherent to power grip.

Therapy resumes once the postoperative dressing is removed around 2 weeks following surgery. At this time, range of motion to the unaffected joints, edema management, and wound care are initiated. A custom or prefabricated volar wrist orthosis in approximately 40 degrees of extension is provided once the post-op dressing is removed. However, because the PIN is likely impacted as well, a standard wrist orthosis leaves the finger and thumb extensors unsupported and thus potentially vulnerable to overlengthening, which could ultimately hinder movement and strength outcomes [8, 9]. If the PIN is injured, a forearm-based orthosis with the finger MCPs in extension/IPs free and thumb MCP/IP in extension may be fabricated for comfort and protection (Image 3). A reasonable scenario is to wear the orthosis with the fingers/thumb included for night and the standard wrist-only orthosis during the day. Sutures are removed approximately 10–14 days after surgery. Once sutures are removed, scar management techniques are implemented.

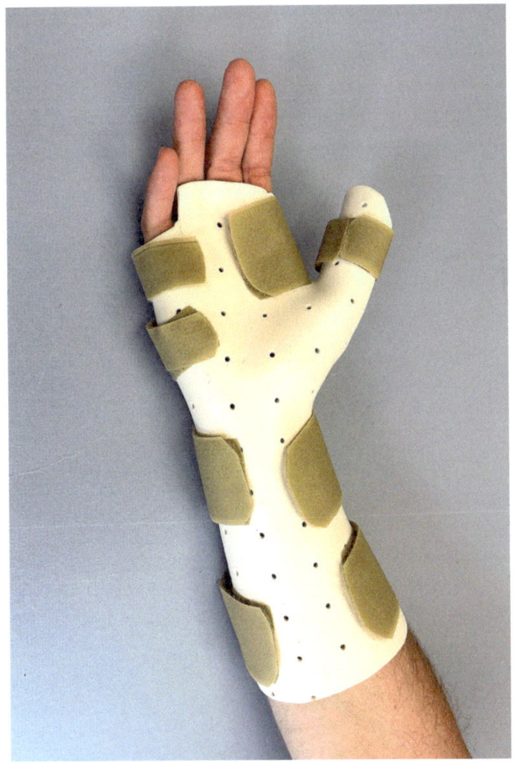

Image 3 A custom forearm-based orthosis that supports the wrist, finger MCPs, and thumb in extension (a "P1 block") is recommended for individuals with radial nerve palsy affecting both wrist and digits to wear at night and to wear a wrist orthosis during the day

Exercises

- Donor Activation
  The FDS contributes to finger PIP joint flexion. Early-phase donor activation includes active composite flexion and may begin around 2 weeks, which is typically when the postoperative dressing transitions to an orthosis (outlined above).
- Combined Donor with Passive Recipient Exercise
  To combine donor with recipient movement at this stage, the patient actively flexes the fingers and passively extends the wrist. This can easily be completed by using the unaffected hand to block the finger MCP joints in extension during active IP flexion while passively extending the wrist (Image 4). Alternatively, passive wrist extension with FDS activation may be achieved with "elbow raises." The palm remains in contact with the edge of a table. The finger IP joints flex over the edge as the elbow is raised (Image 5). After 1 month, resisted donor activation using therapy putty or a gripper tool may be useful to provide additional resistance to the donor. The wrist should be manually supported if resistance is added to the FDS. Phase 1 exercises are completed up to ten repetitions every hour: low repetitions, high frequency [10].

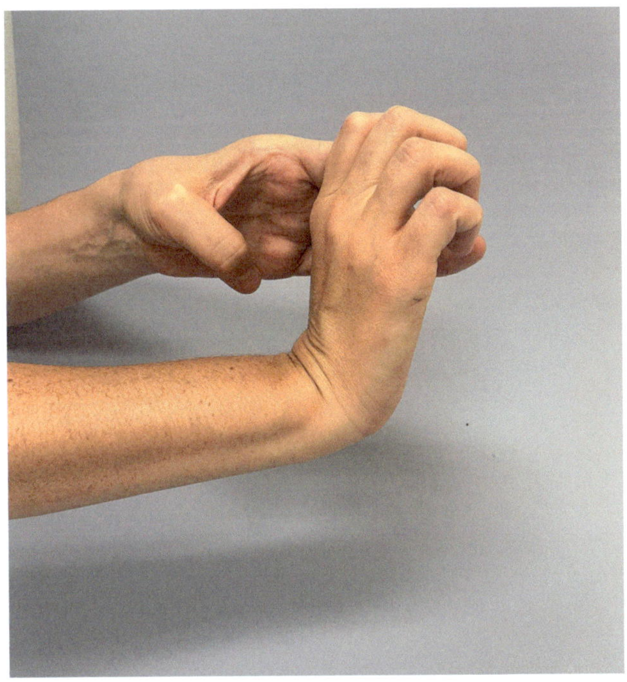

Image 4 Combined donor with passive recipient muscle pairing is achieved by having the individual flex the IP joints while supporting the wrist in extension

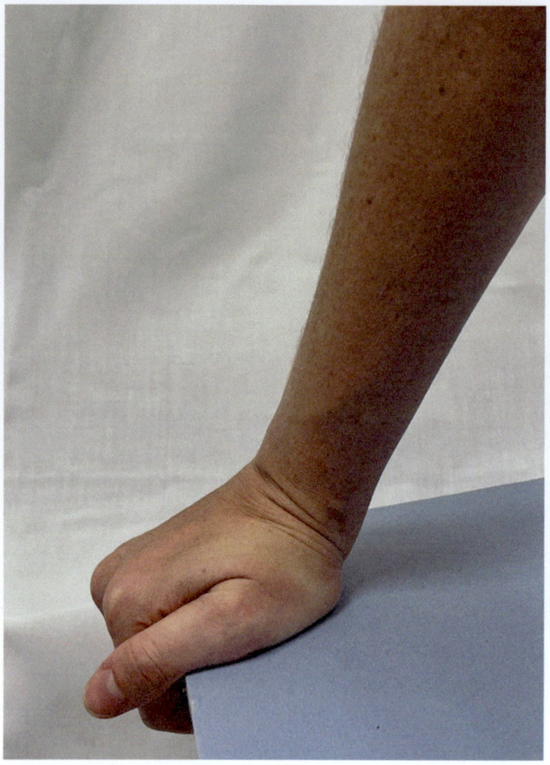

Image 5 Combined donor with passive recipient muscle pairing can also be achieved with the palm on the edge of a table. The individual is instructed to grasp the table edge while raising the elbow, which places the wrist in extension

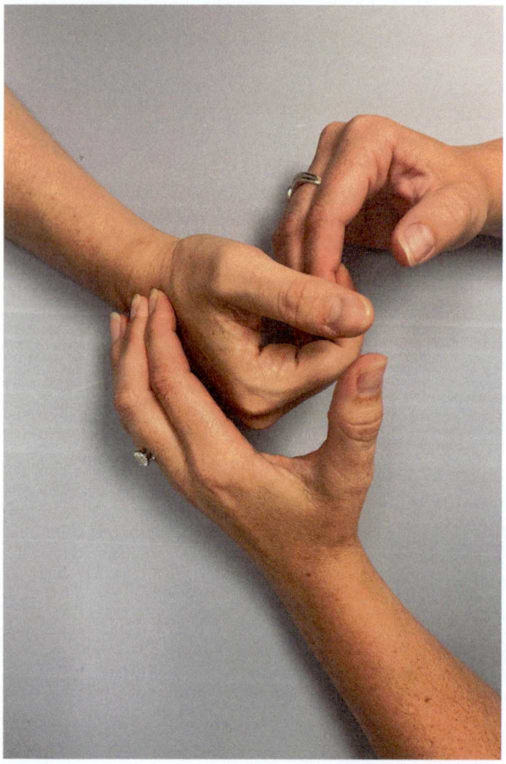

Image 6 Monthly assessment of recovery is performed by manually resisting finger flexion while palpating in the region of the distal ECRB tendon. Changes in tension in the tendon may be noted in the second dorsal extensor compartment or at the base of the third metacarpal where the tendon inserts

Assessment of Recovery

To identify initial recipient muscle contraction, the examiner resists finger flexion while palpating over the ECRB muscle or the distal tendon where it inserts on the base of the third metacarpal (Image 6). This is initially performed in a gravity-minimized plane. Strength should be assessed at each treatment session (or at least monthly) to monitor motor recovery and determine appropriate exercises.

Therapy Frequency

Frequency of therapy visits may be one time per week. Monthly visits become appropriate once the wound is healed, the patient shows understanding of the donor-recipient relationship, and any soft tissue restrictions are resolved.

Phase 2

2−/5 to 3/5 MMT in the Recipient Muscle

Precautions

Avoid prolonged positioning in wrist flexion. Avoid high-intensity exercise of the ECRB. Intense exercise leading to recipient muscle fatigue may impair the regeneration of axons, inhibiting reanimation of the recipient muscle.

Orthosis

The wrist orthosis should continue throughout phase 2 of therapy to not only preserve the length of the wrist extensors but also provide rest to this recovering muscle. The patient should be removing it for light activity to intuitively strengthen wrist extension. However, if light resistance overpowers wrist extension, the orthosis should continue to be used during functional activities. Once the patient can reliably achieve and maintain wrist extension against gravity with use, the orthosis may be discontinued.

Exercises

- **Active Donor with Active-Assisted Recipient**
  ECRB MMT = 2−/5 to 2/5
  The patient is positioned in a gravity-minimized plane, i.e., seated with the arm resting on a table with the forearm in neutral rotation. The hand may be placed under a slick cloth to facilitate wrist movement. The patient makes a fist while trying to independently extend the wrist, and the contralateral hand assists the wrist into end-range extension (Image 7).
- **"Place and Hold" Exercise**
  ECRB MMT = 2+/5
  Once the patient can actively extend the wrist through partial movement against gravity, a "place and hold" exercise may begin. The patient passively places the wrist into extension (while pronated) and actively flexes the fingers.

The contralateral hand slowly removes support of the wrist, and the patient attempts to maintain active extension (while still demanding a strong contraction of the FDS donor).

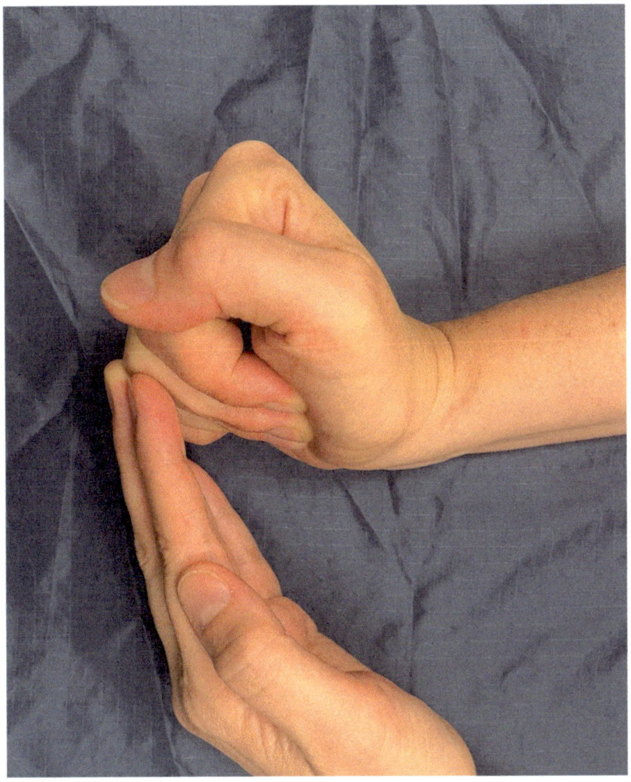

Image 7 Active donor with active-assisted recipient exercise is performed on a slick nylon cloth to reduce friction and make it easier for the wrist to move. The individual is instructed to perform "straight fist" while gentle assist is given into wrist extension as needed

- **Active Donor with Active Recipient**
  ECRB MMT = 3–/5 to 3/5
  The patient performs active finger flexion with active wrist extension while the forearm is pronated. This nerve transfer is very intuitive as it relies on the natural, synergistic motion of the wrist and fingers.
- **Functional Activity**
  Once antigravity wrist extension is consistent, patients should try to incorporate this movement into functional tasks throughout the day. For example, with the fingers resting on a playing card, the patient flexes the fingers. As the card slides toward the palm, the wrist intuitively extends. The playing card decreases the friction between the fingers and table, assisting into further wrist extension (Image 8). Additionally, the patient may stack lightweight plastic cups, which naturally places the wrist into extension while flexing the fingers (Image 9). Both tasks require grasp of light objects, as resistive activity is contraindicated until phase 3 of therapy.

Patients may progress to phase 2 of rehabilitation once they can partially extend the wrist in a gravity-minimized plane. At this point in recovery, the patient should be reliable with his or her home exercise program and demonstrate a good understanding of the donor-recipient muscle relationship. Phase 2 exercises advance from passive to active movement of the wrist. Exercises begin in a gravity-minimized plane and advance to antigravity movement as ECRB strength improves.

Assessment of Recovery

Continue to assess MMT strength of the ECRB with resisted donor activation (finger IP flexion). Measuring active wrist extension, with or without donor activation, in a gravity-

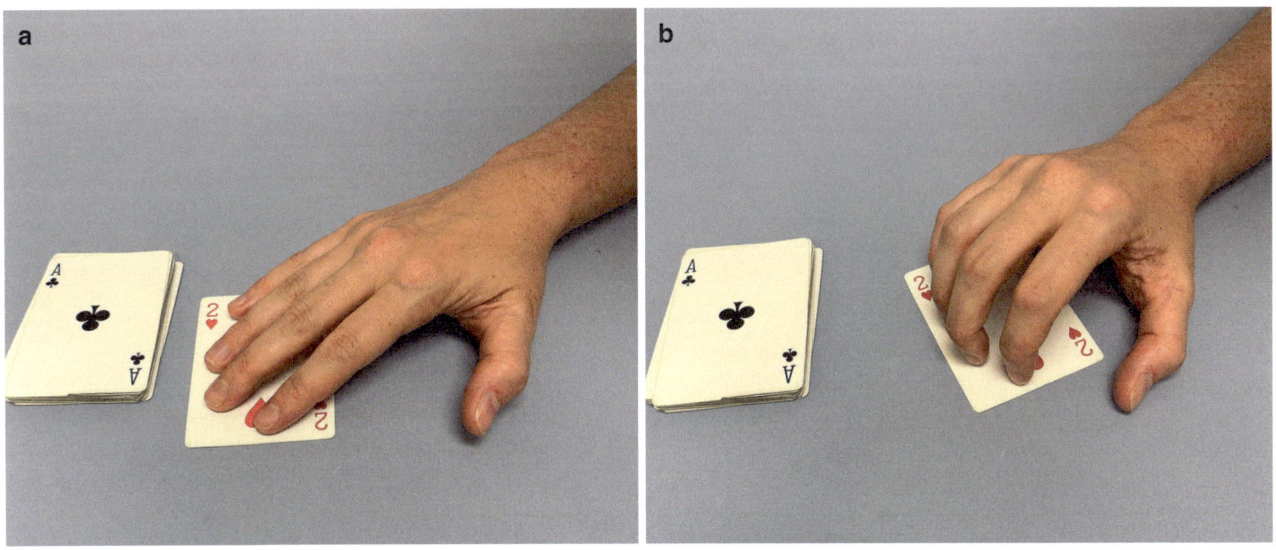

Image 8 Playing cards provide a slick surface to incorporate active-assisted wrist extension with donor FDS activation. The individual is instructed to slide the card toward the palm by flexing the PIP joints while attempting to pull the wrist into extension

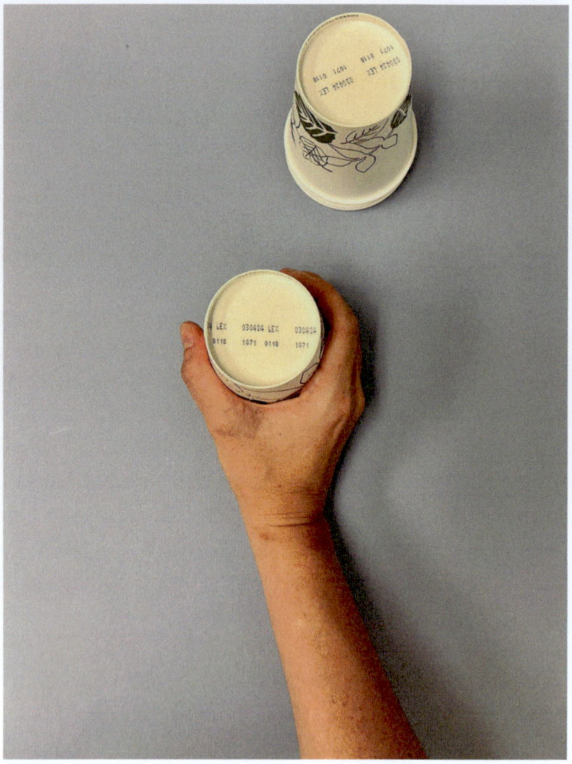

Image 9 Functional activities such as grasping and stacking paper cups encourage combined donor finger flexion with active recipient/wrist extension

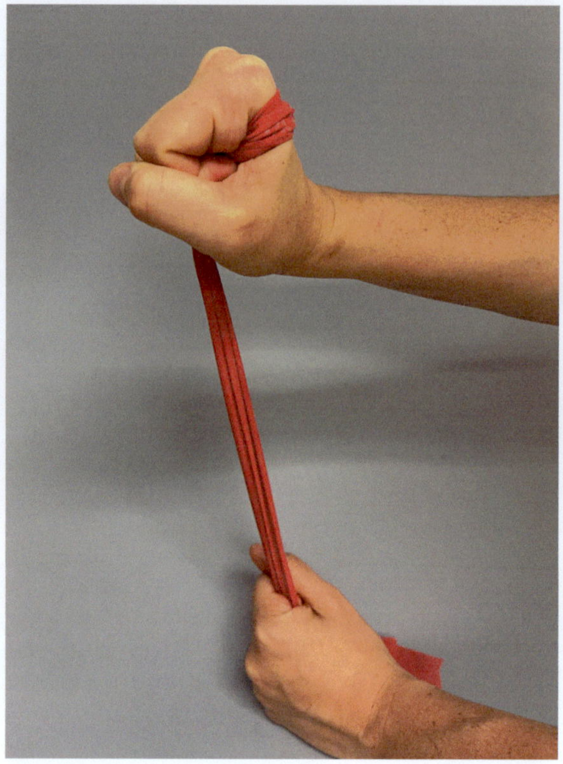

Image 10 In phase 3, combined resisted donor with resisted recipient wrist extension is introduced gradually. A resistance band provides resisted wrist extension with the hand firmly in a fist

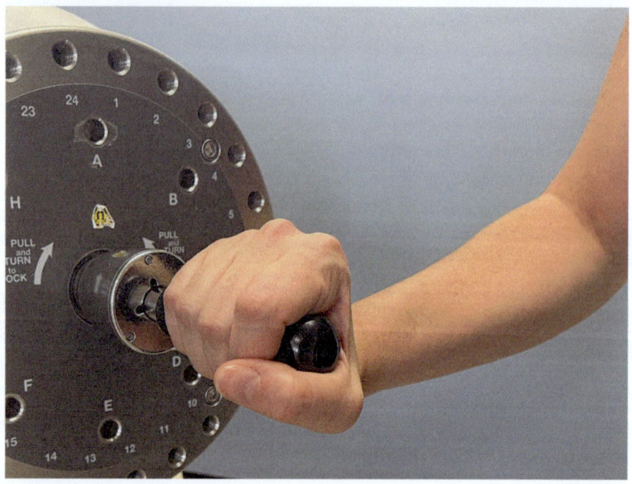

Image 11 When available, BTE tool # 502 is useful for strengthening wrist extension with resisted donor/grasp

lessened plane and eventually against gravity, may be useful to track progress over the prolonged recovery period. Grip strength should also be assessed monthly as wrist extension strength recovers.

Therapy Frequency

Frequency of therapy may be increased to once per week or every other week. This is dependent on patient needs, home exercise compliance, and accessibility to therapy (geographically and financially).

Phase 3

3+/5 MMT and above

Orthosis

An orthosis is no longer required. It may be useful, however, during high-demand activity if fatigue is noted.

Exercises

- **Resistive Recipient Activity with Donor Contraction**
  Exercises continue to pair recipient activity with donor contraction: resisted wrist extension with resisted finger flexion. This can be accomplished with weights or theraband (Image 10). When available, Baltimore Therapeutic Equipment™ (BTE) tool #504 incorporates resisted wrist extension with resisted finger flexion (Image 11).
- **Resistive Recipient Activity Without Donor Contraction**
  Once patients demonstrate reliable wrist extension with resistance, they may learn to de-emphasize the inclusion of the finger flexors (Image 12).

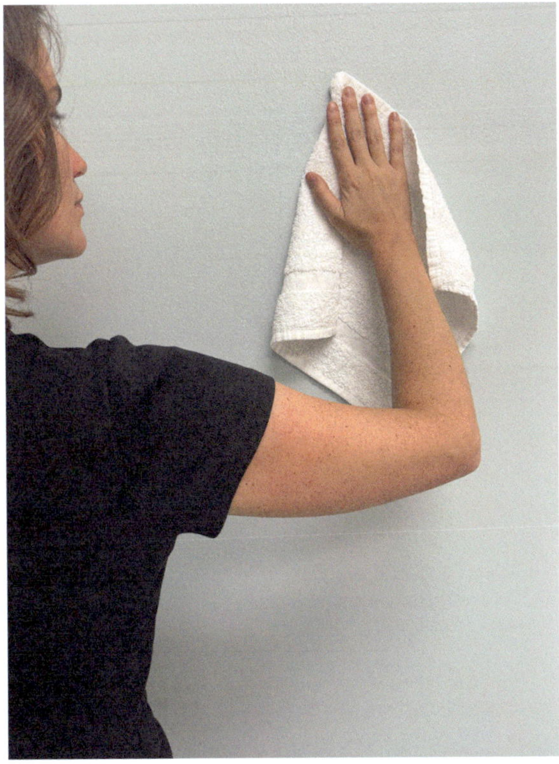

Image 12 De-emphasizing the donor FDS with wrist extension may be achieved with functional activities such as wiping a surface with the fingers and wrist extended

Once the ECRB can begin to withstand some resistance against gravity, exercise instruction should reflect this. Initially, exercise should continue to combine resisted donor and recipient activity. The patient may incorporate more challenging strengthening and functional tasks into his or her daily routine.

Therapy Frequency

Therapy every other week is appropriate, depending on the patient's goals, progress, and other factors.

FDS-to-ECRB nerve transfer

Nerve transfer overview					
Donor nerve	Donor action	Recipient nerve	Recipient action	Indications for functional restoration	Approximate months to functional movement
FDS branch of the median nerve	Finger (PIP) flexion	ECRB branch of the radial nerve	Wrist extension	High radial nerve palsy; loss of wrist extension	12–18 months [4–7, 11]

	Preoperative therapy	Early phase	Middle phase	Late phase
Criteria	Before surgery	0/5 to 1/5 MMT	2−/5 to 3/5 MMT	>3/5 MMT
Purpose of phase	Educate and establish baseline function	Understand donor and recipient relationship Begin pairing donor and recipient muscles to aid in cortical plasticity	Consistently activate recipient in gravity-lessened planes	Strengthen recipient through resistance and gradually separate from donor activation
Precautions	Prevent shortening of wrist and finger flexors Prevent overlengthening of wrist extensor muscles	Limit wrist motion for 2–3 weeks Avoid prolonged resting in wrist flexion	Respect fatigue	Respect fatigue
Frequency of visits (considerations)	1–2 pre-op visits May increase if PROM limitations are present	1×/week until finger and wrist extension PROM is restored, and patient is independent with donor activation; then 1× monthly	1×/week to 1×/month based on patient needs and accurate, consistent demonstration of exercise program	1× every 1–2 weeks based on progress toward patient-specific goals
Orthosis considerations	Custom or prefabricated wrist orthosis for function and prevention of flexor shortening If the PIN is also injured, a low-profile radial nerve palsy in wrist and finger extension is appropriate	Volar wrist orthosis for 2–3 weeks to protect the nerve coaptation Resume use of the wrist brace during the protracted length of recovery to avoid overlengthening of the ECRB. This may be removed for hygiene, exercises, and light activity	Continue intermittent use of the wrist brace if fatigue is an issue	NA unless functional grasp overpowers grip and limits function
Interventions	Wrist extension PROM	**Donor activation**: Finger flexion **Donor-recipient pairing**: Active finger flexion with passive wrist extension	**Active/resisted donor with active assist recipient**: Finger flexion with the forearm in neutral, resting on a slick surface. Active wrist extension is performed, with contralateral hand assist to complete extension **Place and hold**: In an antigravity position, passively place the wrist in extension while the fingers are in a fist. Release the support and attempt to maintain this position	**Resisted donor and recipient**: Putty gripping, maintaining wrist extension Concentric wrist extension using light weights or theraband **Resisted recipient**: With theraband looped around bilateral hands with the wrist and fingers in extension, shoulder external rotation is performed
Additional interventions			Limited E-stim may be appropriate at the end of this phase to aid patients who struggle to isolate the ECRB while grasping light objects	

**During all phases, it is essential to continue cortical reorganization and psychological and psychosocial interventions and progress to incorporate donor/recipient with ADLs

FDS-to-ECRB Nerve Transfer

Goals of Surgery: (1) Restore wrist extension, (2) improve wrist position to grasp objects and provide wrist stability while gripping

Recipient Movement = Bend wrist back (wrist extension)

Recipient Muscle: Extensor carpi radialis brevis (ECRB)

Recipient Nerve: Radial nerve

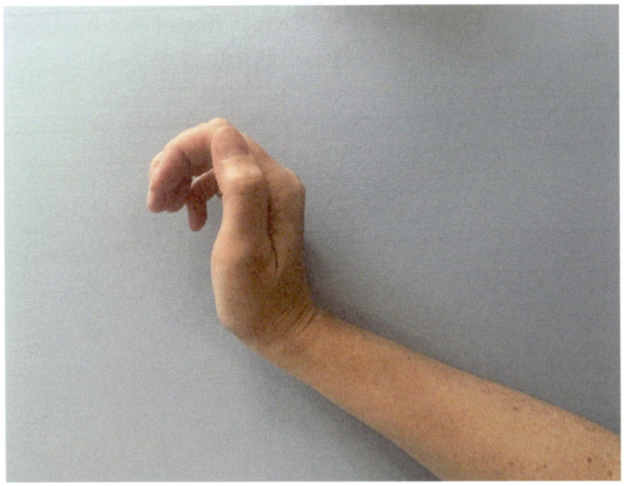

Pull wrist back (wrist extension)

Donor Movement = Bend fingers (finger flexion)
Donor Muscle: Flexor digital superficialis (FDS)
Donor Nerve: Median nerve

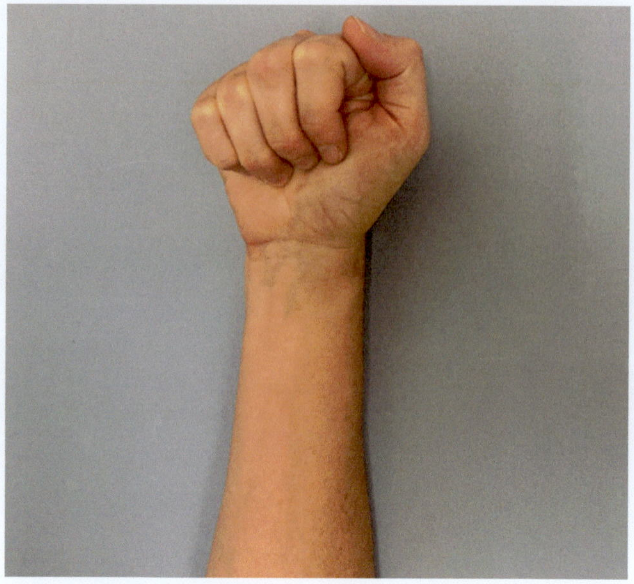

Bend fingers into a fist (finger flexion)

Phase 1 FDS-to-ECRB Nerve Transfer Exercises

☐ **Active or Resisted Donor Movement**:

- Bend your fingers into a fist. You may need to support the wrist by wearing your splint or using your other hand to stabilize the wrist.

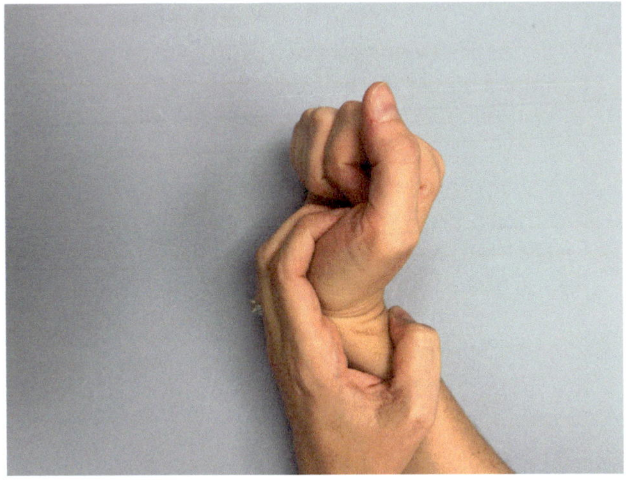

  – One month after surgery, you may use therapy putty or a gripper tool while completing this exercise, but you will need to support the wrist during this exercise.

Complete <u>10</u> repetitions, every waking hour.

☐ **Active Donor + Passive Recipient Movement**:

Complete one of the below exercises <u>10</u> repetitions, <u>3</u> times per day.

1. Use your opposite hand to pull your wrist back. At the same time, bend your fingers toward the palm. Try to keep the big knuckles straight while focusing on bending the rest of the fingers.

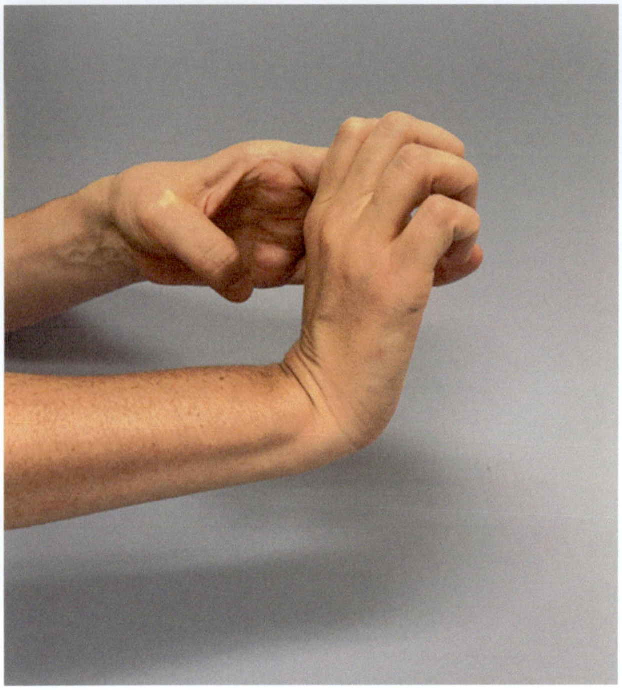

2. Begin with your forearm resting palm down on a table with the fingers resting off the table edge. Bend the fingers into the table edge. At the same time, raise your elbow toward the ceiling, keeping your palm touching to the table. Return to the start position, and repeat.

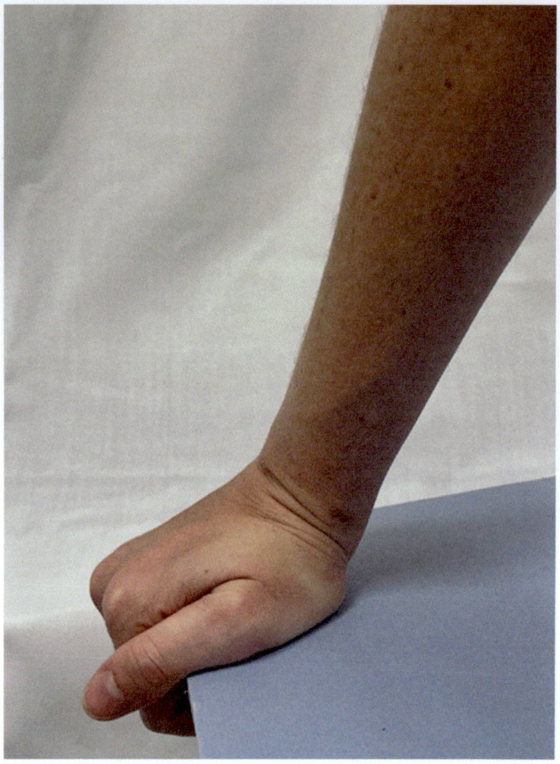

Phase 2 FDS-to-ECRB Nerve Transfer Exercises

☐ **Active Donor + Active-Assisted Recipient Movement**:

- Begin with your forearm resting on a table with the thumb side of the hand toward the ceiling. The hand may rest on a slick cloth such as a pillowcase. Bend your fingers into a fist. At the same time, pull the wrist back. Allow the other hand to help bend the wrist back as far as it will comfortably go. Return to the start position, and repeat.

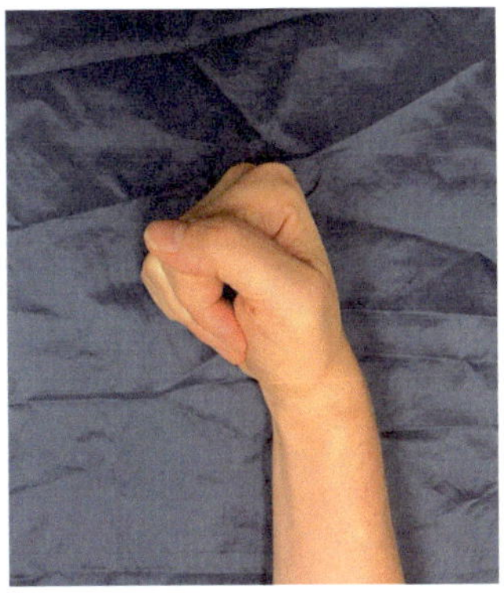

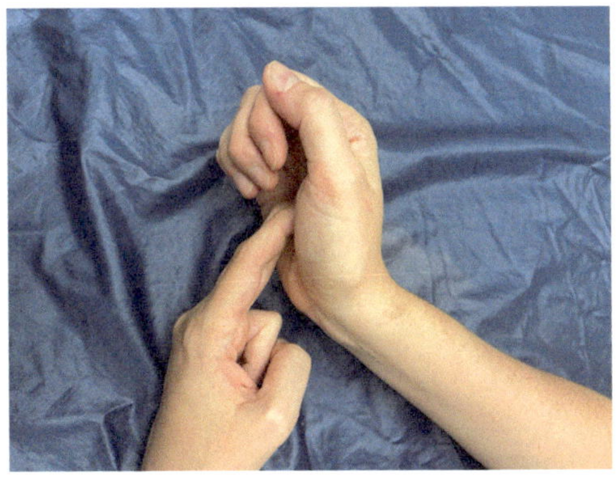

Complete 10 repetitions, 3 times per day.

☐ **"Place and Hold"**

- Begin with your forearm resting on a table. Using your other hand, pull the wrist back as you bend your fingers into a fist. Keep your fingers in a fist, and SLOWLY let go of the wrist support as you try to keep the wrist back **without the help of your other hand**. Return to the start position. Hold for 1–5 s.

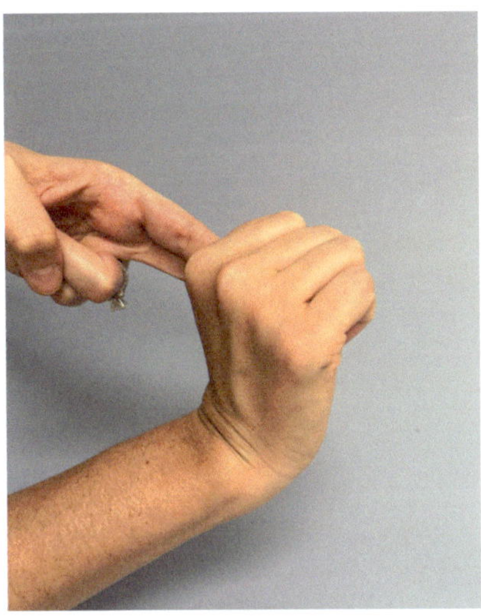

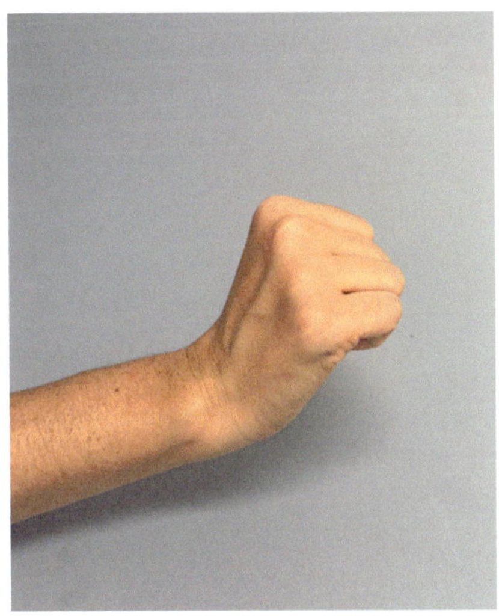

Complete 1–10 repetitions, 2–3 times per day.

☐ **Active Donor + Active Recipient Movement**:

- Bend your fingers into a fist. At the same time, pull your wrist back. Return to the start position, and repeat.

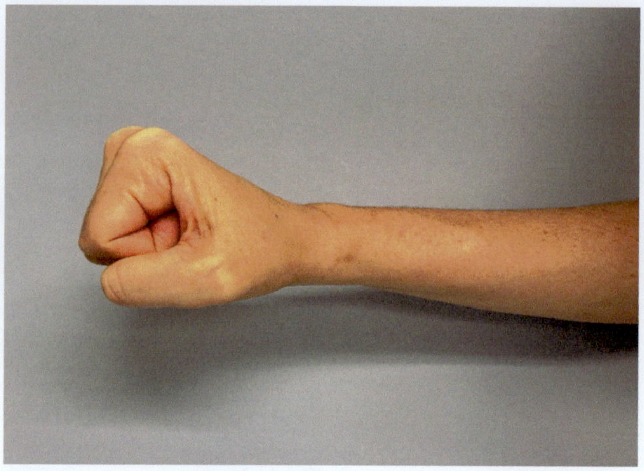

Complete 5–10 repetitions, 3 times per day.

Phase 3 FDS-to-ECRB Nerve Transfer Exercises

☐ **Resisted Donor + Resisted Recipient Movement**:

- Wrist curls: with the forearm supported on a table and your hand over the table edge, make a tight fist holding a ________ pound weight or a therapy band. Bend your wrist back toward the ceiling. Return to the start position, and repeat.

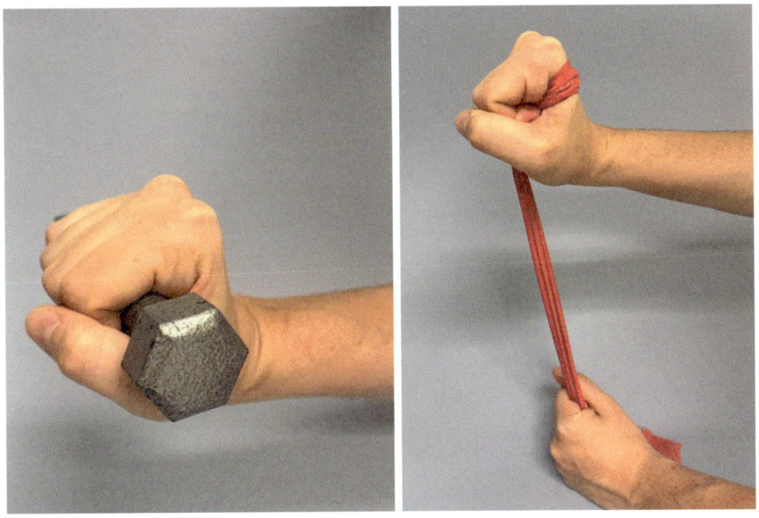

Complete 3–10 repetitions, 2 times per day.

☐ **Resisted Recipient Movement**:

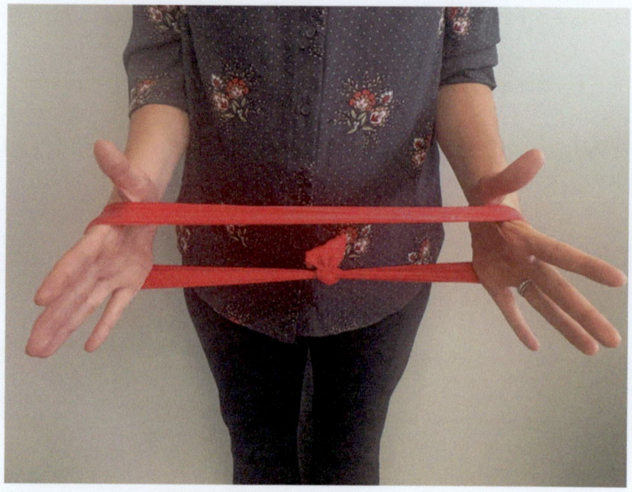

- With your elbows bent by your sides and palms facing each other, wrap a therapy band loop around both hands with your wrists and fingers straight. Keep your elbows close to your body as you pull your hands away from each other, against the resistance. Be sure to keep your wrist and fingers straight throughout this movement. Return to the start position, and repeat. Hold for 3–5 s.

Complete 10 repetitions, 2 times per day

References

1. Pet MA, Lipira AB, Ko JH. Nerve transfers for the restoration of wrist, finger, and thumb extension after high radial nerve injury. Hand Clin. 2016;32(2):191–207.
2. Brown J, Tung T, Mackinnon S. Median to radial nerve transfer to restore wrist and finger extension: technical nuances. Neurosurgery. 2010;61(1):75–83.
3. Lowe JB III, Tung TR, Mackinnon SE. New surgical option for radial nerve paralysis. Plast Reconstr Surg. 2002;110:836–43.
4. Ukrit A, Leechavengvongs S, Malungpaishrope K, Uerpairojkit C, Chongthammakun S, Witoonchart K. Nerve transfer for wrist extension using nerve to flexor digitorum superficialis in cervical 5, 6, and 7 root avulsions: anatomic study and report of two cases. J Hand Surg Am. 2009;34(9):1659–66.
5. Ray WZ, Mackinnon SE. Clinical outcomes following median to radial nerve transfers. J Hand Surg Am. 2011;36(2):201–8.
6. Bertelli JA, Ghizoni MF. Transfer of a flexor digitorum superficialis motor branch for wrist extension reconstruction in C5–C8 root injuries of the brachial plexus: a case series. Microsurgery. 2013;33(2):39–42.
7. Gossman MR, Sahrmann SA, Rose SJ. Review of length-associated changes in muscle: experimental evidence and clinical implications. Phys Ther. 1982;62(12):1799–808.
8. Goldspink G, Tabary C, Tabary JC, Tardieu C, Tardieu G. Effect of denervation on the adaptation of sarcomere number and muscle extensibility to the functional length of the muscle. J Physiol. 1974;236(3):733–42.
9. Kahn L, Moore A. Donor activation focused rehabilitation approach: maximizing outcomes after nerve transfers. Hand Clin. 2016;32(2):263–77.
10. Hill JL, Turner LC, Jones RD, Jimulia DT, Miller C, Power DM. The stages of rehabilitation following motor nerve transfer surgery. J Musculoskelet Surg Res. 2019;3:60.

Rehabilitation Guidelines for Specific Nerve Transfers: Hand

Median Nerve Branch to the Flexor Carpi Radialis (FCR) to the Posterior Interosseous Nerve (PIN) Transfer

Amy M. Young

FCR-to-PIN Nerve Transfer

Background

The posterior interosseous nerve (PIN) is a branch of the radial nerve and innervates the extensor carpi ulnaris (ECU), extensor digitorum communis (EDC), extensor digiti minimi (EDM), abductor pollicis longus (APL), extensor pollicis longus (EPL), extensor pollicis brevis (EPB), and extensor indicis proprius (EIP) muscles [1]. A PIN deficit limits one's ability to extend the fingers and thumb. Wrist extension with excess radial deviation is also noted due to ECU weakness with preserved extensor carpi radialis brevis and longus (ECRB and ECRL) function [1]. The flexor carpi radialis (FCR)-to-PIN nerve transfer has the ability to reinnervate all of the PIN-innervated musculature [2]. The goal of this nerve transfer is to restore the ability to open the hand for functional grasp and fine motor dexterity. However, the functional priority is finger MCP extension (EDC) and thumb MCP and IP (EPL) extension.

The FCR-to-PIN transfer may be performed for isolated PIN impairment or combined with an additional nerve transfer to simultaneously restore wrist extension for more proximal injuries such as high radial nerve injury and brachial plexus injuries to the posterior cord [2–6]. The pronator teres (PT)-to-ECRB *tendon* transfer is frequently combined with a nerve transfer for high radial nerve palsy to provide more immediate correction of wrist extension [3, 7–9].

Outcomes

Garcia-Lopez et al. [4] performed a retrospective study of six patients with radial nerve palsy or brachial plexus injury to the posterior cord following combined FCR-to-PIN and PT-to-ECRL nerve transfers. Approximately 20 months following surgery, all six patients achieved manual muscle testing (MMT) grade 4/5 EPL strength. Four patients achieved MMT grade 4/5 MCP extension strength, and two patients achieved MMT grade 3/5 MCP extension strength. On average, grip strength was 93% of the unaffected side.

Ray and Mackinnon [5] conducted a retrospective review of 19 patients with radial nerve injuries where the median nerve was utilized as a donor. At least eight of those patients underwent FCR-to-PIN and FDS-to-ECRB nerve transfer with or without PT-to-ECRB *tendon* transfer to address high radial nerve palsy. At nearly 20 months post-surgery, four patients demonstrated MMT grade 4/5 or greater finger extension strength, one patient achieved MMT grade 3/5 finger extension strength, and three patients had minimal to no improvement with finger extension. For wrist extension strength, seven patients achieved MMT grade 4/5, and one patient had no improvement. Bertelli [6] completed a prospective study of 29 patients with radial nerve palsy or brachial plexus injury to the posterior cord who underwent either nerve or tendon transfers. Outcomes for 14 patients

A. M. Young (✉)
Northwestern Medicine Center for Surgery of the Hand, Chicago, IL, USA
e-mail: Amy.Young@nm.org

L. C. Kahn et al. (eds.), *Rehabilitation for Nerve Transfers of the Upper Extremity*, https://doi.org/10.1007/978-3-031-92008-0_18

following FCR-to-PIN and AIN-to-ECRB nerve transfers were available. At an average follow-up of 26 months post-surgery, 12 patients achieved MMT grade 4/5 finger extension strength, and only two patients did not recover finger extension. A 30° thumb MCP joint extensor lag was observed in 13 of the 14 patients in this group. On average, grip strength was 58% of the unaffected side.

FCR-to-PIN transfer has the potential benefit of allowing individual finger extension in comparison to tendon transfer outcomes [2, 5, 9]. Following nerve transfers to restore radial nerve function, simultaneous wrist and finger extension is possible [3, 6]. The FCR-to-PIN nerve transfer is typically performed within 10 months of injury to avoid motor end-plate degeneration and promote optimal outcomes [3, 10].

Surgical Description

A curvilinear incision is made along the volar aspect of the proximal two-thirds of the forearm. The brachioradialis muscle is identified, and the superficial radial nerve is dissected on the undersurface of the brachioradialis muscle. The superficial radial nerve is used as a guide to dissect retrograde (distal to proximal) to identify the posterior interosseous nerve and the radial nerve proper. A handheld nerve stimulator is used to confirm that the PIN is not functioning. It is important to perform this evaluation within 30 min of the tourniquet being inflated (if one is being used) and to ensure that the anesthesia team is not using any muscle paralytics. After doing so, the lacertus fibrosus is identified, and after releasing the lacertus fibrosus, the median nerve is identified deep to the lacertus fibrosus and along the inner surface of the flexor pronator mass. After decompressing the median nerve, the branching pattern of the median nerve is identified. It is helpful to decompress the FDS arch, and subsequently identify the anterior interosseous nerve coming off the median nerve proper, being sure to protect the AIN. A handheld nerve stimulator is used to identify the branches of the median nerve to the FCR, again ensuring that this is done within 30 min of the tourniquet being inflated (if one is being used) and that there are no muscle paralytics being used by the anesthesia team. After doing so, the FCR branch of the median nerve is dissected as distally as possible, being sure to identify any additional branch of the median nerve that innervates the flexor-pronator mass. A complete decompression of the radial tunnel is performed to free the PIN. The donor nerve is divided distally, and the recipient nerve is divided proximally after dissecting the PIN from the radial nerve proper as proximally as possible. Coaptation of the FCR branch from the median nerve to the PIN is performed using microsurgical technique.

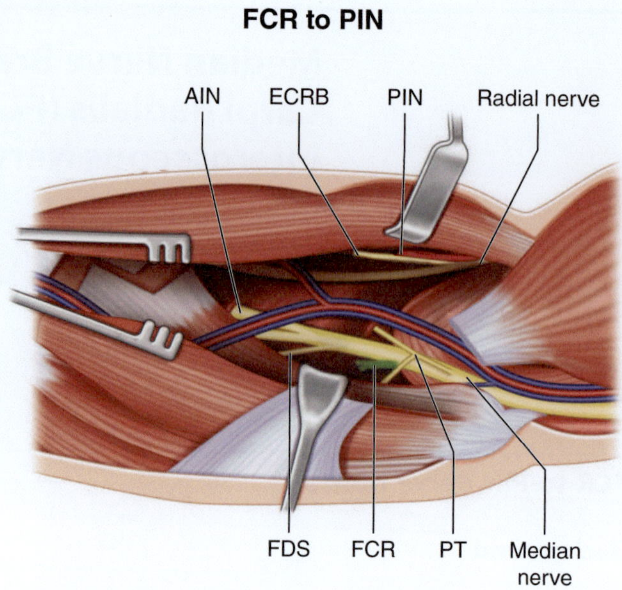

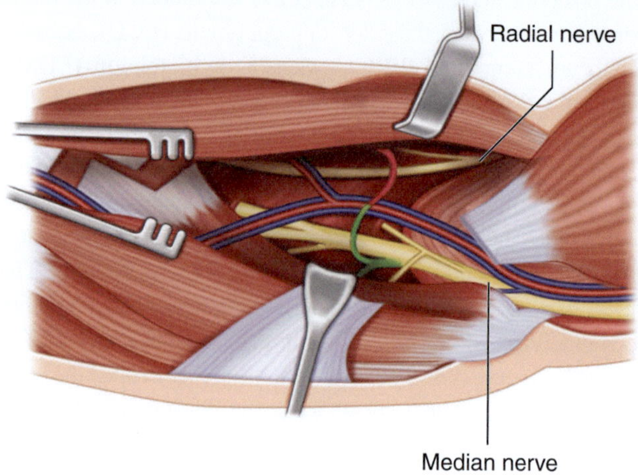

Phases of Rehabilitation

Phase 1

Preoperative to 1/5 MMT in the Recipient Muscles

Precautions

Patients should avoid prolonged positioning in composite finger flexion and composite thumb flexion (especially with wrist flexion), which promotes both flexor tightness and overlengthening of the extensor musculature. According to the length-tension relationship of muscle, overlengthening may contribute to biomechanical failure of the muscle to produce desired movement and strength once reinnervation of the recipient muscles occurs [11–13]. A general rule to follow is to preserve recipient muscle length whenever possible. If a pronator teres (PT)-to-extensor carpi radialis brevis (ECRB) *tendon* transfer is completed at the time of the nerve transfer surgery, priority is given to the more conservative postoperative *tendon* transfer protocol precautions [7, 8]. This would include full-time immobilization in maximum wrist extension (40° or more) for 4 weeks.

Orthosis

For an isolated PIN injury, the patient may be fit with a prefabricated BENIK™ hand-based finger and thumb extension orthosis (Image 1) or similar custom orthosis to preserve muscle length and promote function preoperatively. For high radial nerve injury, the patient may be fit with a prefabricated BENIK™ forearm-based finger and thumb extension orthosis (Image 2) or a similar custom orthosis due to wrist involvement.

Postoperatively, a custom, volar forearm-based orthosis with the wrist in extension, finger MCP joints in extension (IP joints excluded), and thumb MCP and IP joints in extension is fabricated to wear for protection of the nerve coaptation and to minimize edema [7] (Image 3). Around 2–3 weeks post-surgery, the patient may discontinue the custom orthosis during the day and resume the use of the BENIK™ orthosis to promote functional use and preserve muscle length while awaiting recipient muscle reinnervation. At this point, many patients are encouraged to continue the use of the custom thermoplastic orthosis at night for positioning/comfort.

Exercises

- Donor Activation

  Donor muscle activation in phase 1 includes active and isometric wrist flexion exercises. In cases of high radial nerve injury, *isometric* wrist flexion exercises are preferred over active wrist flexion exercises to avoid overlengthening of the wrist and finger extensor musculature. Within the postoperative orthosis, the patient may begin isometric wrist flexion exercises with the instructions to meet the resistance of the orthosis, but not overpower it. Ten to twelve days following surgery, the patient may initiate isometric wrist flexion outside the orthosis with the hand resting palm down on a supportive surface. Active wrist flexion exercises can be completed by those patients with isolated PIN impairment and intact wrist extension. Early-phase donor activation exercises are completed with low resistance, high repetitions, and high frequency to maximize neural signals to the donor muscle [3, 7].

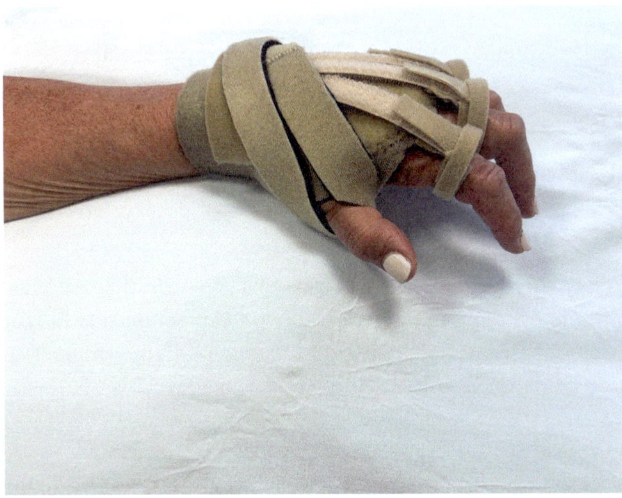

Image 1 A prefabricated BENIK™ hand-based finger and thumb extension orthosis or a similar custom orthosis may be used both pre- and postoperatively (following FCR-to-PIN nerve transfer) to preserve muscle length and promote function

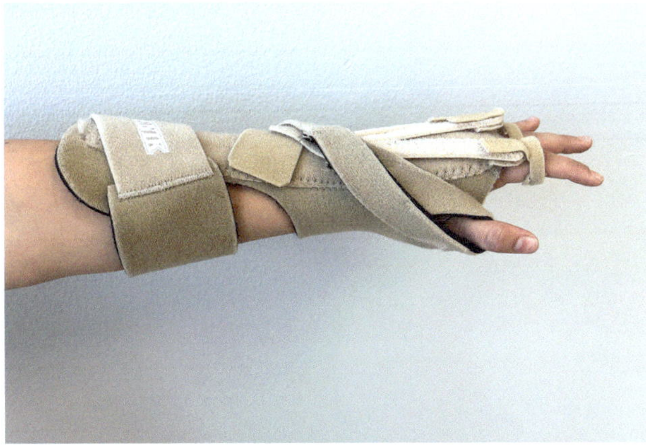

Image 2 For individuals with high radial nerve injury where wrist extension weakness is present, a prefabricated BENIK™ *forearm*-based finger and thumb extension orthosis or a similar custom orthosis is recommended to rest the involved recipient muscles and provide functional extension

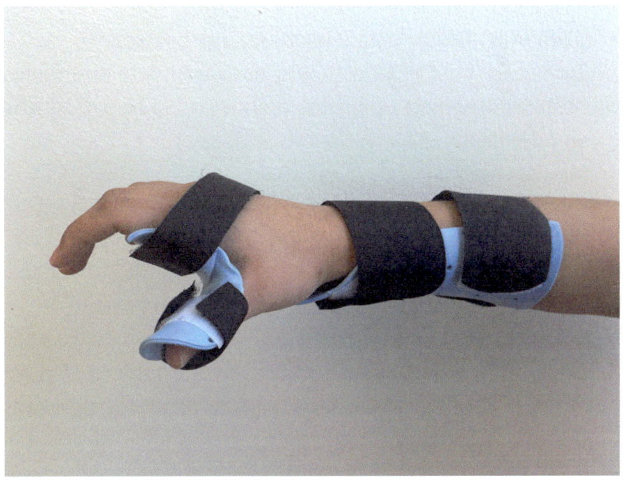

Image 3 A custom, volar, forearm-based orthosis that positions the wrist in extension, finger MCP joints in extension (IP joints excluded), and thumb MCP and IP joints in extension is fabricated to wear for protection in the first few weeks postoperatively. Continued use at night is recommended until phase 2 to maintain recipient muscle length

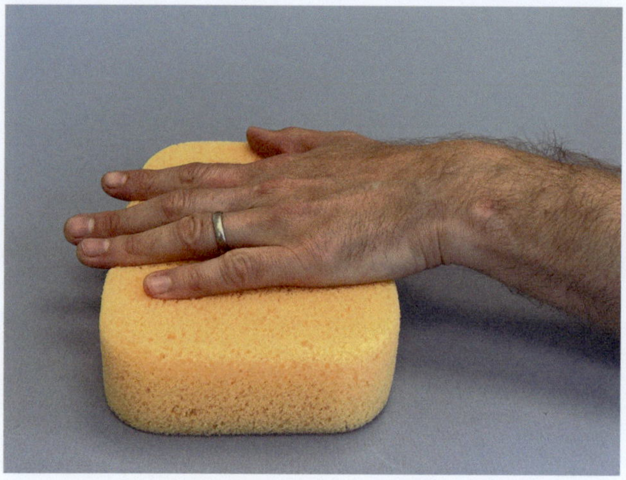

Image 4 An example of active or isometric donor with passive recipient exercise is demonstrated here. The individual presses the palm down into the sponge as the resistance from the sponge passively extends the fingers and thumb

- Combined Donor with Passive Recipient Exercise
  Isometric wrist flexion should be paired with simultaneous passive finger extension. It should also be paired with simultaneous passive thumb extension. For example, patients may rest their palm on light-resistive foam or therapy putty and press the palm down, as the foam or putty passively extends the fingers and thumb (Image 4). Alternatively, they can rest the hand on a piece of paper and slide it back and forth on the table with pressure to the volar MCP region of the palm. For passive ECU exercises, they would rest the hand on the table and press down to activate wrist flexors while passively deviating the wrist ulnarly.

Assessment of Recovery

MMT strength and range of motion measurements of the recipient muscles (EDC, EPL, and ECU), donor muscle (FCR), and other affected muscles and joints will be helpful for pre- and postoperative comparisons. Grip strength measurements should also be obtained.

To identify initial muscle contractions, the therapist should resist wrist flexion (FCR donor activation) while palpating over the EDC and EPL muscle or tendon in the forearm or wrist (Image 5). Look and/or palpate for trace finger MCP and thumb extension. MMT strength may initially be evaluated in a gravity-minimized plane. Technically, gravity will have less influence on the fingers and thumb compared to larger, heavier proximal segments of the upper extremity [14]. The therapist should assess strength at least monthly to determine the appropriate exercise program. Trace muscle contractions may not be observed for up to 6 months [3]. At that point, it may be helpful to track MCP extension lag in a consistent position of 0–30 degrees of wrist extension to monitor progress. It generally takes 12–18 months to achieve functional movement in the PIN muscles [15].

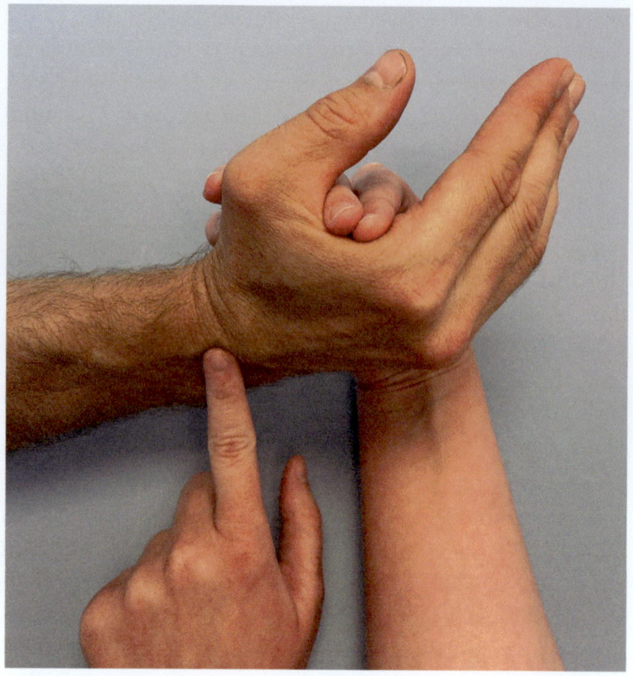

Image 5 Recovery of PIN innervated muscles is assessed in neutral to slight wrist extension. (The position of the wrist should be measured, so it can be replicated each month for greater accuracy of assessment of the recipient without tenodesis contributions.) Resistance is applied against wrist flexion while palpating for tension at the dorsal extensor compartments or their muscle bellies in the dorsal forearm

Therapy Frequency

Frequency of therapy visits is initially one time per week. Once the patient shows understanding of the donor-recipient relationship and any soft tissue restrictions are resolved, the patient should continue therapy one time per month.

Phase 2

From 2−/5 MMT to 3/5 MMT in the Recipient Muscles

Precautions

Avoid high-intensity exercises that involve the recipient muscles. Intense exercise leading to recipient muscle fatigue may impair the regeneration of axons, inhibiting reinnervation of recipient musculature [7].

Orthosis

Patients should continue to wear orthoses for positioning with removal for therapy exercises, hygiene, and light activity (if needed). The orthosis may be discontinued once the patient achieves and maintains full finger and thumb extension against gravity. However, orthoses during functional activities may be beneficial if light resistance easily overpowers finger and thumb extension.

In instances where the strength of the wrist extensors is limited (or results of additional transfers for wrist extension are poor to fair), attention should be given to the recovery of the PIN muscles. If the PIN muscles recover greater strength in the setting of a weak wrist, they will substitute for the wrist extensors resulting in nonfunctional "hook fist" posturing with unbalanced wrist flexion. These individuals will need wrist extension support with a strong orthosis once this pattern is noted to maintain functional grasp.

Exercises

Once partial range of motion is noted in the recipient muscle(s), the patient progresses to phase 2 of therapy. In this phase, the patient begins active-assisted recipient activation as well as "place and hold" exercises [3]. Exercises may begin in a gravity-minimized plane for the recipient muscles and progress to against gravity planes as MMT strength improves.

- Active Donor with Active-Assisted Recipient
  EDC and EPL MMT = 2−/5 to 2/5
  Active wrist flexion is paired with active-assisted finger and thumb extension. For example, the patient may rest the fingers or thumb on a playing card. As the patient presses the palm down to the table (active wrist flexion to neutral), the playing card decreases the friction between the fingers and table, assisting the fingers into MCP extension (Image 6).
- Resisted Donor Activation with Active-Assisted Recipient
  EDC and EPL MMT = 2/5

Resisted wrist flexion with active-assisted digital extension can be achieved by having the patient roll therapyputty into a cylinder. This provides active-assisted finger and thumb extension [3, 7]. The cylinder is then turned 90° so it "stands tall," and the patient is instructed to press the hand into the cylinder while keeping the wrist and forearm in contact with the table. This provides resistance to wrist flexion while assisting the EDC as the patient attempts to actively extend the fingers and thumb (Image 7a, b). Therapy putty resistance may be increased for greater challenge to the donor muscle.

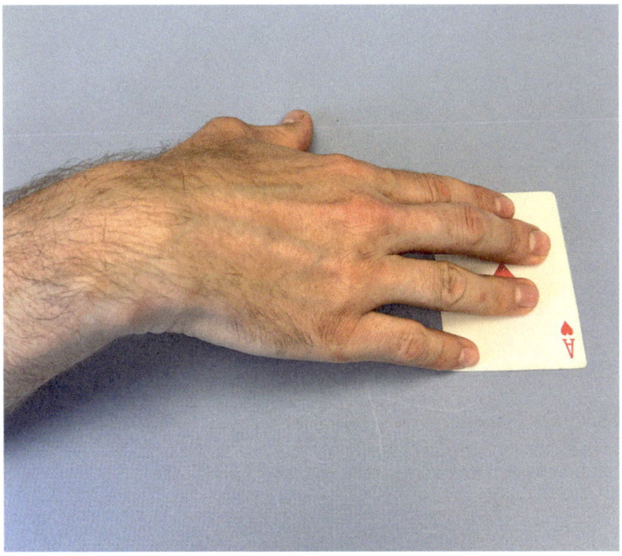

Image 6 Active donor with active-assisted recipient exercises are performed in phase 2. For example, as the patient presses the palm down on the table (active wrist flexion to neutral), the playing card decreases the friction between the fingers and table assisting the fingers into extension

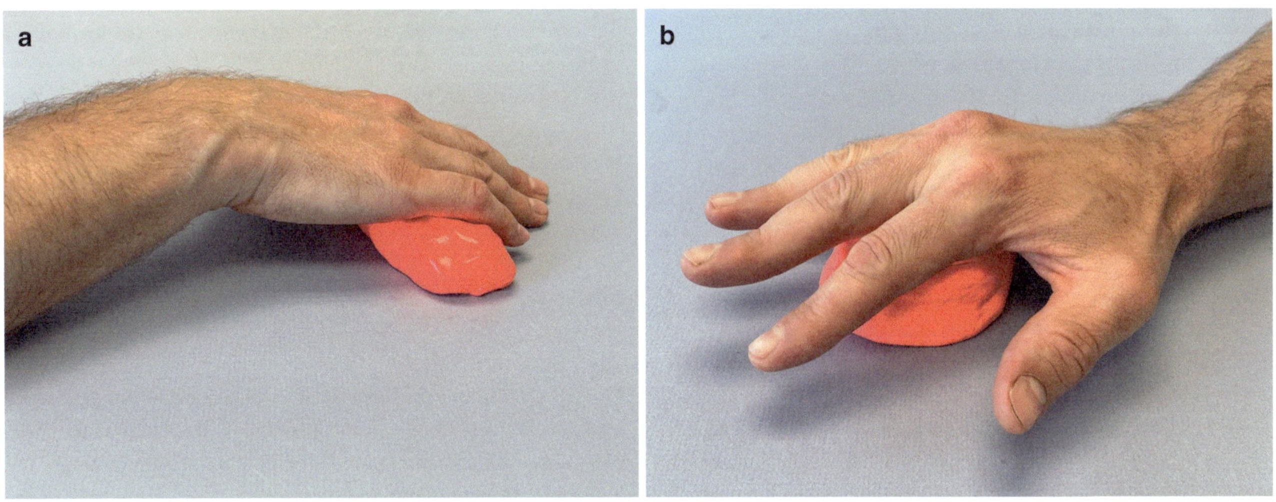

Image 7 (**a**) Resisted donor wrist flexion with active-assisted recipient EDC and EPL is performed with therapy putty. As the individual log rolls the putty, resistance is provided to wrist flexion while passively assisting finger and thumb extension. (**b**) The cylinder is rotated 90°, and the top is placed against the distal palm while the forearm and wrist remain on the table. As the palm presses into the cylinder, the FCR is resisted and the fingers are assisted into extension

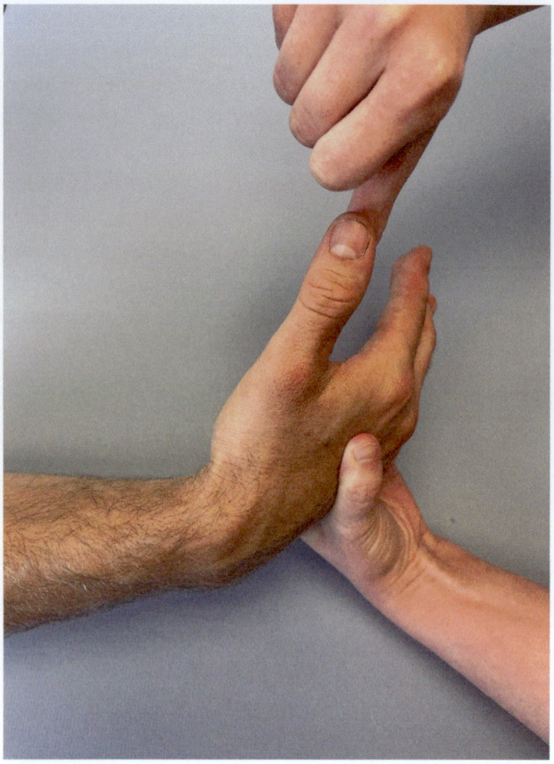

Image 8 "Place and hold" exercise for the EPL is performed by assisting the thumb to end-range thumb extension and releasing the support while maintaining resistance to the donor wrist flexors

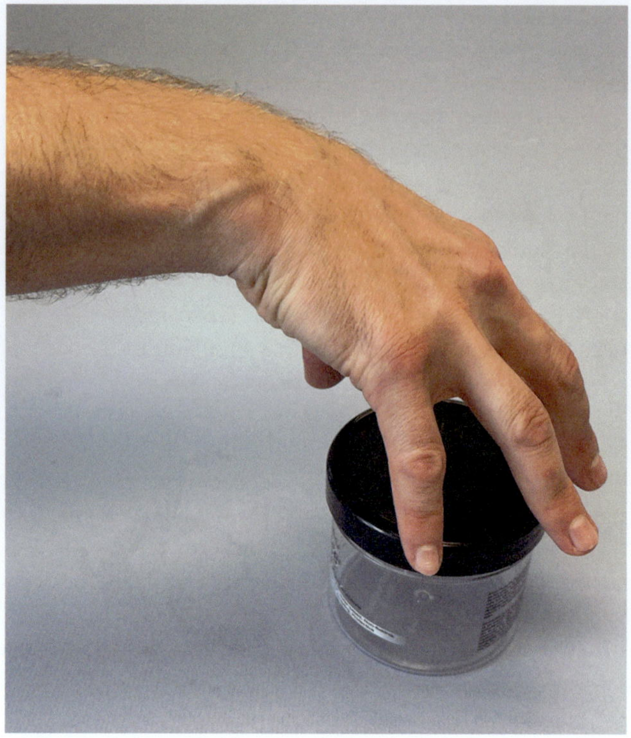

Image 9 Functional tasks such as reaching and opening the hand to retrieve a jar are encouraged in phase 2 as active finger extension improves

- "Place and Hold" Exercise
  EDC and EPL MMT = 2+/5
  When the EDC and EPL achieve 2+/5 MMT (partial range against gravity or more than 50% of the range), "place and hold" exercises begin. The thumb and/or fingers are manually placed in full extension. The therapist (or the patient's contralateral hand) resists wrist flexion as the patient attempts to maintain thumb and/or finger extension while the assistance is removed (Image 8).
- Active Donor with Active Recipient
  EDC and EPL MMT = 3−/5 to 3/5
  As strength improves, the patient may progress to active wrist flexion with active finger and thumb extension. The patient may hold a lightweight ball and then throw it to the floor, resulting in simultaneous wrist flexion and finger extension.
- Functional Activities
  - The patient may successfully begin functional tasks such as opening the hand to grasp containers (Image 9).
  - Wiping a tabletop with a cloth while the palm is flat and the wrist is neutral (in a seated position) will encourage active digit extension with active/resisted wrist flexion.

If the patient is struggling with the donor/recipient co-contraction, mirror therapy may be appropriate at this time.

Assessment of Recovery

Therapists should continue to assess MMT strength of EDC and EPL with resisted donor activation (FCR, wrist flexion). Measuring finger and thumb active extension while detailing the wrist angle, with or without donor activation, may be useful to highlight small changes over the prolonged recovery. Grip strength may also be assessed.

Frequency

Frequency of therapy may be increased to one time per week or every other week in phase 2.

Phase 3

3+/5 MMT and Above

Once the recipient muscles (EDC and EPL) can begin to withstand some resistance against gravity, the patient may incorporate more challenging strengthening and functional tasks.

Precautions

Endurance will take a long time to develop. Avoid excessive fatigue to the finger and thumb extensor muscles.

Orthosis

No orthosis is required unless fatigue is still present. Patients may benefit from a part-time functional orthosis if finger extension fatigue persists during the day. This may include starting the day without an orthosis and then wearing it in the afternoon if any loss of digital extension is noted throughout the day.

Exercises

- Resistive Recipient Activity with Donor Contraction
  The patient continues to combine recipient activity with donor contraction, including exercises requiring resisted finger and thumb extension with resisted wrist flexion. Baltimore Therapeutic Equipment™ (BTE) tool #302 requires finger MCP joint extension paired with resisted wrist flexion when set at the appropriate height (Image 10).
- Resistive Recipient Activity Without Donor Contraction
- The patient may eventually progress to digital extension exercise without the assistive component of the FCR, to improve finger extension with a neutral or extended wrist.
  - The patient can complete isometric finger and thumb extension in a neutral wrist position.
  - Rubber bands are useful to provide resistance to digital extension in wrist neutral or extension (Image 11).
  - Therapy-putty will provide resistance to EPL and EDC with "finger push" and "thumb lift" exercises while maintaining a neutral wrist.

Assessment of Recovery

MMT strength of EDC and EPL with and without donor activation (resisted wrist flexion) should be assessed. The greatest strength will likely be noted during co-contraction of donor (FCR) and recipient (EDC or EPL) muscle activation for 1–2+ years post-surgery [3].

Frequency

Frequency of therapy may continue one time per week or every other week in the late phase 3 until functional goals are met or until the individual has plateaued in functional gains.

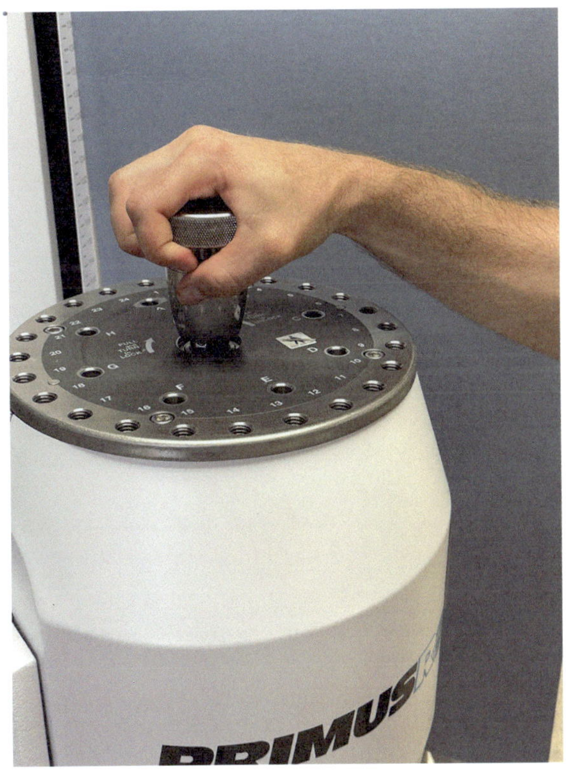

Image 10 When available, the BTE tool 302 is useful for strengthening and functional tasks such as opening a jar as it provides resistance to both the wrist flexors and the EDC and some thumb extensors

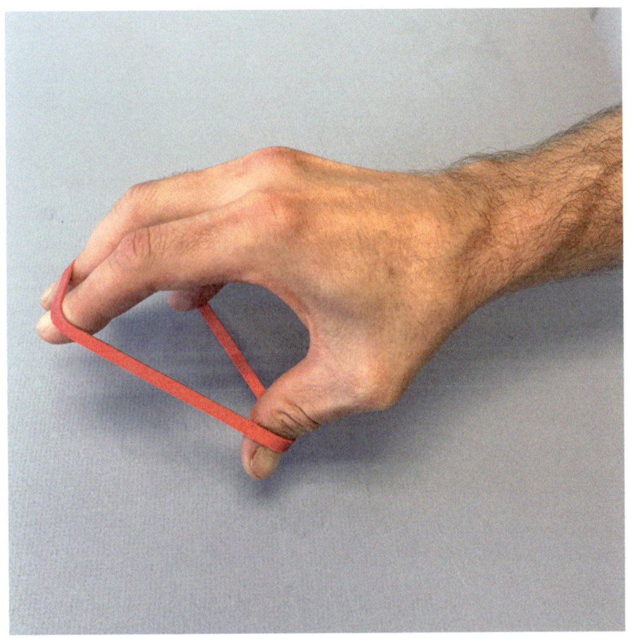

Image 11 Resisted EDC and thumb extension can be performed with rubber bands while the wrist is extended to separate the function from the donor

FCR-to-PIN nerve transfer

Nerve transfer overview					
Donor nerve	Donor action	Recipient nerve	Recipient action	Indications for functional restoration	Approximate months to functional movement
Median nerve to the flexor carpi radialis	Wrist flexion	Posterior interosseous nerve (PIN)	Finger MCP extension and thumb extension	Restore ability to open the hand for functional grasp	12–18 months [15]

Information below is suggested guidelines. Precautions may vary according to surgeon preferences and patient factors

	Preoperative therapy	Early phase	Middle phase	Late phase
Criteria	Before surgery	0/5 to −1/5 MMT	2−/5 to 3/5 MMT	>3/5 MMT
Purpose of phase	Educate and establish baseline function	Understand donor-recipient relationship Activate donor: wrist flexion	Activate nerve transfer for light functional activities requiring hand-opening	Isolate recipient through resistance Separate from donor activation
Precautions	NA	No wrist ROM for the first 2 weeks Avoid prolonged finger and thumb composite flexion to prevent flexor tightness and/or overlengthening of the extensors	Avoid high-intensity exercise Minimize fatigue and force placed on the weak finger and thumb extensors	Resistive exercise should not be performed before the PIN muscles demonstrate 3/5 MMT Avoid fatigue with resistance training
Frequency of visits (considerations)	1–2 visit(s); more if PROM limitations are present	1×/week until PROM is restored, and the patient is independent with the HEP Decrease to 1×/month based on progress	1×/month unless patient requires more guidance If additional nerve transfers were performed, more frequent therapy is warranted	1×/month
Orthosis considerations	Hand-based radial nerve palsy orthosis: either custom thermoplastic or BENIK™ W-700 series The purpose of this is to facilitate finger extension while allowing for functional grasp	Custom or prefabricated wrist orthosis for 2 weeks to protect the nerve coaptation. Some surgeons may prefer to have the finger MP joints in extension and thumb in extension to prevent drag on the PIN A hand-based radial nerve palsy orthosis may be resumed after 2 weeks	Hand-based radial nerve palsy orthosis during activity for function and to limit fatigue in recovering PIN muscles	No orthosis needed except for activities where the extensors are easily fatigued
Interventions		**Donor activation**: Wrist flexion (isometric, active, and resisted) 10× every hour **Donor-recipient pairing**: Active wrist flexion with passive finger MCP extension and thumb composite extension 10–20 reps, 6–8×/day	**Active/resisted donor with active assist recipient**: Passive progresses to active-assisted finger and thumb extension (with active and/or resisted wrist flexion) **Place and hold**: Place fingers and thumb in composite extension. Remove the support and maintain this position (while flexing the wrist)	**Resisted donor and recipient**: Resisted finger and thumb extension with the wrist flexed. Resistance may include therapy putty, a rubber band, or isometric pressure from the opposite hand **Resisted recipient without donor contraction**: Resisted finger and thumb extension while the wrist is in extension or neutral
Additional intervention considerations			Respect fatigue	Initially focus on high-frequency, low-resistance exercises

**During all phases, it is essential to continue cortical reorganization and psychological and psychosocial interventions and progress to incorporate donor/recipient with ADLs

FCR-to-PIN Nerve Transfer

Goal of Surgery: Restore the ability to open the hand to grasp and release objects

Recipient Movement = Lift fingers and thumb up (finger and thumb extension)

Primary Recipient Muscles: Extensor digitorum communis (EDC) and extensor pollicis longus (EPL)

Secondary Recipient Muscle: Extensor carpi ulnaris (ECU)

Recipient Nerve: Posterior interosseous nerve (PIN)

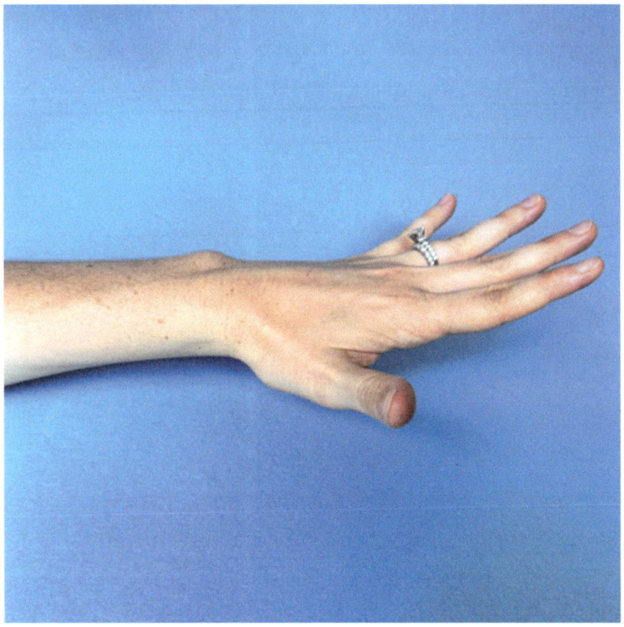

Lift fingers and thumb up (finger and thumb extension)

Donor Movement = Bend wrist forward (wrist flexion)

Donor Muscle: Flexor carpi radialis (FCR)

Donor Nerve: Median nerve

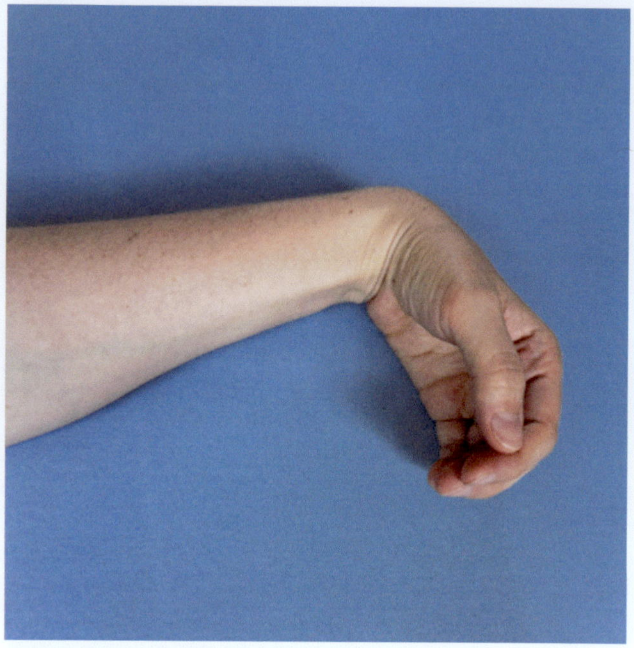

Bend wrist forward (wrist flexion)

Phase 1 FCR-to-PIN Nerve Transfer Exercises

☐ **Isometric Donor Activation:**

- Support the wrist by wearing your splint or resting your forearm palm down on a tabletop. Keep your wrist straight. Press your palm into the splint or press the fist down onto a tabletop. Gently meet the resistance of the splint or tabletop keeping your wrist straight. Hold for 3–5 seconds.

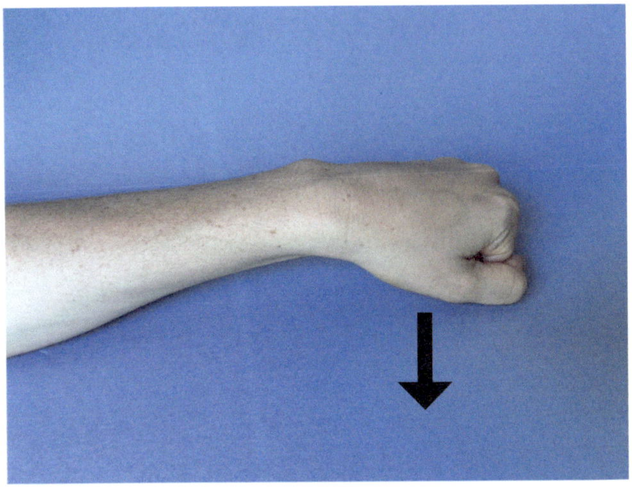

Complete 10 repetitions, every waking hour.

☐ **Isometric Donor + Passive Recipient Movement:**

- Begin with your forearm on a table and your palm resting on light-resistive foam or therapy putty. As you press your palm down into the resistance, the table will straighten your fingers and thumb. Hold for 3–5 seconds.

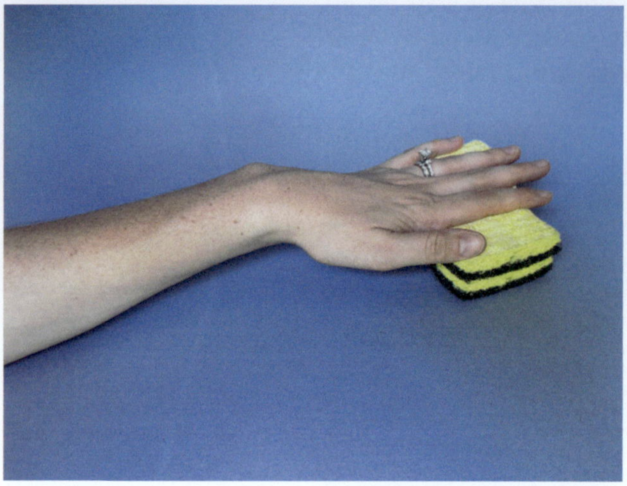

Complete 10 repetitions, 3 times per day.

Phase 2 FCR-to-PIN Nerve Transfer Exercises

☐ **Active Donor + Active-Assisted Recipient Movement**:

Complete the below exercises 10 repetitions, 3 times per day.

1. Begin with your forearm resting palm down on a table. Rest your fingertips on a playing card in a bent position. Press your palm down into the table as you attempt to slide the card away from you to flatten your hand.

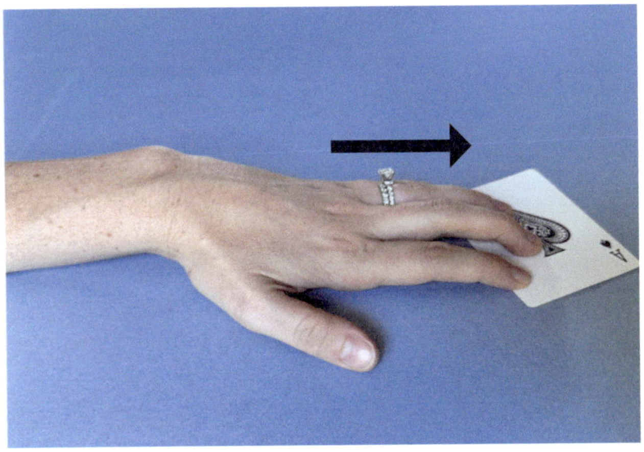

2. Try the same exercise with the thumb. As you press your palm into the table, move your thumb out to the side. Use your other hand to help slide the card out to the side if needed.

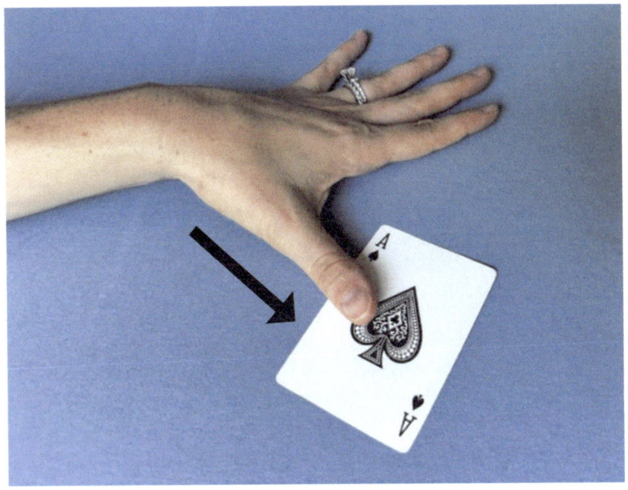

3. Begin with your forearm on a table with your hand resting on a piece of paper. As you gently press your palm down into the paper, move your hand side to side like a windshield wiper.

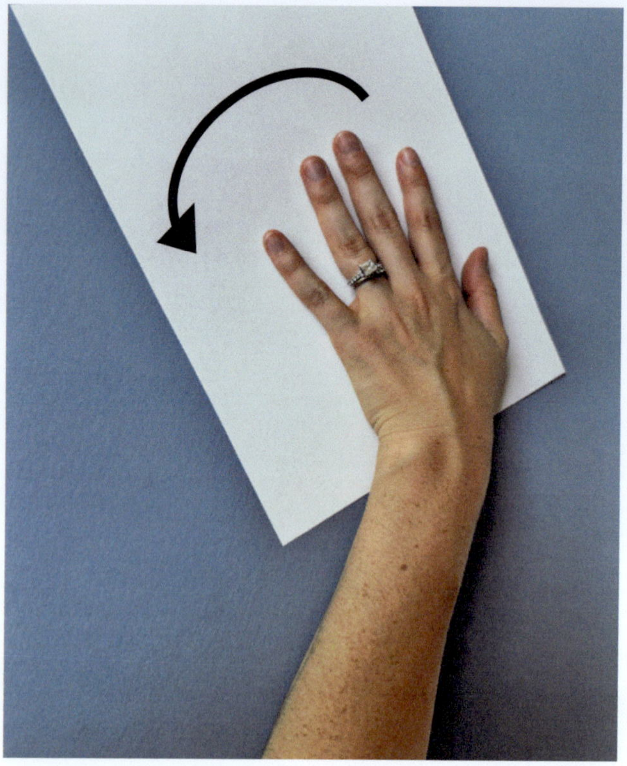

☐ **Resisted Donor + Active-Assisted Recipient Movement**:

- On a tabletop, roll therapy putty into a cylinder. Rest your palm on top of the putty cylinder, and press your palm down into the table as you try to lift your fingers and thumb up (with your own muscles). You may then assist with the opposite hand as needed.

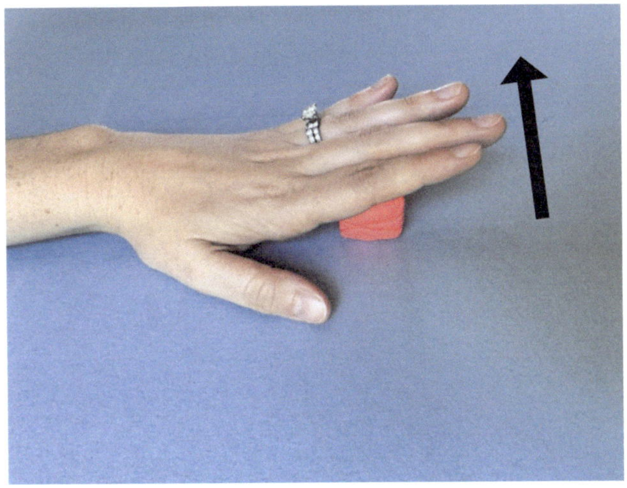

Complete 10 repetitions, 3 times per day.

☐ **Isometric Donor + "Place and Hold"**

Complete the below exercises <u>1–10</u> repetitions, <u>2–3</u> times per day.

Hold for <u>3–5</u> seconds.

1. Rest your forearm and palm on a table with your fingers and thumb relaxed over the edge. Keep your wrist a little bent. Using your other hand, **lift your fingers up**. Press your palm down into the table. SLOWLY let go of your **fingers** as you try to hold them up without the help of your other hand.

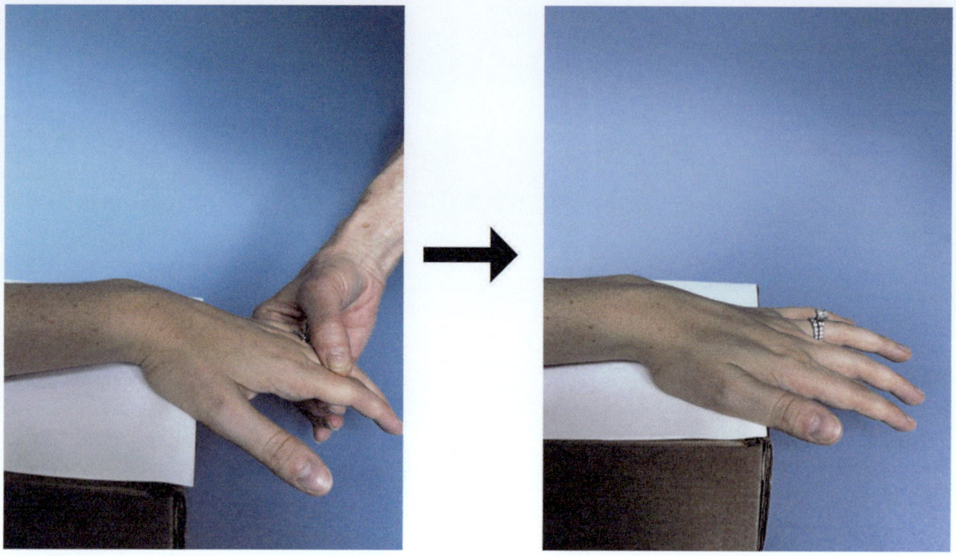

2. Repeat the same exercise with the thumb. Using your other hand, **lift your thumb up**. Press your palm down into the table. SLOWLY let go of your **thumb** as you try to hold it up without the help of your other hand.

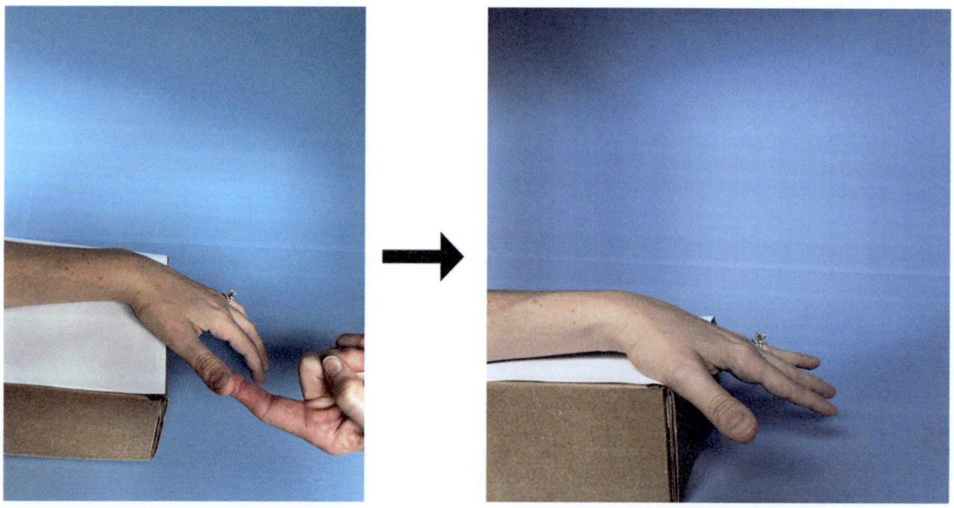

☐ **Active Donor + Active Recipient Movement**:

- Begin with your elbow bent by your side with your palm facing down. Bend your wrist forward toward the ground. At the same time, try to lift your fingers and thumb up toward the ceiling. Gradually try to straighten the thumb and fingers with less wrist bending.

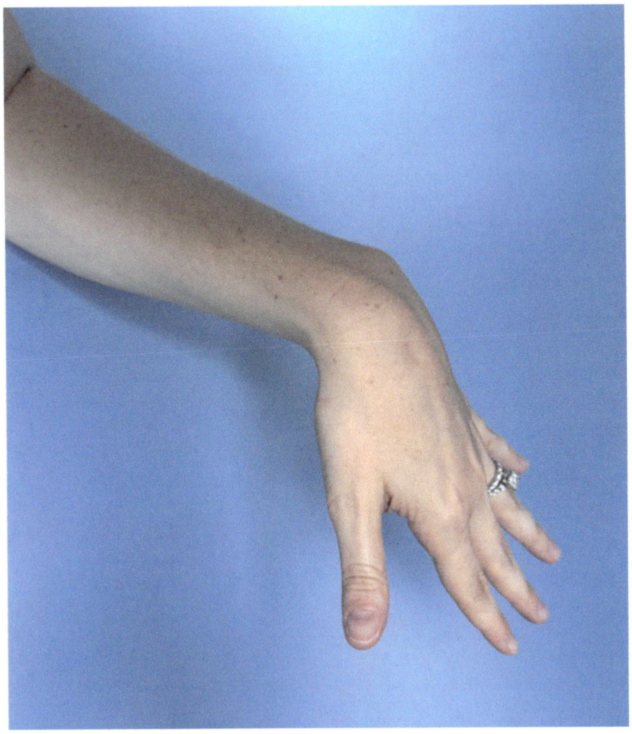

Complete 5–10 repetitions, 3 times per day.

Phase 3 FCR-to-PIN Nerve Transfer Exercises

☐ **Resisted Donor + Recipient Movement**:

- Open a wide jar lid. As your fingers are placed in wide, open position (extension), push your wrist forward and twist the lid open.

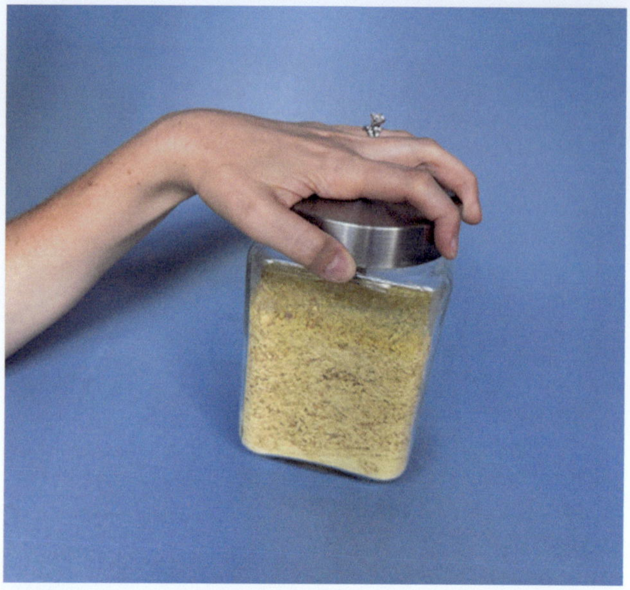

Complete 3–10 repetitions, 2 times per day.

☐ **Isometric Recipient Movement**:

Complete the below exercises 10 repetitions, 2 times per day.

Hold for 3–5 s.

- Begin with your forearm on a table and your fingers resting over the edge. Keep your wrist straight. **Lift your fingers up**. Keeping your fingers up, use your other hand to provide resistance in the **downward direction** across the back of your fingers. Only push hard enough to meet the resistance of your lifted fingers but not enough to overpower them. Your fingers should stay lifted against the resistance you provide.

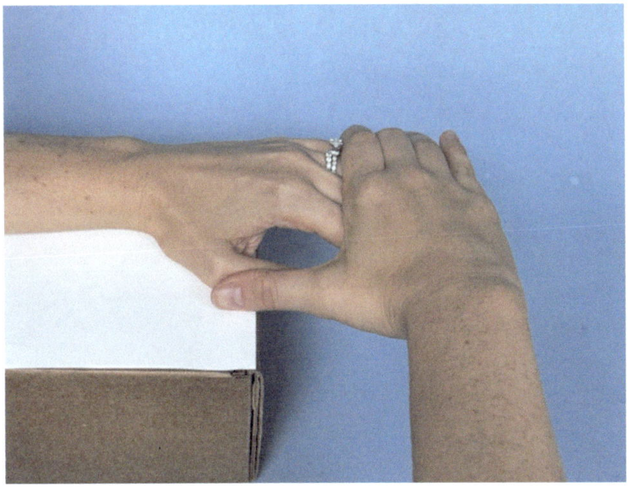

☐ **Resisted Recipient Movement**:

Complete one or more of the below exercises <u>10</u> repetitions, <u>2</u> times per day.

1. Place a rubber band around your fingers and thumb. Keep your wrist straight. Lift your fingers and thumb up against the resistance of the rubber band, like you are opening your hand to pick up an object.

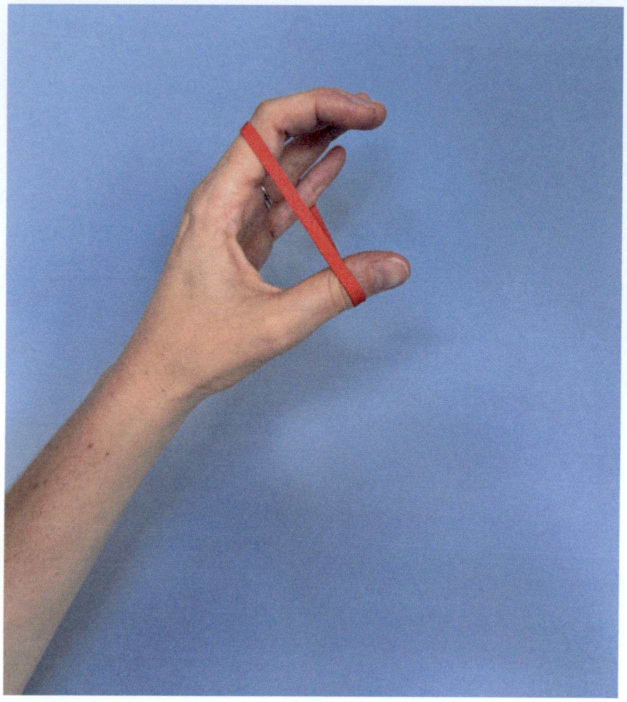

2. Shape therapy putty into a disc. Place fingers and thumb inside the putty, and open the fingers against the resistance of the putty. Keep your wrist straight or slightly backwards. If needed, stabilize your wrist using your opposite hand to prevent the wrist from bending forward.

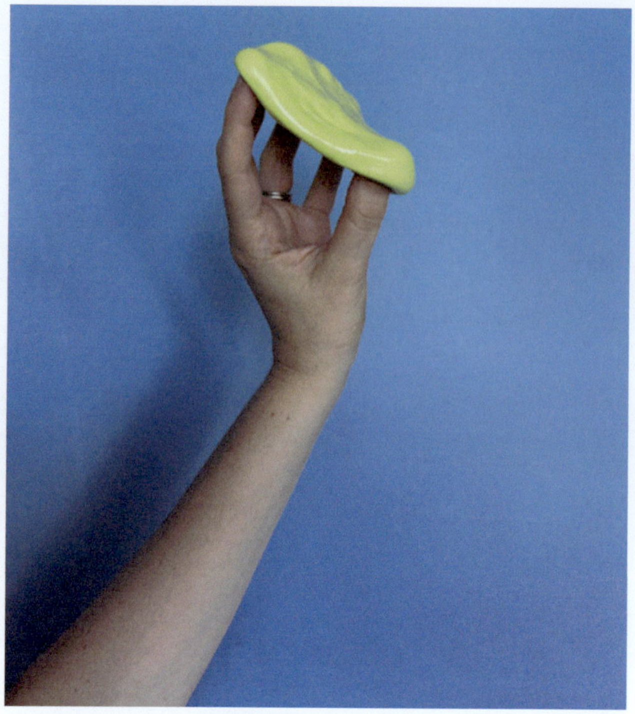

3. Shape therapy putty into a coil, and place it over the back of the thumb. **Lift the thumb UP** as far as it will go. Return to the starting position, and repeat. Keep your wrist straight or slightly backwards (extended). If needed, stabilize your wrist using your opposite hand to prevent the wrist from bending forward.

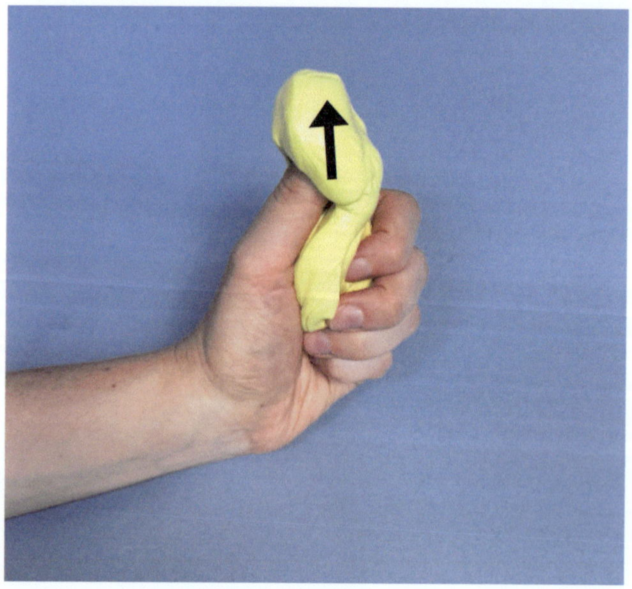

References

1. Sigamoney KV, Rashid A, Ng CY. Management of atraumatic posterior interosseous nerve palsy. J Hand Surg Am. 2017;42(10):826–30. https://doi.org/10.1016/j.jhsa.2017.07.026.
2. Moore AM, Franco M, Tung TH. Motor and sensory nerve transfers in the forearm and hand. Plast Reconstr Surg. 2014;134:721–9. https://doi.org/10.1097/PRS.0000000000000509.
3. Davidge KM, Yee A, Kahn LC, Mackinnon SE. Median to radial nerve transfers for restoration of wrist, finger, and thumb extension. J Hand Surg. 2013;38A:1812–27. https://doi.org/10.1016/j.jhsa.2013.06.024.
4. Garci-Lopez A, Navarro R, Martinez F, Rojas A. Nerve transfers from branches to the flexor carpi radialis and pronator teres to reconstruct the radial nerve. J Hand Surg Am. 2014;39(1):50–6. https://doi.org/10.1016/j.jhsa.2013.10.011.
5. Mackinnon SE, Roque B, Tung TH. Median to radial nerve transfer for treatment of radial nerve palsy. J Neurosurg. 2007;107:666–71. https://doi.org/10.3171/JNS-07/09/0666.
6. Bertelli JA. Nerve versus tendon transfer for radial nerve paralysis reconstruction. J Hand Surg Am. 2020;45(5):418–26. https://doi.org/10.1016/j.jhsa.2019.12.009.
7. Kahn LC, Moore AM. Donor activation focused rehabilitation approach maximizing outcomes after nerve surgery. Hand Clin. 2016;32:263–77. https://doi.org/10.1016/j.hcl.2015.12.014.
8. Brown JM, Tung THH, Mackinnon SE. Median to radial nerve transfer to restore wrist and finger extension: technical nuances. Neurosurgery. 2010;61(1):75–83. https://doi.org/10.1227/01.NEU.0000354364.13224.C8.
9. Ray WZ, Mackinnon SE. Clinical outcomes following median to radial nerve transfer. J Hand Surg. 2011;36A:201–8. https://doi.org/10.1016/j.jhsa.2010.09.034.
10. Pet MA, Lipira AB, Ko JH. Nerve transfers for the restoration of wrist, finger, and thumb extension after high radial nerve injury. Hand Clin. 2016;32:191–207. https://doi.org/10.1016/j.hcl.2015.12.007.
11. Goldspink G, Tabary C, Tabary JC, Tardieu C, Tardieu G. Effect of denervation on the adaptation of sarcomere number and muscle extensibility to the functional length of the muscle. J Physiol. 1974;236(3):733–42.
12. Gossman MR, Sahrmann SA, Rose SJ. Review of length-associated changes in muscle: experimental evidence and clinical implications. Phys Ther. 1982;62(12):1799–808.
13. Lieber RL, Bodine-Fowler SC. Skeletal muscle mechanics: implications for rehabilitation. Phys Ther. 1993;73(12):844–56.
14. Avers D, Brown M. Muscle testing: techniques of manual examination and performance testing. 10th ed. Philadelphia: Saunders; 2018.
15. Hill JL, Turner LC, Jones RD, Jimulia DT, Miller C, Power DM. The stages of rehabilitation following motor nerve transfer surgery. J Musculoskelet Res. 2019;3:60.

Supinator Branch of the Radial Nerve to the Posterior Interosseous Nerve Transfer

Jennifer Q. Farrar and Lorna C. Kahn

Background

Functional grasp begins with opening the hand to reach around an object. The ability to open the hand is controlled by the extrinsic extensor and intrinsic muscles of the hand. In isolation, the extrinsic finger extensor muscles (extensor digitorum communis (EDC), extensor indicis proprius (EIP), and extensor digitorum quinti/minimi (EDQ/M) muscles) extend the MCP joints of the fingers, and the extensor pollicis (EPL), extensor pollicis brevis (EPB), and abductor pollicis longus (APL) extend and abduct the thumb. These muscles, along with extensor carpi ulnaris (ECU), are innervated by the posterior interosseous nerve (PIN) [1]. The extensor carpi radialis brevis (ECRB) is often innervated by the PIN as well [2, 3]. When the extensor carpi radialis longus (ECRL) contracts in isolation, often seen with a PIN palsy, the wrist will extend with a strong radial deviation torque [3, 4].

Injury to the PIN can occur in isolation, as part of a radial nerve injury or with more global paralysis, as part of a brachial plexus injury. Atraumatic PIN palsy may occur due to entrapment neuropathy, Parsonage-Turner syndrome, or spontaneous hourglass constriction [5].

Surgical intervention for PIN palsy in the setting of spinal cord injury or lower plexus injury typically involves a supinator to PIN nerve transfer. There are two muscles that perform supination of the forearm. The biceps brachii is the primary supinator, and the supinator muscle is a secondary supinator [3, 4]. The supinator muscle is innervated by the radial nerve with fibers primarily from the C6 nerve root. Supination function is therefore preserved in a lower plexus injury (C7–T1) [3, 5]. Having a redundant source of supination makes the supinator branch a good donor option to help restore finger and thumb extension [3, 4]. Another benefit is the close proximity of the supinator branch of the radial nerve to the PIN recipient, which coincides with the golden rule of nerve transfers: to have no tension on the coaptation [3, 5]. The similarity in diameter of the donor and recipient nerves (when both medial and lateral branches of the supinator nerve are used), as well as their myelinated fiber counts, makes it an ideal choice for this nerve transfer [4].

The goal of the supinator to PIN transfer is to restore finger and thumb extension [3, 5, 6]. It is also intended to reestablish function in the ECU, so it may rebalance and centralize wrist extension [4, 7]. Additionally, in the absence of abductor pollicis longus, the ability for the thumb to actively open the first web space to grasp and release an object would be impaired [6, 7]. It is imperative to understand that this transfer aims to restore active extension of the finger metacarpophalangeal joints. Due to the extrinsic extensor attachment on the extensor hood mechanism, there may be some extension provided to the interphalangeal joints, but median and ulnar innervated intrinsic muscles are primarily responsible for this movement [4, 6]. When performed in the tetraplegic or lower/mid-plexus injury populations, the tenodesis effect will further assist the individual with digital extension [3].

Outcomes

The coaptation of the supinator to PIN transfer is approximately 3–4 cm from the proximal branching of the PIN muscles [6, 8]. This suggests that patients may detect a flicker of a muscle contraction as early as 3–4 months from surgery [6, 8]. Reinnervation may be noted on electrodiagnostic tests as soon as 4 months after the operation, but active movement is typically seen between 5 and 9 months [5, 6].

J. Q. Farrar (✉)
Vanderbilt Health Belle Meade Clinic, Vanderbilt University Medical Center, Nashville, TN, USA
e-mail: Jennifer.q.farrar@vumc.org

L. C. Kahn
Milliken Hand Rehabilitation Center, WashU Medicine, St. Louis, MO, USA
e-mail: Kahn.lorna.c@wustl.edu

L. C. Kahn et al. (eds.), *Rehabilitation for Nerve Transfers of the Upper Extremity*,
https://doi.org/10.1007/978-3-031-92008-0_19

With the goal of achieving functional hand opening, manual muscle testing (MMT) grade level of a 3/5 for finger and thumb extension, several authors have reported similar outcomes following supinator to PIN nerve transfer. Bertelli and his group reported success in all four patients following a brachial plexus injury at 1 year following surgery that was performed between 5 and 7 months after injury. He also reported achieving hand opening in 12 of 13 individuals with spinal cord injuries following supinator to PIN nerve transfers [4, 6]. Van Zyl and colleagues demonstrated evidence of finger extension in 19 of 21 patients and thumb extension in 17 of those patients [9]. Xu et al. had success with this transfer in nine out of ten patients [10]. Dong et al. also reported attaining "good" results with this transfer. He noted that finger extension was recovered within 5–7 months in three out of four patients [11]. Hahn achieved this result in 11 out of 11 patients within 1 year of surgery [8]. Interestingly, this study included an extensive description of a rehabilitation program specific to this nerve transfer. Fifteen months following injury, Zhang et al. reported success in two out of two cases [12]. However, when the nerve transfer was delayed until 2 years post-injury, Khalifeh and his group reported success in only 7 out of 13 cases [13, 14].

Surgical Description

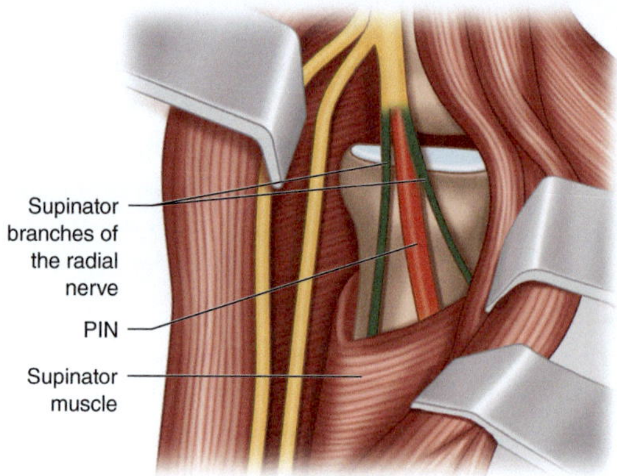

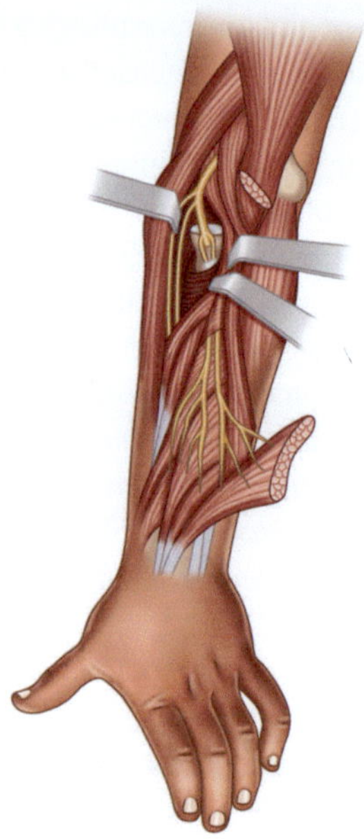

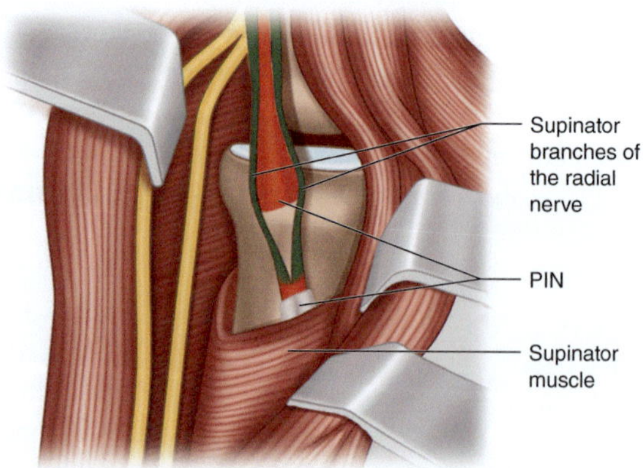

A curvilinear incision is made along the volar aspect of the proximal two-thirds of the forearm. The brachioradialis muscle is identified, and the superficial radial nerve is dissected on the undersurface of the brachioradialis muscle. The superficial radial nerve is used as a guide to dissect retrograde (distal to proximal) to identify the posterior interosseous nerve and the radial nerve proper. The supinator branches are identified proximal to the radial tunnel, with 2–3 branches typically visualized entering the superficial head of the supinator. Intraoperative stimulation is used to confirm isolated supination when stimulating the supinator branches as well as a lack of function in the PIN. It is important to stimulate these branches within 30 minutes of the tourniquet being inflated (if one is being used) and to ensure that the anesthesia team is not using any muscle paralytics. A thorough radial tunnel decompression is performed, preserving the supinator branches. The supinator branches are neurolyzed from the radial nerve proper and divided distally. The PIN is neurolyzed from the radial nerve proper and divided proximally. Coaptation of the supinator branches to the PIN is performed using microsurgical technique.

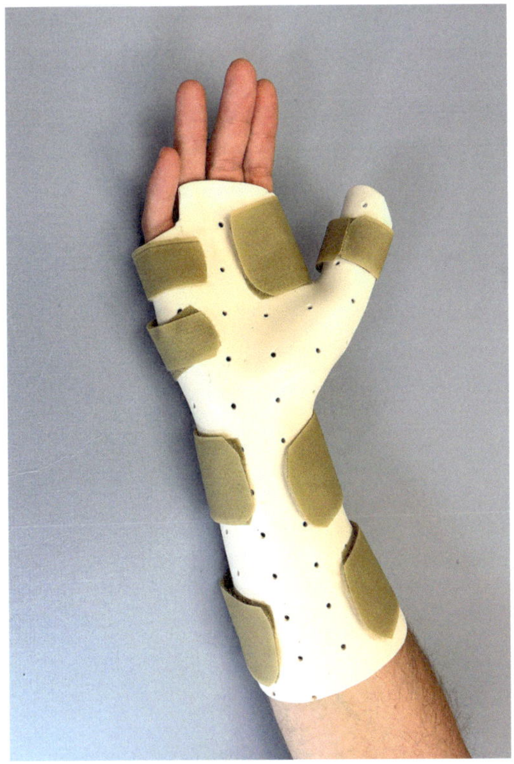

Image 1 A custom fabricated forearm-based P1 block orthosis that supports the wrist, the entire thumb, and the MCP joints of the fingers in extension is recommended for the first 2 weeks after surgery and then at night to maintain muscle length until PIN function returns

Phases of Rehabilitation

Phase 1

Pre-op to 1/5 MMT in the Recipient Muscle

Postoperative care will vary with the patient and the surgeon. In some cases, the patient is positioned with the elbow flexed to 90 degrees with the forearm and wrist in a neutral position [8]. For others, a prefabricated wrist orthosis will suffice. For individuals with an isolated PIN palsy where strong antagonist flexors are intact, a custom fabricated forearm-based wrist extension orthosis with an MCPJ extension block (a P1 block) with composite thumb extension is recommended initially for the first 2 weeks and then reduced to night use until return of PIN function (Image 1). Others have described using a resting hand orthosis with the metacarpal phalangeal joints in 70 degrees of flexion, the interphalangeal joints in 0 degrees of extension, and the thumb supported in radial abduction for individuals with tetraplegia or lower plexus injuries undergoing this nerve transfer [8]. Due to the lack of tension on the repair, combined elbow and wrist extension should not cause strain at the site, and thus some patients may not require postoperative protection [5]. It is important to discuss this with the referring surgeon. Protection of any concurrent nerve or tendon transfers should also be considered.

Patients are typically seen in the surgeon's clinic at 2 weeks after surgery and meet with the therapist soon afterward for initial assessment and treatment. Assessment should include baseline assessment of radial and PIN motor function, grip and pinch strength, and degrees of extension lag at all digits along with assessment of functional deficits related to home, work, and community roles. Patients are educated in protective positioning, behavioral modifications, preservation of passive range of motion (PROM), edema control strategies, and scar management techniques. In rare cases, neuropraxia can occur in muscles in the operative region. These muscles should be supported and monitored for recovery over the following months.

Individuals are instructed to avoid tensioning the nerve for 3–6 weeks following surgery [8]. This has been described as avoiding placing the surgical arm in a position of combined shoulder external rotation and elbow and wrist extension with forearm supination [8]. Technically, radial nerve tension should also be discouraged which means avoiding combined shoulder and elbow extension with pronation and wrist flexion (Image 2).

Motor reeducation, including cortical reorganization, begins within the first postoperative month. Patients are introduced to the new anatomical relationship between the donor (supinator) and recipient (digital extension) muscle functions. The home exercise program should highlight simple donor activation with forearm rotation and combined activation of supination with passive extension of the fingers and thumb for the recipient PIN. Ideally, donor activation should be performed for ten repetitions every hour the patient is awake [15].

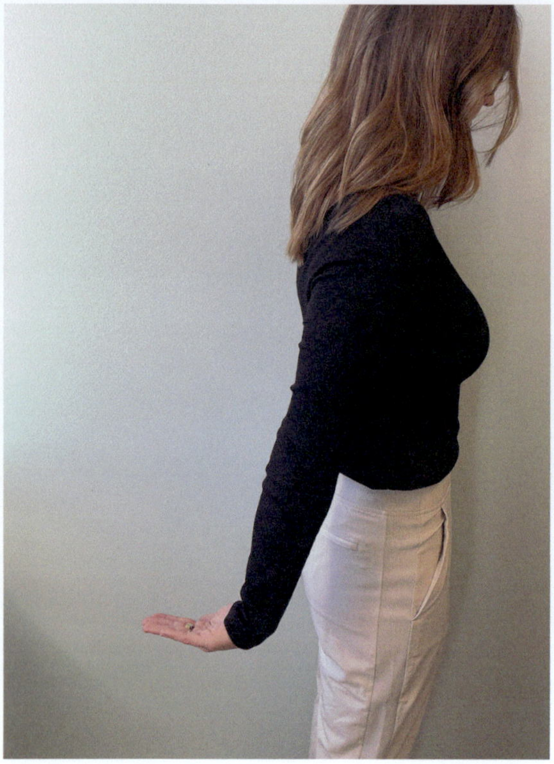

Image 2 Avoid tension to the radial nerve during the initial postoperative 3–6 weeks. This image demonstrates what NOT to do

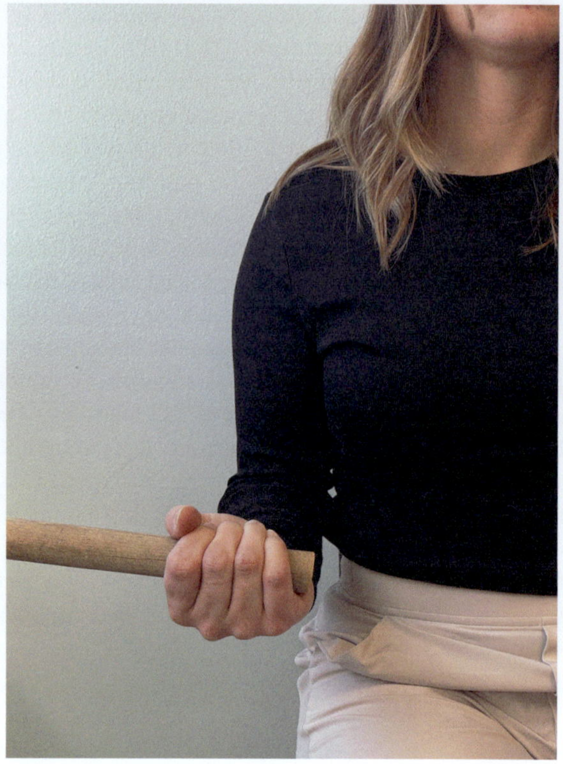

Image 3 Donor activation is performed hourly with active forearm supination

Realistic time frames for recovery should be clearly outlined to help patients set realistic expectations. Evidence of PIN reinnervation has been noted electrodiagnostically at 4 months post-operation, but active motion may not occur until 9 months after surgery [5]. The EDC is usually the first muscle to respond due to the close proximity of the transfer [8]. Bertelli and Ghizoni reported active extension of the fingers and thumb seen as early as 5 months following a brachial plexus injury [4]. Another study reported achieving MMT grade of 3/5 at 6–12 months after surgery [7].

Exercises

- ROM of Uninvolved Joints
  Patients are instructed to perform active range of motion of the uninvolved joints immediately following surgery. This includes shoulder flexion, abduction, and external rotation, as well as elbow ROM. As outlined above, patients should avoid full stretch into combined shoulder extension, elbow extension, pronation, and wrist flexion [8].
- Donor Activation
  The patient is instructed in the concept of "flooding the donor muscle" throughout the day. Donor activation is performed with active forearm supination or lightly resisted supination [4] (Image 3). Ten repetitions each hour throughout the day are recommended.
- Combined Donor with Passive Recipient Exercises
  At follow-up therapy visits, the patient is instructed to combine the donor and recipient muscle actions to encourage cortical plasticity by strengthening the new motor pathways. Exercise includes active (or resistive) supination with passive extension of the fingers and thumb. The passive portion of the exercise may be completed by the contralateral hand or using the underside of a table (Image 4).

Clinical Pearl
Due to lack of thumb extension, patients without PIN function often develop shortening of their thumb flexors and adductor. Attention should be given to stretching these muscles into extension and radial abduction with exercise or an orthosis.

Assessment of Recovery

Monitoring for reinnervation of the target muscles should occur at monthly therapy visits. The patient actively supinates the forearm while attempting to actively extend the fingers and thumb. The examiner provides resistance to the donor supinator while palpating for any contraction in the digital extensors, thumb extensors, or ECU (Image 5). All six dorsal wrist extensor compartments should be palpated as it

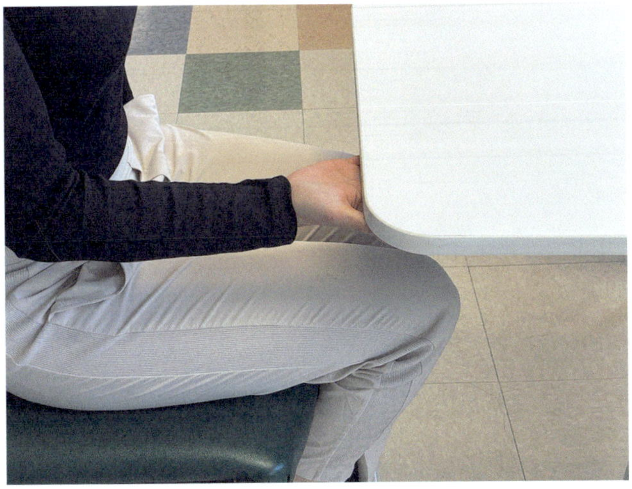

Image 4 Combined active donor with passive recipient exercise may be performed with the hand resting on the underside of a table and sliding it back and forth

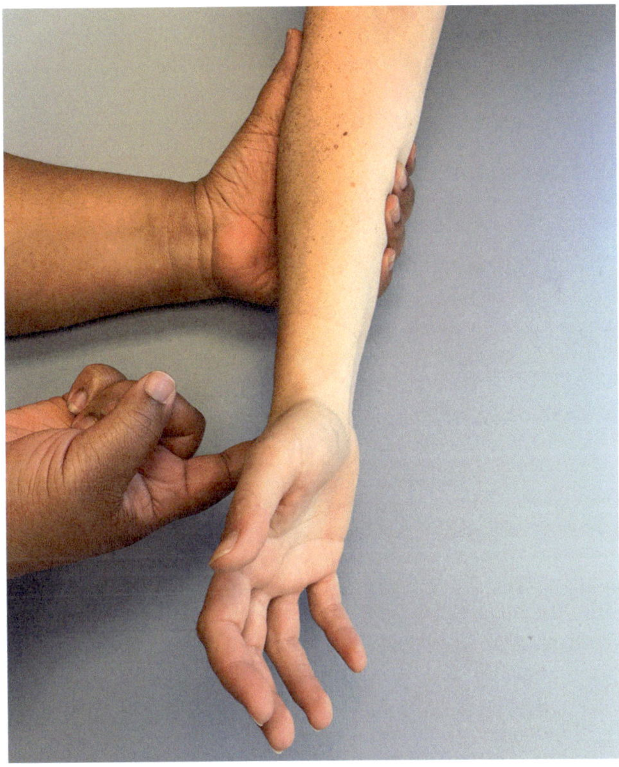

Image 5 Assessment of recovery is performed by resisting forearm supination while palpating along the dorsal wrist compartments to assess for recipient tension

is often easiest to palpate early tension at the tendon, and muscles do not always reinnervate in the pattern one would expect.

Therapy Frequency

The patient is first seen in therapy about 2 weeks after surgery for the initial evaluation. After this, the patient may attend therapy once every 2 weeks until they are able to demonstrate good carryover of recommendations and transfer training exercises. Therapy frequency may vary based on the patient's needs and distance required to travel to the clinic. Patients are seen more frequently if they have passive joint limitations, high pain levels, nerve hypersensitivity, excessive edema, and/or stiffness of uninvolved joints.

Phase 2

2−/5 to 3/5 MMT in the Recipient Muscles

Patients may progress to phase 2 of rehabilitation once they demonstrate some ECU function and/or active extension of the fingers and/or thumb. With so many recipient muscles, each with a different distance from the coaptation of nerve transfer, some muscles may advance to phase 2 before others. At this point in the recovery, the patient should be reliable with the home program and demonstrate a good understanding of the donor-recipient muscle relationship.

Phase 2 exercises advance from passive to active-assistive movement of the recipient muscles. With the forearm in neutral or supinated, resistance is applied in the direction of pronation with cues for a strong donor/supinator response. Forearm resistance is provided by the uninvolved hand, the side of a table, or a wall while simultaneously assisting the digits into MCPJ extension. It can be difficult to provide forearm resistance while assisting the digits. Using an object like a book or disc weight in the hand while resisting forearm supination may be helpful (Image 6). The therapist should cue to the patient not to flex the fingers into the book or disc but rather allow the help of the book or disc to stretch the fingers into extension and open the hand.

A custom-fabricated, hand-based thumb and MCPJ extension orthosis (a "P1 block") may be helpful for some patients to assist recipient extension during exercise [8]. A custom or prefabricated orthosis such as a Benik W711 or 701™ is encouraged during the day to enhance function as it supports the hand in an open position while enabling the hand to flex and grasp items (Image 7). This is not recommended for individuals who have concomitant weakness of the ulnar and median nerves, impairing hand function.

Clinical Pearl

For active-assistive ulnar wrist extension (ECU), the patient can place his or her palm against the underside of a table (in supination) while attempting to slide the hand into ulnar deviation with assist from the uninvolved hand. Additionally, he or she may hold a Frisbee and attempt to "cock it" ulnarly, in supination with assist of the opposite hand pulling the Frisbee.

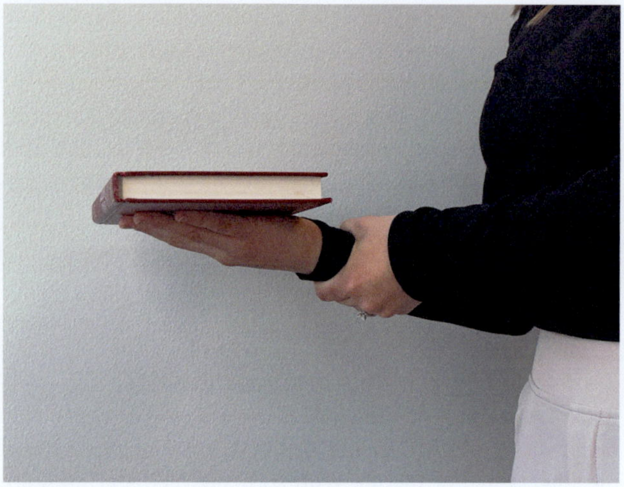

Image 6 A book or disc weight may be used to provide passive thumb and finger extension while manually resisting supination of the forearm

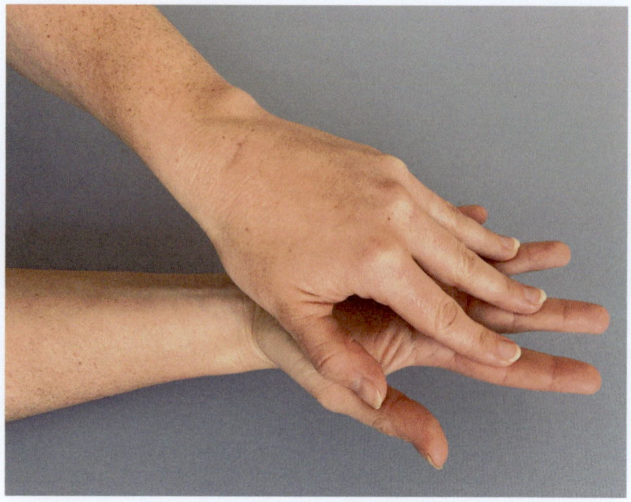

Image 8 Combined active donor supination with the uninvolved hand performing assisted recipient finger and thumb extension

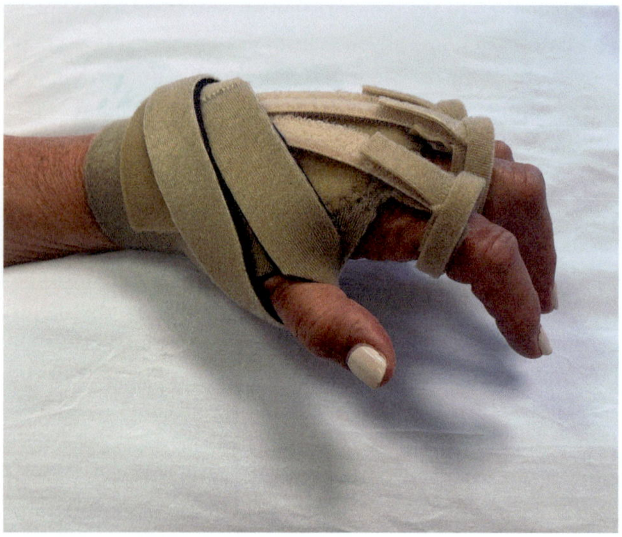

Image 7 A prefabricated orthosis such as the BENIK 701™ will enable the individual to reach and grasp objects without having to manually do so with the uninvolved hand by supporting the fingers and thumb in extension

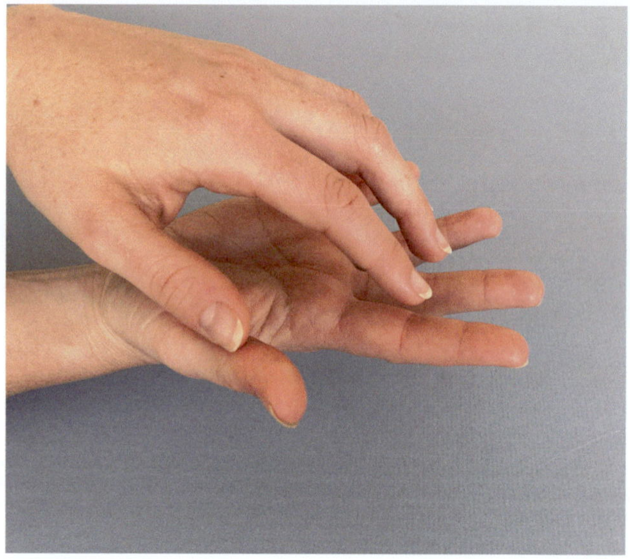

Image 9 The forearm actively supinates while the uninvolved hand places the thumb and fingers in extension and then releases them while cueing the patient to maintain the extended position

Exercises

- Active Donor with Active-Assisted Recipient
  Finger MCPJ and Thumb Extension MMT = 2−/5 to 2/5
  With the affected arm adducted to the side of the body and the elbow flexed to 90°, the patient supinates and attempts to open the hand fully while the contralateral hand assists finger and thumb extension and/or ulnar deviation of the wrist (Image 8). The arm of a chair or a rolled towel on a table may be used to resist forearm supination to increase donor activation and subsequent recipient muscle response.
- "Place and Hold" Exercise
  Finger MCPJ and Thumb Extension MMT = 2+/5
  Once the patient can actively extend the fingers and thumb (or ulnarly deviate and extend the wrist) through partial range of motion, a "place and hold" exercise may be initiated. The patient is instructed to use the opposite hand to position the thumb and fingers into end-range extension while actively supinating. The support to the fingers/thumb is then removed, and the patient is instructed to maintain the position (Image 9).
- Active Donor with Active Recipient
  Finger MCPJ and Thumb Extension MMT = 3−/5 to 3/5

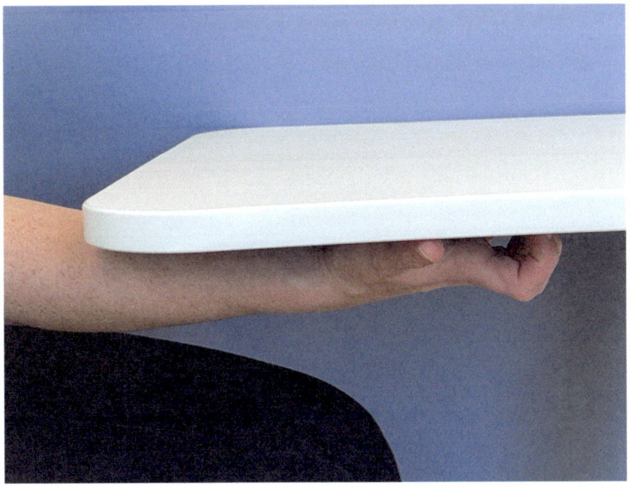

Image 10 The forearm is actively supinated while the patient is cued to "scratch" the undersurface of a table (hook fist) to actively pull into end-range finger MCPJ extension in the digits

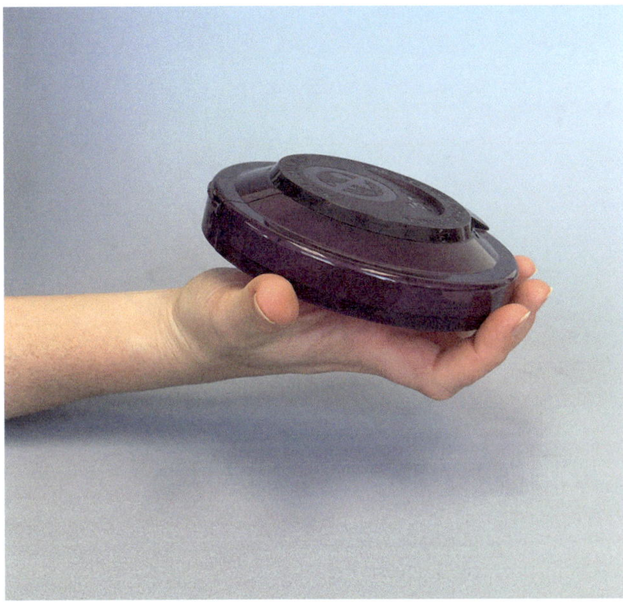

Image 11 A large jar lid may be used to promote intrinsic minus position with MCPJ extension while supinating the forearm

As recipient function improves and the patient can actively extend the fingers and thumb through more than 50% ROM against gravity, exercises advance to primarily active motion with continued co-contraction of the supinator. For example, the patient may "scratch" the undersurface of a table, pulling into a hook fist position while resisting the forearm with a twisting motion to promote a supinator contraction (Image 10). Using a flat object such as a jar lid or light disc, patients can attempt to hold this with their fingertips in intrinsic minus/hook fist while rotating the forearm into supination (Image 11).

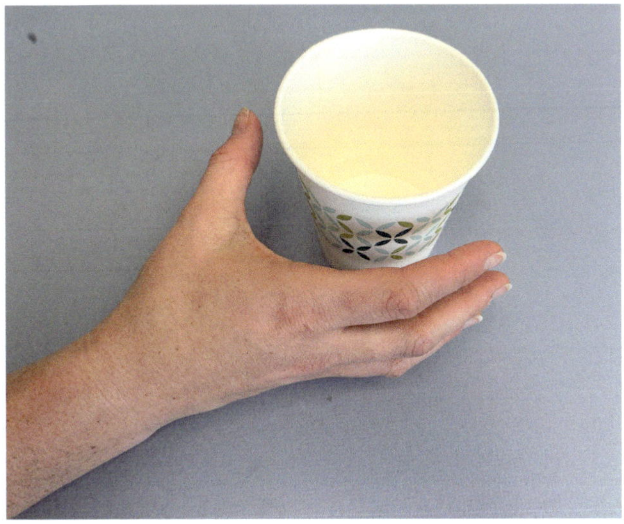

Image 12 Individuals are eventually encouraged to practice actively initiating supination while opening the hand to reach or place an object, such as a cup

- Functional Activity
  As extension of the fingers and thumb improves, the patient should volitionally incorporate this movement into functional tasks throughout the day. Examples of functional activities include extending the fingers and thumb to reach a cup or bottle from a table or placing items on a table, countertop, or shelf by releasing the object (goal of this transfer) (Image 12). Other activities include placing shampoo in the hand, taking change, tossing a ball into the air, flipping playing cards, shaking hands, and clapping. Bilateral activity may also improve motor learning (Image 13).
- Therapy Frequency
  Therapy visits in phase 2 may occur on a weekly, bimonthly, or monthly basis, depending on the patient's needs.

Phase 3

3+/5 MMT in the Recipient Muscle

Phase 3 begins once the thumb, fingers, and wrist (with ulnar deviation) can fully extend and withstand light resistance. It is important that resistive exercises are not initiated before 3/5 MMT strength is obtained as this often leads to fatigue, frustration, substitution, and ineffective recruitment of the target muscles. To prevent fatigue, short bouts of exercise with low resistance are encouraged throughout the day. As recipient muscle strength increases, exercises may slowly exclude the assistive action of the supinator. Remember that by powering the supinator, the patient will typically be able to produce a stronger contraction of the extensor muscles of

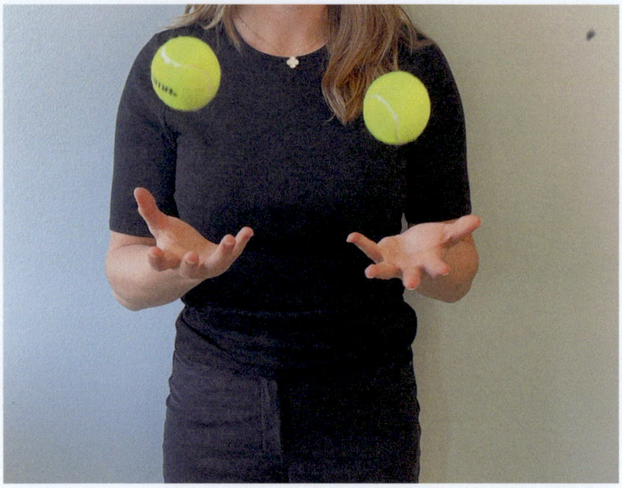

Image 13 Tossing a ball in the air (with the involved only or bilaterally to enhance motor learning) combines active supination with finger and thumb extension

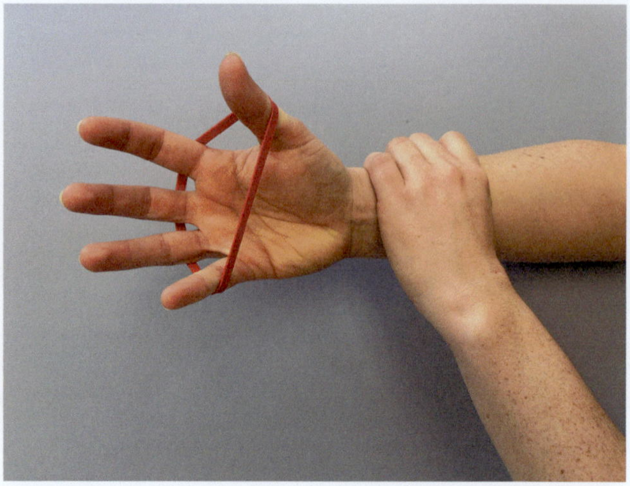

Image 14 Phase 3 resistance is added to the recipient finger and thumb extensor muscles with a rubber band while the forearm is supinated

the fingers and thumb. This may be problematic for some as it may cause unexpected hand opening when they are firmly supinating. Practicing without supination should aid with overcoming this.

This transfer is very synergistic and easy for patients to learn and recover function. When multiple transfers are performed simultaneously, this one may take the least intervention for the individual to demonstrate success.

Exercises

- Resistive Recipient Activity with Donor Contraction
  Resistance may be provided with the contralateral hand, rubber bands, resistance bands, therapy putty, or a Power Web™. A rubber band is placed around the digits as the patient is instructed to supinate the forearm while extending the fingers (Image 14). Additionally, the patient may hold a table tennis racquet and supinate while extending and ulnarly deviating the wrist to strengthen the ECU. This can be advanced by pushing the racquet edge into therapy putty in a supinated, ulnarly deviated direction (Image 15). Contracting the supinator muscle will augment the power of the PIN muscles, which may be functionally useful in situations where this is needed.
- Resistive Recipient Activity Without Donor Contraction
  Once patients demonstrate consistent finger and thumb extensor control, they may learn to de-emphasize the involvement of the supinator. For example, therapy putty is used with the fingertips embedded and the hand on a table in forearm pronation. The patient is cued to push the putty by extending the fingers through it. There are many activities of daily living that involve finger/thumb extension with the forearm in a pronated position. Some examples include wiping a table/wall, typing, and lifting small cans from the top with the fingertips (Image 16).

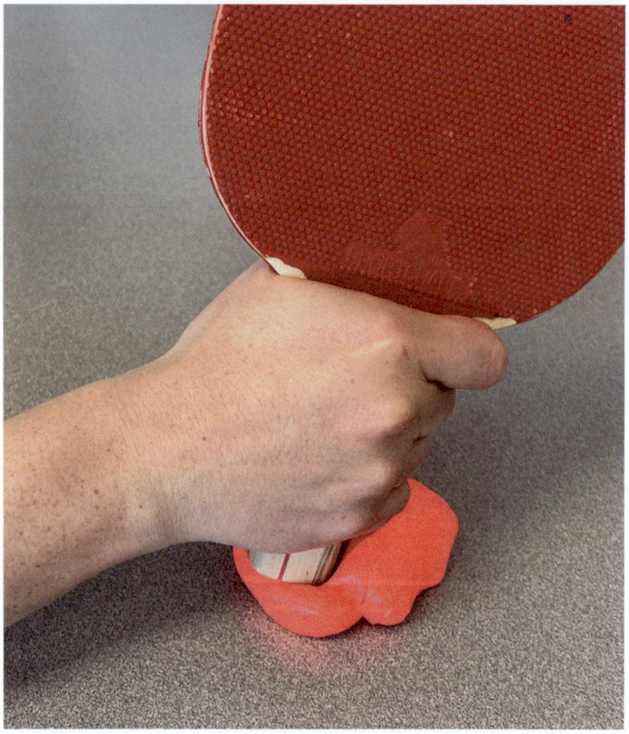

Image 15 ECU strengthening can be performed with active supination by holding a table tennis racquet and pushing it into putty in the direction of ulnar deviation with wrist extension

- Therapy Frequency
  Once a 3+/5 MMT grade is achieved, some individuals may benefit from bimonthly therapy visits. Exercises are reviewed and advanced as appropriate, depending on the strength and coordination of the thumb and finger extensors and the functional needs of the patient. Duration of visits will depend on patient goals, insurance availability, and ability to show functional gains with therapy.

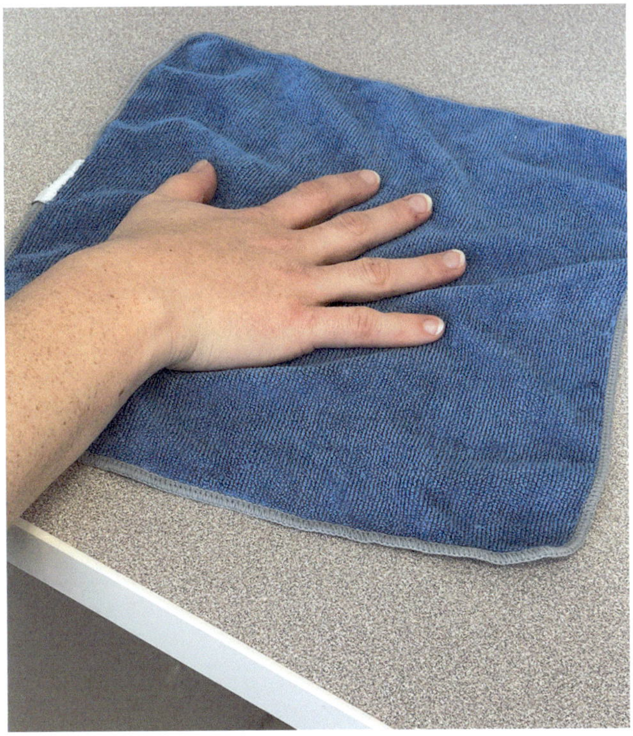

Image 16 Many ADL are performed in pronation and require thumb and finger extension such as wiping a table with a cloth. This will aid in de-emphasizing the supinator from the recipient muscles

Supinator to PIN nerve transfer

Nerve transfer overview					
Donor nerve	Donor action	Recipient nerve	Recipient action	Indications for functional restoration	Approximate months to functional movement
Supinator branch of the radial nerve	Forearm supination	Posterior interosseous nerve (PIN)	Finger MCPJ extension and thumb extension	Restore ability to open the hand for functional grasp	5–9 months [5, 6]

Information below is suggested guidelines. Precautions may vary according to surgeon preferences and patient factors

	Preoperative therapy	Early phase	Middle phase	Late phase
Criteria	Before surgery	0/5 to −1/5 MMT	2−/5 to 3/5 MMT	>3/5 MMT
Purpose of phase	Educate and establish baseline function	Understand the donor-recipient relationship Activate donor: forearm supination	Activate nerve transfer for light functional activities requiring hand-opening	Strengthen recipient muscles with resistance Separate from donor activation
Precautions	NA	No wrist ROM for the first 2 weeks Avoid stress to the nerve coaptation site for 3–6 weeks by avoiding combined shoulder external rotation, elbow extension, pronation, and wrist flexion [8]	Avoid high-intensity exercise Minimize fatigue and force placed on the weak EDC, EPL, and ECU	Resistive exercise should not be performed before the PIN demonstrates 3/5 MMT Avoid fatigue with resistance training
Frequency of visits (considerations)	1–2 visits; more if PROM limitations are present	1×/week until PROM is restored and patient is independent with HEP and then decrease to 1×/month based on patient needs	1–2×/month If additional nerve transfers and/or tendon transfers were performed, more frequent therapy is warranted	1–2×/month depending on the patient's needs

(continued)

	Preoperative therapy	Early phase	Middle phase	Late phase
Criteria	Before surgery	0/5 to −1/5 MMT	2−/5 to 3/5 MMT	>3/5 MMT
Orthosis considerations	Hand-based radial nerve palsy orthosis: either custom thermoplastic or BENIK™ W-701 if finger flexors are intact The purpose of this is to facilitate finger extension, allow for functional grasp/flexion, and limit overlengthening of the PIN muscles If significant tightness of the extrinsic flexors is present, a static P1 block is recommended at night to maintain finger MCP joint and thumb extension range	Custom or prefabricated wrist orthosis for 2 weeks to protect the nerve coaptation Some surgeons may prefer to have the finger MCP joints in extension and thumb in extension to prevent drag on the PIN A functional, hand-based radial nerve palsy orthosis may be resumed after 2 weeks if flexor function is intact	Hand-based MCPJ extension orthosis (P1 block) during heavy activity to limit fatigue in the recovering muscles	No orthosis unless the PIN muscles fatigue easily
Interventions	Education Maintenance of joint PROM	**Donor activation**: Forearm supination (isometric, active, and/or resisted) 10× every hour **Donor-recipient pairing**: Active supination with passive finger MCP extension and thumb composite extension 10–20 reps, 6–8×/day	**Active/resisted donor with active assist recipient**: Passive progresses to active-assisted finger and thumb extension (with active and/or resisted supination) **Place and hold**: Place fingers and thumb in composite extension. Remove the support and maintain this position (while supinated)	**Resisted donor and recipient**: Resisted finger and thumb extension while supinated. Resistance may include therapy putty, rubber bands, or isometric pressure from the opposite hand **Resisted recipient without donor contraction**: Resisted finger and thumb extension while maintaining a pronated or forearm neutral position
Additional intervention considerations		"Scratch" the underside of a table in supination to obtain a hook fist position with MCP joints in extension and IP joints in flexion	Respect fatigue	Begin with low resistance and advance gradually as tolerated

During all phases, it is essential to continue cortical reorganization, psychological and psychosocial interventions, and progress to incorporate donor/recipient with ADL

Supinator to PIN Nerve Transfer

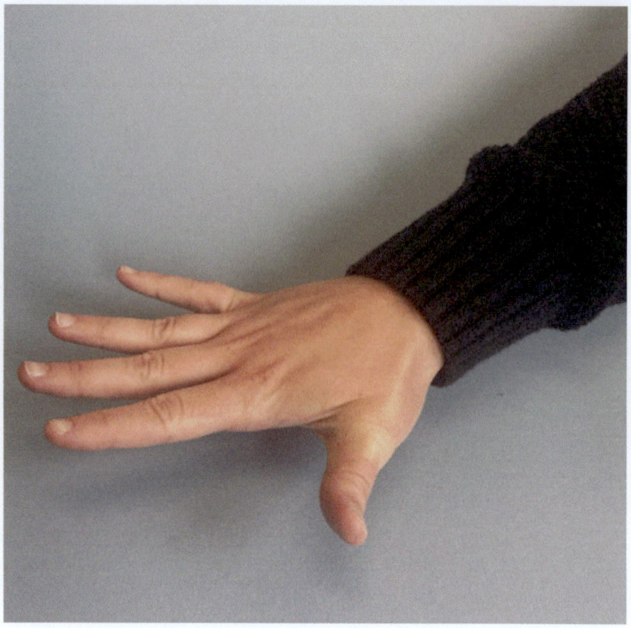

Goal of Surgery: Restore the ability to open the hand to grasp and release objects

Recipient Movement = Lift the Fingers and Thumb Up (Finger and Thumb Extension)

Primary Recipient Muscles: Extensor Digitorum Communis (EDC) & Extensor Pollicis Longus (EPL)

Secondary Recipient Muscle: Extensor Carpi Ulnaris (ECU)

Recipient Nerve: Posterior Interosseous Nerve (PIN)

Donor Movement = Rotate the Forearm Facing Up (Supination)

Donor Muscle: Supinator

Donor Nerve: Supinator Branch of the Radial Nerve

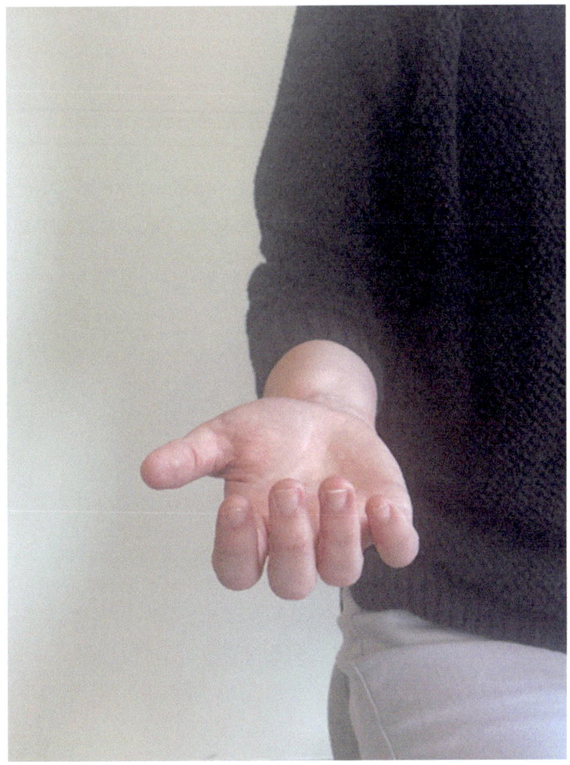

Phase 1 Supinator to PIN Nerve Transfer Exercises

☐ **Active or Resisted Donor Movement**:

- With your elbow resting by your side, rotate the forearm so that your palm is facing up. Rotate the forearm back to a palm-down position, and repeat.

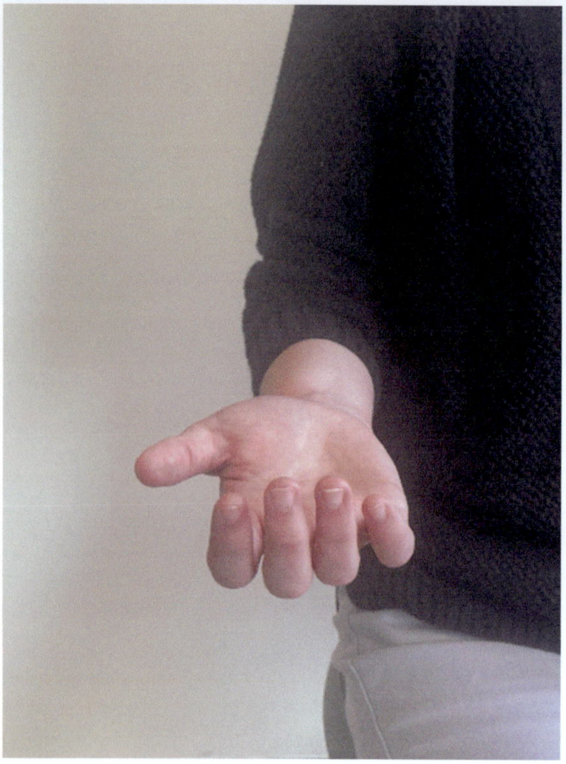

Complete 10 repetitions, every waking hour

- You may also resist forearm rotation (donor movement) isometrically for added challenge.
  - Rotate your forearm into a palm-**up** position while you use your opposite hand to try and rotate the forearm into a palm-**down** position. Hold for 5–10 seconds.

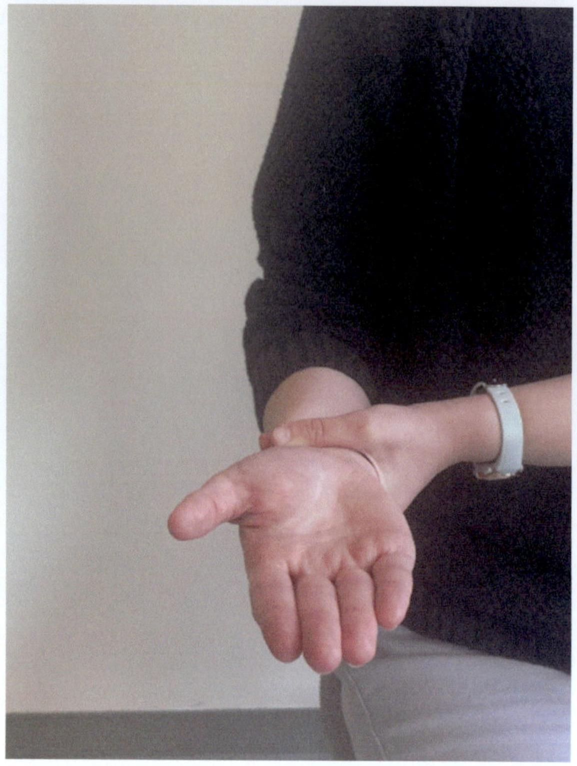

  - With the elbow by your side, hold a lightweight hammer or similar object and slowly rotate it from a palm-down position to a palm-up position.

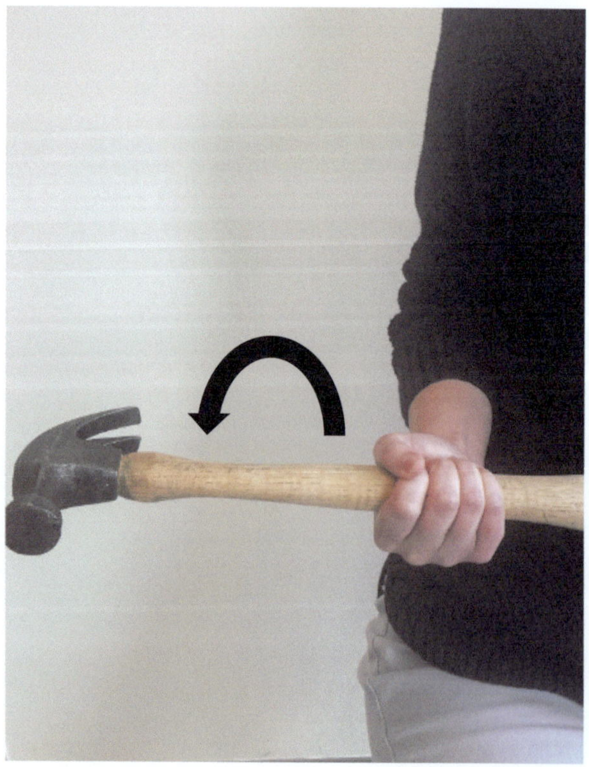

Hold for 3–5 seconds and complete 10 repetitions, 6 times per day

☐ **Combined Donor with Passive Recipient Movement**:

Complete one of the below exercises 10 repetitions, 3 times per day.

- Begin with your elbow by your side and forearm facing down. Rotate the forearm palm-up, and then use your opposite hand to push the fingers into an open or extended position.

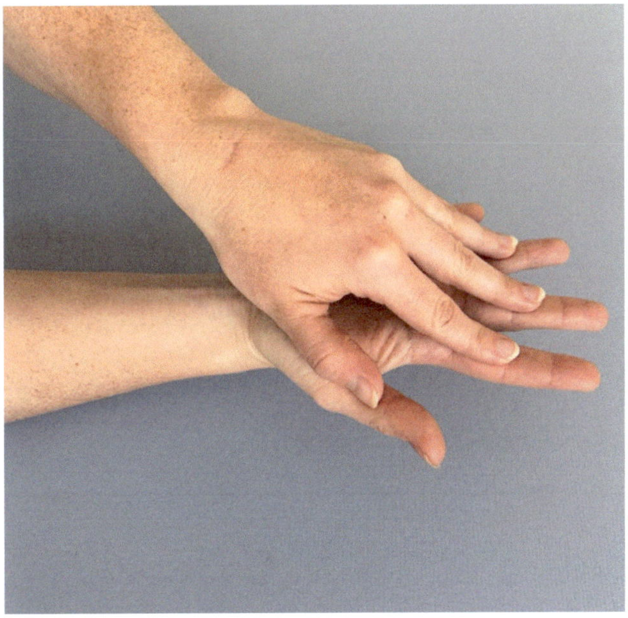

- Begin with your elbow by your side and forearm facing down. Rotate the forearm palm-up, and then use a dowel to roll the fingers into an open or extended position.

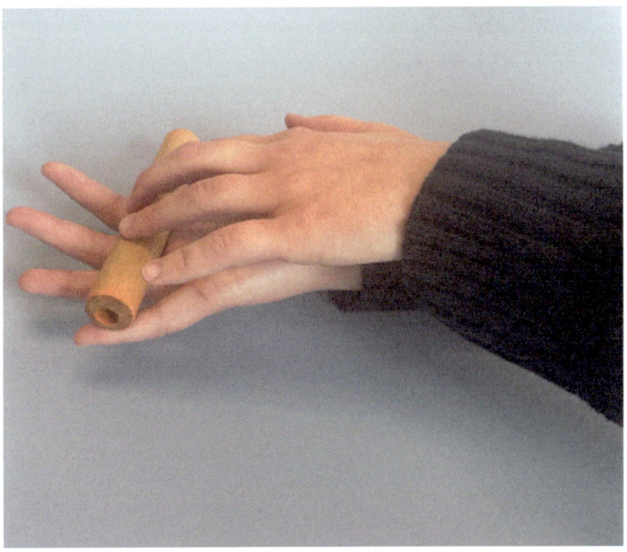

- Sit in front of table with your elbow by your side and forearm facing down. Rotate the forearm palm-up, and use the underside of the table to stretch the fingers open.

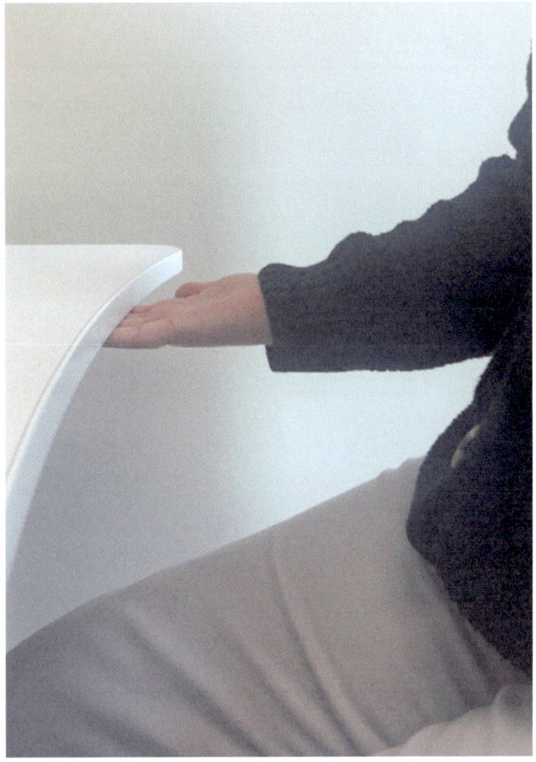

Complete 10 repetitions, 3 times per day.

Phase 2 Supinator to PIN Nerve Transfer Exercises

☐ **Active Donor + Active-Assisted Recipient Movement**:

- Begin with your elbow by your side and forearm facing down. Rotate the forearm palm-up, and try to independently open your fingers as much as you can. Then, assist the fingers open into maximum extension using your other hand.

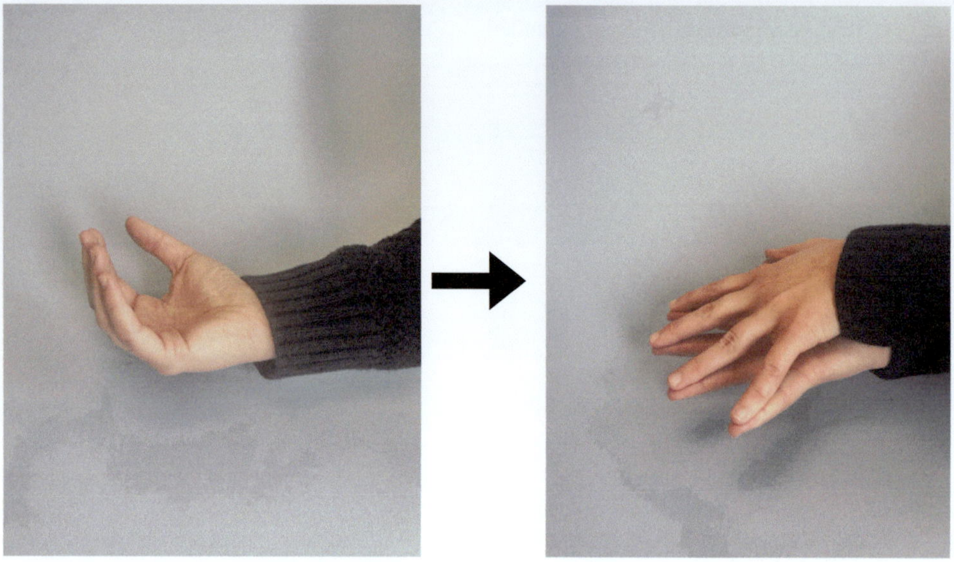

- Sit with your hand underneath a table top with your palm facing up. Lightly "scratch" underneath the table into a "hook" fist. The knuckles at the base of the fingers should stay straight while the tips of the fingers should bend.

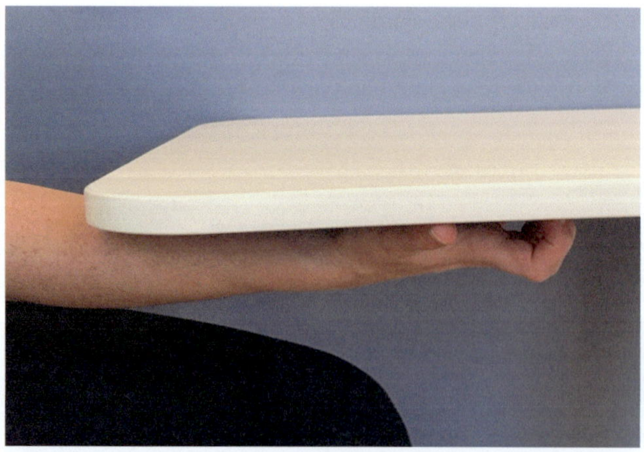

Complete 10 repetitions, 3 times per day.

☐ **Place and Hold Exercises**:

- With the forearm facing palm-up, use your other hand to stretch the fingers into an open or straight position. Then, slowly release the support from your other hand, and try to maintain your fingers in this open position.

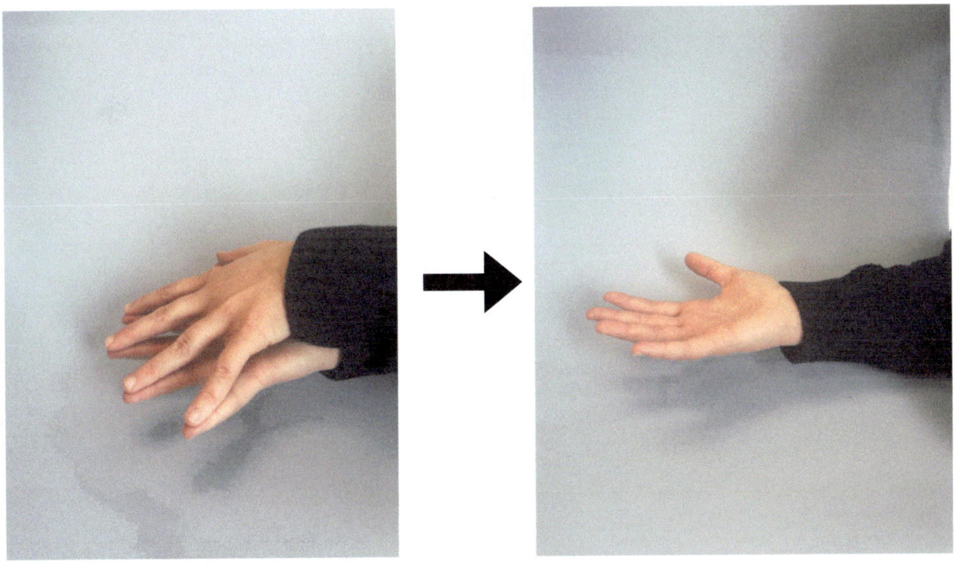

Complete 10 repetitions, 3 times per day.

☐ **Active Donor + Active Recipient Movement**:

- Start with your forearm facing down and your elbow by your side. Twist your forearm palm-up, and open your fingers as if you are trying to catch something or receive change.

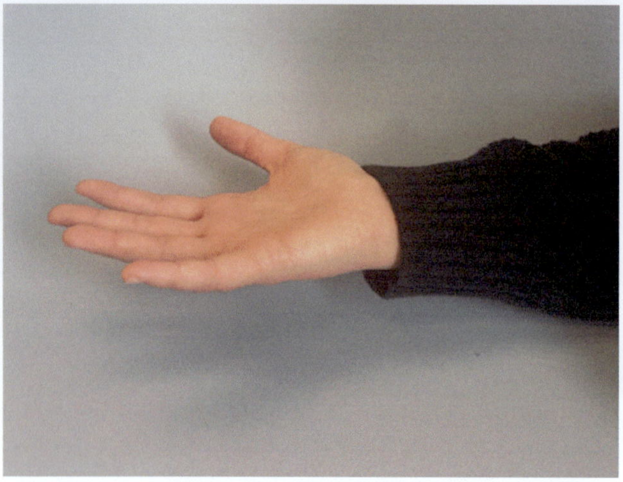

- Place a large jar lid (or something similar) in the hand with your fingertips curled at the edge. Keep this in your hand as you rotate the palm facing up.

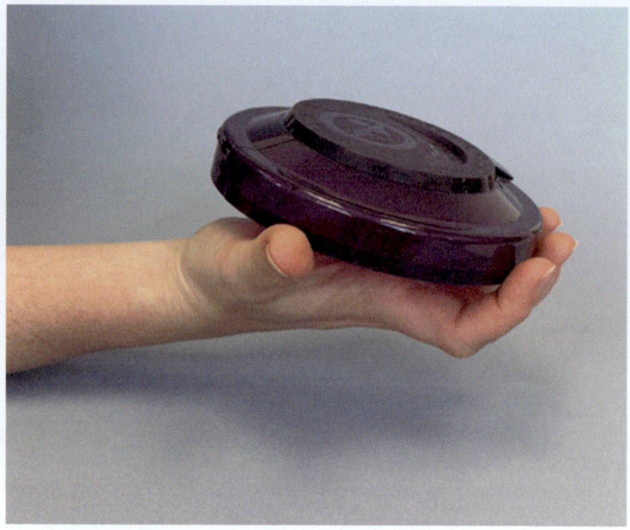

Complete 10 repetitions, 3 times per day.

Phase 3 Supinator to PIN Nerve Transfer Exercises

☐ **Resisted Recipient with Donor Contraction**:

- Start in a palm-up position. Place a rubber band around the base of the fingers and thumb. Open the fingers and thumb against the resistance of the rubber band, and hold for 3–5 seconds.

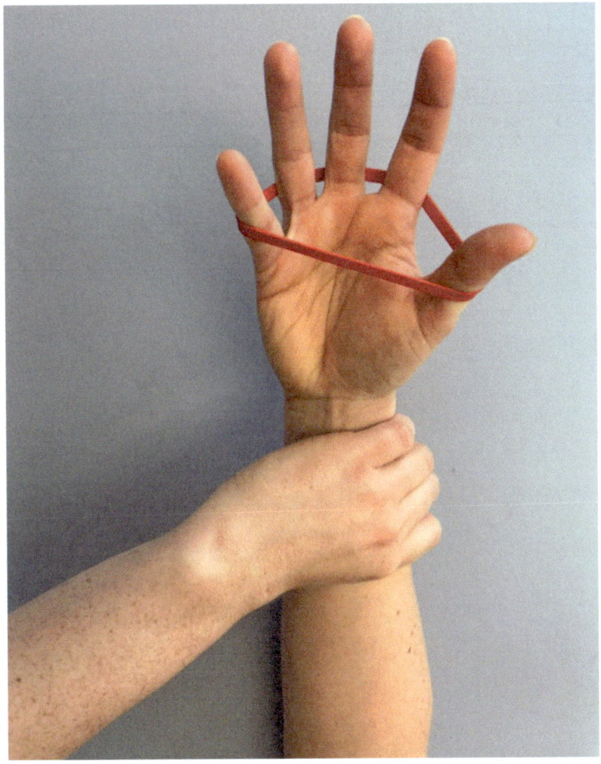

Complete 10 repetitions, 3 times per day.

☐ **Resisted Recipient Without Donor Contraction**:

- Start in a palm-down position. Shape therapy putty into a disc, and place around the fingers. Open the fingers and thumb against the resistance of the putty.

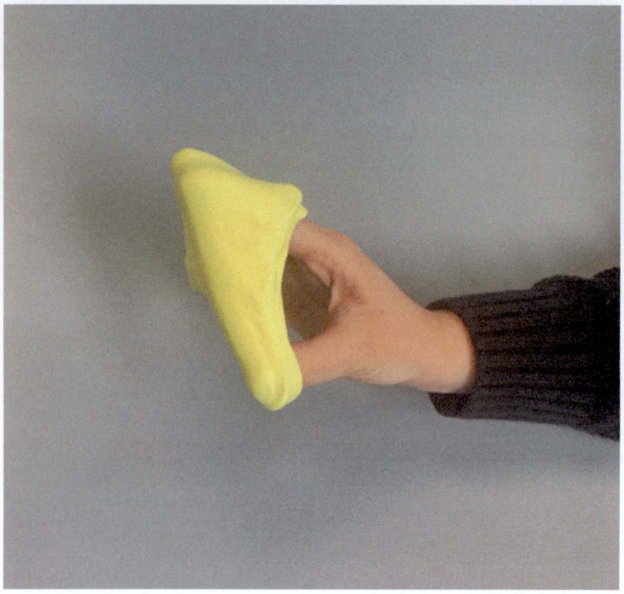

- You may also flatten the putty onto a table. Start with the fingers flexed, and open the fingers against the resistance of the putty.

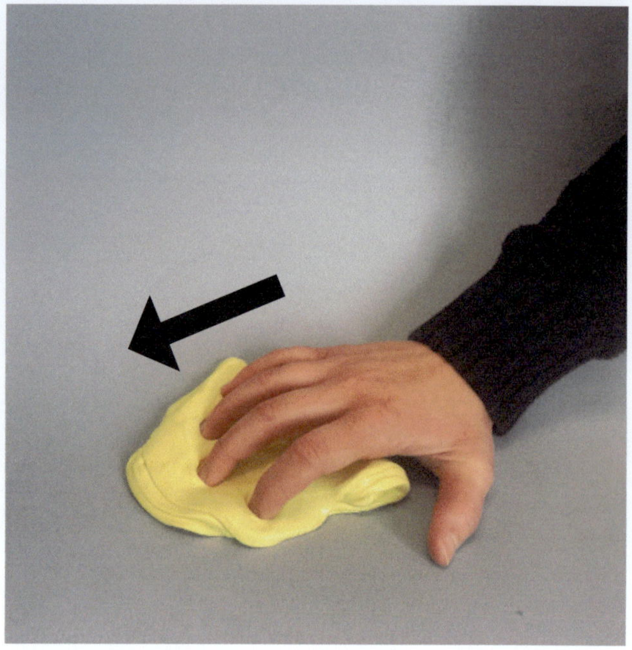

Complete 10 repetitions, hold for 3–5 seconds, 3 times per day

References

1. Sigamoney KV, Rashid A, Ng CY. Management of atraumatic posterior interosseous nerve palsy. J Hand Surg Am. 2017;42(10):826–30.
2. MacKenzie A. Restoration of function after adult brachial plexus injury. In: Osterman AL, Skirven TM, Fedorczyk JM, Amadio PC, Feldscher SB, Shin EK, editors. Rehabilitation of the hand and upper extremity. 7th ed. Elsevier Mosby; 2020.
3. Caetano EB, Vieira LA, Sabongi Neto JJ, Caetano MF, Sabongi RG, Pacileo Cruz BA. Anatomical study of innervation of the supinator muscle to reinnervate the posterior interosseous nerve. Braz J Orthop Surg. 2019;54:253–60.
4. Bertelli JA, Ghizoni MF. Transfer of supinator motor branches to the posterior interosseous nerve in C7-T1 brachial plexus palsy. J Neurosurg. 2010;113:129–32.
5. Bazarek S, Sten M, Nin D, J.M. B. Supinator to posterior interosseous nerve transfer for restoration of finger extension. Oper Neurosurg. 2021;21:408–13.
6. Bertelli JA, Tacca CP, Ghizoni MF, Kechele PR, Santos MA. Transfer of supinator motor branches to the posterior interosseous nerve to reconstruct thumb and finger extension in tetraplegia: a case report. J Hand Surg. 2010;35A:1647–51.
7. Souza FH, Bernardino SN, Cezar AB Jr, et al. Nerve transfers for functional hand recovery in traumatic lower brachial plexopathy. Surg Neurol Int. 2020;11:358.
8. Hahn J, Cooper C, Flood S, Weymouth M, van Zyl N. Rehabilitation of supinator nerve to posterior interosseous nerve transfer in individuals with tetraplegia. Arch Phys Med Rehabil. 2016;96(6):S160–8.
9. van Zyl N, Galea MP, Cooper C, Hahn J, Hill B. Transfer of the supinator nerve to the posterior interosseous nerve for hand opening in tetraplegia through an anterior approach. J Hand Surg Eur Vol. 2021;46(7):717–24.
10. Xu B, Dong Z, Zhang CG, Gu YD. Clinical outcome following transfer of the supinator motor branch to the posterior interosseous nerve in patients with C7–T1 brachial plexus palsy. J Reconstr Microsurg. 2015;31(2):102–6.
11. Dong Z, Gu YD, Zhang CG, Zhang L. Clinical use of supinator motor branch transfer to the posterior interosseous nerve in C7–T1 brachial plexus palsies. Journal of neurosurgery. J Neurosurg. 2010;113(1):113–7.
12. Zhang CG, Dong Z, Gu YD. Restoration of hand function in C7–T1 brachial plexus palsies using a staged approach with nerve and tendon transfer: report of 2 cases. J Neurosurg. 2014;121(5):1264–70.
13. Khalifeh JM, Dibble CF, Van Voorhis A, et al. Nerve transfers in the upper extremity following cervical spinal cord injury. Part 1: systematic review of the literature. J Neurosurg Spine. 2019;31(5):629–40.
14. Khalifeh JM, Dibble CF, Van Voorhis A, et al. Nerve transfers in the upper extremity following cervical spinal cord injury. Part 2: preliminary results of a prospective clinical trial. J Neurosurg Spine. 2019;31(5):641–53.
15. Kahn L, Moore A. Donor activation focused rehabilitation approach: maximizing outcomes after nerve transfers. Hand Clin. 2016;32(2):263–77.

Anterior Interosseous Nerve (AIN) Branch of the Pronator Quadratus to the Posterior Interosseous Nerve (PIN) Transfer

Amy M. Young

Anterior Interosseous Nerve (AIN) (Pronator Quadratus/PQ Branch) to the Distal Posterior Interosseous Nerve (PIN) Transfer

Background

The posterior interosseous nerve (PIN) is a motor branch of the radial nerve that innervates the extensor carpi ulnaris (ECU), extensor digitorum communis (EDC), extensor digiti minimi (EDM), abductor pollicis longus (APL), extensor pollicis longus (EPL), extensor pollicis brevis (EPB), and extensor indicis proprius (EIP) [1]. A PIN deficit limits one's ability to extend the fingers and thumb. Technically, the PIN muscles are responsible for MCP joint extension in the fingers and contribute to some IP joint extension through the dorsal hood mechanism, in addition to composite extension at the thumb. When a PIN deficit is present, dominant radial-directed wrist extension is also noted due to ECU weakness and preserved ECRL function [1]. The goal of the AIN-to-PQ-to-PIN nerve transfer is to restore the ability to open the hand for functional grasp and dexterity. Although the well-known FCR-to-PIN transfer is universally recognized as the gold standard to reinnervate all of the PIN-innervated muscles [2], this transfer often leads to disappointing outcomes for thumb extension power given that its main role is to reinnervate *proximal* PIN function. The literature describes two situations for the use of the AIN-to-PIN transfer. In one scenario, the AIN to PQ is transferred to the proximal portion of the PIN in an attempt to recover all PIN muscle function. More often, however, it is used to augment a second nerve transfer by transferring AIN to PQ to the distal branch of the PIN (DBPIN), which innervates EPL, EPB, APL, and EIP to recover better thumb function. The AIN-to-DBPIN nerve transfer has been described using the most distal aspect of the AIN to primarily restore thumb function, i.e., a more *distal* PIN injury. Additionally, the classic FCR-to-PIN nerve transfer may not be feasible in cases where the FCR branch is not long enough to reach the distal PIN target.

Outcomes

Fairley and Daneshvar detail a case report of AIN-to-PIN nerve transfer for a patient with PIN palsy after undergoing repair of the distal biceps brachii tendon [3]. The authors chose AIN-to-PIN transfer versus FCR to PIN due to the distal nature of the injury and resultant nerve gap of greater than 5 cm. One year and 6 months after transfer, the patient demonstrated what the authors describe as "full" thumb extension and "full" thumb strength. A 20-degree MCP joint extensor lag was noted at the index finger with "almost full strength" and 30-degree MCP joint extensor lag at middle through small fingers with "moderate strength." A more central line of pull was observed into wrist extension through reinnervation of the ECU.

Bertelli completed a prospective study of 29 patients with radial nerve palsy or brachial plexus injury to the posterior cord who underwent either nerve or tendon transfers [4]. At an average follow-up of 26 months post-surgery, 13 of 14 patients who underwent FCR-to-PIN and AIN-to-ECRB

A. M. Young (✉)
Northwestern Medicine Center for Surgery of the Hand, Chicago, IL, USA
e-mail: Amy.Young@nm.org

L. C. Kahn et al. (eds.), *Rehabilitation for Nerve Transfers of the Upper Extremity*,
https://doi.org/10.1007/978-3-031-92008-0_20

nerve transfers demonstrated a 30-degree MCP joint extensor lag at the thumb. Due to the recurrent outcome of thumb MCP joint extensor lag, Bertelli et al. proposed the addition of AIN to PQ to the DBPIN transfer for thumb extension in combination with FCR-to-PIN and PT-to-ECRB nerve transfers for high radial nerve impairment [5]. A cohort of five patients was studied. Two of five patients (40%) demonstrated no extensor lag at the thumb MCP joint, and three patients demonstrated a 15- to 20-degree thumb MCP joint extensor lag at follow-up, ranging from 7 to 29 months postoperatively. All patients achieved independent control of thumb and finger extension, and forearm pronation was preserved. No mention of index finger extension in isolation (EIP) was noted.

Surgical Graphic

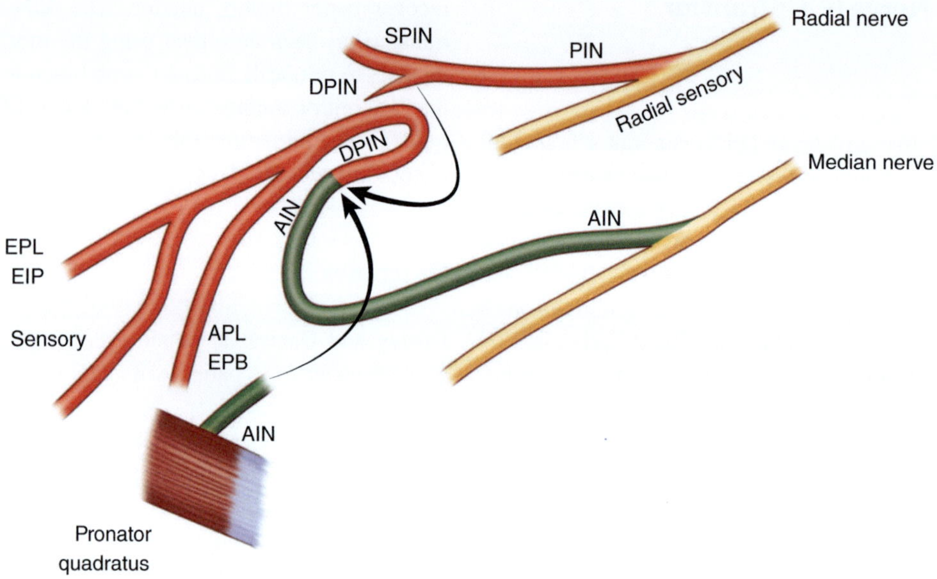

Microsurgical technique of Anterior Interosseous Nerve (Ain) Branch of the Pronator Quadratus to the Posterior Interosseous Nerve (Pin) Transfer

A longitudinal incision is made along the dorsal aspect of the proximal forearm, along the posterior border of the brachioradialis muscle. The PIN is identified, and a thorough decompression of the radial tunnel is performed. At the distal aspect of the released supinator, the deep branch of the PIN is identified. A handheld nerve stimulator is used to confirm the absence of function when stimulating the deep branch of the PIN, ensuring that the anesthesia team is not using muscle paralytics. This stimulation must be performed within 30 min of the tourniquet being inflated if one is being used. The surgeon then works distally and opens the interosseous membrane at the juncture of the middle and distal thirds of the forearm. The anterior interosseous nerve is identified through the window in the interosseous membrane and freed from the surrounding tissue including the pronator quadratus muscle. A handheld nerve stimulator is used to confirm function of the AIN, ensuring that only the PQ responds and that there is no thumb IP flexion or finger DIP flexion with stimulation. This stimulation must also be performed within 30 min of the tourniquet being inflated, if one is being used. If the surgeon prefers, a separate incision on the volar forearm can be used to facilitate identification and mobilization of the AIN. From either approach, the AIN is divided distally and transposed to meet the recipient deep branch of the PIN. Coaptation of the AIN/PQ branch to the PIN is performed using microsurgical technique.

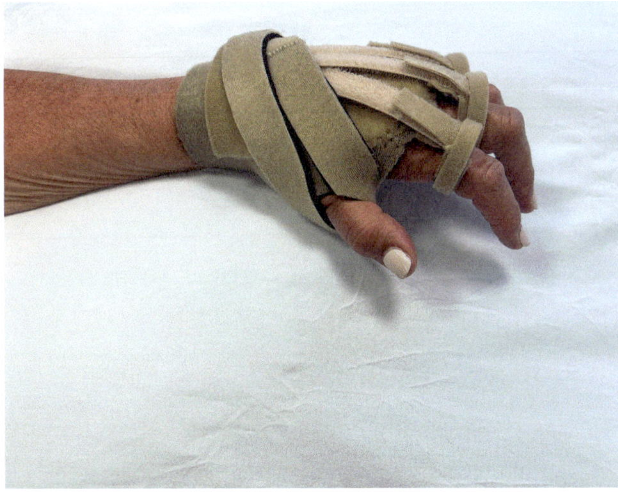

Image 1 Individuals with an isolated PIN palsy would benefit from a hand-based orthosis such as the BENIK™ 701 for functional extension support

Phases of Rehabilitation

Phase 1

Preoperative to 1/5 MMT

Precautions

Patients should avoid prolonged positioning in composite finger flexion and composite thumb flexion, which can promote flexor tightness and overlengthening of the extensor musculature. According to the length-tension relationship of muscle, overlengthening may contribute to biomechanical failure of the muscle to produce desired movement and strength once reinnervation of the recipient muscles occurs [6–8]. A general rule to follow is to preserve recipient muscle length whenever possible.

Orthoses

For isolated PIN injury, the patient may be fit with a prefabricated BENIK™ hand-based finger and thumb extension orthosis (Image 1) or a similar custom orthosis to preserve muscle length and promote hand opening function. For high radial nerve injury, the patient may be fit with a prefabricated BENIK™ forearm-based finger and thumb extension orthosis (Image 2) or a similar custom orthosis due to the additional loss of wrist extension.

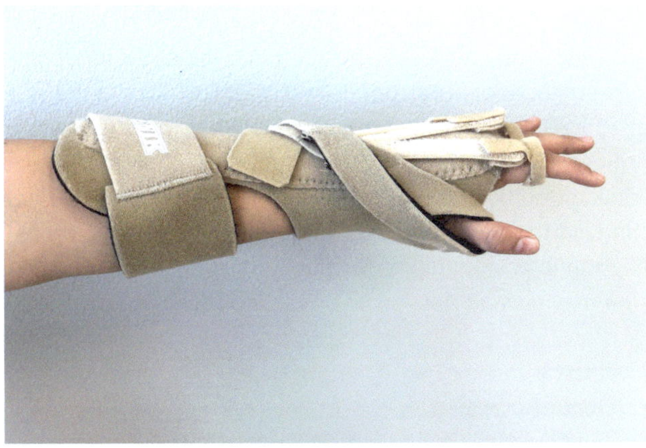

Image 2 A forearm-based prefabricated BENIK™ 711 is recommended for individuals with a radial nerve palsy involving the wrist for functional support to both wrist and finger extension

At 10–14 days post-surgery, the postoperative dressings are removed in the surgery clinic. A protective postoperative orthosis is not always necessary as there is typically no tension across the nerve coaptation [5]. However, a custom volar, forearm-based orthosis with finger MCP joints in extension, IP joints free, thumb MCP/IP joints in extension, and CMC joint in abduction may be fabricated to wear for protection if the surgeon prefers [9] (Image 3). Patients may choose to resume the use of the BENIK™ orthosis (appropriate to the level of injury) following the initial postoperative period (2–3 weeks) to promote functional use and preserve muscle length while awaiting recipient muscle reinnervation.

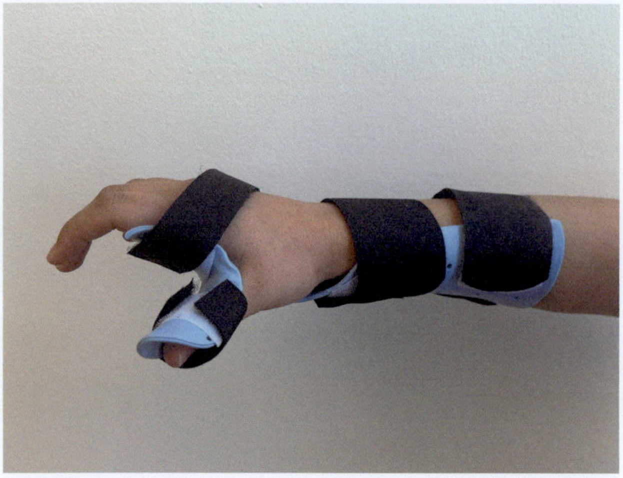

Image 3 A custom forearm-based orthosis that supports the finger MCP joints and thumb in extension with the wrist (in 20–30 degrees of extension) is useful for protection in the first few weeks postoperatively. It may also be used after this at night to maintain soft tissue length while awaiting recipient nerve function

Some individuals may benefit from the abovementioned custom thermoplastic orthosis at night if their PROM is insufficient or if they are not compliant with the daytime orthosis. The unopposed action of the ulnar innervated adductor pollicis and flexor pollicis brevis for pinch function can lead to loss of first web space range of motion (ROM). Nighttime positioning of the thumb in abduction and extension may prevent this.

Exercises

- Donor Activation
  Ten to twelve days following surgery, the patient may initiate donor PQ exercise with active and isometric forearm pronation. Early-phase donor activation exercises are completed with high repetitions and high frequency to maximize neural signals to the donor muscle and promote cortical plasticity [9, 10].
- Combined Donor with Passive Recipient Exercise
  Active forearm pronation should be paired with simultaneous passive finger MCP joint extension and thumb extension (Image 4).

Clinical Pearl

The patient may place a hand on a medium-sized ball and rotate the forearm into pronation against the ball (resisting the donor PQ) while the ball supports the thumb and fingers in extension (Image 5).

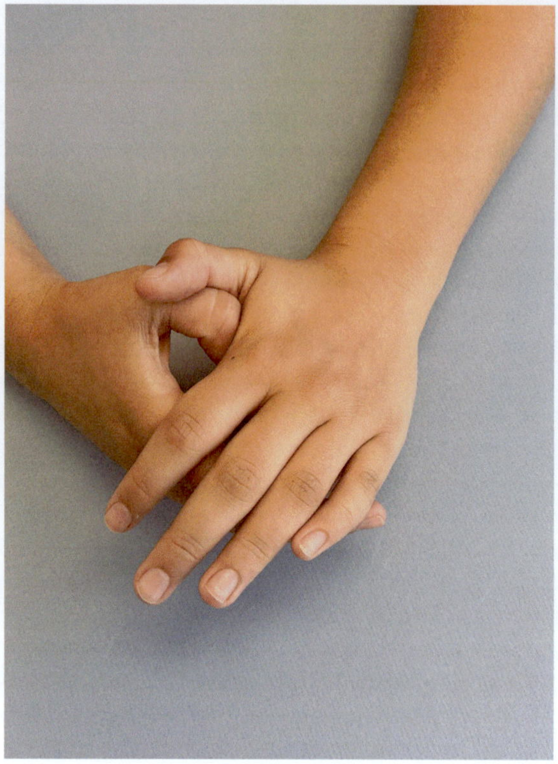

Image 4 Active donor pronation is combined with passive thumb and finger MCP extension in phase 1

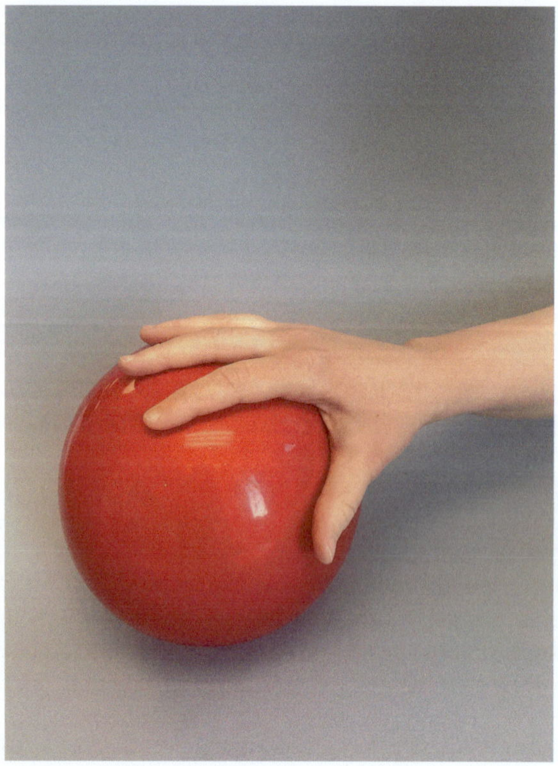

Image 5 A medium-sized ball may be used for resistance to pronation while supporting the fingers and thumb in extension

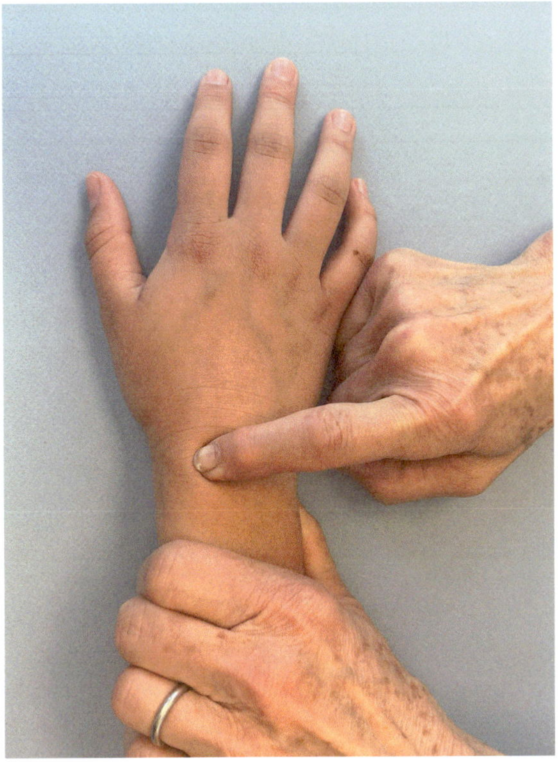

Image 6 Monthly recipient assessment is performed by manually resisting forearm pronation while palpating the PIN-innervated muscles or tendons in the dorsal wrist compartments. Initially, one should palpate for tension in the muscle/tendon while looking for trace finger MCP joint and thumb extension. The wrist should be maintained in neutral to a maximum of 30 degrees of wrist extension to limit tenodesis contributions

Assessment of Recovery

Baseline MMT strength of the recipient muscle actions (finger MCP and thumb MCP/IP extension), donor muscle action (forearm pronation), and other affected muscles as well as active/passive range-of-motion (A/PROM) measurements are helpful for pre- and postoperative comparisons. Other outcome measures such as pinch and grip strength measurements should also be obtained.

To identify early postoperative recipient muscle contraction, the therapist should resist forearm pronation (donor activation) while palpating over the PIN innervated muscles or tendons in the dorsal wrist compartments (Image 6). The therapist feels for tension in the muscle/tendon while looking for trace finger MCP joint and thumb extension. The wrist should be maintained in neutral to a maximum of 30 degrees of wrist extension to limit tenodesis contributions. MMT strength should be assessed at least monthly to determine the phase of recovery and appropriate therapeutic exercises. Trace muscle contractions may be observed at the thumb 4–8 months following surgery beginning at the APL and progressing to the EPL, EPB, and lastly EIP following transfer of AIN to PQ to the DBPIN [5]. In addition to monthly assessment of recipient muscle contraction, the recovery may also be monitored with goniometric measurements of extensor lag at the MCP joints. Again, be sure to maintain the same amount of wrist extension while taking measures to avoid contributions from tenodesis effect.

Therapy Frequency

Initially, frequency of therapy visits may be one time per week. Once the patient demonstrates understanding of the donor-recipient relationship and any soft tissue restrictions are resolved, continuing therapy at a frequency of one time per month is recommended.

Phase 2

2−/5 to 3/5 MMT in the Recipient Muscle(s)

Precautions

The patient should avoid high-intensity digital extension exercises. Intense exercise leading to recipient muscle fatigue may impair the regeneration of axons, inhibiting effective reinnervation of recipient musculature [9].

Orthoses

Patients may continue the orthosis described in phase 1 to wear during the day and night with removal for therapy exercises and hygiene. Orthosis use may be intermittently beneficial until at least 3/5 MMT strength is achieved for finger MCP and thumb extension.

Exercises

Once partial active finger MCP joint and thumb extension are noted, the patient progresses to phase 2 of rehabilitation. In this phase, exercises transition from passive to active-assisted motion in the recipient muscles. The patient first begins active-assisted finger MCP and thumb extension as well as "place and hold" exercises [10]. Phase 2 of therapy is typically characterized by movement in a gravity-minimized plane, yet this is more relevant for larger, heavier joints that are more vulnerable to gravity and antagonistic forces.

- Active Donor with Active-Assisted Recipient
  The patient performs active forearm pronation paired with active-assisted finger and thumb extension. The forearm begins in supination and then pronates while the patient is instructed to attempt independent active digital extension. Assistance is given using the contralateral hand to complete the motion.
- Resisted Donor Activation with Active-Assisted Recipient
  The patient combines isometric forearm pronation with active-assistive finger and thumb extension by rolling therapy putty into a cylinder focusing on pressing the radial palm into the putty while rolling [9, 10] (Image 7). As strength improves, therapy putty resistance is increased for a greater challenge.

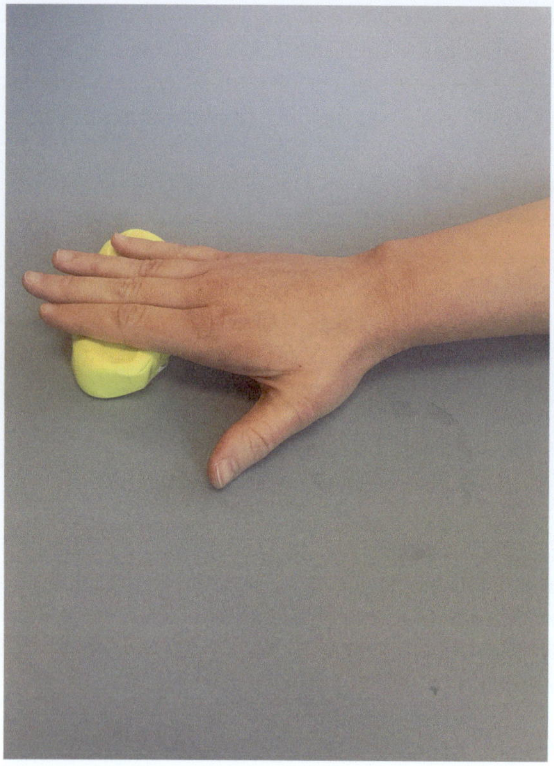

Image 7 Resisted donor with assisted recipient exercises may be performed by combining isometric forearm pronation with finger and thumb extension over a cylinder of therapy putty. The individual is cued to press the radial aspect of the palm into the putty while rolling the hand back and forth over it

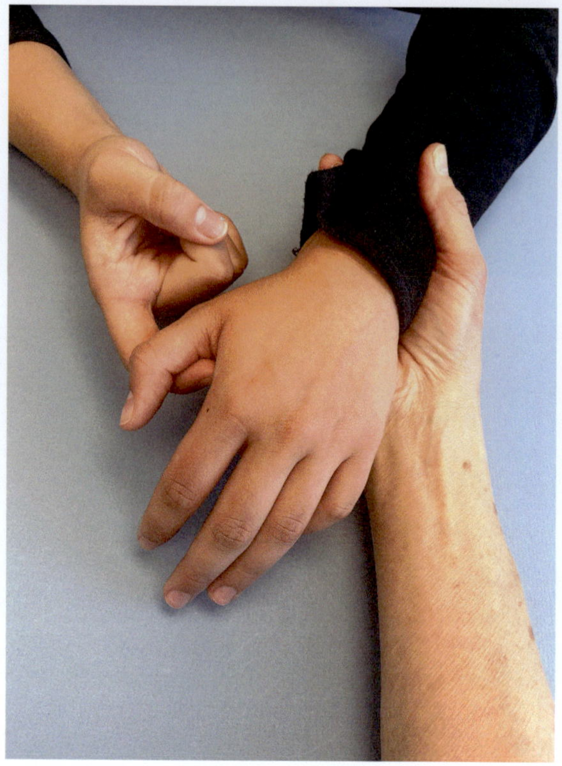

Image 8 Resisted donor activation with active-assisted recipient exercises may also be performed by manually resisting forearm pronation while manually assisting thumb and/or finger extension

The therapist may also resist forearm pronation and support the thumb (and/or fingers) in midrange extension while the patient attempts independent extension (Image 8).

- "Place and Hold" Exercise
  When finger MCP joint and thumb extension achieve 2+/5 MMT, "place and hold" exercises may begin. The patient manually places the fingers in midrange MCP joint extension. The therapist then resists forearm pronation as the patient attempts to maintain finger extension without assistance (Image 9a, b). The thumb may also be placed in midrange extension while resisting forearm pronation as the patient attempts to maintain thumb extension without assistance. As strength improves, the finger MCP joints and thumb may be placed in end-range (full) extension to enhance the challenge.
- Active Donor with Active Recipient
  The patient actively pronates the forearm while simultaneously extending fingers and thumb (Image 10).
- Functional Activity
  Once finger MCP joint and thumb extension reach a 3−/5 MMT grade, the patient may begin functional tasks such as opening the hand to grasp containers, which typically requires some degree of pronation force (Image 11).

Assessment of Recovery

The therapist continues to assess pinch, grip, and MMT strength of finger MCP joint and thumb extension with resisted donor activation (forearm pronation). Measuring finger MCP and thumb extension (extensor lag) with and without forearm pronation (in a consistent wrist extension position) may provide useful information regarding donor influence.

Therapy Frequency

Frequency of therapy may be increased to one time per week or every other week during phase 2 based on the patient's needs.

Phase 3

3+/5 MMT and Above

Once finger MCP joint and thumb extension reach full range and can withstand some resistance, patients may incorporate more challenging strengthening and functional tasks into their daily therapy home program. There are no orthoses or precautions in phase 3 unless the patient experiences fatigue and/or extensor lag. Patients may consider wearing the orthosis later in the day until fatigue is no longer an issue. Exercises should not lead to fatigue with resistance training.

Exercises

- Resistive Recipient Activity with Donor Contraction
  The patient continues paired recipient activity with donor contraction, including exercises requiring resisted finger MCP and thumb extension with resisted forearm pronation. Baltimore Therapeutic Equipment™ (BTE) tool #302, at head tilt 1, requires finger MCP joint extension paired with the forearm in pronation [10] (Image 12).
- Resistive Recipient Activity Without Donor Contraction
  There may be instances in which patients need to de-emphasize the assistive component of the donor PQ. He or she may eventually progress to resistive digital extension without forearm pronation. To strengthen the PIN muscles without the donor, the therapist can change the BTE tool #302 from head tilt 1 to head tilt 5 to place forearm in neutral versus pronation. The patient may also work on functional activities requiring supination with finger extension such as holding a tray or holding the hand open to receive change. Therapy putty and/or a rubber band may also be useful to strengthen the digital extensors in a supinated or forearm-neutral position (Image 13).

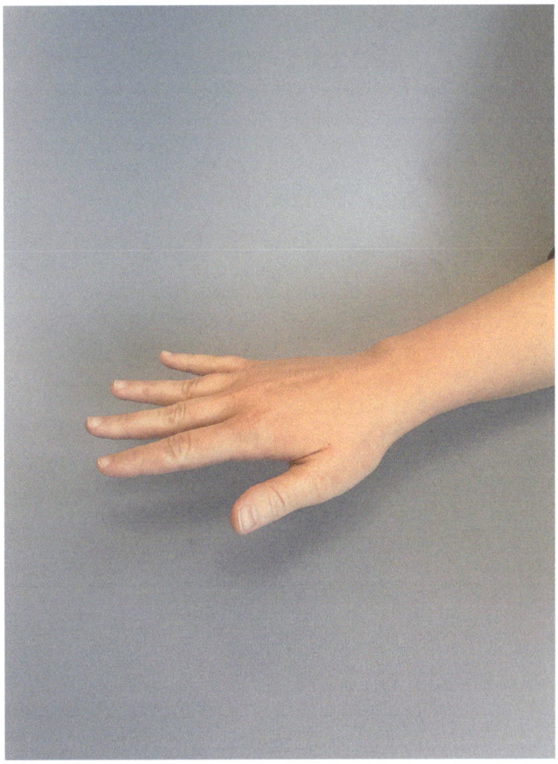

Image 10 Active donor forearm pronation is paired with active finger and thumb extension

Clinical Pearl
The patient may roll the hand back and forth over a dowel with cues to isometrically press into pronation while attempting to hold the thumb and fingers in extension as the dowel rolls proximally.

Assessment of Recovery

The therapist should assess MMT strength of finger MCP joint and thumb extension with and without donor activation (active or resisted forearm pronation). Maximum strength will likely be noted with co-contraction of pronation and digital extension activation for 1–2+ years post-surgery [10].

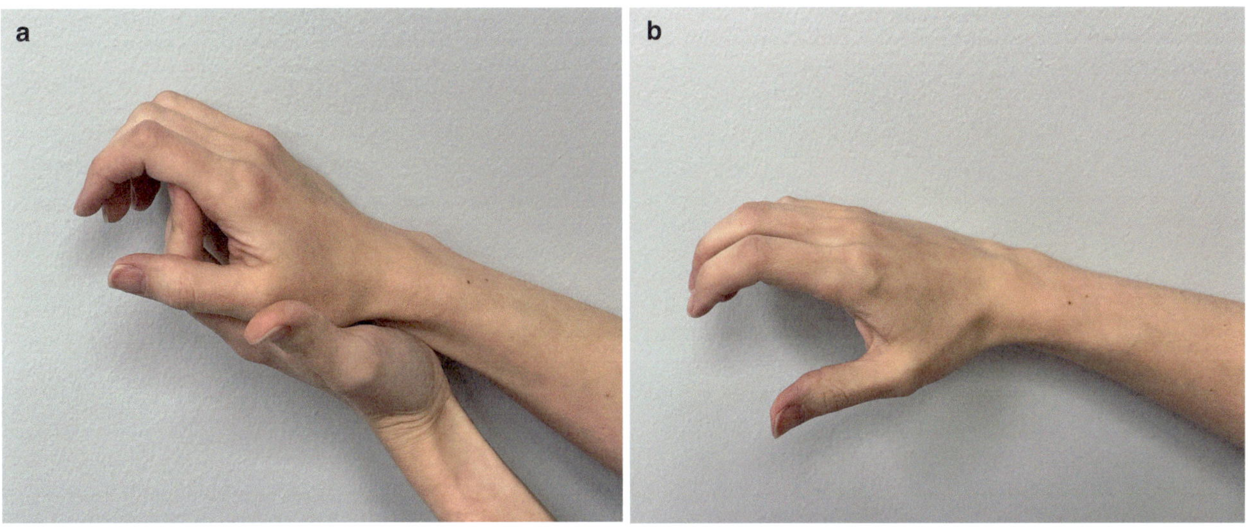

Image 9 (**a**, **b**) Place-and-hold exercises are performed by manually placing the fingers and thumb in midrange MCP joint extension. Resistance is applied to forearm pronation as the individual attempts to maintain finger/thumb extension without assistance

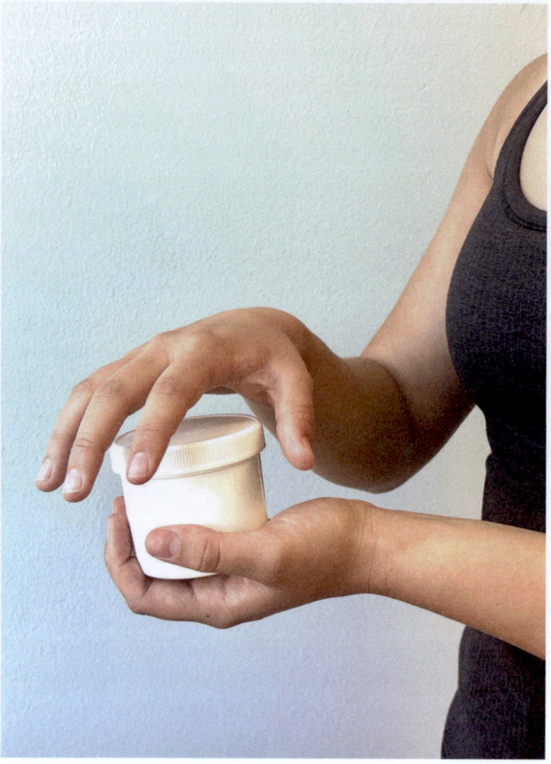

Image 11 Functional activities that combine pronation and active finger/thumb extension are encouraged towards the end of phase 2. In this image, the individual practices opening the hand to grasp the lid of a jar

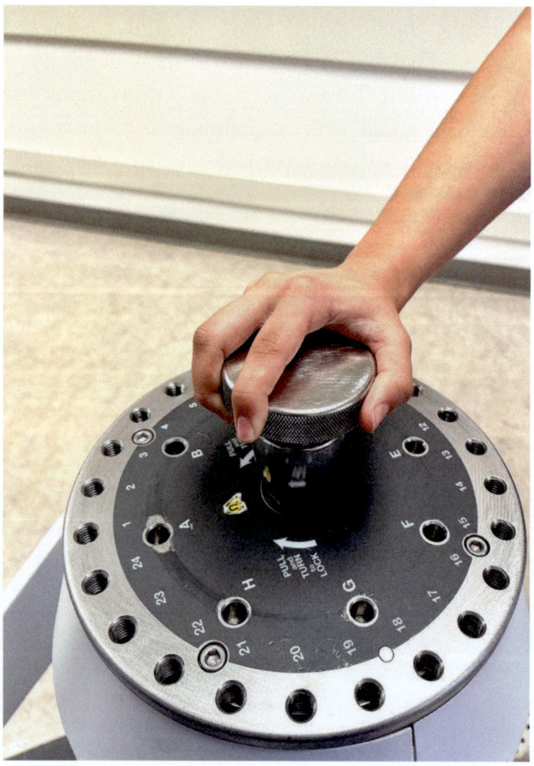

Image 12 In phase 3, resisted recipient and active donor exercises may be achieved with Baltimore Therapeutic Equipment™ (BTE) tool #302, at head tilt 1. This requires finger MCP joint extension paired with forearm pronation

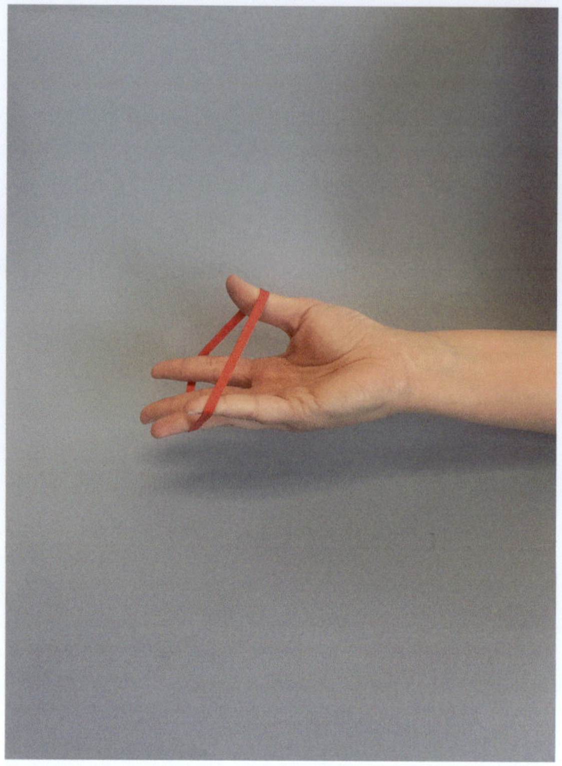

Image 13 To de-emphasize donor activation while strengthening PIN muscles, rubber bands are used to provide resistance to finger extension with the forearm in a supinated position

Therapy Frequency

Frequency of therapy visits may continue one time per week or every other week in phase 3.

AIN (PQ)-to-PIN nerve transfer

Nerve transfer overview					
Donor nerve	Donor action	Recipient nerve	Recipient action	Indications for functional restoration	Approximate months to functional movement
Anterior interosseous nerve (AIN) to the pronator quadratus (PQ)	Forearm pronation	Posterior interosseous nerve (PIN)	Finger MCP extension and thumb extension	Restore ability to open the hand for functional grasp	Data not available

Information below is suggested guidelines. Precautions may vary according to surgeon preferences and patient factors

	Preoperative therapy	Early phase	Middle phase	Late phase
Criteria	Before surgery	0/5 to −1/5 MMT	2−/5 to 3/5 MMT	>3/5 MMT
Purpose of phase	Educate and establish baseline function	Understand donor-recipient relationship and begin patterning the two to aid with cortical plasticity Activate donor: forearm pronation	Activate nerve transfer for light functional activities requiring hand-opening	Strengthen recipient muscles with resistance Separate digital extension from the donor PQ
Precautions	NA	No wrist ROM for the first 2–3 weeks Avoid prolonged finger and thumb composite flexion to prevent flexor tightness and/or overlengthening of the extensors	Avoid high-intensity exercise Minimize fatigue and force placed on the weak PIN-innervated muscles	Resistive exercise should not be performed before the PIN-innervated muscles demonstrate 3/5 MMT Avoid fatigue with resistance training
Frequency of visits (considerations)	1–2 visits; more if PROM limitations are present	1×/week until PROM is restored, and patient is independent with HEP Decrease to 1×/month based on progress and goals	1×/month If additional nerve transfers were performed, more frequent therapy is warranted	1×/month based on patient needs and goals
Orthosis considerations	Hand-based orthosis: either custom thermoplastic MCP extension assist or BENIK™ W-700 series The purpose of this is to facilitate finger extension while allowing for functional grasp/flexion	Custom or prefabricated wrist orthosis for 2 weeks to protect the nerve coaptation. Some surgeons prefer a "P1 blocking" orthosis, with the finger MCP joints in extension and thumb in extension to prevent drag on the PIN A hand-based radial nerve palsy orthosis may be resumed after the post-op protective phase. The static P1 blocking orthosis may continue to be used at night, as needed	Hand-based radial nerve palsy orthosis during heavy activities	No orthosis
Interventions		**Donor activation**: Forearm pronation (isometric, active, and resisted) 10× every hour **Donor-recipient pairing**: Active pronation with passive finger MCP extension and thumb composite extension 10–20 reps, 6–8×/day	**Active/resisted donor with active assist recipient**: Passive progresses to active-assisted finger and thumb extension (with active and/or resisted pronation) **Place and hold**: With the forearm in pronation, place fingers and thumb in composite extension. Remove the support and maintain this position	**Resisted donor and recipient**: Resisted finger and thumb extension while pronated. Resistance may include therapy putty, a rubber band, or isometric pressure from the opposite hand **Resisted recipient without donor contraction**: Resisted finger and thumb extension while maintaining a supinated or forearm neutral position
Additional intervention considerations		Rolling the fingers onto a dowel or medium-size ball is an intuitive way to activate the donor in pronation while the ball assists digital extensors	Respect fatigue	Respect fatigue Advance resistance gradually

**During all phases, it is essential to continue cortical reorganization and psychological and psychosocial interventions and progress to incorporate donor/recipient with ADLs

AIN-to-PQ-to-PIN Nerve Transfer

Goal of Surgery: Restore the ability to open the hand to grasp and release objects

Recipient Movement = Lift fingers and thumb up (finger and thumb extension)

Primary Recipient Muscles: Extensor digitorum communis (EDC) and extensor pollicis longus (EPL)

Secondary Recipient Muscle: Extensor carpi ulnaris (ECU)

Recipient Nerve: Posterior interosseous nerve (PIN)

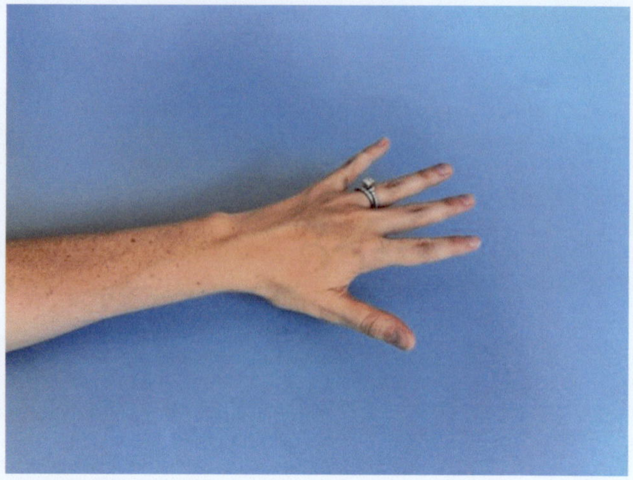

Lift fingers and thumb up (finger and thumb extension)

Donor Movement = Turn palm down (forearm pronation)

Donor Muscle: Pronator quadratus (PQ)

Donor Nerve: Anterior interosseous nerve (AIN)

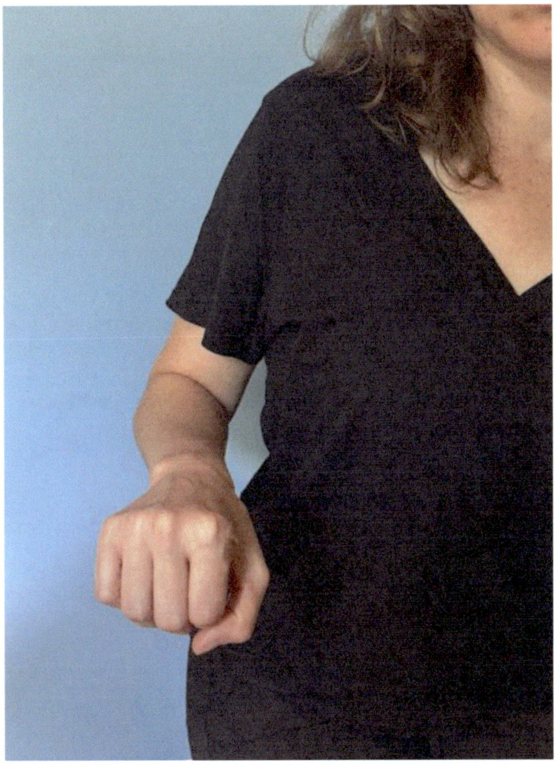

Rotate the forearm palm down (pronation)

Phase 1 AIN-to-PQ-to-PIN Nerve Transfer Exercises

☐ **Active or Resisted Donor Movement**:

Complete one of the below exercises <u>10</u> repetitions, every waking hour.

1. Begin with your elbow bent by your side and forearm palm up. Turn your palm down. Return to the start position, and repeat.

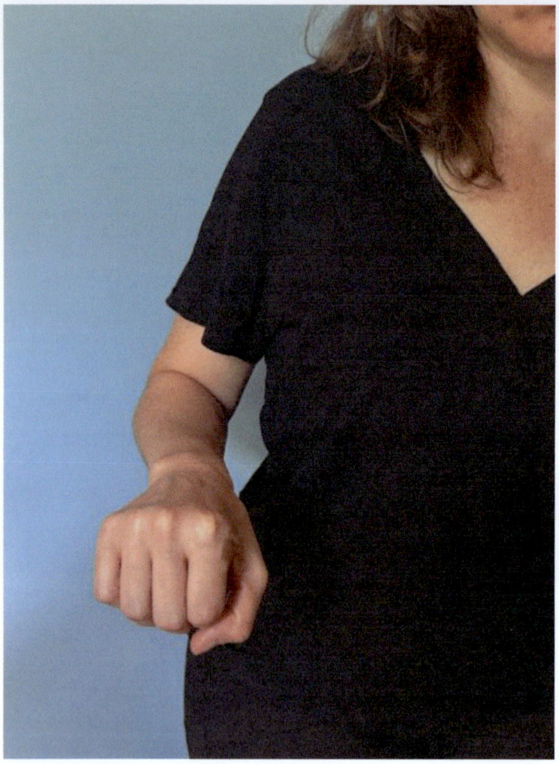

2. Begin with your forearm facing palm down. Use your opposite hand to manually try to rotate the forearm palm up. Resisting the pressure from your opposite hand, maintain a palm down position. Hold for <u>3–5</u> seconds.

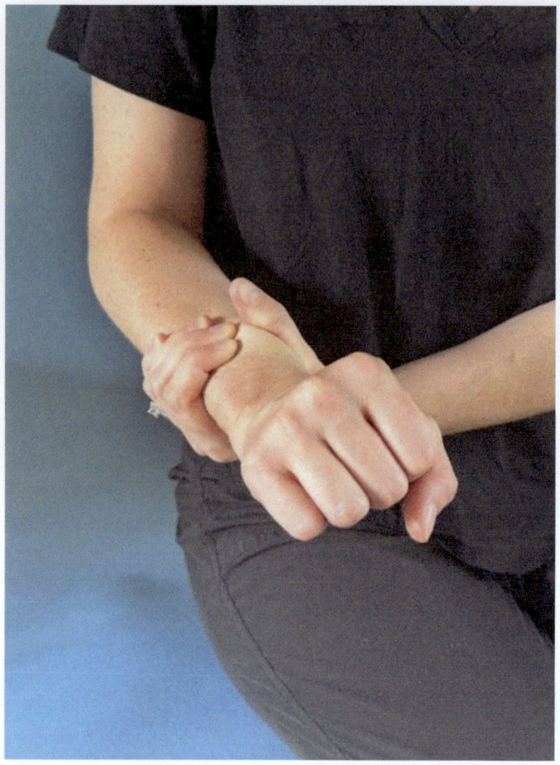

☐ **Active Donor + Passive Recipient Movement**: **Complete 10 repetitions, 3 times per day.**

- Begin with your elbow bent by your side and forearm palm up. Turn your palm down, and at the same time, use your other hand to lift the fingers and thumb up.

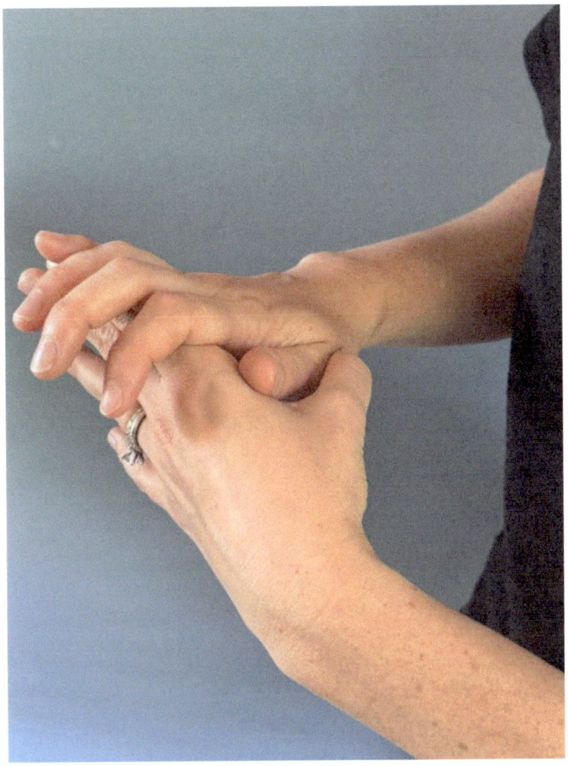

Phase 2 AIN-to-PQ-to-PIN Nerve Transfer Exercises

☐ **Active Donor + Active-Assisted Recipient Movement**:

- Begin with your elbow bent by your side and forearm palm up. Turn your palm down as you attempt to lift your fingers and thumb up. Then, use your other hand to help lift your fingers and thumb **the rest of the way up**.

Complete 10 repetitions, 3 times per day.

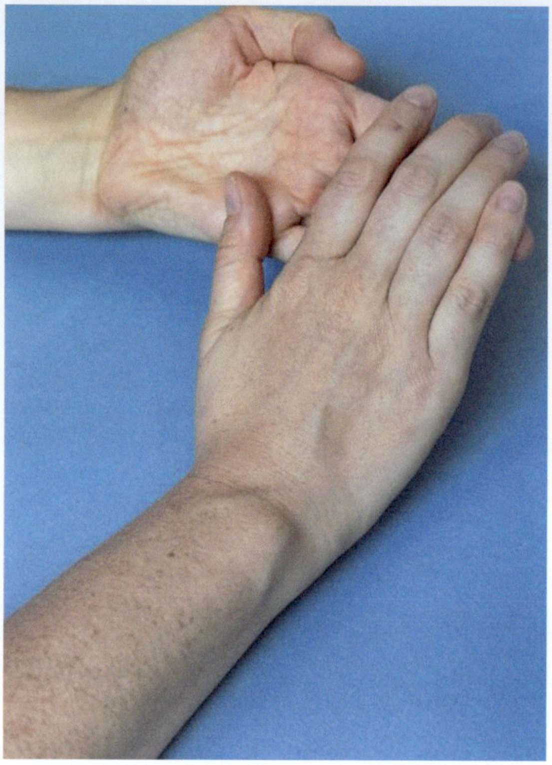

☐ **Isometric Donor + Active-Assisted Recipient Movement**:

- Begin with your forearm resting palm down on a table and your hand resting on therapy putty. As you roll the therapy putty into a cylinder, press the thumb side of your hand into the putty. Allow the therapy putty to lift your fingers and thumb up as you roll the putty toward you.

Complete <u>10</u> repetitions, <u>3</u> times per day.

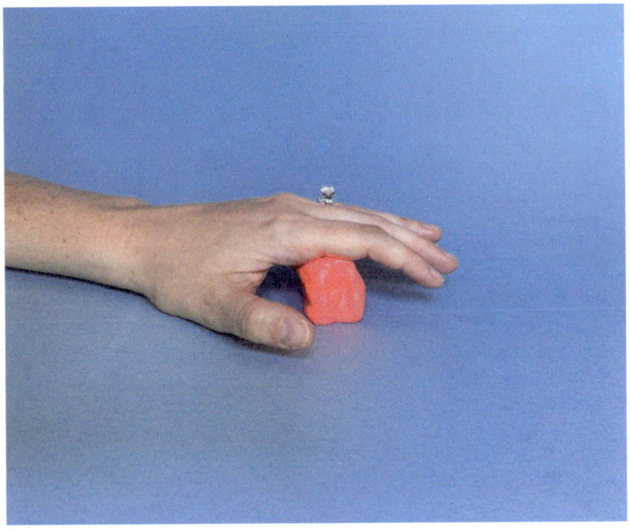

☐ **Isometric Donor + "Place and Hold":**

Complete the below exercises <u>1–10</u> repetitions, <u>2–3</u> times per day.

Hold for <u>3–5</u> s.

1. Begin with your forearm resting on a table and your fingers and thumb relaxed over the edge. Using your other hand, **lift your fingers up**. Press the thumb side of your forearm down into the table. SLOWLY let go of your **fingers** as you try to hold them up without the help of your other hand.

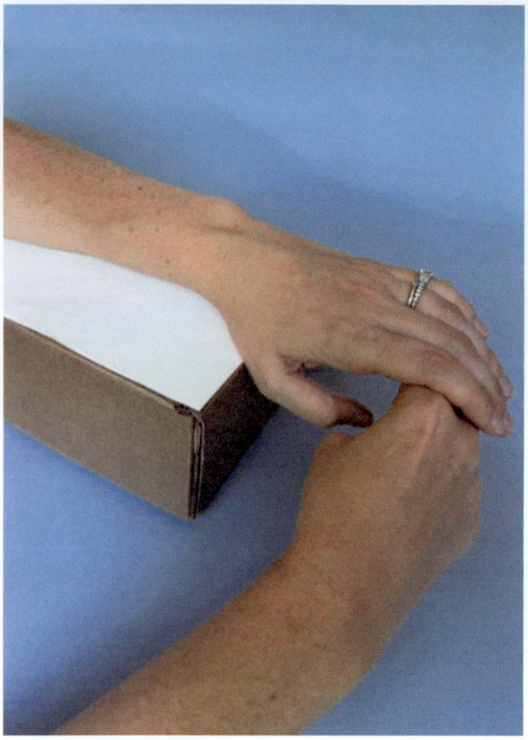

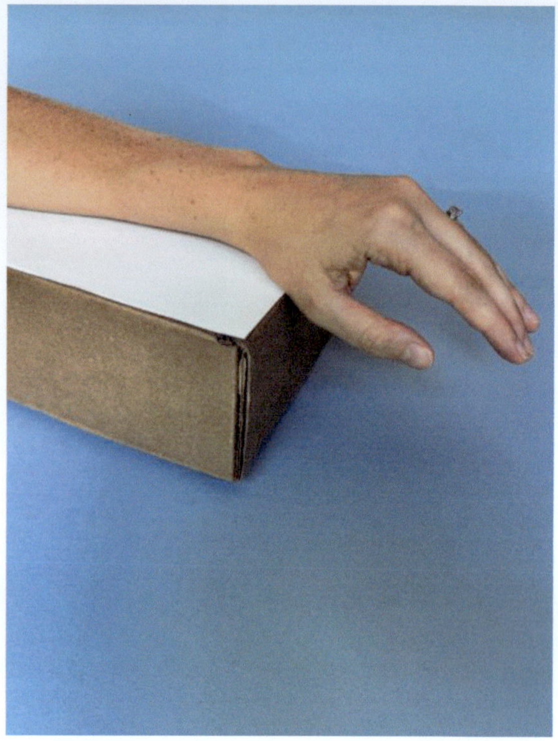

2. Begin with your forearm resting on a table and your fingers and thumb relaxed over the edge. Using your other hand, **lift your thumb up**. Press the thumb side of your forearm down into the table. SLOWLY let go of your **thumb** as you try to hold it up without the help of your other hand.

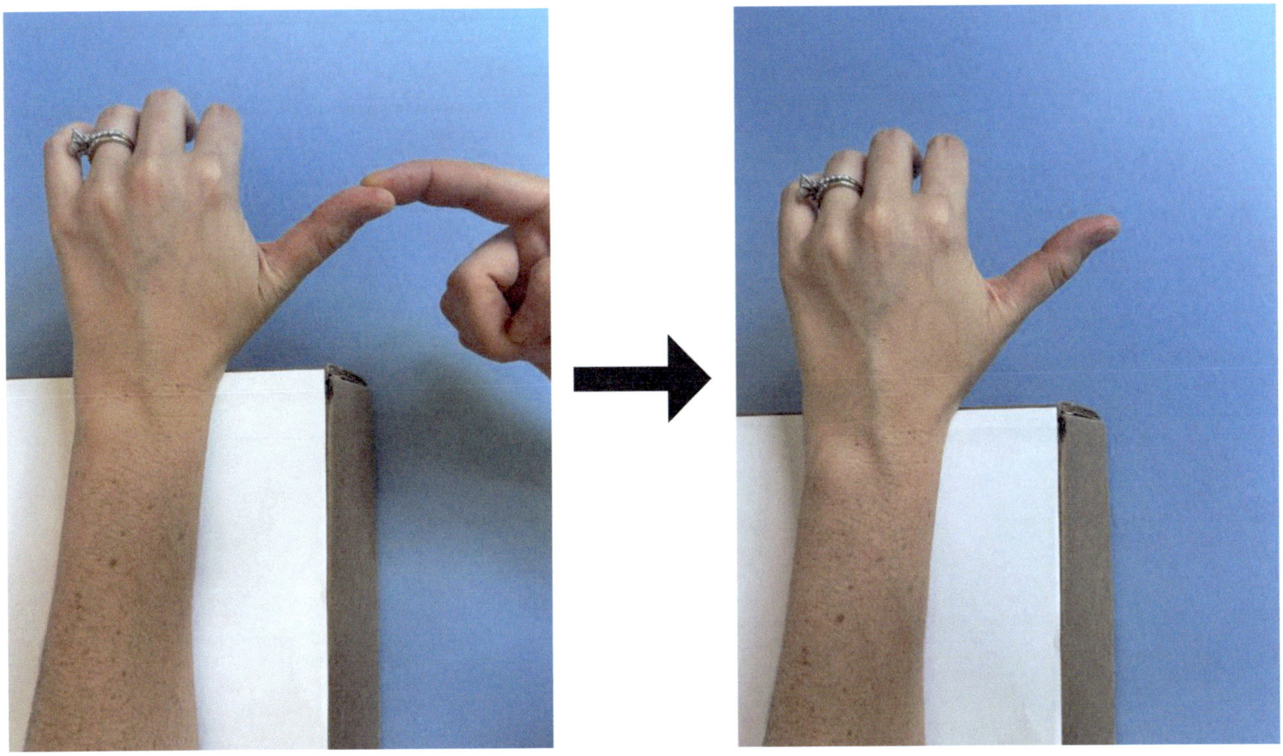

☐ **Active Donor + Active Recipient Movement**:

- Begin with your elbow bent by your side and forearm palm up. Turn your palm down. At the same time, **lift your fingers and thumb up**. Return to the start position, and repeat.

Complete 5–10 repetitions, 3 times per day.

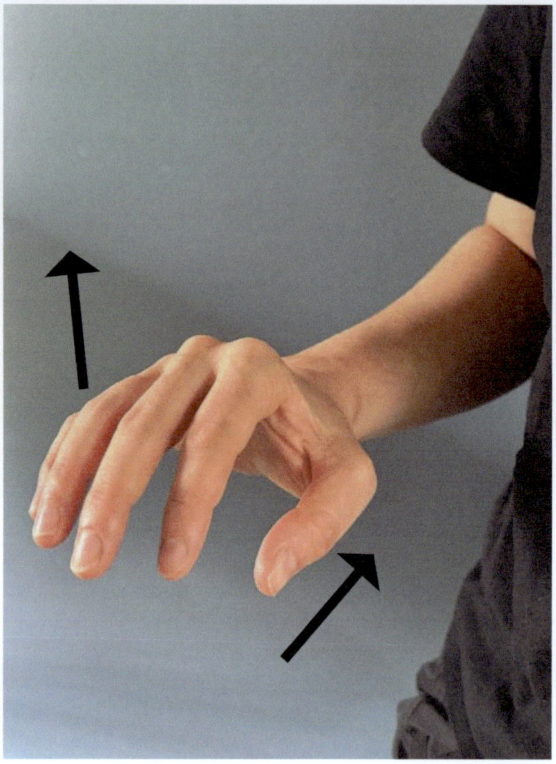

Phase 3 AIN-to-PQ-to-PIN Nerve Transfer Exercises

☐ **Resisted Donor + Resisted Recipient Movement**:

- Open a wide jar lid. With your fingers straight and the hand open (extension), maintain your forearm in a palm-down (pronated) position while you twist the jar lid open.

  Complete 3–10 repetitions, 2 times per day.

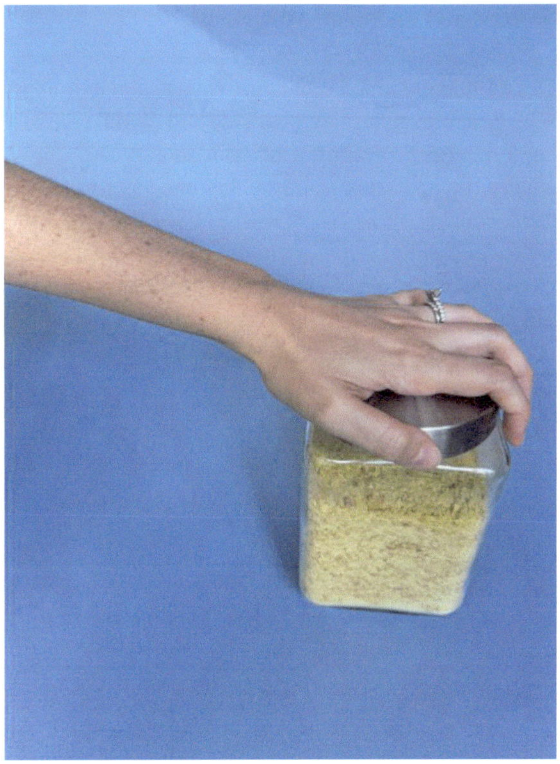

☐ **Resisted Recipient Movement**:

- Place a rubber band around your fingers and thumb. Begin with your elbow bent by your side and thumb side of your hand facing the ceiling. Lift your fingers and thumb up against the resistance of the rubber band as you open your hand.

  Complete 10 repetitions, 2 times per day.

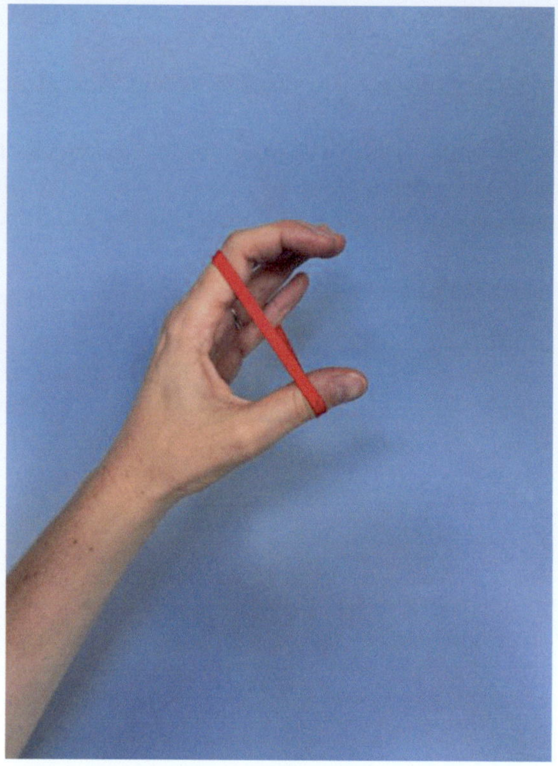

References

1. Sigamoney KV, Rashid A, Ng CY. Management of atraumatic posterior interosseous nerve palsy. J Hand Surg Am. 2017;42(10):826–30. https://doi.org/10.1016/j.jhsa.2017.07.026.
2. Moore AM, Franco M, Tung TH. Motor and sensory nerve transfers in the forearm and hand. Plast Reconstr Surg. 2014;134:721–9. https://doi.org/10.1097/PRS.0000000000000509.
3. Fairley JA, Daneshvar P. AIN to PIN transfer for PIN palsy following distal biceps tendon repair: a case report. Case Rep Plast Surg Hand Surg. 2022;9(1):173–8. https://doi.org/10.1080/23320885.2022.2096614.
4. Bertelli JA. Nerve versus tendon transfer for radial nerve paralysis reconstruction. J Hand Surg Am. 2020;45(5):418–26.
5. Bertelli JA, Nehete S, Duarte ECW, Ghizoni MF. Transfer of the distal anterior interosseous nerve for thumb motion reconstruction in radial nerve paralysis. J Hand Surg Am. 2020;45(9):877.e1–e10.
6. Goldspink G, Tabary C, Tabary JC, Tardieu C, Tardieu G. Effect of denervation on the adaptation of sarcomere number and muscle extensibility to the functional length of the muscle. J Physiol. 1974;236(3):733–42.
7. Gossman MR, Sahrmann SA, Rose SJ. Review of length-associated changes in muscle: experimental evidence and clinical implications. Phys Ther. 1982;62(12):1799–808.
8. Lieber RL, Bodine-Fowler SC. Skeletal muscle mechanics: implications for rehabilitation. Phys Ther. 1993;73(12):844–56.
9. Kahn LC, Moore AM. Donor activation focused rehabilitation approach maximizing outcomes after nerve surgery. Hand Clin. 2016;32:263–77. https://doi.org/10.1016/j.hcl.2015.12.014.
10. Davidge KM, Yee A, Kahn LC, Mackinnon SE. Median to radial nerve transfers for restoration of wrist, finger, and thumb extension. J Hand Surg. 2013;38A:1812–27. https://doi.org/10.1016/j.jhsa.2013.06.024.

Extensor Carpi Radialis Brevis (ECRB) Branch of The Radial Nerve to the Flexor Digitorum Superficialis (FDS) Nerve Transfer

Jamie Findeiss

Background

The flexor digitorum superficialis (FDS) muscle is responsible for flexion of the proximal interphalangeal (PIP) joints of the hand and assists with flexion of the metacarpophalangeal (MP) joints and wrist [1]. The FDS is therefore a major contributor to functional grasp. The FDS is innervated by a branch of the median nerve that is derived from C8 and T1 nerve roots. This branch of the median nerve arises from the medial cord of the brachial plexus. Injury or dysfunction of the FDS can occur through a variety of mechanisms, including trauma, compressive neuropathy, transection of the median nerve, iatrogenic injuries, C8 and/or T1 root injuries, and medial cord injuries [2].

Many hand surgeons and therapists will agree that *flexion is function*. Finger flexion (in addition to elbow flexion) is often prioritized in the restoration of function following pan-brachial plexus injury. Even with intact ulnar nerve function (i.e., ring and small finger FDP, lumbricals, and interossei assisting with grip), the loss of the FDS innervation results in deficient grip strength, typically 40–43% of the contralateral side [3, 4]. It is well documented that patients with tetraplegia rank hand function as significantly more important to quality of life compared to walking, sexual function, bladder function, and pain relief [5]. The inability to close the hand limits a person's ability to hold objects, manipulate tools, open containers, and sustain any functional grip. This results in tremendous disability in all aspects of life: self-care, work, sports, social participation, community engagement, and more.

The restoration of finger flexion can be achieved via a nerve transfer using the synergistic donor extensor carpi radialis brevis (ECRB). The ECRB is innervated by the radial nerve and arises from C5–C6 root levels. The ECRB is responsible for wrist extension in combination with the extensor carpi radialis longus (ECRL) and the extensor carpi ulnaris (ECU), making the ECRB an expendable donor.

High median nerve injuries are relatively uncommon as they account for 0.1% of injuries affecting upper extremity peripheral nerves [6]. Therefore, there are few studies of the ECRB-to-FDS nerve transfer, making it difficult to interpret outcomes without large-scale data. Jitpun describes a case report of a patient with C8–T1 spinal cord injury who underwent ECRB-to-FDS nerve transfer, in combination with brachialis-to-AIN nerve transfer to restore digital flexion [7]. This case yielded a highly successful outcome of 4/5 manual muscle testing (MMT) strength in finger flexion of the MCP and PIP joints at 18 months. The authors attribute the success of this nerve transfer to the synergistic nature of the donor and recipient and cortical plasticity. Tenodesis has a natural effect on finger flexion, and this combination of donor and recipient capitalizes on that effect [7].

There is a clear need for higher-level data to illustrate the successful restoration of grasp following ECRB-to-FDS transfer in the context of brachial plexus injury. Our team has found this transfer to be effective, intuitive, and relatively easy to rehabilitate due to its synergistic nature.

J. Findeiss (✉)
Athletico Physical Therapy, St. Louis, MO, USA

L. C. Kahn et al. (eds.), *Rehabilitation for Nerve Transfers of the Upper Extremity*,
https://doi.org/10.1007/978-3-031-92008-0_21

Surgical Description

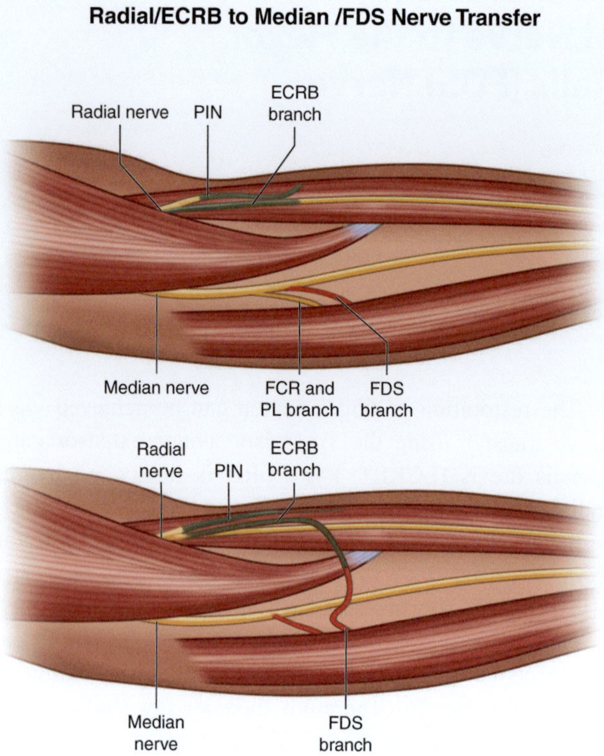

Microsurgical technique of Extensor Carpi Radialis Brevis (ECRB) Branch of the Radial Nerve to the Flexor Digitorum Superficialis (FDS) Nerve Transfer

A curvilinear incision is made along the volar aspect of the proximal two-thirds of the forearm. The brachioradialis muscle is identified, and the superficial radial nerve (SRN) is dissected on the undersurface of the brachioradialis muscle. The superficial radial nerve is used as a guide to dissect retrograde (distal to proximal) to identify the posterior interosseous nerve (PIN) and the radial nerve proper. There is typically a branch to the ECRB identified close to the point where the PIN and SRN branch from the radial nerve proper. Intraoperative stimulation is used to confirm function of the ECRB branch. It is important to stimulate the ECRB branch within 30 min of the tourniquet being inflated (if one is being used) and to ensure that the anesthesia team is not using any muscle paralytics. After doing so, the lacertus fibrosus is identified, and after releasing the lacertus fibrosus, the median nerve is identified deep to the lacertus fibrosus and along the inner surface of the flexor pronator mass. After decompressing the median nerve, the branching pattern of the median nerve is identified. It is helpful to decompress the FDS arch and subsequently identify the anterior interosseous nerve (AIN) coming off the median nerve proper, being sure to protect the AIN. The FDS branches are visualized as entering the muscle belly distal to the released FDS arch. A handheld nerve stimulator is used to confirm that the FDS branches are not functioning, again ensuring that this is done within 30 min of the tourniquet being inflated (if one is being used) and that there are no muscle paralytics being used by the anesthesia team. After doing so, the FDS branches of the median nerve are neurolyzed proximally from the median nerve proper and dissected as proximally as possible. The donor nerve/ECRB nerve is divided distally, and the recipient nerve is divided proximally after dissecting the FDS branch as proximally as possible. Coaptation of the ECRB branch of the radial nerve to the FDS branch of the median nerve is performed using microsurgical technique.

Phases of Rehabilitation

Phase 1

Preoperative to 1/5 MMT in Recipient Muscle

Preoperative

It is important to educate patients using simple and concise terms regarding the donor and recipient actions, stages of healing, expectations, and timeline for recovery. If there are joint contractions present, therapy should prioritize passive finger motion at all joints. The patient should ideally have full passive flexion of the fingers prior to surgery. This is important so that a weak, recovering muscle is not limited by stiff, contracted joints or short extrinsic extensor muscles.

Postoperative

Following surgery, the wrist is immobilized for up to 2 weeks in a postoperative dressing. At that time, the patient is seen in the surgery clinic for suture removal (pending MD preference), wound care as needed, and referral to therapy. The patient transitions to a prefabricated wrist orthosis to protect the nerve coaptation until 3–4 weeks from surgery. The wrist orthosis should be in slight extension, which will place the finger flexors at a mechanically advantageous position. It is important to educate patients to avoid resting in full digit extension. Resting in this position could contribute to both shortening of the digital extensors and overstretching of the recipient flexors, making it difficult to generate sufficient power as the FDS strength returns. Patient education is a recurring theme in phase 1, including the overview of timeline/expectations, donor activation, and initiation of donor and recipient co-contraction [8].

Exercises

- Donor Activation
  Donor activation begins with active or isometric wrist extension against gravity. Performance of 10–20 repetitions every hour is recommended. If the patient lacks lumbrical function and thus MCP flexion (in addition to known lack of IP flexion), it may be difficult to avoid

substitution with the digital extensors during donor activation.

Clinical Pearl

The use of a four-finger anti-claw orthosis places the MCP joints in flexion, thus helping to prevent excessive MCP joint extension (extensor digitorum communis/EDC compensation) while trying to isolate the ECRB during nerve transfer training. The anti-claw places the fingers in a position of opportunity for finger flexion (Image 1).

- Combined Donor with Passive Recipient Exercise
  Active wrist extension should be simultaneously paired with passive finger flexion to strengthen the new neural pathway (Image 2). As mentioned above, it is important to prevent excessive MCP joint extension. During passive recipient exercise, the patient should stretch not only the IP joints into flexion but the MCP joints as well.

Assessment of Recovery

To assess for return of the FDS, the therapist stabilizes the MCP joint and the wrist in neutral. Pressure is applied to the back of the hand to elicit an isometric contraction of the donor ECRB, and the patient is cued to attempt to make a fist while the therapist monitors for flexion in the PIP joint(s). The flexion arc should be measured and tracked for improvement. An MMT score of 2−/5 is achieved when the patient can partially flex the PIP joints. Care should be taken to ensure that the patient is not inadvertently using tenodesis to produce active finger flexion. To avoid this, the wrist must be maintained in neutral to avoid wrist extension motion, which would allow the fingers to flex by the passive tension in the extrinsic flexor muscles (Image 3).

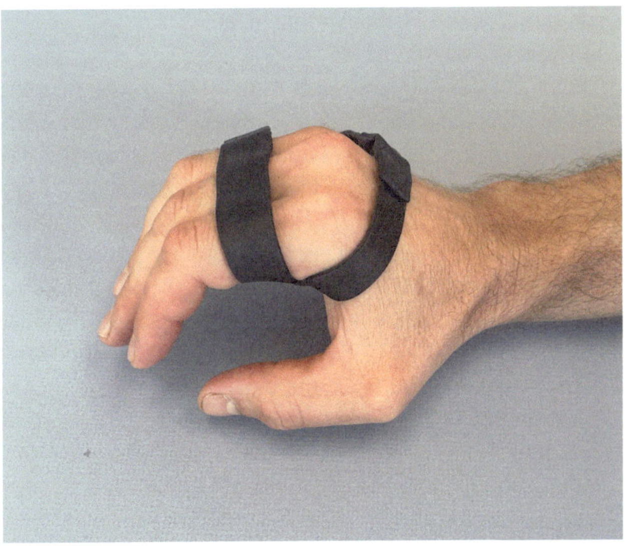

Image 1 An anti-claw orthosis which includes all four fingers is recommended in phase 1 and early in phase 2 to encourage finger flexion and limit antagonist EDC influence

Frequency of Visits

Weekly visits are appropriate until the patient has full passive motion of all joints, is proficient with donor activation, and has a good understanding of the donor-recipient relationship. At each postoperative visit, ROM and manual muscle testing (MMT) should be assessed to determine the appropriate exercise program.

Phase 2

2−/5 to 3/5 MMT in Recipient Muscle

Precautions

Avoid high-intensity exercises that involve the recipient muscles. Intense exercise leading to recipient muscle fatigue may impair the regeneration of axons, inhibiting reinnervation of recipient musculature during early reinnervation [8–10].

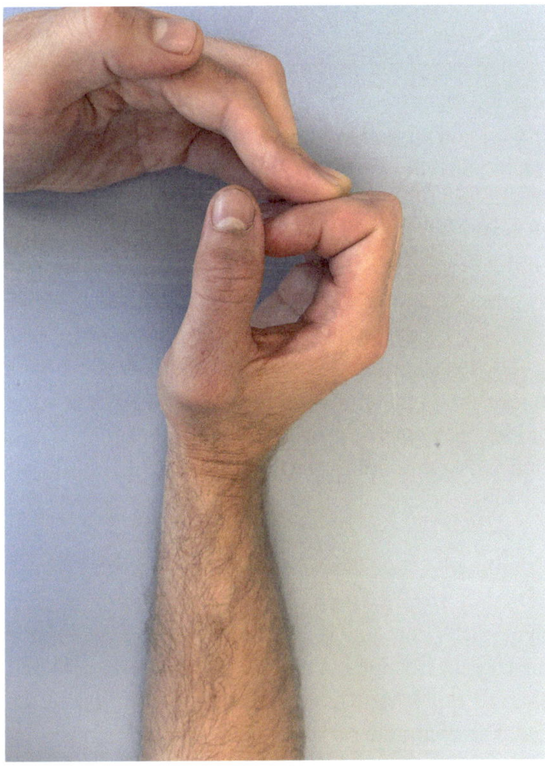

Image 2 Patterning active wrist extension with passive finger flexion is performed in phase 1 to promote the new neural pathway

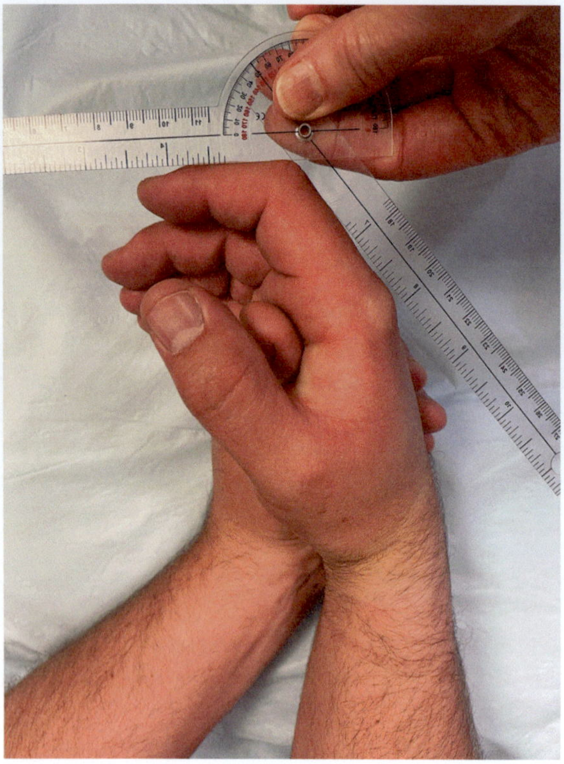

Image 3 Assessment of recovery of FDS function is performed by blocking wrist extension to limit tenodesis effect while resisting active wrist extension. The PIP is measured with a goniometer to quantify any new motion

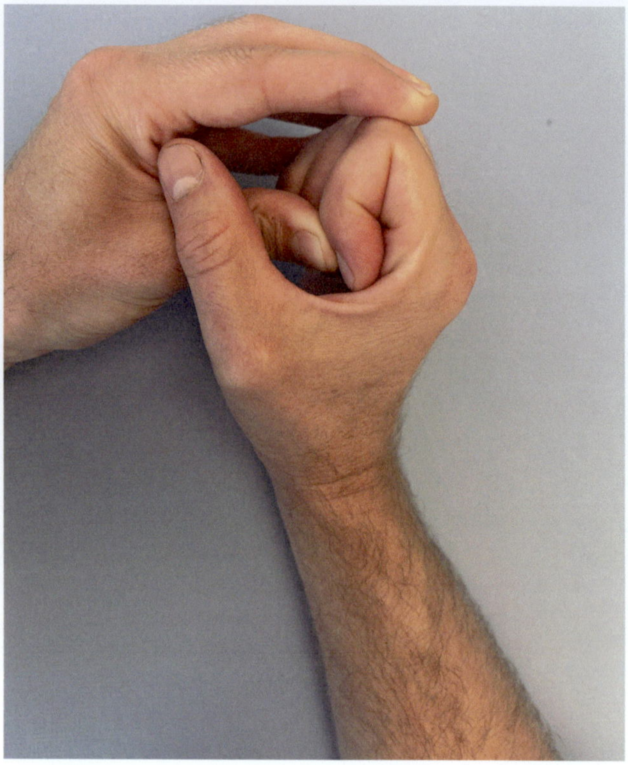

Image 4 Combined active donor/ECRB with active-assisted recipient/ FDS is achieved with the opposite hand completing finger flexion

Orthosis

Continued use of the anti-claw orthosis may be helpful if the patient has excessive MCP joint extension (EDC substitution) while trying to work on donor activation and/or donor-recipient pairing.

Exercises

Once the patient can produce any active joint flexion at the PIP joints, treatment advances to phase 2 of rehabilitation. Phase 2 is characterized by active-assisted and gravity-lessened exercises for the recipient FDS. Gravity-lessened exercises are typically more relevant for larger, heavier joints (shoulder, elbow, wrist) compared to finger joints, so positioning is less important for finger exercises [10]. However, gravity-lessened exercises are still described below.

- Combined Active Donor with Active-Assisted Recipient
  FDS MMT = 2−/5 to 2/5
  Synergistic motion in a gravity-lessened position: With the forearm resting in neutral rotation, the patient actively extends the wrist while simultaneously trying to make a fist. The contralateral hand then assists the fingers further into a full composite fist (Image 4).
- "Place and Hold" Finger Flexion
  FDS MMT = 2+/5
  The patient passively places the fingers into composite flexion while the wrist actively extends. The contralateral hand is removed while the patient attempts to hold this position for 5 s. Manual resistance to donor wrist extension may be helpful to increase the response in the recipient.
- Active Donor with Active Recipient
  FDS MMT = 3−/5 to 3/5
  In an antigravity plane, such as the wrist resting over the table edge, the patient will actively extend the wrist while actively flexing the fingers into the palm. He or she will then relax the wrist while the fingers extend.
- Functional Activity
  Functional activities are encouraged during this phase to optimize grip. This may include grasping and/or stacking plastic cups. Holding a cup automatically places the wrist and fingers in a gravity-lessened plane (forearm neutral) while the patient extends the wrist and flexes the fingers (Image 5). Having the patient practice grasping handfuls of dried beans or cotton balls, extending the wrist, and transferring them from one container to another is another useful and functional activity. To increase the challenge, the patient may perform this exercise with both hands by squeezing and twisting a soft object while forcefully extending the involved wrist, such as with squeezing water out of a rag.

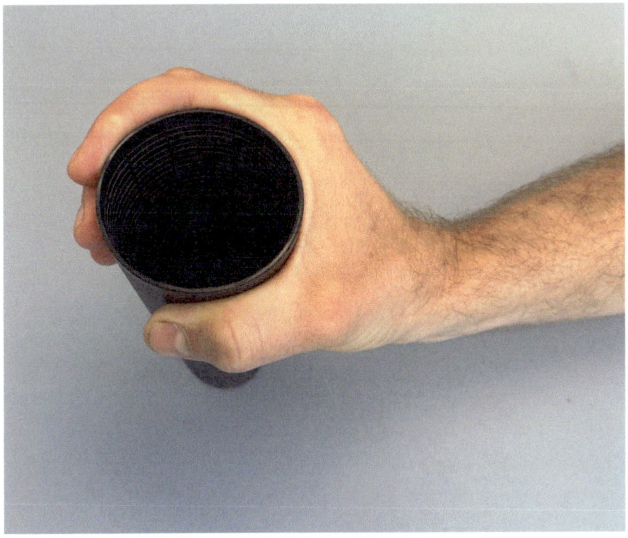

Image 5 Holding a cup or cone positions the wrist and fingers in a gravity-lessened, forearm neutral plane. Instruct the patient to extend the wrist and flex the fingers while grasping it

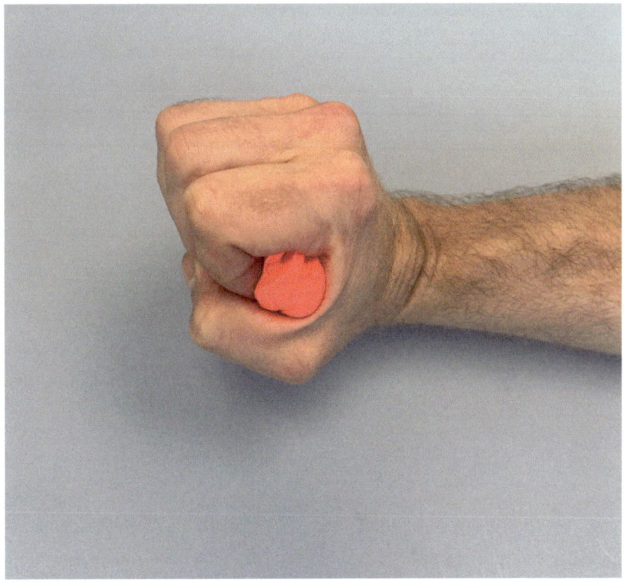

Image 6 Recipient FDS strengthening is achieved by squeezing therapy putty. Adding resisted donor/ECRB action will increase the response

Assessment of Recovery

To assess for return of the FDS, the therapist stabilizes the MCP and wrist joints in neutral. Pressure is applied to the dorsal surface of the hand. Have the patient resist wrist extension while trying to flex the PIP joint of each finger. An MMT score of 3/5 is achieved if the patient can actively flex the PIP joints through full available passive range. Resistance should not be applied to the recipient muscle until the patient demonstrates full active PIP flexion. Care should be taken to ensure that the patient is not inadvertently using tenodesis to produce active finger flexion. This is why blocking the patient's wrist in neutral to avoid extension is so important, as it would allow the fingers to bend with passive tension from the flexor tendons.

Frequency of Visits

It is appropriate for patients to attend therapy two to three times per month at this stage in recovery. However, there is a large emphasis on consistent home exercises. Some individuals may need more frequent therapy sessions if they are not compliant with home therapy or if they struggle with other factors, including insufficient passive finger motion, persistent edema, cognition, or complex regional pain syndrome (CRPS).

Phase 3

3+/5 MMT in the Recipient Muscle

Once the patient can achieve full finger flexion, treatment advances to regaining functional grasp and improving strength for daily tasks.

Exercises

- Resistive Recipient Activity with Donor Contraction
  Gripping therapy putty in the position of wrist extension will inherently recruit the donor with resistance to the recipient (Image 6). The patient may also grasp a dowel, place it in therapy putty on a table, and attempt to pull the dowel towards them or in the direction of wrist extension to demand more from the donor while maintaining grasp. Using a resistance band for resisted wrist extension will increase demand on the donor while grasping a foam handle to encourage finger flexion with the FDS (Image 7).
- Resistive Recipient Activity Without Donor Contraction
  For many nerve transfers, there may be instances in which recipient muscle strength is needed without donor recruitment. However, due to the synergistic nature of wrist extension and finger flexion, it is not as helpful to completely de-emphasize the assistive component of the ECRB while strengthening grasp. Eventually, one may gradually reduce the degrees of wrist extension during a grasping activity, such as holding a small weight in neutral wrist while performing a biceps curl (Image 8). Alternatively, one can challenge the patient to maintain grasp on a light weight while performing a wrist flexion curl with the forearm supinated. Resistive finger flexion (such as using a hand gripper) with the wrist in flexion may be advantageous in some situations, such as for personal hygiene.

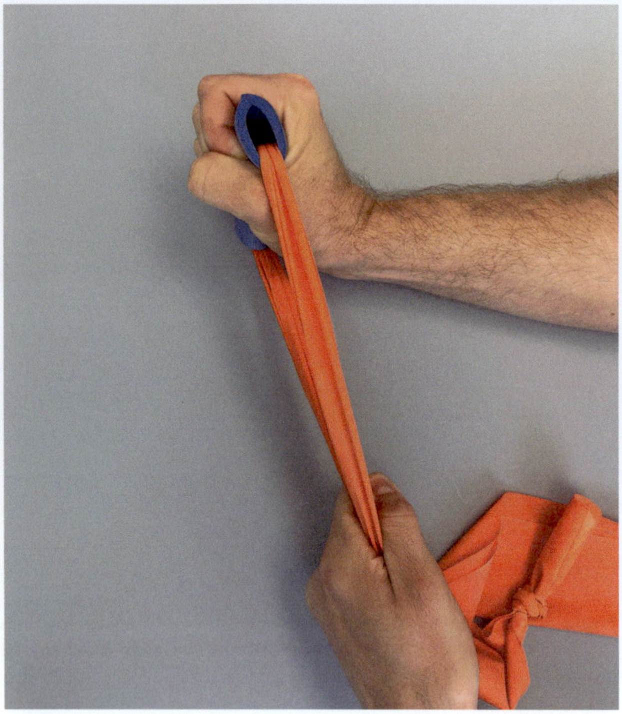

Image 7 To increase donor contribution with grip strengthening, resistance bands may be used with a foam tube handle to encourage grasp

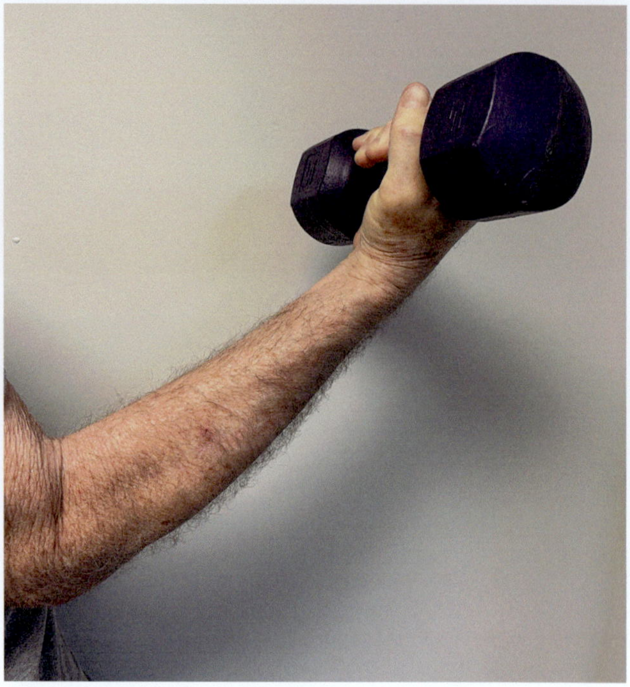

Image 8 To advance grip strength without donor contribution, hand weights may be added to biceps curls with the wrist flexed and the forearm supinated

Neuromuscular electrical stimulation (NMES) at this stage may be helpful to increase muscle strength [11]. Performing functional grasping while participating in NMES is also helpful in reeducating the neuromuscular pathway. It is important to note that NMES is only indicated in either innervated or partially innervated muscle.

ECRB-to-FDS nerve transfer

Nerve transfer overview					
Donor nerve	Donor action	Recipient nerve	Recipient action	Indications for functional restoration	Approximate months to functional movement
Radial nerve	Wrist extension	Median nerve to the FDS	Finger flexion	Grasp of objects and grip strength	18 months [7] (limited data)

Information below is suggested guidelines; precautions may vary according to surgeon preferences and patient factors

	Preoperative therapy	Early phase	Middle phase	Late phase
Criteria	Before surgery	0/5 to 1/5 MMT	2−/5 to 3/5 MMT	>3/5 MMT
Purpose of phase	Educate and establish baseline function	Understand donor and recipient relationship Activate donor	Consistently activate recipient in gravity-lessened planes	Isolate recipient against gravity and with resistance
Precautions	Avoid excessive lengthening of the FDS and shortening of the digital extensors	Prevent hyperextension of the MCP and PIP joints to avoid stiffness	Respect fatigue Protect recipient length	Respect fatigue
Frequency of visits (considerations)	1–2 visits; may increase if PROM limitations are present	1×/week until PROM is full and patient is independent with donor activation; then 1× monthly	1× week to 1× month based on patient needs and demonstration of accuracy and compliance of exercise program	1× every 1–2 weeks based on progress toward patient-specific goals
Orthosis considerations	NA	Wrist immobilization for 2–3 weeks for protection Once the rest period has ended, consider an anti-claw orthosis to prevent excessive MCP joint extension while trying to simultaneously isolate the ECRB and FDS	Continue anti-claw orthosis to block MCP hyperextension and place the fingers in a position of opportunity for flexion during transfer training	NA
Interventions		**Donor activation**: Wrist extension **Donor-recipient pairing**: Active or resisted wrist extension with passive composite finger flexion Consider an elastic flexion strap placing the fingers in passive flexion while working on donor activation	**Active/resisted donor with active-assisted recipient**: Wrist extension with active-assisted finger flexion **Place and hold**: Place the fingers in full composite flexion. Remove the support, and maintain this position (with simultaneous wrist extension)	**Resisted donor and recipient**: Resisted finger flexion with the wrist extended Therapy putty, resistance bands, or light weights may be used **Resisted recipient**: Resisted finger flexion with the wrist in neutral or slight flexion when needed
Additional intervention considerations		During recovery, patients often posture the fingers rigidly in extension due to absence of the flexors. Dynamic/static-progressive orthoses and flexion gloves/straps may be helpful	Functional tasks are encouraged, such as stacking cones, picking up cups, and wringing out a washrag	Combined finger and wrist flexion is not often mechanically advantageous, but it may be useful for some functional tasks

During all phases, it is essential to continue cortical reorganization and psychological and psychosocial interventions and progress to incorporate donor/recipient with ADLs

ECRB-to-FDS Nerve Transfer

Goal of Surgery: Restore the ability to bend your fingers

Recipient Movement = Finger flexion

Recipient Muscle: Flexor digitorum superficialis (FDS)

Recipient Nerve: Median nerve

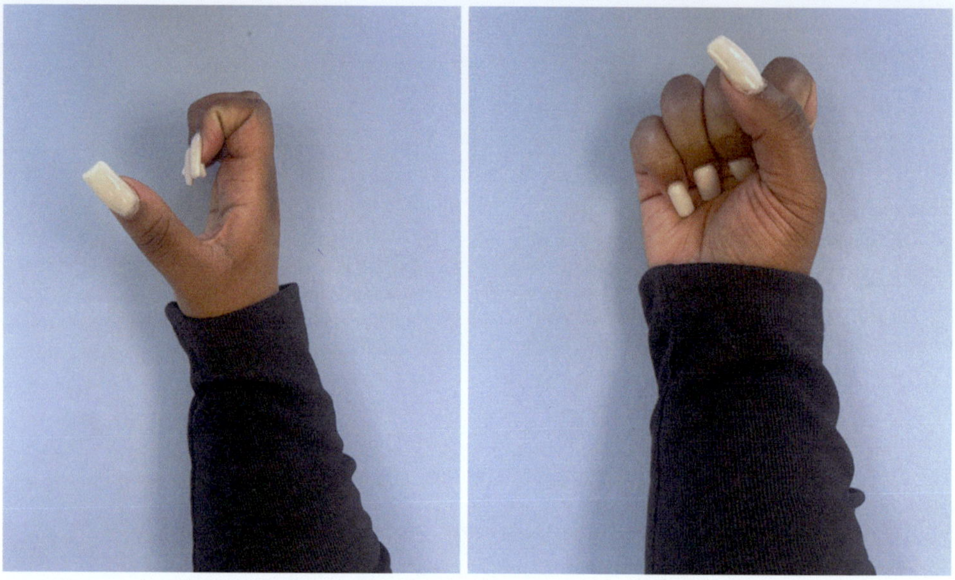

Bend fingers into a claw (hook fist flexion); Bend fingers into a fist (finger flexion)

Donor Movement = Wrist extension
Donor Muscle: Extensor carpi radialis brevis (ECRB)
Donor Nerve: Radial nerve

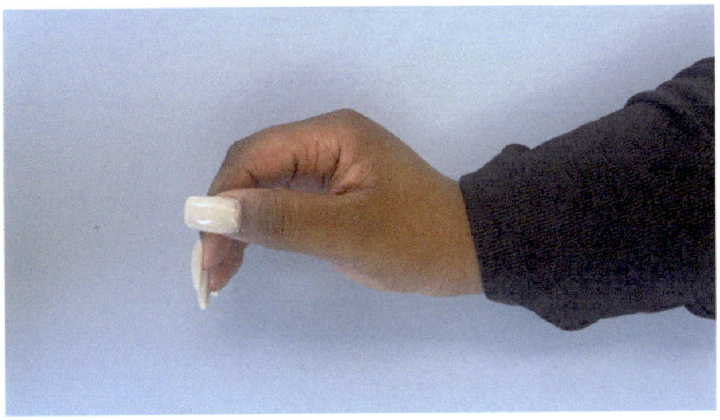

Pull wrist back (wrist extension)

Phase 1 ECRB-to-FDS Nerve Transfer Exercises

☐ **Active or Resisted Donor Movement**:

- Begin with your forearm facing down, resting on a table. Actively extend your wrist, and hold this position for 3–5 s.

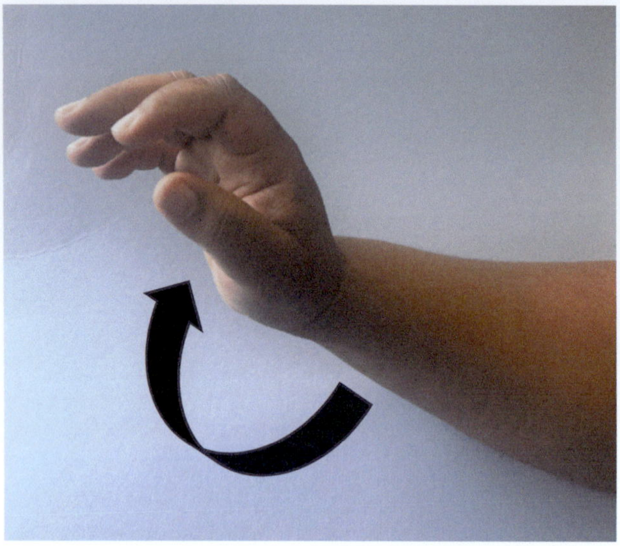

Complete 10 repetitions every waking hour.

- You may also add resistance using pressure from your opposite hand. Push down onto the back of your hand, and resist for 5 s. Perform 6 repetitions, 4 times per day.

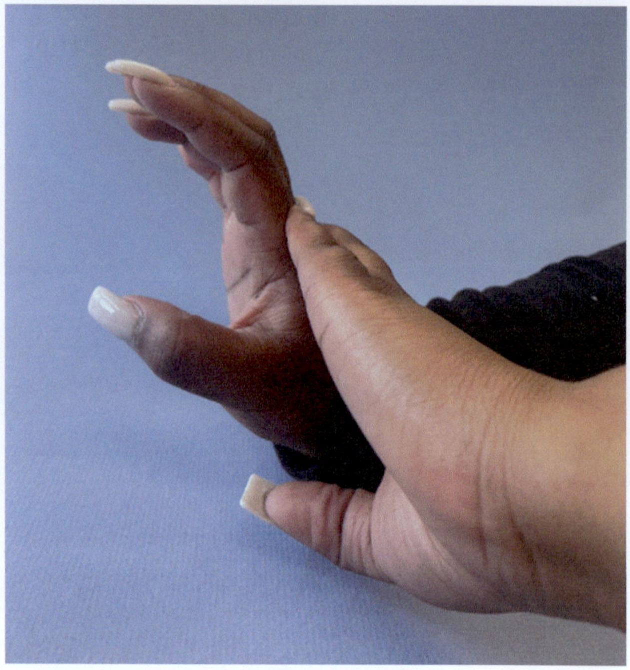

- Your therapist may suggest wearing an anti-claw splint during this exercise if you are having a difficult time relaxing the fingers.

☐ **Combined Donor + Pasvsive Recipient Movement**:

- Pull your wrist back, and use your other hand to bend the fingers into the palm. Hold for 3–5 s. Then bring your wrist forward, and let your fingers naturally straighten out.

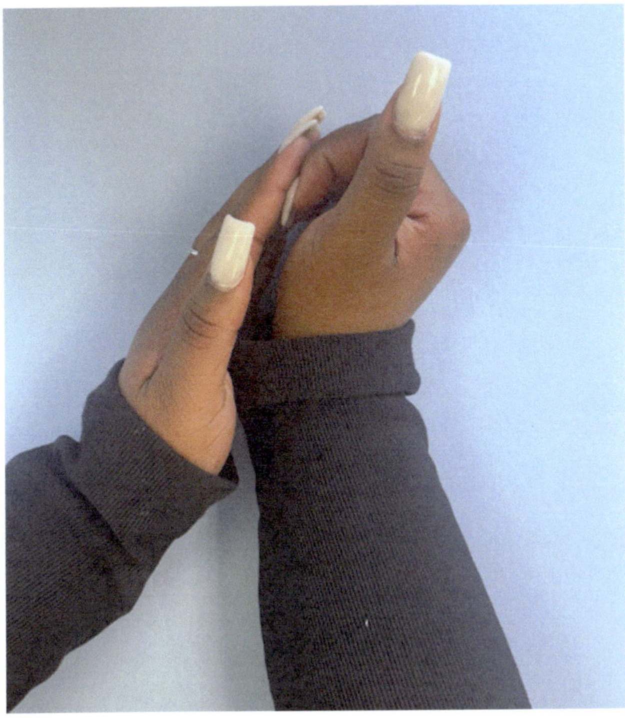

- If your fingers are very stiff, your therapist may provide you with a simple elastic strap that places your fingers into a fist. While this is on your hand, bend the wrist back and forth.

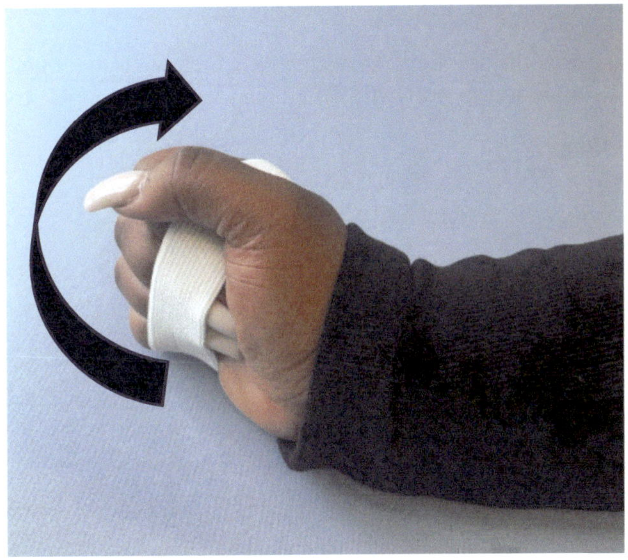

Phase 2 ECRB-to-FDS Nerve Transfer Exercises

Complete all checked exercises for 1–10 repetitions, 2–3 times per day.

☐ **Combined Donor + Active-Assisted Recipient**:

- Sit with your forearm resting on a table with the thumb facing up. Actively slide/bend your wrist back as you try to curl your fingers into a fist. As you reach the point where you cannot bend the fingers anymore on your own, use your opposite hand to bend the fingers further into a tight fist.

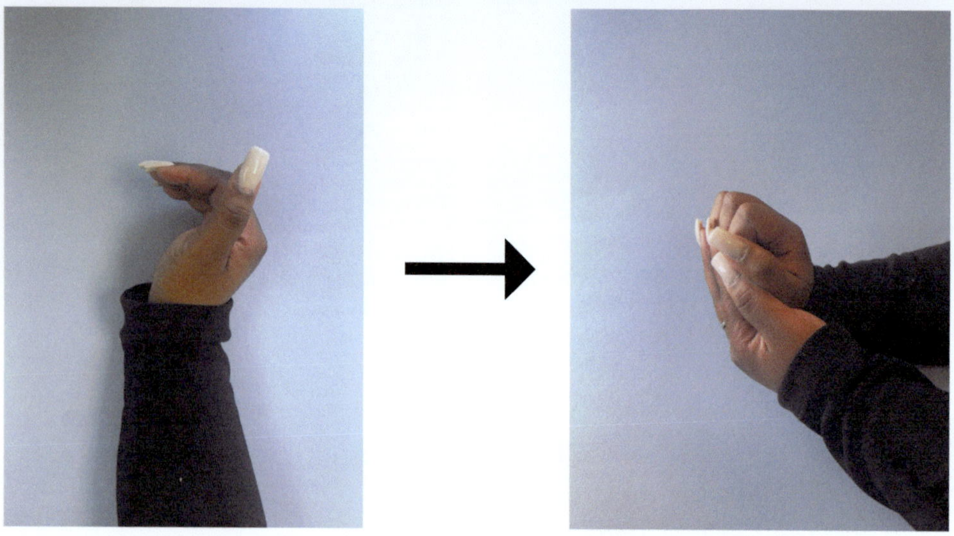

- If you are having a hard time relaxing the big knuckles of your fingers, your therapist may fabricate you an anti-claw splint, which will help keep these knuckles (MCP joints) bent so you can more easily work on bringing the rest of your fingers into the palm.

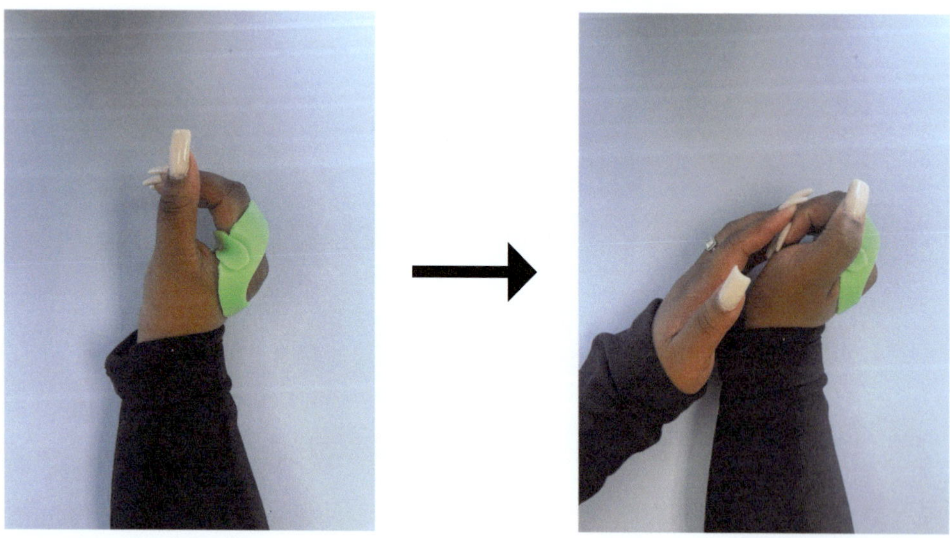

□ **"Place-and-Hold" Exercise**

- Bend your wrist back as you assist in curling your fingers into a fist with your other hand. Release the support, and attempt to maintain this position for 3–5 s. Relax and repeat. You will become more successful at maintaining this position as the recipient muscle becomes stronger.

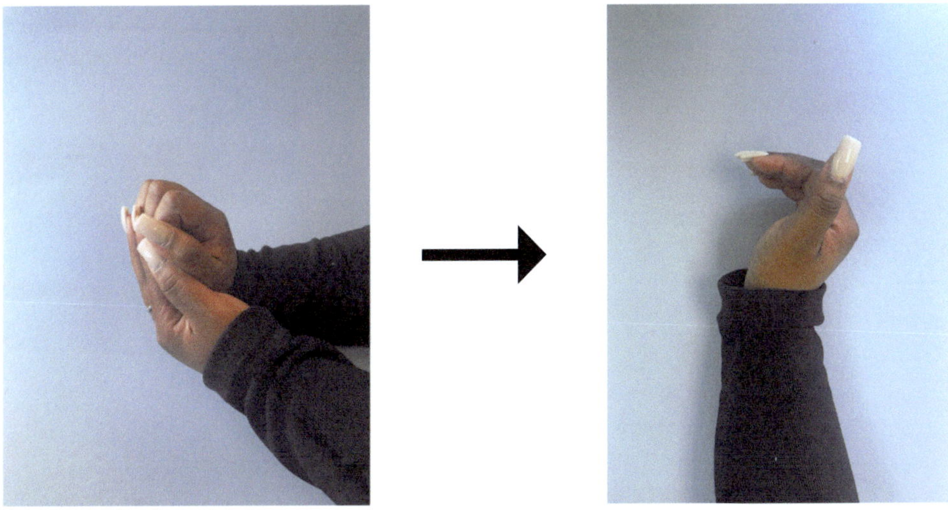

☐ Active Donor + Active Recipient

- Work on actively lifting your wrist up while curling your fingers into a fist (without assistance). Then bend the wrist, and open the fingers. Repeat.

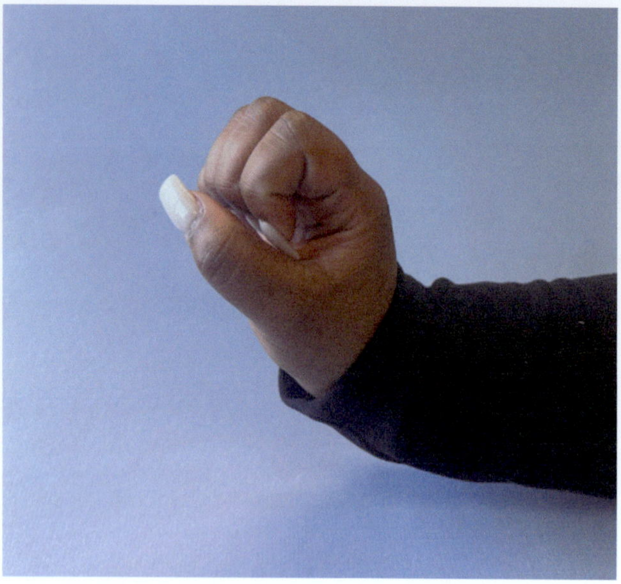

☐ Functional Activities

Complete daily activities such as holding a water bottle or stacking plastic cups. Transferring light objects such as cotton balls into a container or turning the top of a pepper mill encourages active finger bending/flexion. You can increase the challenge by wringing out a kitchen towel with both hands. The key is to activate the muscles that lift your wrist back during these activities.

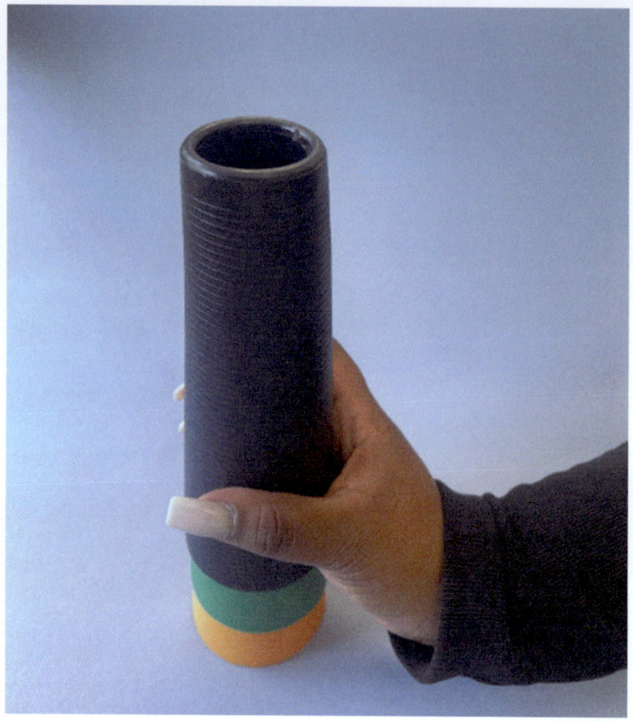

Phase 3 ECRB-to-FDS Nerve Transfer Exercises

Complete all checked exercises for 10 repetitions, 2–3 times daily.

☐ **Resisted Recipient with Donor Contraction**:

- Place a looped end of a resistance band around your hand. Use your **opposite** hand to pull the band downward as you bring the **injured** wrist up and squeeze the band with your fingers. Relax and repeat. To improve finger bending, consider using a foam handle around the resistance band.

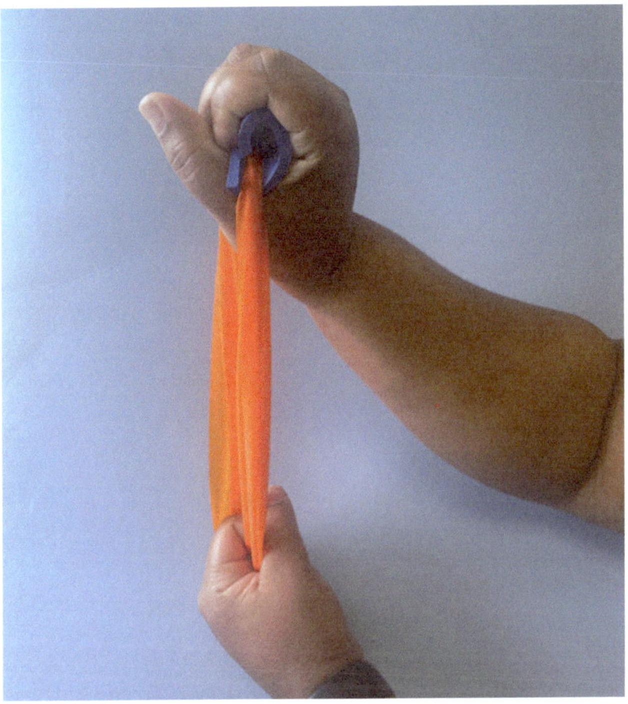

- Using therapy putty, gently squeeze the putty with all of your fingers equally while keeping your wrist pulled back. Try to hold for 3–5 s, relax, and repeat.

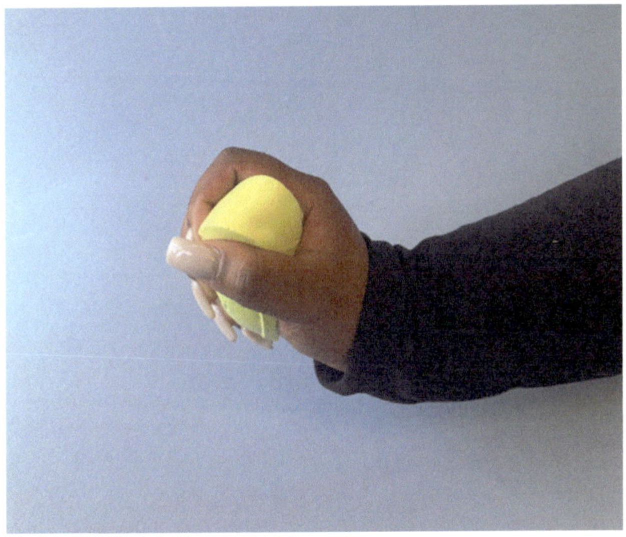

☐ **Resisted Recipient Without Donor Contraction**:

- Hold onto a light weight prescribed by your therapist with your wrist in a straight or slightly flexed position. Complete slow elbow curls while keeping the weight firmly grasped in your hand.

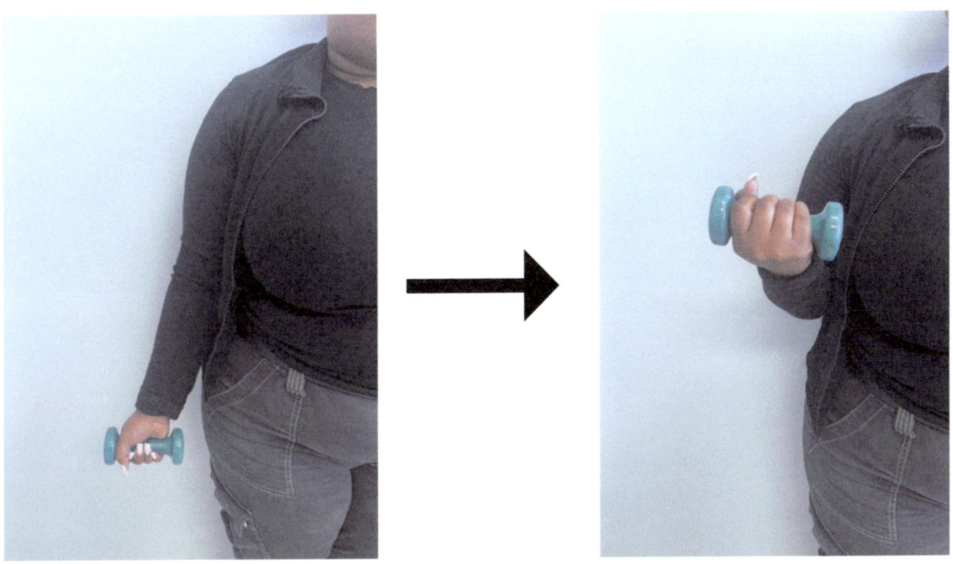

- Begin with your palm facing up and your wrist hanging off the table edge. Using a lightweight dumbbell, slowly flex the wrist while holding the weight and then slowly lower it back down.

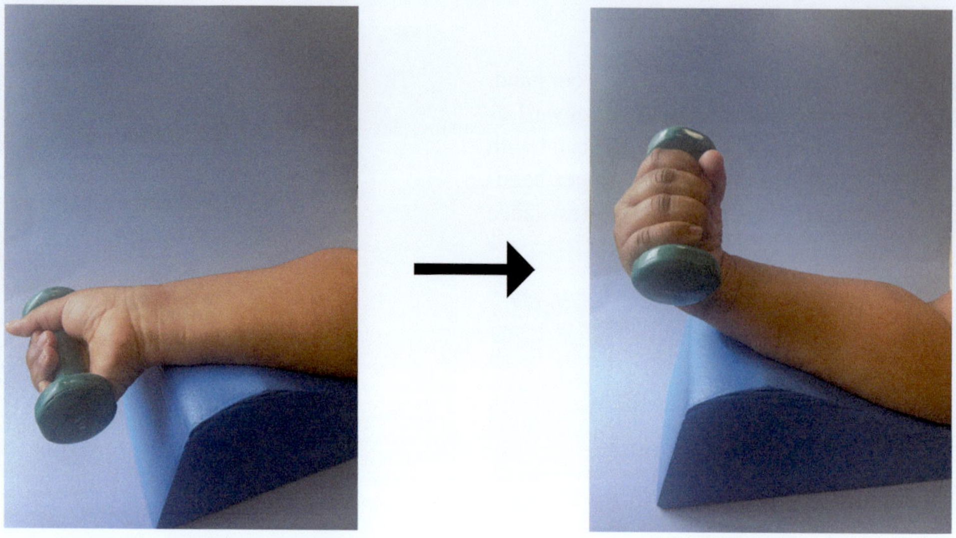

References

1. Kendall FP, McCreary EK, Provance PG, Rodgers MM, Romani WA. Muscles: testing and function with posture and pain, vol. 5. Lippincott Williams & Wilkins; 2005.
2. Mackinnon SE. Nerve surgery. Thieme; 2015.
3. Bertelli JA, Soldado F, Lehn VL, Ghizoni MF. Reappraisal of clinical deficits following high median nerve injuries. J Hand Surg Am. 2016;41(1):13–9.
4. Soldado F, Bertelli J, Ghizoni M. High median nerve injury: motor and sensory nerve transfers to restore function. Hand Clin. 2016;32:209–17.
5. Lo C, Tran Y, Anderson K, Craig A, Middleton J. Functional priorities in persons with spinal cord injury: using discrete choice experiments to determine preferences. J Neurotrauma. 2016;33(21):1958–68.
6. Boswick JA, Stromberg WB. Isolated injury to the median nerve above the elbow: a review of thirteen cases. J Bone Joint Surg. 1967;49(4):653–8.
7. Jitpun E, Rojanawatsirivej A, Tangviriyapaiboon T. Single-stage double motor nerve transfer for all finger flexion in iatrogenic C8-T1 spinal nerve injury: a case report and review of literature. Acta Neurochir. 2022;164(10):2683–8.
8. Kahn L, Moore A. Donor activation focused rehabilitation approach: maximizing outcomes after nerve transfers. Hand Clin. 2016;32(2):263–77.
9. Tam SL, Archibald V, Tyreman N, Gordon T. Tetrodotoxin prevents motor unit enlargement after partial denervation in rat hindlimb muscles. J Physiol. 2002;543(2):655–63.
10. Kahn LC, Stonner MM, Dy CJ. Key concepts for nerve transfer rehabilitation after surgical reconstruction for brachial plexus and peripheral nerve injuries. J Hand Surg Am. 2023;49:160.
11. Limthongthang R, Muennoi P, Phoojaroenchanachai R, Vathana T, Wongtrakul S, Songcharoen P. Effectiveness and safety of home-based muscle electrical stimulator in brachial plexus injury patients. J Med Assoc Thail. 2014;97(9):S56–61.

Extensor Carpi Radialis Brevis (ECRB) Branch of the Radial Nerve to the Anterior Interosseous Nerve (AIN) Transfer

Amy M. Young

Background

The anterior interosseous nerve (AIN) is a branch of the median nerve and innervates the flexor pollicis longus (FPL), index and middle finger flexor digitorum profundus (FDP), and pronator quadratus (PQ) muscles. An AIN deficit limits one's ability to make the "OK" sign or flex the thumb interphalangeal joint and index finger DIP joint tip-to-tip [1, 2]. Weakness of middle-finger DIP joint flexion and forearm pronation (in elbow extension) is also noted. Pinch, grasp, and fine-motor dexterity are severely impaired when an individual is unable to flex the thumb to the index fingertip. The extensor carpi radialis brevis (ECRB)-to-AIN nerve transfer is a reliable procedure that promotes the restoration of functional pinch and grasp. This transfer may be performed for isolated AIN impairment or combined with other nerve transfers to address more extensive deficits from proximal injuries such as high median nerve injury, C7–T1 brachial plexus root avulsion, or C6–C7 cervical spinal cord injury [3–5].

Outcomes

Solaja et al. describe the outcomes of ten patients who underwent supercharged end-to-side (SETS) ECRB-to-AIN transfer for Parsonage-Turner syndrome specifically impairing the AIN [3]. Preoperatively, median FPL strength was manual muscle testing (MMT) grade 1.5/5, and median index finger FDP strength was grade 1/5. At a mean follow-up of nearly 15 months post-surgery, this group of patients achieved a median MMT grade of 4/5 for thumb FPL strength and 5/5 for index finger FDP strength. Grip and pinch strength measurements were only available for four of the ten patients. Compared to the unaffected side, a mean grip strength of 92% and a mean lateral pinch strength of 79% were achieved. However, this appeared to be highly variable. Bertelli also performed the ECRB-to-AIN transfer on two patients with high median and ulnar nerve injuries and two patients with C7–T1 brachial plexus root avulsions [4]. Other nerve transfers were also performed simultaneously based on individual patient needs. At approximately 13-month follow-up, all four patients demonstrated the ability to make a full composite fist, touching all fingertips to the palm. Mean grip strength for this group was approximately 11 pounds, and mean lateral pinch strength, approximately 4.4 pounds. Additionally, Bertelli [4] noted improvement in the ability to flex all the fingers, not just the median nerve-innervated index and middle. All four patients who underwent ECRB-to-AIN transfer achieved MMT grade 4/5 strength in the FPL and the FDP of the index, middle, and ring fingers. Strength recovery in the small finger was more varied; two patients achieved grade 4/5 strength, and two patients achieved grade 3/5 strength.

In a group of three patients with C6 and C7 cervical spinal cord injuries, Bertelli and his group performed ECRB-to-AIN nerve transfers in five limbs [5]. MMT grade of 4/5 for finger flexion strength was achieved at an average of 17 months following surgery. In four limbs, restoration of finger flexion at the ulnar-innervated ring and small fingers was also observed. It is hypothesized that this phenomenon may be due to tendon interconnections between the radial and ulnar fingers or neural interconnections between the median nerve and musculature traditionally thought to be innervated by the ulnar nerve [5]. In an anatomical study by Sanapanich et al. [6], it was found that nearly 1/3 of cadavers studied had branches from the AIN to the FDP of the ulnar fingers.

Following surgery in the Bertelli study described above, wrist extension movement and strength were maintained [3, 5]. To promote optimal outcomes, the ECRB-to-AIN nerve transfer should be performed no later than 6 months post-injury [2, 4].

A. M. Young (✉)
Northwestern Medicine Center for Surgery of the Hand, Chicago, IL, USA
e-mail: Amy.Young@nm.org

L. C. Kahn et al. (eds.), *Rehabilitation for Nerve Transfers of the Upper Extremity*,
https://doi.org/10.1007/978-3-031-92008-0_22

Surgical Graphic

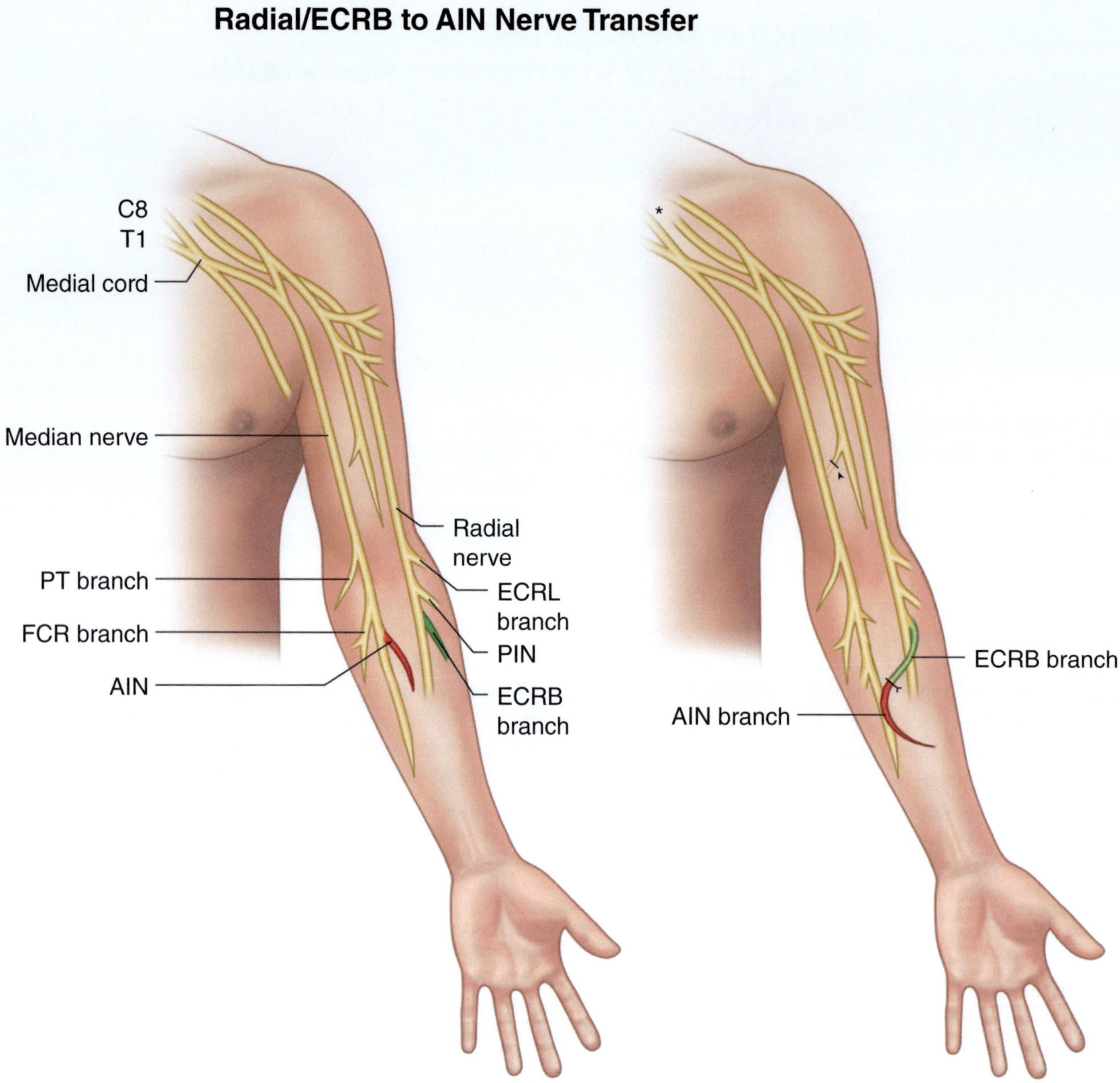

A curvilinear incision is made along the volar aspect of the proximal two-thirds of the forearm. The brachioradialis muscle is identified, and the superficial radial nerve is dissected on the undersurface of the brachioradialis muscle. The superficial radial nerve is used as a guide to dissect retrograde (distal to proximal) to identify the posterior interosseous nerve and the radial nerve proper. There is typically a branch to the ECRB identified close to the point where the posterior interosseous nerve (PIN) and superficial radial nerve (SRN) branch from the radial nerve proper. Intraoperative stimulation is used to confirm the function of the ECRB branch. It is important to stimulate these branches within 30 min of the tourniquet being inflated (if one is being used) and ensure that the anesthesia team is not using any muscle paralytics. After doing so, the lacertus fibrosus is identified, and after releasing the lacertus fibrosus, the median nerve is identified deep to the lacertus fibrosus and along the inner surface of the flexor pronator mass. After decompressing the median nerve, the branching pattern of the median nerve is identified. It is helpful to decompress the FDS arch and subsequently identify the anterior interosseous nerve coming off the median nerve proper. A handheld nerve stimulator is used to confirm that the AIN is not functioning, again ensuring that this is done within 30 min of the tourniquet being inflated (if one is being used) and that there are no muscle paralytics being used by the anesthesia team. After doing so, the AIN is dissected from the median nerve as proximally as possible and divided. The donor ECRB branch nerve is dissected as proximally as possible from the radial nerve proper, divided distally, and then transposed to meet the recipient AIN. Coaptation of the ECRB branch to the AIN is performed using microsurgical technique.

Phases of Rehabilitation

Phase 1

Preoperative to 1/5 MMT in the Recipient Muscle(s)

Precautions

The thumb IP joint and index finger DIP joint are at high risk of joint stiffness following AIN impairment [7]. Passive joint motion of thumb IP joint and index finger DIP joint flexion should be maintained while awaiting reinnervation of the FPL and index finger FDP.

Prolonged, unbalanced hyperextension at these joints can lead to stiffness as well as overlengthening of FPL and index finger FDP. According to the length tension relationship of muscle, overlengthening may contribute to biomechanical failure of the muscle to produce desired movement and strength once reinnervation of the recipient muscles occurs [7–9]. A general rule to follow is to preserve recipient muscle length whenever possible.

Orthoses

The patient may wear a sling for the first week after surgery if needed for comfort. Many physicians prefer wrist immobilization for the first 2–3 weeks to protect the nerve coaptation. Once postoperative edema is resolved, finger-based orthoses that hold the index finger DIP and thumb IP joints in slight flexion (Image 1) may be worn during the day to help promote functional pinch and preserve muscle length. A thumb IP joint orthosis in neutral extension may be worn at night to avoid unopposed EPL tension into hyperextension and maintain muscle length (Image 2).

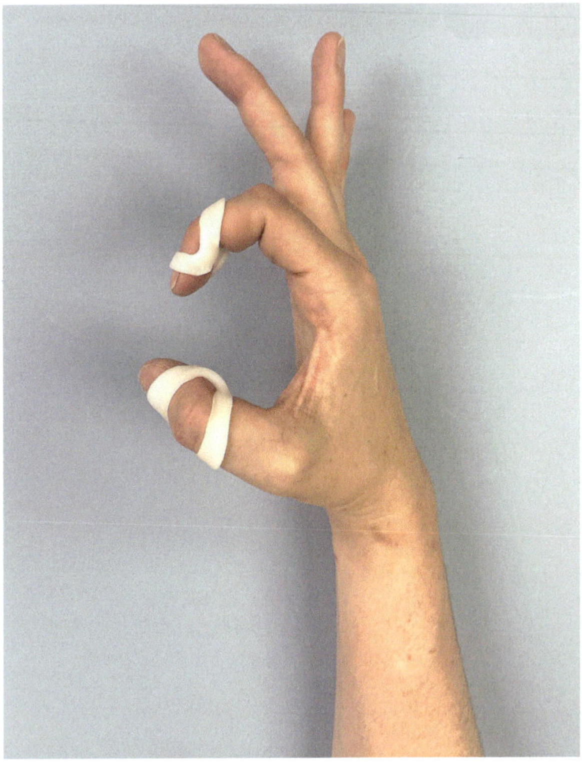

Image 1 Finger-based orthoses which maintain the thumb IP and index finger DIP joints in slight flexion are useful prior to surgery and postoperatively (once edema is resolved) to limit excessive hyperextension and improve function

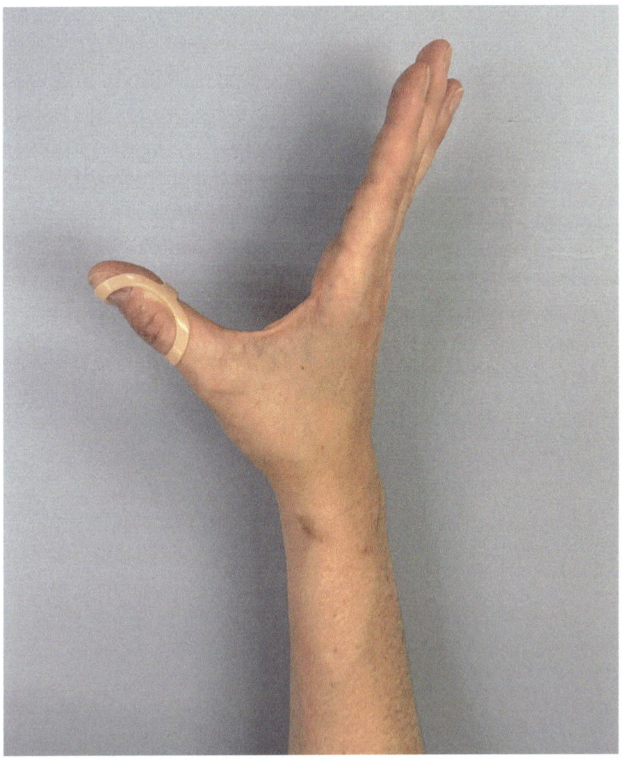

Image 2 A neutral prefabricated finger-based orthosis is demonstrated for use at night to limit hyperextension posturing

Exercises

- Passive Range of Motion
  Passive composite flexion of the thumb and index finger as well as isolated thumb IP flexion and index DIP flexion will help prevent and reduce joint stiffness [7]. Passive isolated index finger DIP flexion is necessary to stretch the often shortened oblique retinacular ligament (ORL).
- Donor Activation
  Donor muscle activation exercises in phase 1 include active and isometric wrist extension. After a rest period of 10–12 days following surgery, the patient may initiate donor muscle activation. Early-phase donor activation

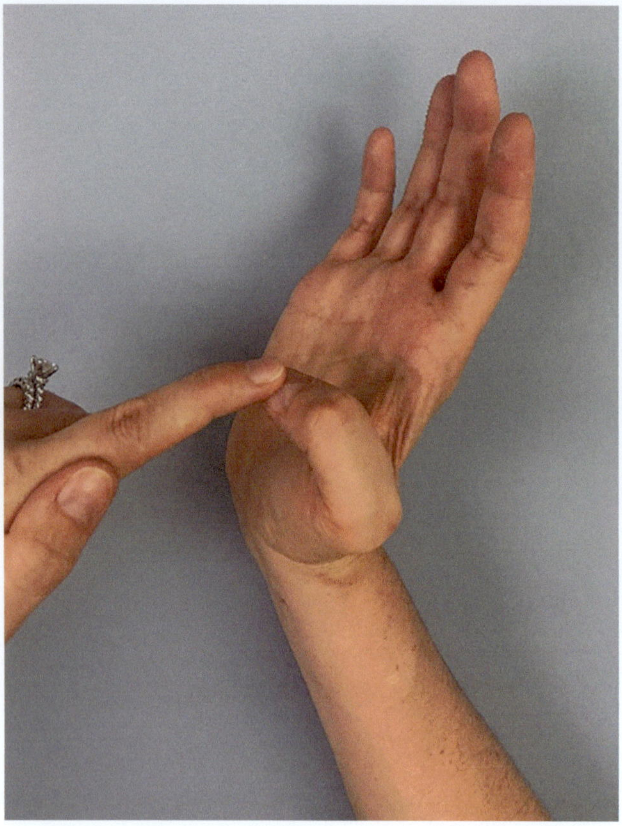

Image 3 In phase 1, active donor wrist extension is combined with passive recipient FPL activation to promote the new neural pathway and train the individual on how the nerve transfer will work

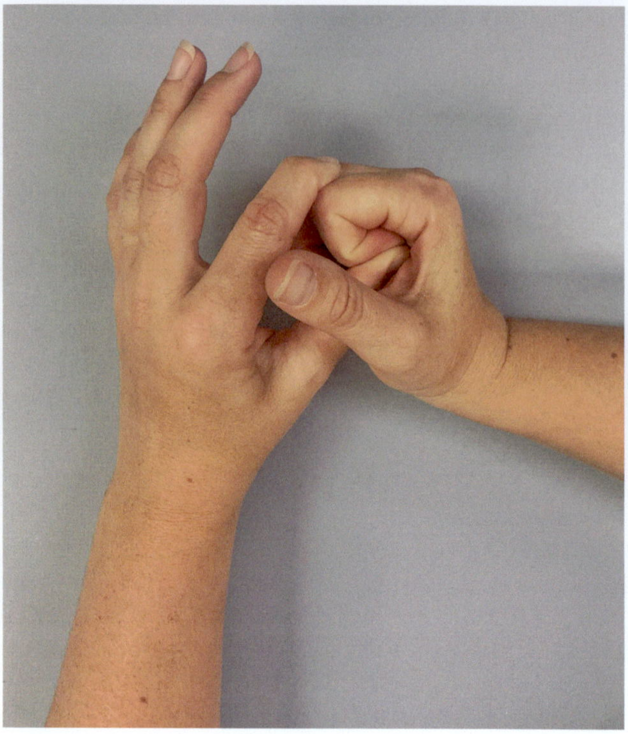

Image 4 Patterning of active donor wrist extension is also combined with passive FDP/finger flexion in phase 1

exercises are completed with high repetitions and high frequency to maximize neural signals to the donor muscle [10].

- Combined Donor with Passive Recipient Exercise
  Active wrist extension should be paired with simultaneous passive thumb flexion (Image 3). Active wrist extension should separately be paired with simultaneous passive index finger flexion (Image 4).

Clinical Pearl

To achieve accurate pairing wrist extension with passive thumb flexion, a simple exercise orthosis may be fabricated using a wrist strap, rubber band, and a sewing hook glued to the thumbnail. The rubber band is attached from the wrist cuff to the thumbnail hook. As the patient performs active wrist extension, the thumb passively flexes via the increased tension in the rubber band. This exercise orthosis can enhance proper completion of the paired donor with passive recipient movement and adherence to the home exercise program (Image 5).

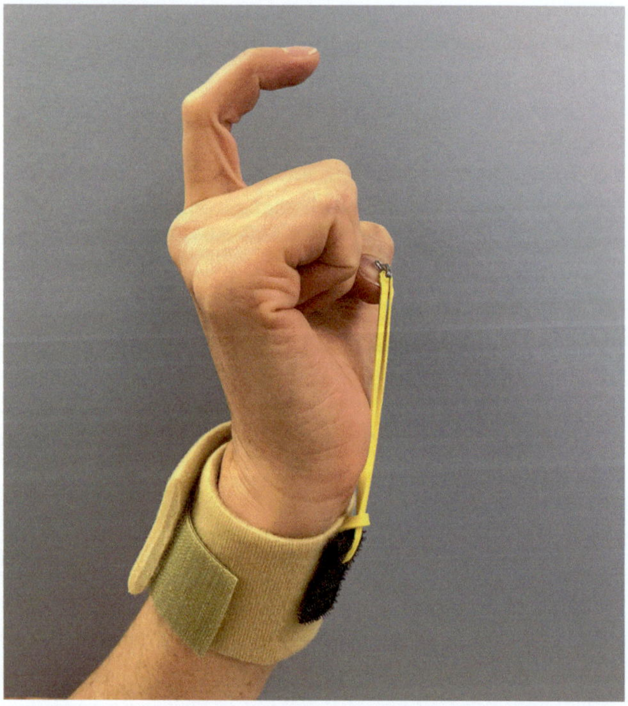

Image 5 This Kleinert-style device is simple and inexpensive to make and allows the individual to easily perform repetitive patterning exercises of active donor with passive recipient one-handed

Assessment of Recovery

Routine strength and range-of-motion measurements of the recipient muscles (FPL and index finger FDP), donor muscle (ECRB), and other affected muscles and joints provide helpful pre- and postoperative comparisons. The therapist should assess recipient MMT strength at least monthly to monitor recipient muscle recovery and determine appropriate therapeutic exercises and potential changes to home instructions. Grip and pinch strength measurements should also be obtained at these intervals.

To identify initial muscle contractions, the examiner resists wrist extension (donor activation) while the patient attempts to flex the thumb IP joint. Palpation over the volar aspect of the thumb proximal phalanx or volar radial forearm is performed to feel for FPL contraction (Image 6). Look for trace thumb IP joint flexion with the MCP joint blocked. (If no thumb function exists, then unblock the MCP as thumb flexion may occur at the CMC or MCP prior to the IP joint.) The same procedure should be performed to evaluate for index finger flexion. If the FDS is intact, the PIP joint should be blocked in extension to assess DIP flexion. Palpate over the volar aspect of index finger middle phalanx while monitoring index finger DIP joint for trace signs of flexion (Image 7). Trace muscle contraction may initially become evident at the FPL 3–4 months postoperatively with reinnervation of the hand progressing from the radial to ulnar side [4, 10]. At this point, goniometric measures of isolated thumb IP and index DIP flexion will provide more accurate assessment of monthly progress. It may take 12–24 months to achieve functional movement [1, 10].

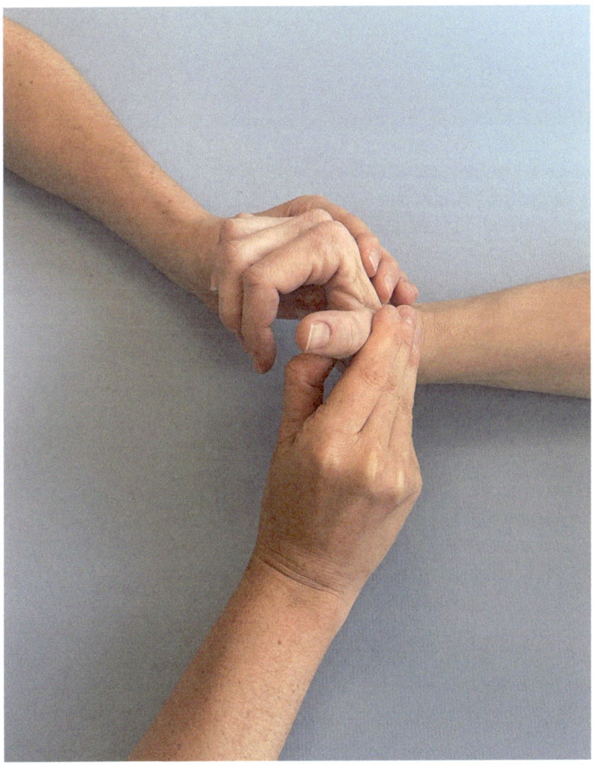

Image 6 To assess for recipient response in the FPL, donor wrist extension is resisted while the volar aspect of the thumb proximal phalanx is palpated. Early on, one is feeling for change in muscle-tendon tension, which often develops before actual movement of the IP joint

Clinical Pearl

Thumb EPL tension is unopposed without antagonist FPL activity. Therefore, thumb IP hyperextension may be observed. A patient may become skilled at relaxing the EPL from hyperextension to neutral extension, making it appear as if the FPL is contracting. When observing for muscle contraction of FPL, look for thumb IP flexion beyond 0 degrees of extension and palpate for muscle contraction. This compensatory movement pattern may also be observed at the index finger DIP joint due to unopposed tension at the terminal extensor tendon.

Therapy Frequency

Initially, frequency of therapy visits is generally one time per week. Once the patient demonstrates an understanding of the donor-recipient relationship and any soft tissue restrictions are resolved, the patient may benefit from continuing therapy one time per month.

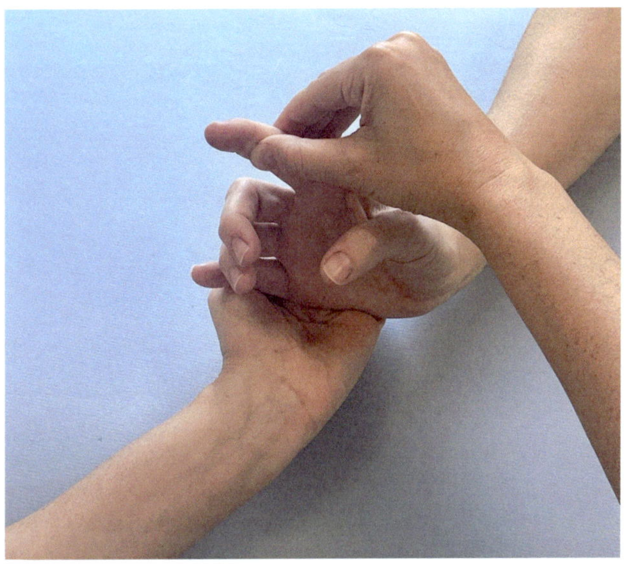

Image 7 To assess for recipient response in the index FDP, donor wrist extension is resisted while palpating the volar aspect of the index finger middle phalanx for tension changes in the FDP while the PIP is blocked

Phase 2

2–/5 to 3/5 MMT in the Recipient Muscle(s)

Orthoses

Patients may continue to use a finger-based orthosis (also called "oval-8" orthosis) that holds the thumb IP joint and index finger DIP joint in slight flexion during the day. Orthoses may be discontinued once the patient is able to achieve and maintain enough thumb IP flexion and index DIP flexion to overcome extensor tension. However, orthosis use during functional activities may be beneficial to enhance stability with functional pinch.

Exercises

Once the recipient muscle(s) can move in a partial range of movement, the patient progresses to phase 2 of rehabilitation. In this phase, the patient will begin active-assisted recipient activation as well as "place and hold" exercises [11]. Exercises may begin in a gravity-lessened plane and progress to an antigravity plane as strength improves. However, gravity may have less influence on thumb and finger flexion compared to larger and heavier proximal segments of the upper extremity [12].

- Active Donor with Active-Assisted Recipient
  FPL and Index FDP MMT = 2–/5 to 2/5
  Active wrist extension with simultaneous active-assisted index finger flexion is performed (Image 8). The patient may also continue to use the exercise cuff to pair active wrist extension with active-assisted thumb flexion. However, the focus will change from the thumb being a passive participant to an active participant. During active wrist extension, the patient initiates active thumb flexion, and the rubber band will assist into further IP flexion.
- "Place and Hold" Exercise
  FPL and Index FDP MMT = 2+/5
  The thumb and index finger are manually placed in a "C" shape or "OK sign" for midrange flexion (Image 9a), and the patient attempts to hold this position while actively extending the wrist (Image 9b). As strength progresses,

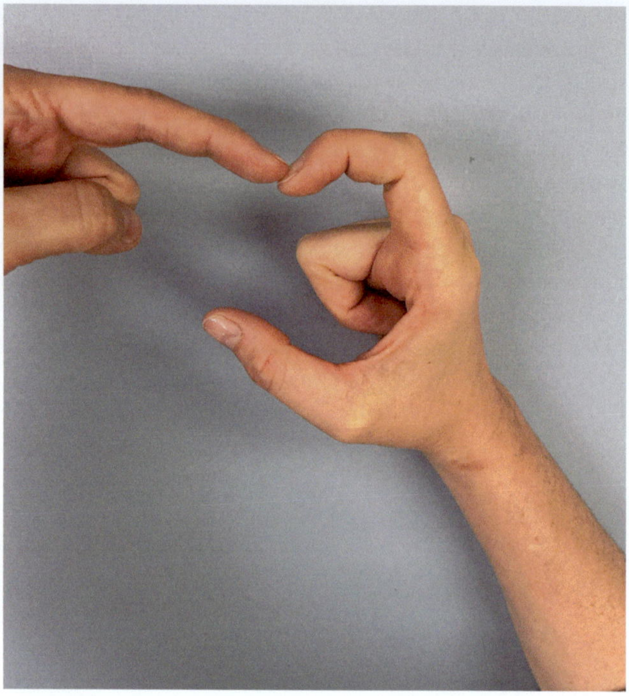

Image 8 Active donor with assisted recipient FDP is demonstrated. The individual is instructed to flex as far as they can, and gentle assistance is provided to complete the motion

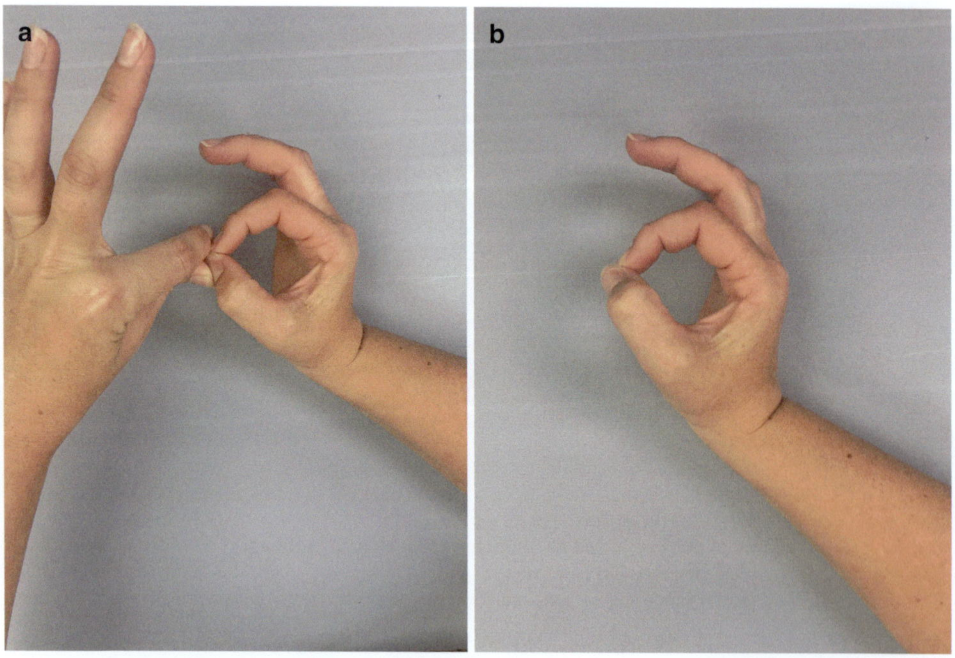

Image 9 (**a**) Place-and-hold exercises are performed with assistance to the available end range of motion for thumb and index finger flexion. (**b**) The support is then released, and the individual is instructed to attempt to maintain this position while keeping the wrist in full extension

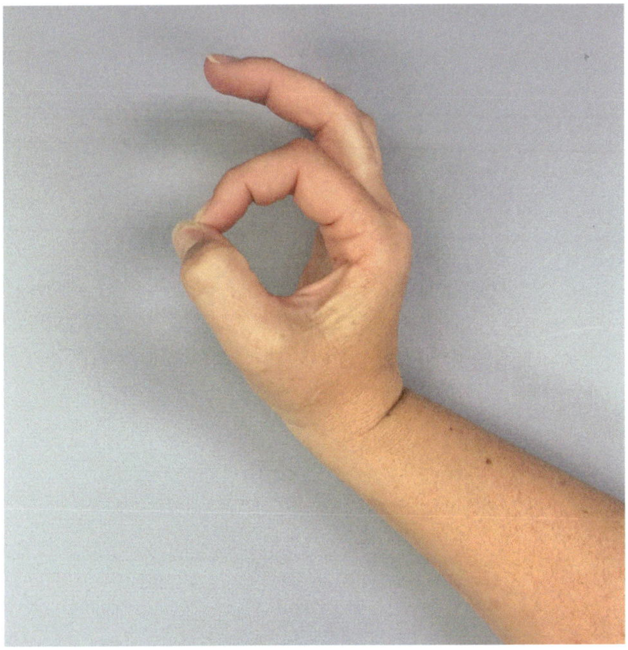

Image 10 Active donor with active recipient exercise is demonstrated with the individual pulling the wrist into full extension while making the "OK" sign

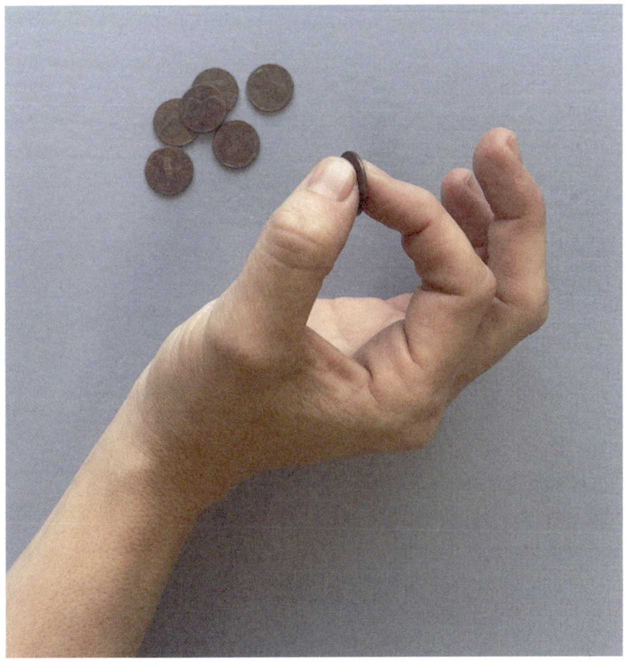

Image 11 Functional activities that involve tip-to-tip pinch are encouraged as strength and movement return

the exercise advances by placing the thumb IP joint and index finger DIP joint in end-range composite flexion during the "place and hold." At this time, isolated flexion exercises for the thumb IP and index finger DIP during resisted wrist extension will be required to accommodate end-range flexion at each joint.

- Active Donor with Active Recipient
  FPL and Index FDP MRC = 3/5 to 3−/5
  The patient actively extends the wrist while simultaneously trying to make a "C" or "OK sign" (Image 10).
- Functional Activity
  Patients are encouraged to perform functional activities that combine thumb and finger flexion with wrist extension such as wringing out a washcloth, pulling a door handle, and twisting a screwdriver. A buddy strap that holds the index and middle fingers together will improve participation of the index finger in functional grasp.
  Pinching activities initially involve picking up cotton balls or coins using tip-to-tip pinch (Image 11). Wider and spherical grasp patterns may be useful with grasp activities [7]. Patients may progress to more complex functional tasks based on individual goals such as buttoning, zipping, or writing.

Assessment of Recovery

The therapist should assess MMT strength of the FPL and index finger FDP with active or resisted wrist extension (donor activation). ECRB strength should be monitored to ensure that wrist extension does not bias to the ulnar side, which would indicate donor weakness and subsequent ECU compensation [4]. Measuring active thumb IP flexion and index finger DIP flexion with and without donor activation may be useful to highlight small changes over a prolonged period of time. Routine grip and pinch strength assessments are recommended. Fine-motor coordination assessments such as the 9-hole peg test will also provide objective measures of functional outcomes [13, 14].

Frequency

Frequency of therapy may be increased to one time per week or every other week in phase 2 based on patient needs.

Phase 3

3+/5 MMT and Greater

Once the recipient muscles (FPL and index finger FDP) begin to withstand some resistance, the patient may incorporate more advanced strengthening and functional tasks.

Exercises

- Resistive Recipient Activity with Donor Contraction
  Exercise prescription should continue to pair recipient activity with donor contraction, including exercises requiring resisted thumb and index finger flexion with resisted wrist extension. Pinching and pulling items (such as beads, marbles, or buttons) from therapy putty is one example of isolated resisted tip-to-tip pinch while still demanding a strong contraction of the donor

ECRB. Baltimore Therapeutic Equipment™ (BTE) tool #504 and #102 (at head tilt 5) and tool #302 (at head tilt 2–3) combine resisted thumb and finger flexion with resisted wrist extension as well (Image 12).

- Resistive Recipient Activity Without Donor Contraction
  The patient may progress to digital flexion exercises without donor contraction, if needed. The patient may complete tip-to-tip or three-point pinching into resistive therapy putty with the wrist in neutral or flexion (Image 13). Holding a pen in the hand while attempting to "click" the top button is another simple way to regain isolated functional strength (Image 14).

Assessment of Recovery

The therapist should assess MMT strength of the FPL and index finger FDP with and without resisted wrist extension (donor activation). Greatest strength will likely be noted during co-contraction of donor (ECRB) and recipient (FPL and index finger FDP) muscle activation for 2+ years post-surgery [11]. Therapists should continue to monitor grip and pinch strength and fine-motor coordination throughout the final phase of rehabilitation.

Frequency

Frequency of therapy may continue one time per week or every other week in phase 3.

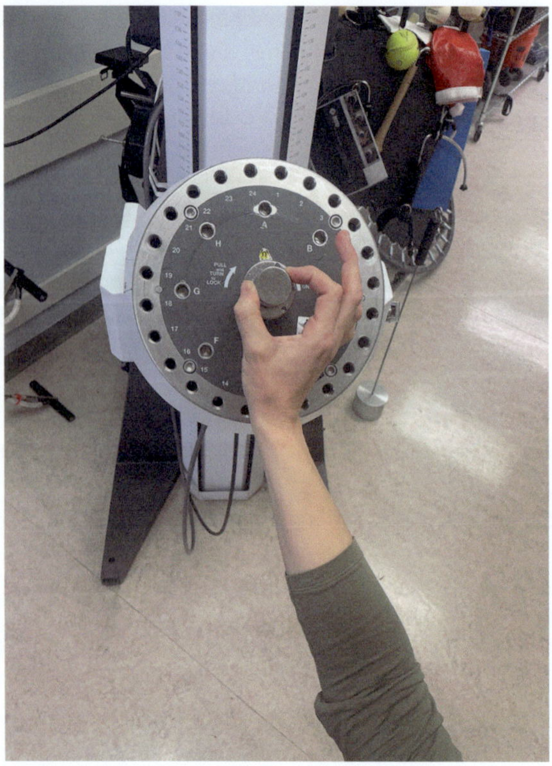

Image 12 Baltimore Therapeutic Equipment (BTE) tool 102, when available, is used to provide combined resistance to both donor wrist extensors and recipient FPL and index FDP

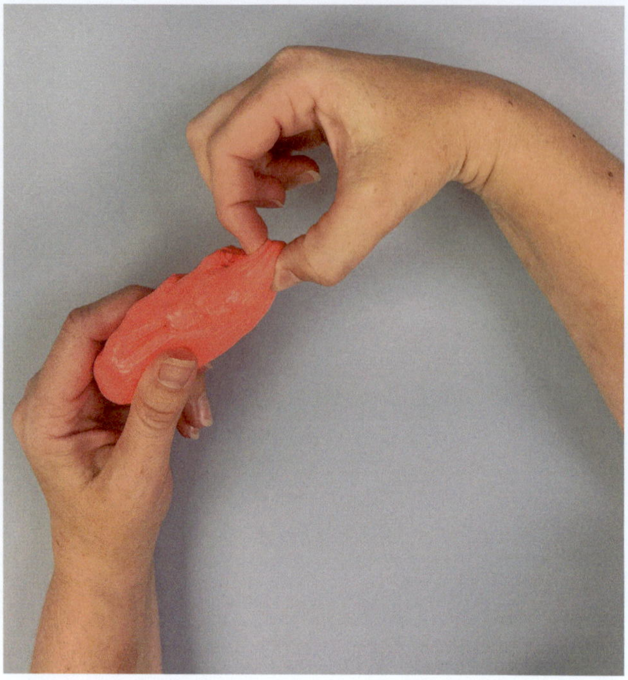

Image 13 Once adequate strength is achieved in the recipient muscles, de-emphasizing donor contributions may begin. The wrist is maintained in flexion, while resistance from therapy putty is applied to the FPL and index FDP during a pinch exercise

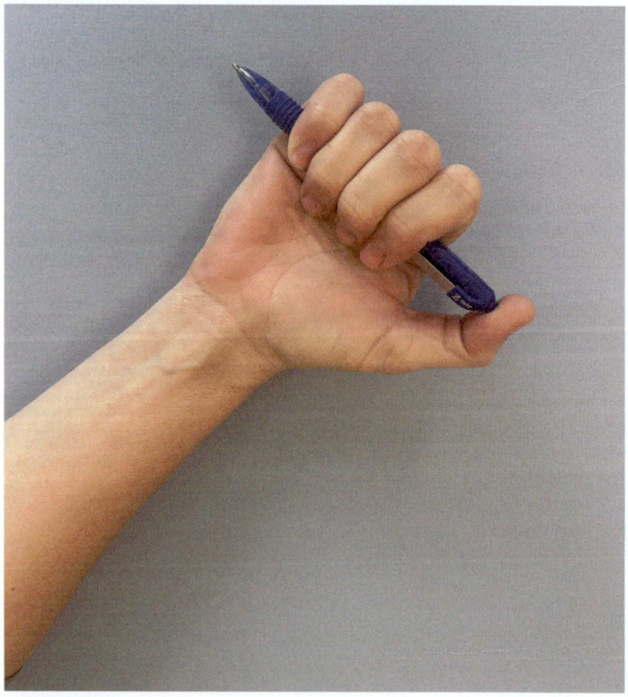

Image 14 Clicking the end of a pen while the wrist is held in neutral to slight flexion is a simple way to improve FPL strength and isolation

ECRB-to-AIN nerve transfer

Nerve transfer overview					
Donor nerve	Donor action	Recipient nerve	Recipient action	Indications for functional restoration	Approximate months to functional movement
Radial nerve	Wrist extension	Anterior interosseous nerve	Thumb IP and index DIP (and composite) joint flexion	Pinch, grasp, and fine motor dexterity	13–17 months [3–5]

Information below is suggested guidelines; precautions may vary according to surgeon preferences and patient factors

	Preoperative therapy	Early phase	Middle phase	Late phase
Criteria	Before surgery	0/5 to 1/5 MMT	2–/5 to 3/5 MMT	>3/5 MMT
Purpose of phase	Educate and establish baseline function	Understand donor and recipient relationship Activate donor	Activate nerve transfer for functional activities requiring light pinch	Isolate recipient through resistance Separate pinch function from donor activation (wrist extension)
Precautions	Avoid excessive lengthening of FPL and FDP	Prevent hyperextension of thumb IP and index DIP to limit stiffness and overlengthening	Respect fatigue Protect recipient length	Respect fatigue
Frequency of visits (considerations)	1–2 pre-op visits; may increase if PROM limitations are present	1×/week until PROM is full and patient is independent with donor activation; then 1× monthly	1×/week to 1×/month based on patient needs and accurate, consistent demonstration of exercise program	1× every 1–2 weeks based on progress toward patient-specific goals
Orthosis considerations	Consider finger-based orthoses with thumb IP and index DIP in slight flexion during the day	Wrist immobilization for 3 weeks for post-op protection Finger-based orthoses, maintaining thumb IP and index DIP in slight flexion, once the post-op period has ended	Continue finger-based orthoses with thumb IP and index DIP in slight flexion during day until active thumb IP and index DIP flexion can overcome extensor tension	NA
Interventions		**Donor activation**: Wrist extension **Donor-recipient pairing**: Active wrist extension with passive thumb IP and index DIP flexion	**Active/resisted donor with active assist recipient**: Wrist extension with active-assisted thumb/index flexion Optional use of exercise cuff in chapter (see Image 5) **Place and hold**: Place thumb and index into an "OK" position. Remove the support, and maintain this position with the wrist extended	**Resisted donor and recipient**: Wrist extension with resisted thumb IP and index DIP flexion **Resisted recipient**: Tip-to-tip or three-point pinching into resistance putty, holding pen to "click" top with wrist in neutral or flexion
Additional intervention considerations		See clinical pearl section of chapter—Image 5	**MMT 3–/5 to 3/5** Simultaneous "C" or "OK" sign with wrist extension Functional tasks such as wringing out washcloth, pulling door handle, twisting a screwdriver Pick up cotton balls using tip-to-tip pinch and progress to wider grasp patterns	Therapist facilitation of movement due to prolonged time of nonuse (may still need to activate donor for stronger contraction but continue to work on selective activation) Maximum strength and functional use may take 2–3 years to gain

**During all phases, it is essential to continue cortical reorganization and psychological and psychosocial interventions and progress to incorporate donor/recipient with ADLs

ECRB-to-AIN Nerve Transfer

Goal of Surgery: Restore ability to pinch and grasp

Recipient Movements = Bend thumb and index finger (thumb IP and index DIP flexion)

Recipient Muscles: Flexor pollicis longus (FPL) and flexor digitorum profundus (FDP)

Recipient Nerve: Anterior interosseous nerve (AIN)

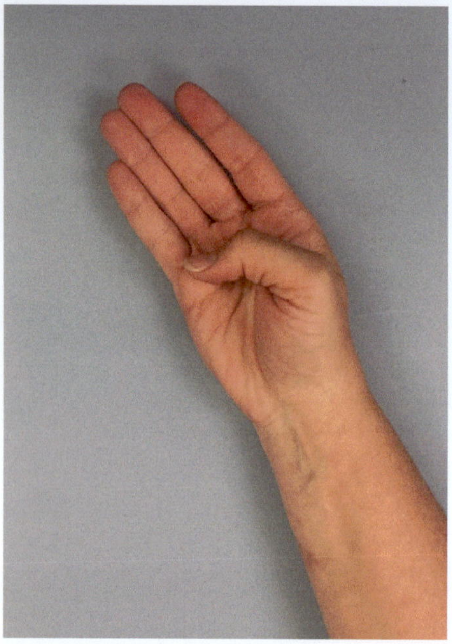

Bend thumb (thumb IP flexion)

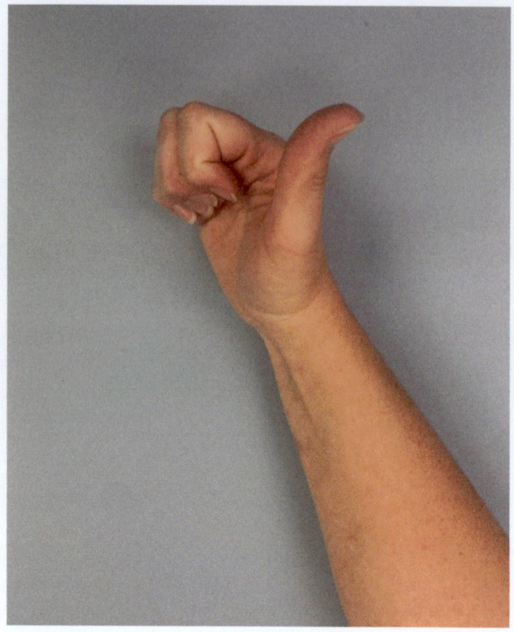

Bend index finger (index DIP flexion)

Donor Movement = Bend wrist back (wrist extension)
Donor Muscle: Extensor carpi radialis brevis (ECRB)
Donor Nerve: Radial nerve

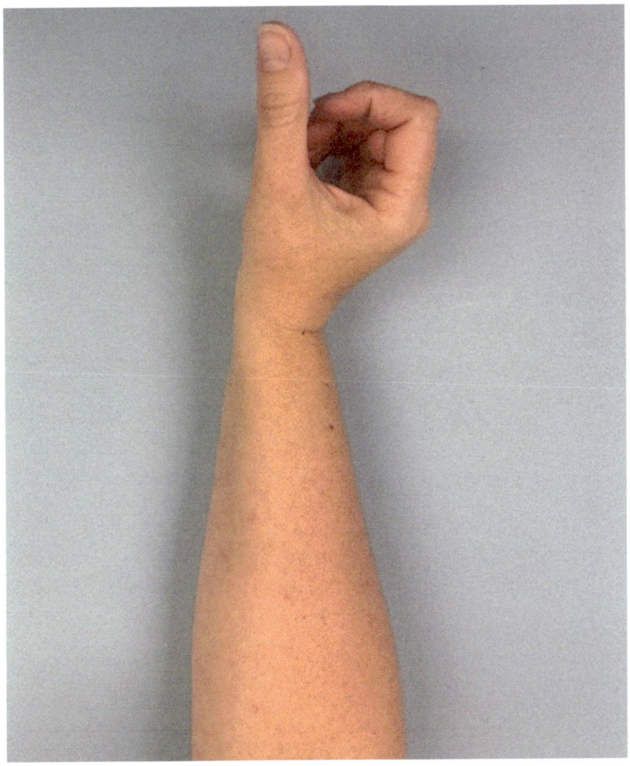

Bend wrist back (wrist extension)

Phase 1 ECRB-to-AIN Nerve Transfer Exercises

☐ **Passive Range of Motion**:
Complete each of the below exercises 3–5 repetitions, 3–5 times per day.
Hold for 10–30 seconds.

1. Using your other hand, push your entire thumb into a bent position.

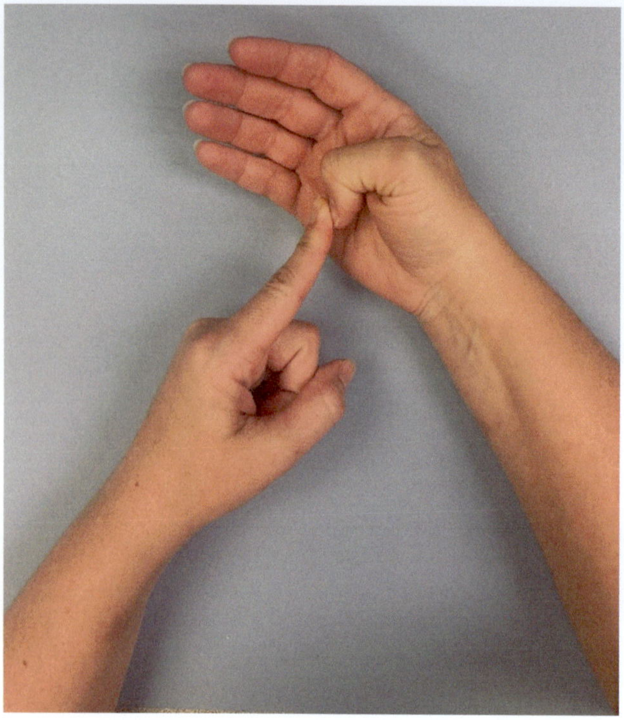

2. Using your other hand, bend just the tip of the thumb.

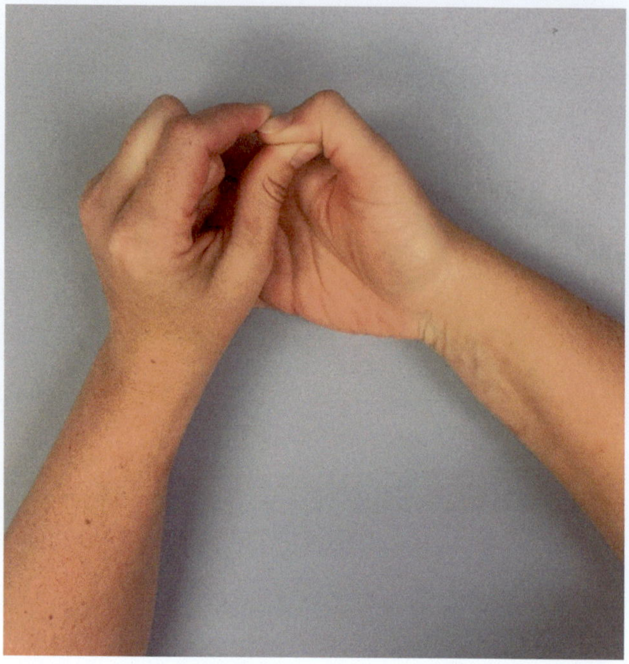

3. Using your other hand, push your index finger into a tightly bent position.

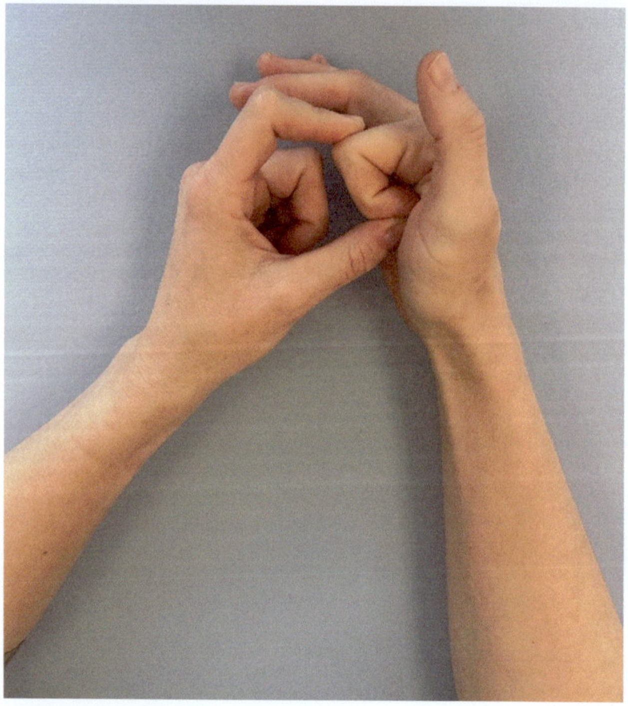

4. Using your other hand, push the tip of your index finger into a bent position keeping the rest of the index finger straight.

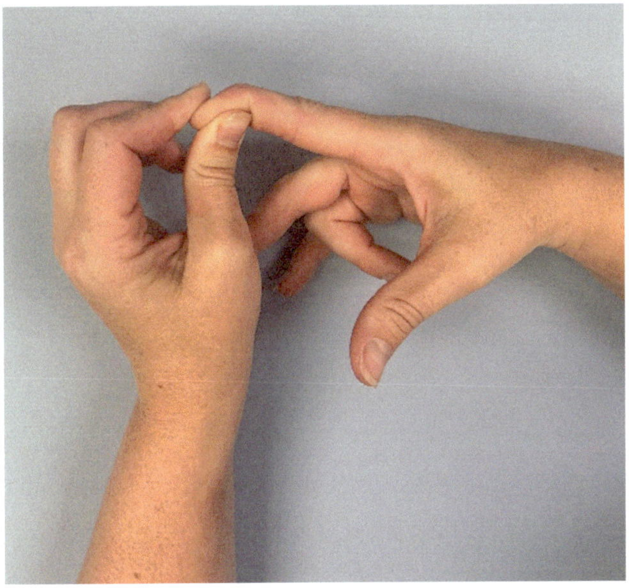

☐ **Active or Resisted Donor Movement**:

- Rest your hand over the edge of a table with your palm down. Bend your wrist back.

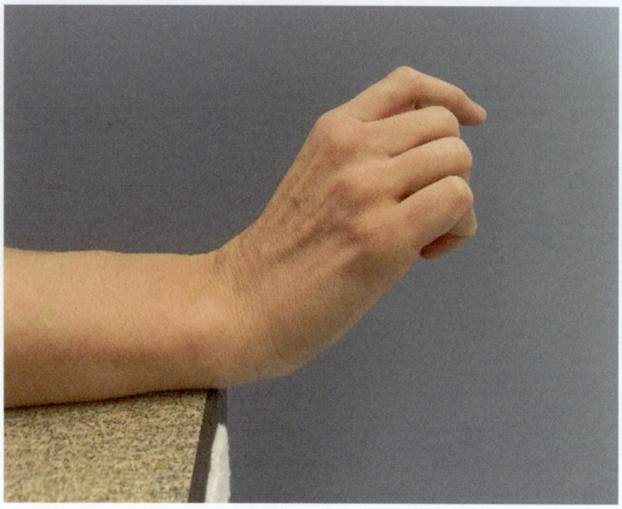

- One month after surgery, you may provide resistance to your wrist using your opposite hand while completing this exercise. Hold for 3–5 seconds. Return to the start position, and repeat.

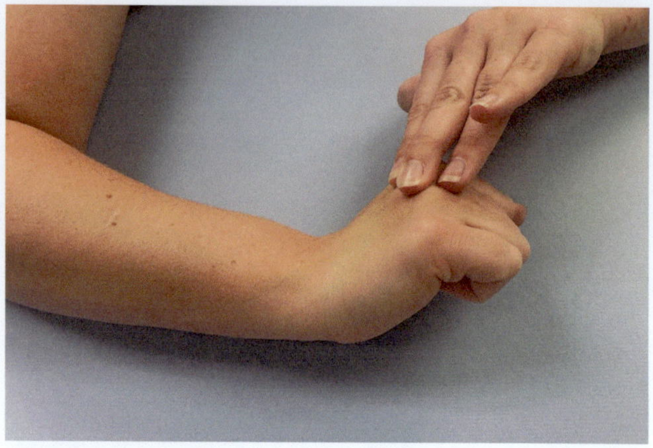

Complete 10 repetitions, every waking hour.

☐ **Active Donor + Passive Recipient Movement**:
Complete each of the below exercises <u>10</u> repetitions, <u>3</u> times per day.

1. Bend your wrist back. At the same time, use your other hand to push your **thumb** into a bent position. Focus on bending the tip of the thumb.

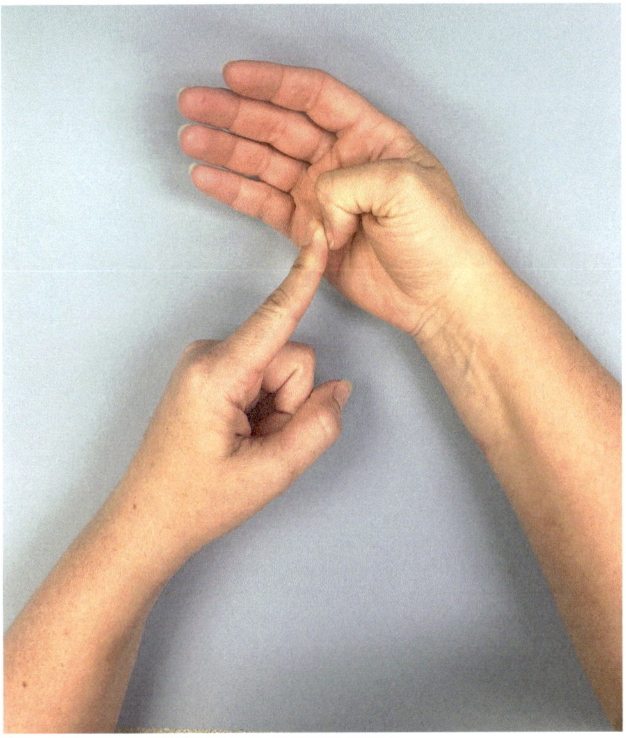

• Alternatively, wear an exercise cuff with a rubber band attached to your **thumb nail** when recommended by your therapist. Bend your wrist back, and the rubber band will pull your thumb tip into a bent position.

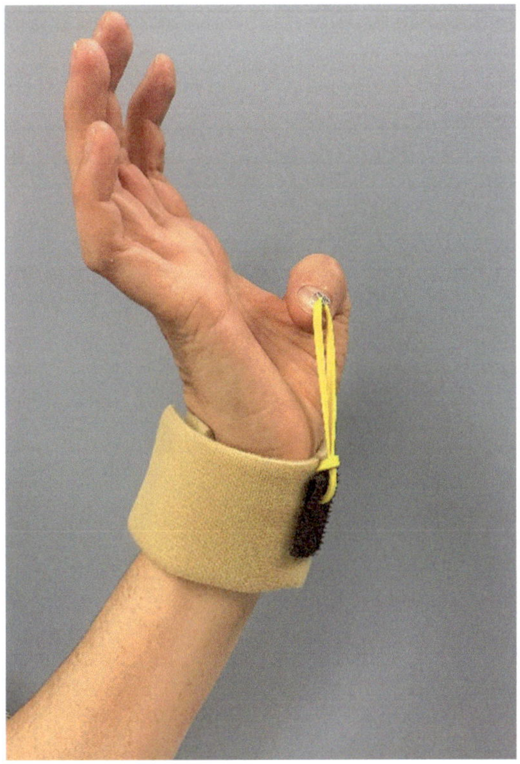

2. Bend your wrist back. At the same time, use your other hand to push your **index finger** into a tightly bent position. Focus on bending the tip of the index finger.

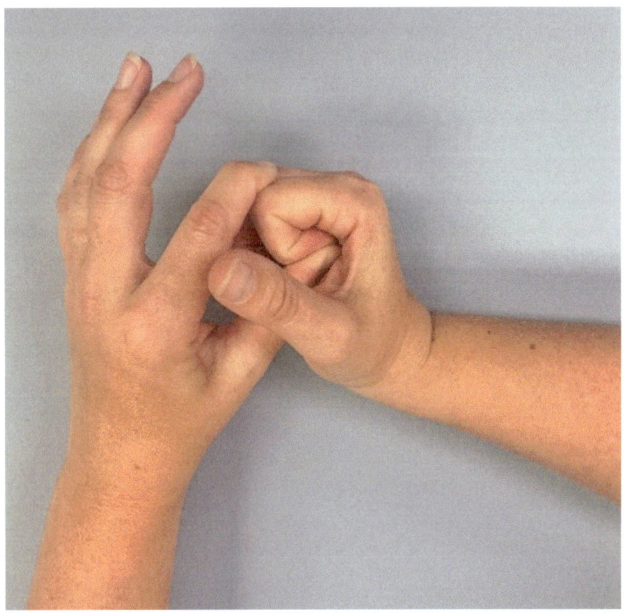

Phase 2 ECRB-to-AIN Nerve Transfer Exercises

☐ **Active Donor + Active-Assisted Recipient Movement**:

Complete each of the below exercises <u>10</u> repetitions, <u>3</u> times per day.

1. Bend your wrist back while attempting to bend your thumb forward. Then, allow the other hand to help bend the **thumb** forward as far as it will comfortably go.

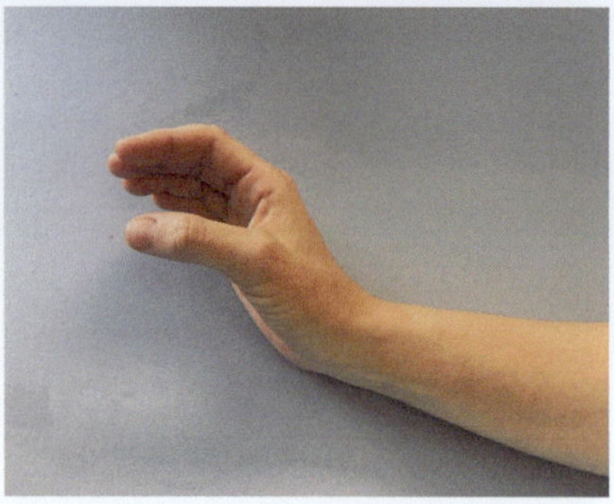

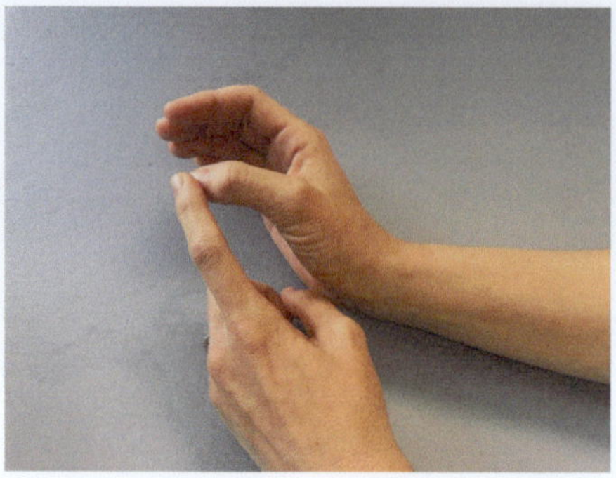

2. Bring your wrist back while attempting to bend the fingers. Then, allow the other hand to help push the **index finger** into a tightly bent position as far as it will comfortably go.

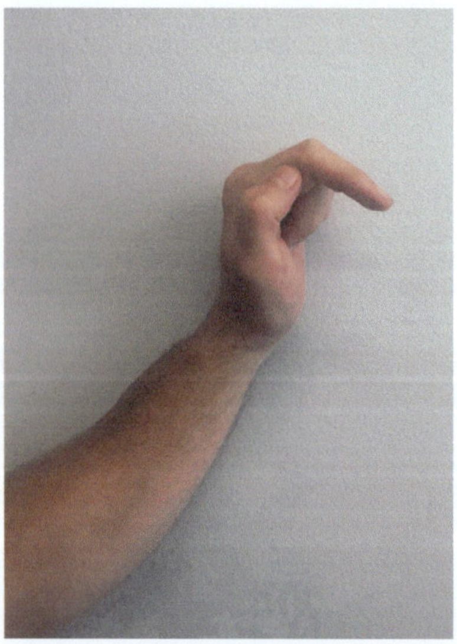

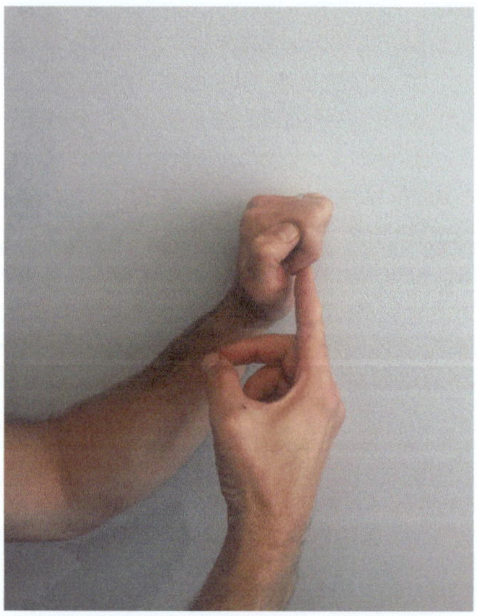

☐ **"Place and Hold" Recipient Movement**:

- Using your other hand, place the **thumb and index finger** in a "C" shape or "OK sign." Then, bend your wrist back. Keeping the wrist back, SLOWLY let go with your other hand as you try to keep the "C" or "OK sign" shape at your thumb and index finger. Hold for 3–5 seconds.

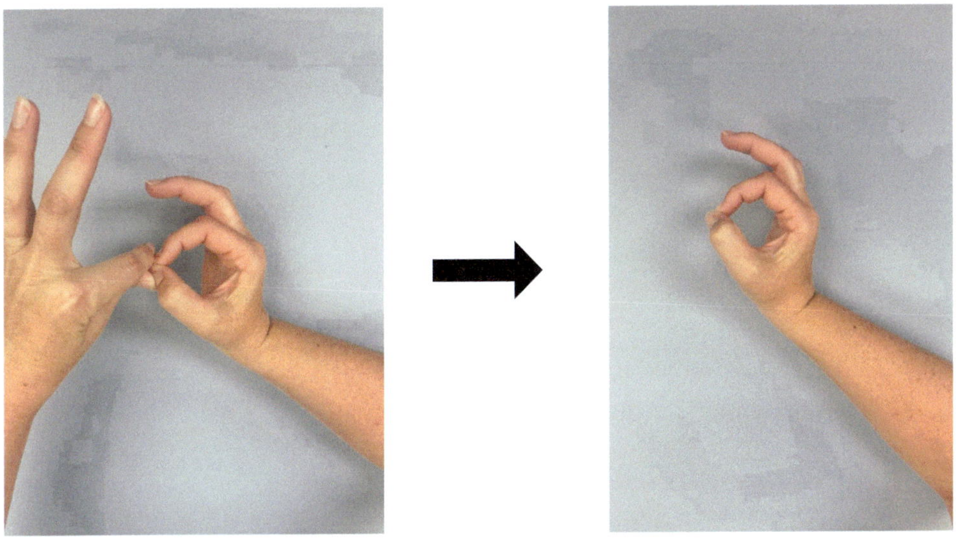

- Place your **thumb** into a bent position as far as it can comfortably go using your other hand to help. Then, bend the wrist back. Keeping the wrist back, SLOWLY let go with your other hand while you try to keep the thumb bent.

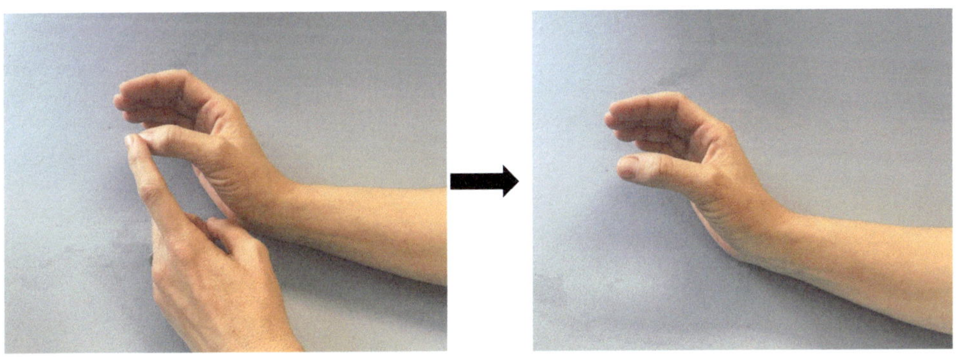

- Place your **index finger** into a tightly bent position as far as it can comfortably go using your other hand to help. Then, bring the wrist back. Keeping the wrist back, SLOWLY let go with your other hand while you try to keep the index finger bent.

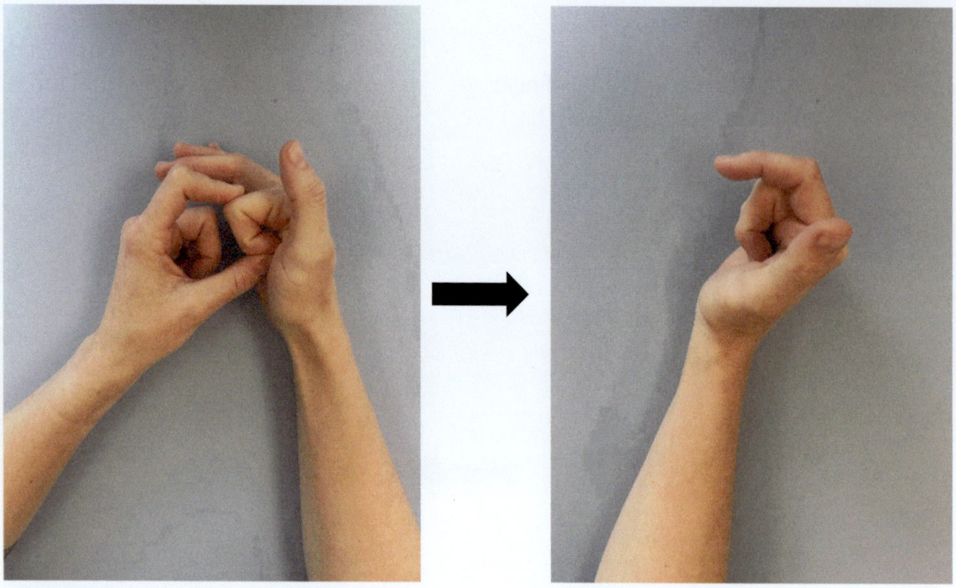

Complete 5–10 repetitions, 2–3 times per day

☐ **Active Donor + Active Recipient Movement**:

- Rest your hand over the edge of a table with your palm down. Bend your wrist back, and at the same time, try to make an "OK sign" with your thumb and index finger. You may also try to pick up lightweight items between the thumb and index finger while also bending your wrist back.

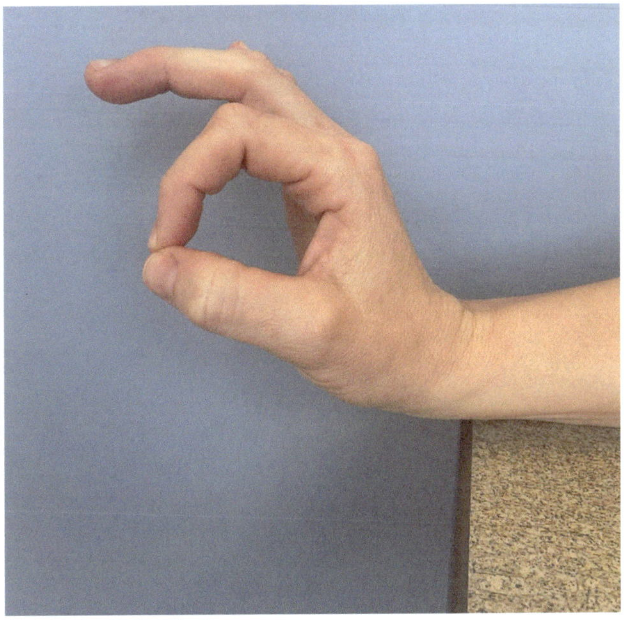

Complete 5–10 repetitions, 3 times per day.

Phase 3 ECRB-to-AIN Nerve Transfer Exercises

☐ **Resisted Donor + Resisted Recipient Movement: Complete one or more of the below exercises 10 repetitions, 2 times per day**

- With your palm down, pull coins, marbles, or other small items out of therapy putty using thumb to index finger pinch.

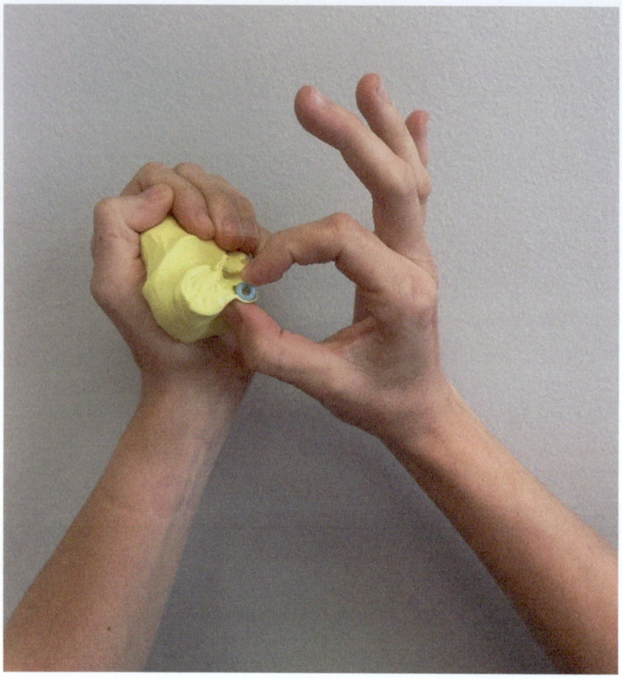

Complete 3–10 repetitions, 2 times per day.

- Hold therapy putty in your hand. Allow your thumb to bend into therapy putty like you are pressing a game show buzzer.

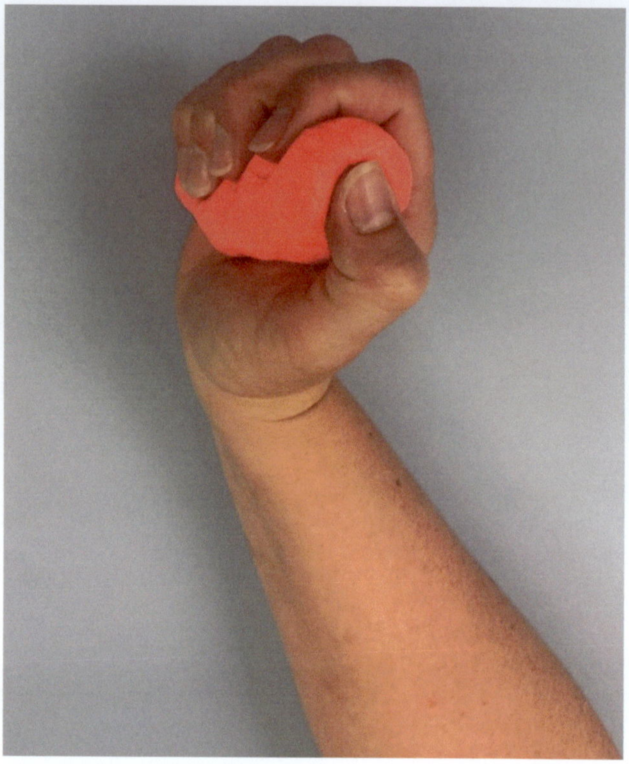

☐ **Resisted Recipient Movement**:

- Grasp the putty with both hands. Pinch the therapy putty between your thumb and index fingertips while you stabilize with the other hand. Your wrist should be in a slightly bent position.

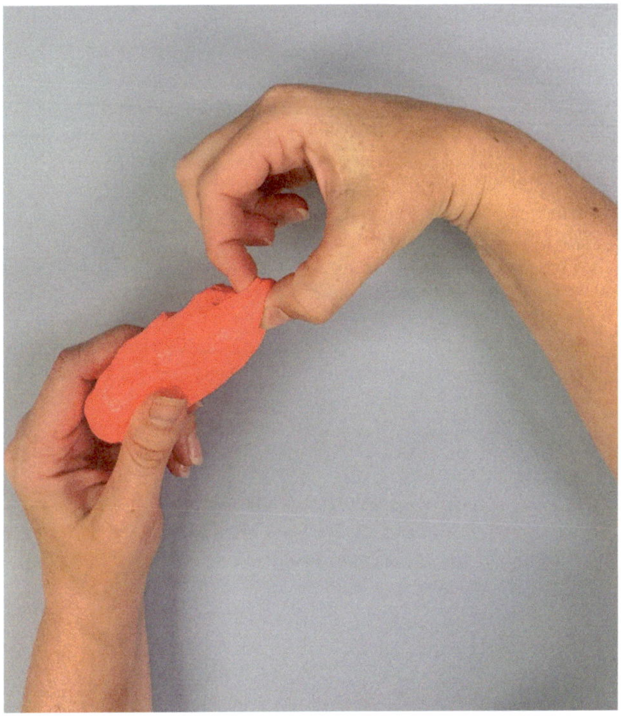

References

1. Westrup A, Prather K, Zhao X, Stephens M, Jea A. Transfer of extensor carpi radialis brevis branch of radial nerve to anterior interosseous nerve for lower trunk brachial plexopathy after motor vehicle accident. Neurosurg Focus Video. 2023;11(1):8.
2. Soldado F, Bertelli J, Ghizoni M. High median nerve injury: motor and sensory nerve transfers to restore function. Hand Clin. 2016;32:209–17.
3. Solaja O, Baergen A, Head L, Wolff G, Boyd K. Clinical outcomes of upper extremity nerve transfers in neuralgic amyotrophy. J Plast Reconstr Surg. 2023;152:1072e.
4. Bertelli JA. Transfer of the radial nerve branch to the extensor carpi radialis brevis to the anterior interosseous nerve to reconstruct thumb and finger flexion. J Hand Surg Am. 2015;40(2):323–8.
5. Bertelli JA, Ghizoni MF. Nerve transfers for restoration of finger flexion in patients with tetraplegia. J Neurosurg Spine. 2017;26:55–61.
6. Sananpanich K, Kraisarin J, Siriwittayakorn W, Tongprasert S, Suwansirikul S. Double motor nerve transfer for all finger flexion in cervical spinal cord injury: an anatomical study and a clinical report. J Hand Surg Am. 2018;43(10):920–6.
7. Goldspink G, Tabary C, Tabary JC, Tardieu C, Tardieu G. Effect of denervation on the adaptation of sarcomere number and muscle extensibility to the functional length of the muscle. J Physiol. 1974;236(3):733–42.
8. Gossman MR, Sahrmann SA, Rose SJ. Review of length-associated changes in muscle: experimental evidence and clinical implications. Phys Ther. 1982;62(12):1799–808.
9. Lieber RL. Skeletal muscle structure, function, and plasticity. Lippincott Williams & Wilkins; 2002.
10. Kahn L, Moore A. Donor activation focused rehabilitation approach: maximizing outcomes after nerve transfers. Hand Clin. 2016;32(2):263–77.
11. Davidge KM, Yee A, Kahn LC, Mackinnon SE. Median to radial nerve transfers for restoration of wrist, finger, and thumb extension. J Hand Surg Am. 2013;38(9):1812–27.
12. Avers D, Brown M. Muscle testing: techniques of manual examination and performance testing. 10th ed. Saunders; 2018.
13. Campodonico A, Pangrazi PP, De Francesco F, Riccio M. Reconstruction of a long defect of the median nerve with a free nerve conduit flap. Arch Plast Surg. 2020;47(2):187–93.
14. Wang YC, Bohannon RW, Kapellusch J, Garg A, Gershon RC. Dexterity as measured with the 9-hole peg test (9-HPT) across the age span. J Hand Ther. 2015;28(1):53–60.

Brachialis Branch of the Musculocutaneous Nerve to the Anterior Interosseous Nerve Transfer

Macyn M. Stonner

Background

The anterior interosseous nerve (AIN) is a motor branch of the median nerve that innervates the pronator quadratus, flexor pollicis longus, and lateral half of the flexor digitorum profundus. The main deficit that arises after AIN injury is the loss of pinch function due to lack of thumb interphalangeal (IP) joint flexion and index finger distal interphalangeal (DIP) joint flexion. The classic clinical sign of AIN palsy is the inability to make an "OK" sign with the thumb and index finger. The index finger and thumb will typically rest in extension. AIN palsy can occur at any level of the nerve (from the lower trunk of the brachial plexus to the median nerve in the forearm) and from many mechanisms, including a plexus stretch injury [1], radiation-induced brachial plexopathy [2], a sharp neurotmetic injury to the median nerve, Parsonage-Turner syndrome (brachial neuritis), and compressive AIN syndrome [3].

Given the lengthy regenerative distance from the brachial plexus to the forearm, restoration of distal hand function in lower plexus injuries where radial and ulnar function is absent or limited has historically been unattainable via nerve transfer. Finger flexion has typically been restored using tendon transfers (when there are appropriate donors) or free functional muscle transfers, both of which have challenges, including prolonged immobilization, donor-site morbidity, and transfer failure [4]. The brachialis (branch of the musculocutaneous nerve) to the AIN nerve transfer provides a reliable option to improve thumb and finger flexion in lower plexus injuries. The brachialis branch of the musculocutaneous nerve can usually be mobilized for a significant length and thus transferred easily to the forearm musculature [5, 6]. The brachialis-to-AIN transfer has gained popularity in the past decade for both spinal cord injury and brachial plexus injury [7].

Outcomes

The original report of brachialis-to-AIN nerve transfer was in 2004 by Gu and colleagues who described the surgical technique in 32 cadaveric arms followed by a report of one case. This case resulted in MMT strength grade 2/5 for FPL and 2/5 for FDP [5]. Outcomes have greatly improved since these initial findings. In 2012, Ray et al. reported on four patients with lower plexus injuries, demonstrating 4/5 MMT strength for both FPL and FDP in three out of the four cases [8]. The majority of documented studies on brachialis-to-AIN transfer are in the context of tetraplegia. Mackinnon and colleagues published a single tetraplegic case that achieved 3/5 MMT strength of the FPL and FDP at 15 months postoperatively [9]. Their team has found that early reinnervation begins at around 12 months and continues to strengthen for up to 4 years [8]. Bertelli and Ghizoni performed eight cases in 2017, three of which led to MMT grade 3/5, and one led to 4/5 MMT grade. Four of the eight scored between 0/5 and 2/5 MMT grades, yet these cases were noted to have lengthy nerve coaptation distances (>15 cm) [10]. There remains a need for more evidence documenting outcomes for this nerve transfer in the context of brachial plexus injuries.

M. M. Stonner (✉)
Milliken Hand Rehabilitation Center, WashU Medicine,
St. Louis, MO, USA
e-mail: macyn.stonner@wustl.edu

L. C. Kahn et al. (eds.), *Rehabilitation for Nerve Transfers of the Upper Extremity*,
https://doi.org/10.1007/978-3-031-92008-0_23

Surgical Description

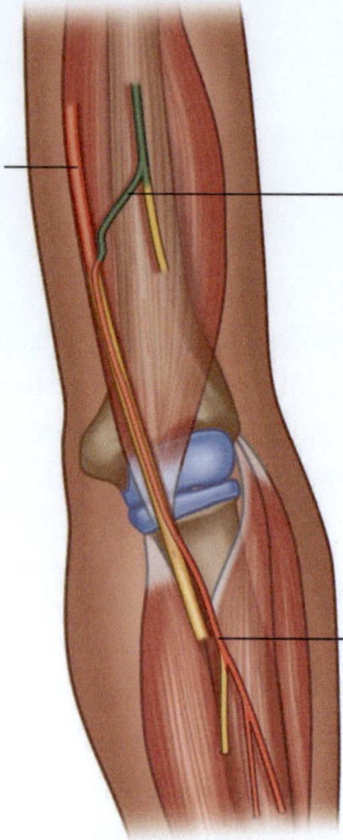

Microsurgical technique of Brachialis Branch of the Musculocutaneous Nerve to the Anterior Interosseous Nerve Transfer

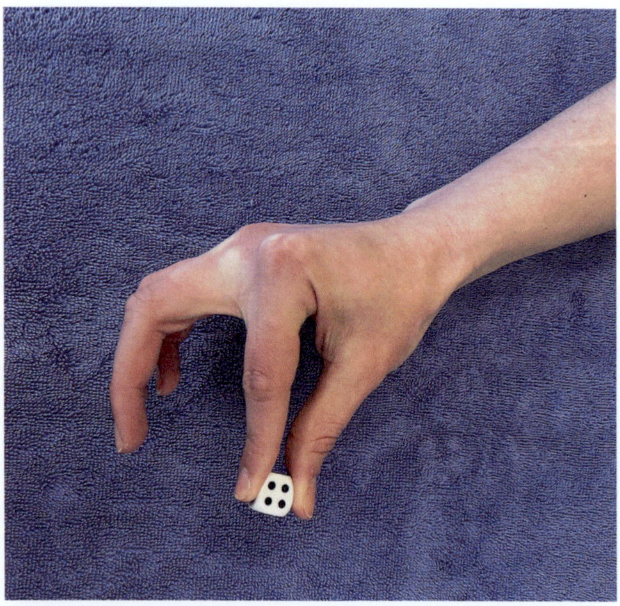

Image 1 Lack of AIN function can result in inefficient or faulty pinch patterns such as this hyperextension posturing of the thumb IP and index DIP joints

A longitudinal incision is made along the mid-brachial sulcus. The musculocutaneous nerve is identified deep to the biceps muscle, in the intramuscular interval between the biceps and brachialis. The branch from the musculocutaneous nerve to the brachialis is identified. Intraoperative stimulation is used to confirm robust function of the brachialis branch. It is important to ensure that there are no muscle paralytics being used by the anesthesia team. The median nerve is then identified adjacent to the brachial artery. Intraoperative stimulation is used to confirm that there is no AIN response when interrogating the entire circumference of the median nerve, ensuring that there are no muscle paralytics being used by the anesthesia team. A separate curvilinear incision is made along the volar aspect of the proximal two-thirds of the forearm. The lacertus fibrosus is identified, and after releasing the lacertus fibrosus, the median nerve is identified deep to the lacertus fibrosus and along the inner surface of the flexor pronator mass. After decompressing the median nerve, the branching pattern of the median nerve is identified. The AIN is identified branching from the median nerve proper. Intraoperative stimulation is used to confirm that there is no AIN response. The AIN is then neurolyzed as proximal as possible from the median nerve proper and divided proximally. The donor brachialis branch is neurolyzed from the musculocutaneous nerve proper, divided distally, and transposed to meet the AIN. Coaptation of the brachialis branch of the musculocutaneous nerve to the AIN is performed using microsurgical technique.

Phases of Rehabilitation

Phase 1

Preoperative to 1/5 MMT in the Recipient Muscle

Both the surgeon and therapist should provide thorough yet simplified education about the anatomy involved in the nerve transfer and therapy/timeline expectations. Patients should be educated on thumb mechanics as they often pinch using an inefficient posture with the thumb IP joint and index DIP joint in extension (or hyperextension) (Image 1). If patients lack *passive* thumb IP flexion and/or index DIP flexion, they should be referred to hand therapy preoperatively to address this through passive range-of-motion (PROM) exercises and static progressive splinting, if needed.

After surgery, the patient may be placed in a dressing that protects the elbow in flexion and wrist in neutral. The fingers do not have to be included in the initial postoperative dressing as the nerve coaptation is proximal to the elbow in the medial aspect of the upper arm. The dressing is typically removed around 2 weeks after surgery. Patients may be referred to a therapy visit at this time, often in conjunction with their appointment with the surgeon. The patient may transition to a custom or prefabricated neutral wrist orthosis for another 1–2 weeks depending on the patient's discomfort and surgeon's preference. Between 10 days and 3 weeks (pending wound healing and surgeon preference), sutures are removed or, in the case of internal sutures, the ends are clipped. Scar management may begin once the wound is fully healed. Instrument-assisted soft tissue mobilization (IASTM) is not recommended after nerve surgery. The therapist may provide a general timeline about the anticipated timeframe for functional return of thumb pinch, which has been published to be around 16 months [11]. At the completion of the first therapy visit, the patient should be able to identify the action of the donor (elbow flexion in forearm pronation) and demonstrate an understanding that performing this movement amplifies neural messages to the thumb (flexor pollicis longus/FPL) and index finger (flexor digitorum profundus/FDP) [12, 13].

Exercises

- ROM of Uninvolved Joints

  Patients are instructed to perform active range of motion (AROM) of uninvolved joints immediately following surgery (if they have active function of these joints). ROM of the shoulder, elbow, forearm, wrist, and digits is encouraged to prevent swelling and joint stiffness. If the patient has tightness of the thumb IP joint and/or index finger DIP joint, passive isolated and composite flexion stretches should be prioritized.
- Donor Activation

  As early as 2 weeks from surgery, patients should be instructed in "flooding the donor" exercises [12]. Donor activation is performed with active or isometric elbow flexion with the forearm in pronation to bias brachialis function over biceps, at a frequency of ten repetitions every hour (Image 2).
- Combined Donor with Passive Recipient Exercise

  At follow-up therapy visits, the patient is instructed in combined donor-recipient exercises to strengthen the new motor pathway. This would include active elbow flexion with passive or "assisted" digit flexion (thumb IP and index DIP) (Image 3), performed at a high frequency (10–20 repetitions, six to eight times per day).

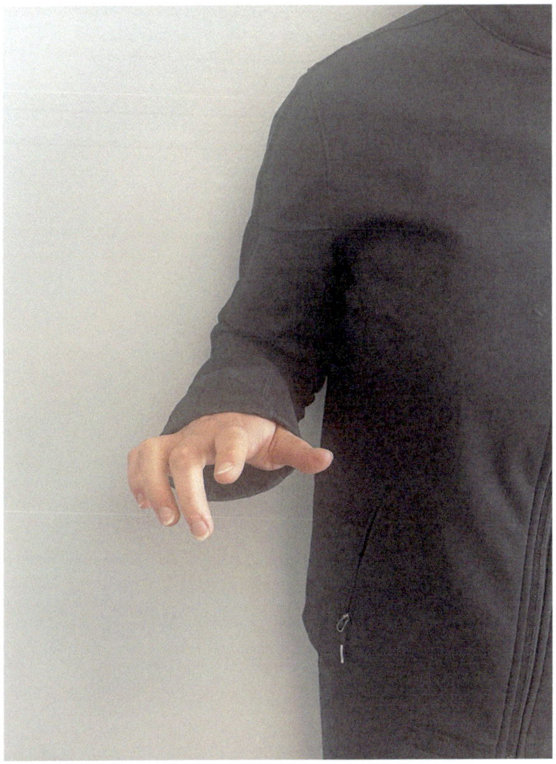

Image 2 Donor activation exercises are performed by flexing the elbow with the forearm in pronation to bias the brachialis function over the biceps.

Clinical Pearl

During this phase, custom oval-8 orthoses are beneficial to place the thumb IP and index DIP joints in slight flexion (Image 4) [14]. This may help reduce the maladaptive hyperextension posture during pinch and place the recipient muscles in a shortened and thus protected position.

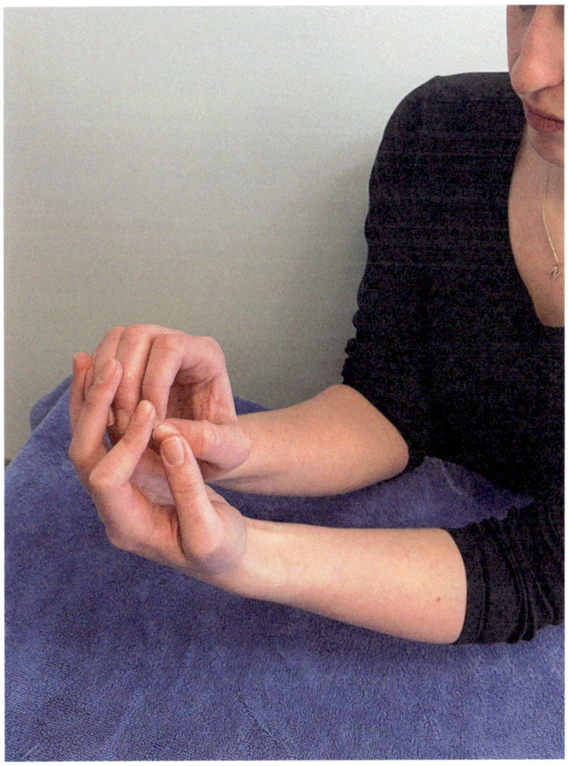

Image 3 Passive flexion of the thumb and index finger is performed with active flexion of the elbow during phase 1

Clinical Pearl

For patients with no finger flexion function, an ActiveHand™ brace may be useful to promote passive finger flexion and for performing resisted elbow flexion with the fingers held in flexion (Image 5).

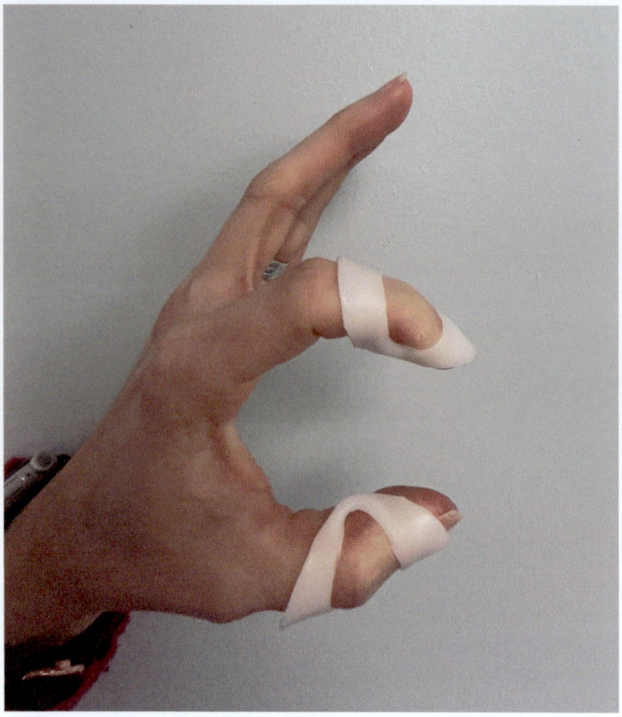

Image 4 Finger-based splints to block index DIP and thumb IP hyperextension will limit excessive lengthening of the recipient muscle and reduce the faulty pinch movement pattern

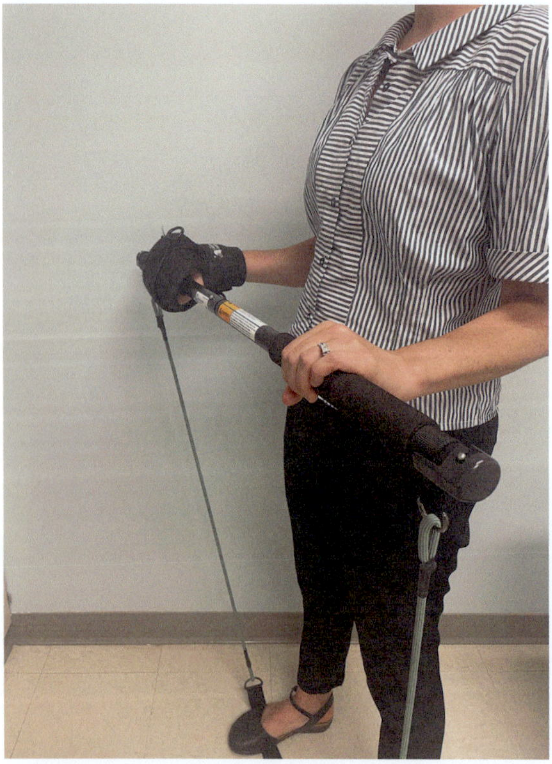

Image 5 An ActiveHand™ device is useful to maintain the hand in flexion during resisted elbow flexion exercises

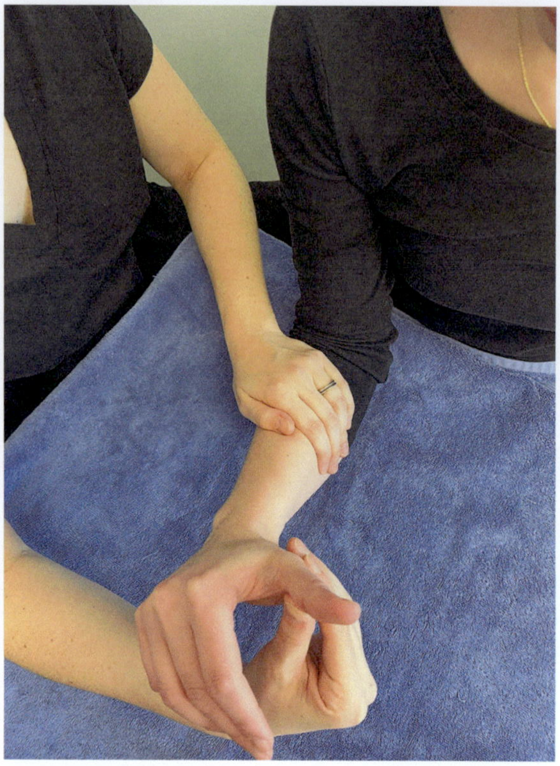

Image 6 Assessment of recovery of the FPL is performed by resisting elbow flexion in a pronated position while bracing the wrist in neutral and supporting the base of the thumb. Any movement of the IP joint into flexion is considered a positive sign of recovery. IP flexion may be measured to more accurately track recovery of motion

Assessment of Recovery

AIN function is assessed after a few months during therapy visits. FDP and FPL reinnervation are assessed separately. As the examiner resists elbow flexion (in pronation) and supports the thumb, the patient is cued to try to flex the IP joint of the thumb (Image 6). Typically, MMT strength is evaluated in a gravity-minimized plane. However, gravity has less influence on the fingers and thumb compared to larger and heavier proximal segments of the upper extremity [15]. The examiner palpates along the volar thumb proximal phalanx to evaluate for any tension in the FPL tendon while also looking for active IP joint flexion. The same process is used to evaluate for FDP function of the index finger. Elbow flexion is resisted as the therapist supports the index finger middle phalanx, palpating for FDP tension while looking for DIP flexion (Image 7). Often, the FDS is also denervated, and any IP movement of digit is considered positive as the FDP crosses both joints.

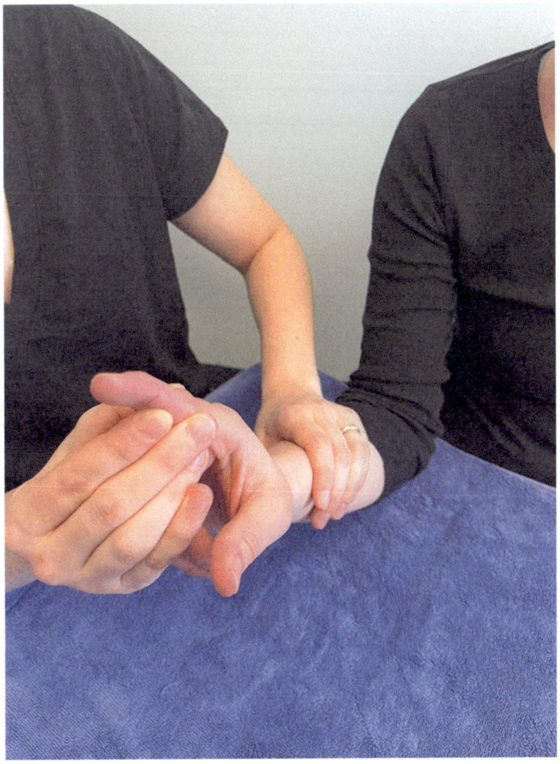

Image 7 Assessment of recovery of the index FDP is performed by resisting elbow flexion with the forearm in a pronated position, bracing the wrist in neutral and supporting the base of the index finger while monitoring for any active DIP flexion in the index finger

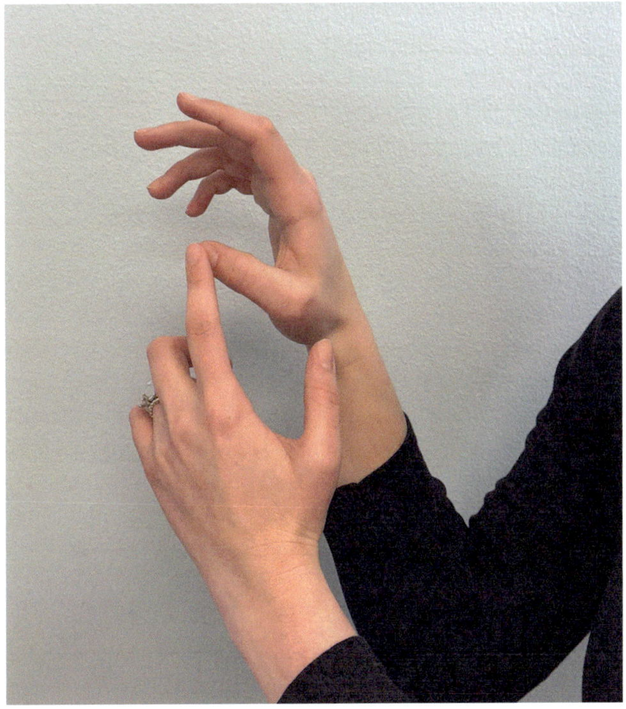

Image 8 During phase 2, active donor with active-assisted recipient exercises are achieved by flexing the elbow while the contralateral hand *assists* thumb IP flexion to complete the range

Clinical Pearl

Care should be taken to ensure that the patient is not inadvertently using tenodesis to produce active finger flexion. To avoid this, the wrist must be firmly maintained in a neutral position, avoiding extension, which would allow the fingers to flex by the passive tension in the extrinsic flexor muscles.

Therapy Frequency

Frequency of therapy visits is initially one time per week. Once the patient shows understanding of the donor-recipient relationship and any soft tissue restrictions are resolved, limiting therapy visits to one time per month is advised.

Phase 2

2−/5 to 3/5 MMT in the Recipient Muscle

Patients may progress to phase 2 of rehabilitation once they demonstrate active flexion of the thumb IP joint and index finger DIP joint. Exercises typically begin in a gravity-minimized plane for wrist, elbow, and shoulder conditions. However, the role of antigravity versus gravity-minimized planes is not an important factor with digital movement. At this point in recovery, the patient should be reliable with his or her home exercise program and demonstrate a good understanding of the donor-recipient muscle relationship. Throughout this phase, assisted motion is emphasized in the FPL and index FDS while gradually increasing resistance to the donor to increase a response in these recipient muscles. Additionally, suppleness of the thumb IP and index DIP joints should be maintained.

Exercises

- Active Donor with Active-Assisted Recipient
  FPL and Index FDP MMT = 2−/5 to 2/5
  Phase 2 exercises advance from passive to active-assisted thumb IP and index DIP flexion while simultaneously contracting the brachialis. The patient should attempt independent IP flexion while the flexing the elbow. The contralateral hand *assists* further thumb IP flexion after the initial attempt of independent active flexion (Image 8). The same exercise is performed for index DIP flexion.
- "Place and Hold" Exercise
  FPL and Index FDP MMT = 2+/5
  At this point in recovery, "place and hold" exercises may begin. The patient passively places the thumb in IP flexion and then attempts to hold this position for 5 seconds while the elbow is simultaneously contracted (with or without resistance). The same exercise is performed separately for index DIP flexion.

- Active Donor with Active Recipient
  FPL and Index FDP MMT = 3−/5 to 3/5
  As the AIN muscle strength increases and they can flex through mid to full range, the patient may work on active pinch between the thumb tip and index fingertip (Image 9), with cues to make an "OK" sign which would lead to some degree of thumb IP and index DIP flexion.
- Functional Activity
  Patients are encouraged to activate their nerve transfer for functional activities requiring light pinch. Basic pinch activities may include picking up cotton balls and threading beads on a string (Image 10). Activities that require more dexterity would include sewing or putting in earrings. These tasks intuitively contract the donor brachialis by flexing the elbow. Patients should make their best attempt to avoid collapsing their thumb IP and index DIP joints into extension or hyperextension during attempted pinch.

Therapy Frequency

If they are compliant with their home program and making progress, patients may only need to attend formal therapy once per month in phase 2. High emphasis is placed on short, frequent independent exercises at home.

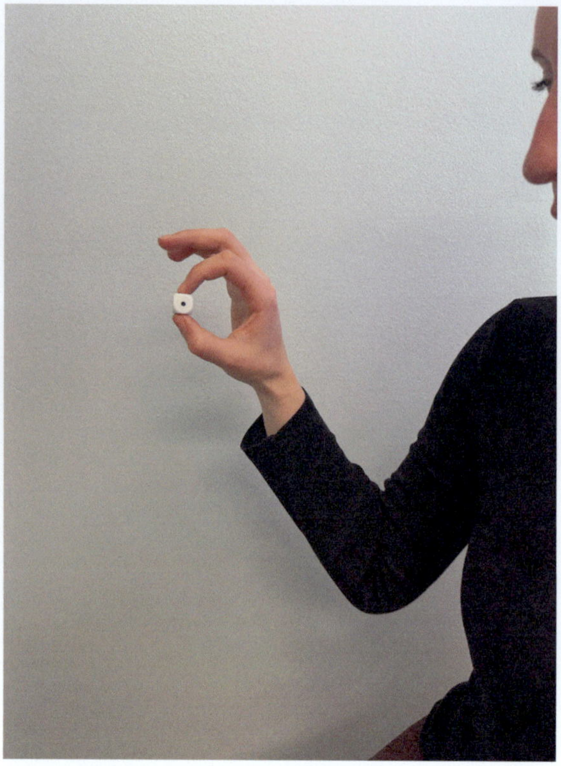

Image 9 As the AIN muscles increase in strength and can flex through mid to full range, the patient may work on active pinch between the thumb tip and index as with holding a small object like a die cube

Phase 3

3+/5 or Greater in the Recipient Muscle

Late-phase therapy begins once the thumb IP and index DIP joint can flex through full range against some resistance. Phase 3 is characterized by resistive exercise, which should not be initiated before the FPL and index FDP demonstrate a 3/5 MMT strength grade as this would likely result in the thumb IP and index DIP joints collapsing into extension (or hyperextension) during pinch. To prevent fatigue, low resistance should remain an important concept during this time with repetition based on activity or exercise tolerance.

Exercises

- Resistive Recipient Activity with Donor Contraction
  Resistive thumb IP flexion (and index DIP flexion) begins with simultaneous contraction of the brachialis. With the elbow flexed to 90° and the forearm pronated, the patient can pinch and pull therapy putty while trying to maintain an "OK" sign with the thumb and index finger (Image 11). Patients can also isometrically hold a golf ball or marble between their fingers to replicate pinch stabilization for daily tasks. Engaging the brachialis will augment tip to tip contact of the thumb and index finger, which will be functionally useful as additional pinch strength is needed.

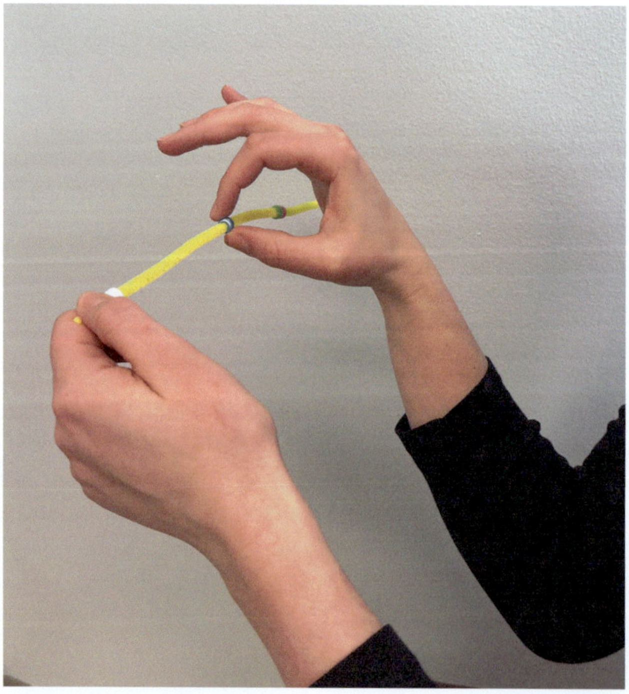

Image 10 Functional activities in phase 2 include pinch activities, such as threading beads on a string

- Resistive Recipient Activity Without Donor Contraction
  Once patients demonstrate reliable activation of their transfer using simultaneous elbow flexion, they may learn

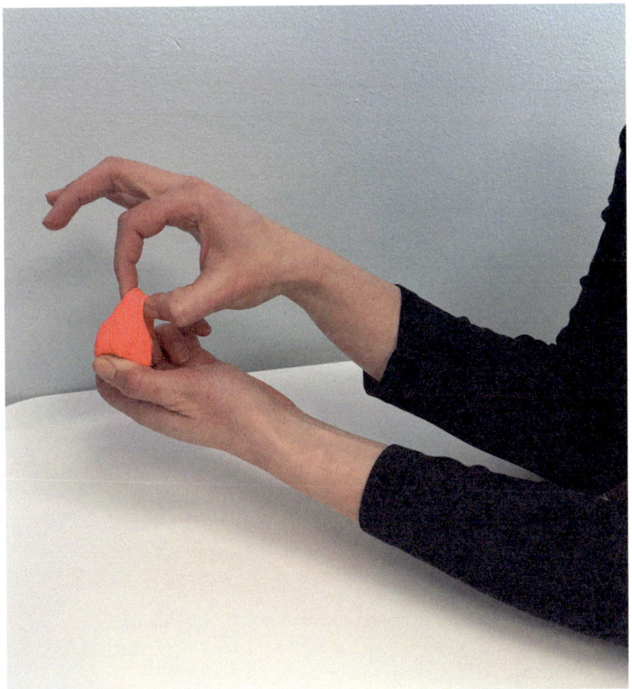

Image 11 Resistive recipient activity with donor contraction can be achieved by having the patient pinch and pull therapy putty while maintaining the thumb and index finger in a flexed position

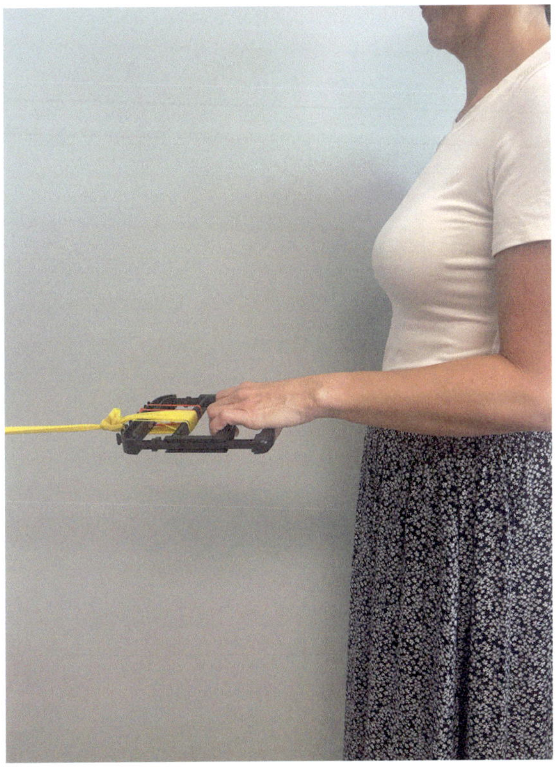

Image 12 Resisting the donor and recipient muscles simultaneously can be achieved by securing a long piece of resistance band to a gripper tool, such as the Hand Helper. The opposite end of the band is attached to a doorknob or secure post. The patient holds the gripper and attempts to make a tight fist while pulling the elbow back into flexion against the resistance of the band

Clinical Pearl
Resisted exercises can be advanced to both the donor and recipient muscles. The therapist can demonstrate a helpful home exercise by securing a long piece of resistance band to a gripper tool, such as the Hand Helper. The opposite end of the band is attached to a doorknob, and the patient sits across from it while holding the gripper. The patient is cued to squeeze the gripper while flexing the elbow in a pronated position against the resistance of the band (Image 12).

to separate the two functions. Patients may begin to work on resistive tasks with the thumb and index finger while the elbow is in extension, such as reaching away from the body while pinching (Image 13). Examples may include reaching to place a power cord in a wall, twisting a doorknob open, or pushing a thumbtack into a corkboard.

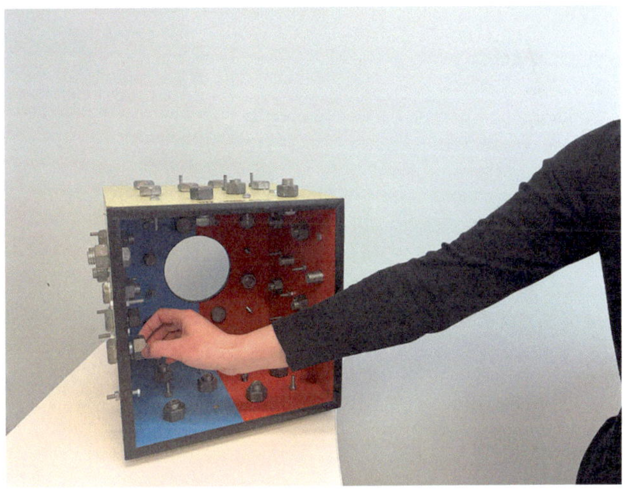

Image 13 Advancing strength training to de-emphasize the donor is achieved by performing resistive pinch tasks while the elbow is in extension, such as reaching away from the body while unscrewing a bolt

Therapy Frequency

Patients may only need to attend formal therapy three to four times in phase 3. High emphasis is placed on frequent independent exercises at home.

Brachialis-to-Anterior Interosseous Nerve (AIN) transfer

Nerve transfer overview					
Donor nerve	Donor action	Recipient nerve	Recipient action	Indications for functional restoration	Approximate months to functional movement
Brachialis branch of the musculocutaneous nerve	Elbow flexion in forearm pronation	Anterior interosseous nerve (AIN) branch of the median nerve	Thumb IP and index DIP (and composite) joint flexion	Pinch strength and coordination	12–16 months [8, 9]

Information below is suggested guidelines. Precautions may vary according to surgeon preferences and patient factors

	Preoperative therapy	Early phase	Middle phase	Late phase
Criteria	Before surgery	0/5 to −1/5 MMT	2−/5 to 3/5 MMT	>3/5 MMT
Purpose of phase	Educate and establish baseline function	Understand donor-recipient relationship Activate donor	Activate nerve transfer for functional activities requiring light pinch	Isolate recipient through resistance Separate pinch function from donor activation (elbow flexion)
Precautions	Prevent hyperextension of thumb IP and index DIP to avoid stiffness	Prevent hyperextension of thumb IP and index DIP to avoid stiffness	Respect fatigue	Respect fatigue
Frequency of visits (considerations)	1–2 pre-op visits; more if PROM limitations are present	1×/week until PROM is full, and patient is independent with donor activation and motor re-education concepts; then 1× monthly	1×/week to 1×/month based on patient needs, compliance, and accuracy of the exercise program	1× every 1–2 weeks based on progress toward patient-specific goals
Orthosis considerations	Finger-based IP extension block orthoses if hyperextension posturing is present	Dressing that protects the elbow in flexion and wrist neutral until 2 weeks post-op and then transition to a wrist orthosis until 3–4 weeks (per surgeon preference and patient comfort) Consider finger-based orthosis maintaining thumb IP and index DIP in slight flexion after rest period is complete	Continue finger-based orthoses for thumb IP and index DIP in slight flexion during day. This is to help with functional pinch and reinforce the new motor pattern Discontinue orthoses once active thumb IP and index DIP flexion can overcome extensor tension	None
Interventions		**Donor activation**: Elbow flexion with forearm in pronation (isometric, active, and resisted) 10× every hour **Donor-recipient pairing**: Active elbow flexion with passive thumb IP and index DIP flexion 10–20 reps, 6–8×/day	**Active/resisted donor with active assist recipient**: Passive progresses to active-assisted thumb IP and index DIP flexion with (active and/or resisted) elbow flexion **Place and hold**: Place thumb and index into an "OK" position. Remove the support and maintain this position (with simultaneous elbow flexion in pronation)	**Resisted donor and recipient**: Resisted elbow flexion and forearm pronation while maintaining "OK" sign with resistance (holding golf ball, marble, or putty) **Resisted recipient without donor contraction**: Tip-to-tip or three-point pinching into resistance with the elbow extended (putty, holding pen to "click" top, pushing plug into wall socket, twisting doorknob, pushing tack into corkboard)
Additional intervention considerations		See clinical pearl section of chapter, Image 4	**MMT 3− to 3/5**: Simultaneous "OK" sign with elbow flexion **Functional tasks**: Picking up cotton balls, threading beads through string while bending the elbow, buttoning a shirt, and putting on earrings	Therapist facilitation of movement is encouraged due to prolonged time of disuse (may still need to activate donor for stronger contraction but continue to work on selective activation) Focus on high repetitions, low resistance Maximum strength and functional use may take 2–3 years to regain

During all phases, it is essential to continue cortical reorganization and psychological and psychosocial interventions and progress to incorporate donor/recipient with ADLs

Brachialis-to-AIN Nerve Transfer

Goal of Surgery: Restore the ability to bend the thumb and index finger together for pinch

Recipient Movements = Bend index fingertip (DIP joint flexion)
Bend thumb tip (IP joint flexion)
Pinch index and thumb together

Recipient Muscles: Flexor digitorum profundus (FDP), flexor pollicis longus (FPL)

Recipient Nerve: Anterior interosseous nerve

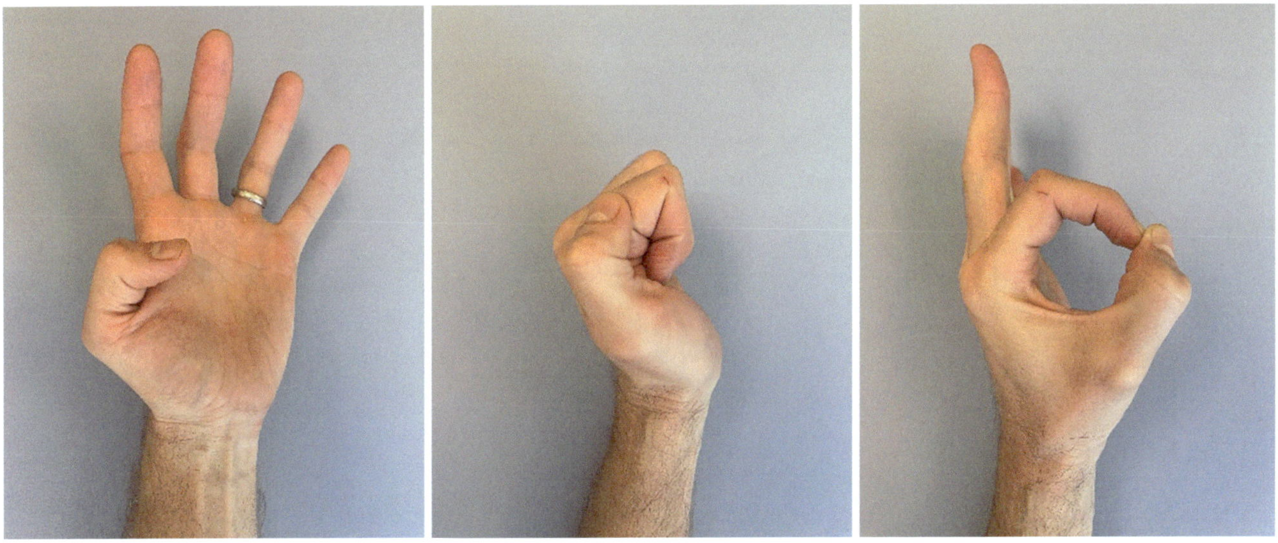

Donor Movement = Bend the elbow (elbow flexion) with the forearm facing down

Donor Muscle: Brachialis

Donor Nerve: Anterior interosseous nerve

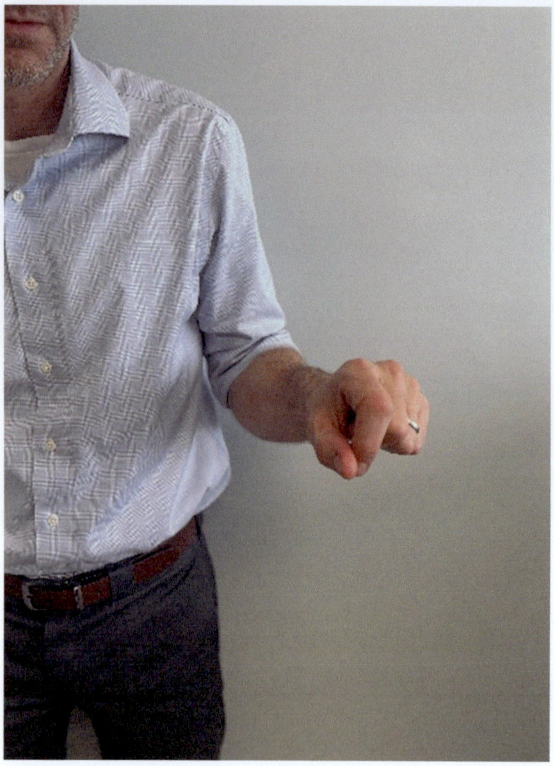

Phase 1 Brachialis-to-AIN Nerve Transfer Exercises

☐ **Passive Range of Motion**:

Complete the below exercises 3–5 repetitions, 2–3 times per day.

1. Using your opposite hand, manually stretch the thumb into a bent position across the palm. Make sure to emphasize the tip of the thumb (the IP joint).
2. Using your opposite hand, manually stretch the index finger into the palm. Make sure to emphasize the tip of the index finger (the DIP joint).

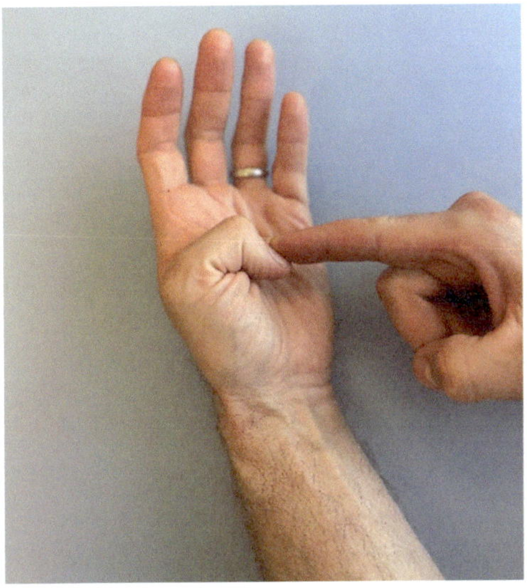

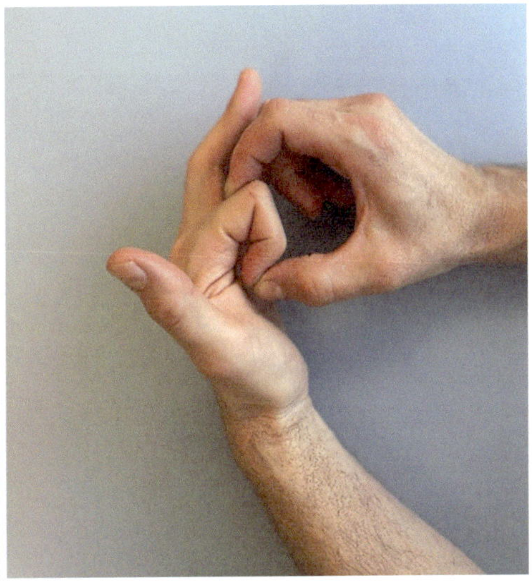

☐ **Active or Resisted Donor Movement**:
Complete <u>10</u> repetitions, every waking hour.

1. Beginning with the arm down by your side, bend the elbow while the palm is facing down.

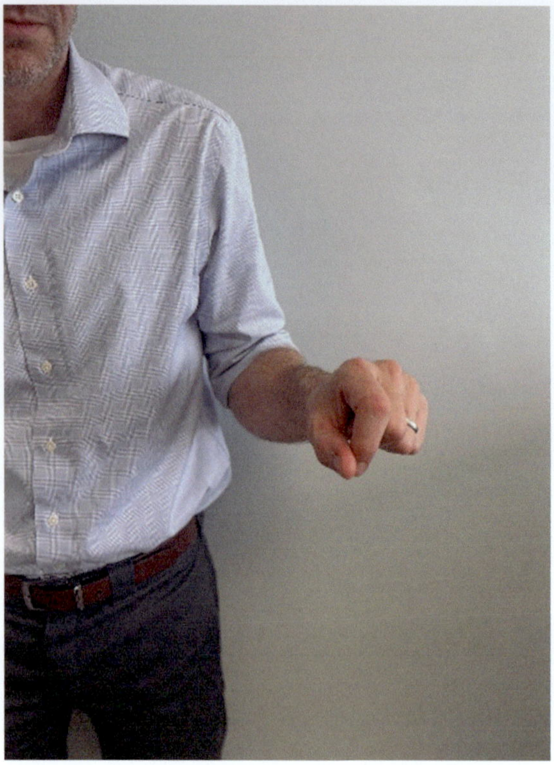

2. If advised by your therapist, hold a ___ pound weight in your hand. Beginning with the arm down by your side, bend the elbow while the palm is facing down (pronated).
   Complete <u>10</u> repetitions, <u>2–3</u> times per day.

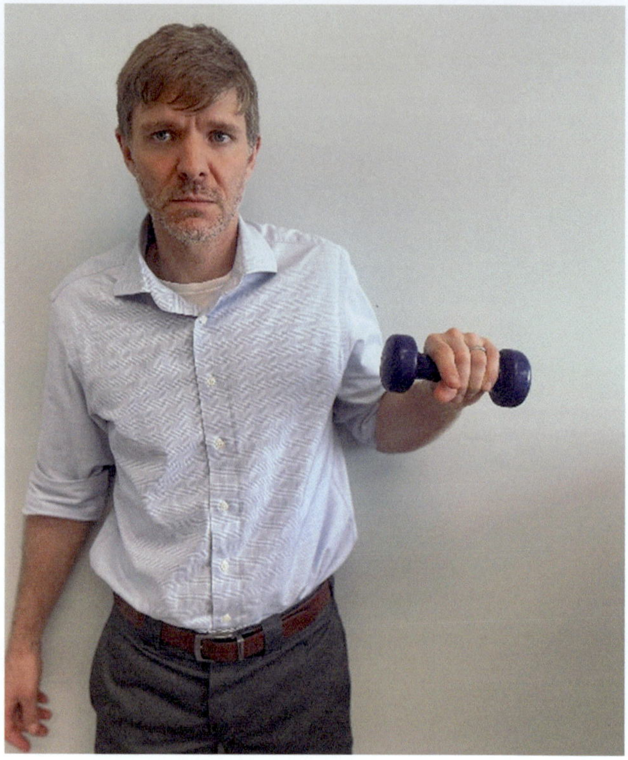

☐ **Isometric Donor Activation**:

1. Begin with your palm facing down and elbow bent to about 90°. Bend the elbow while simultaneously using your opposite hand to push down on the forearm.

Hold for 5 seconds, complete 10 repetitions, 2–3 times per day.

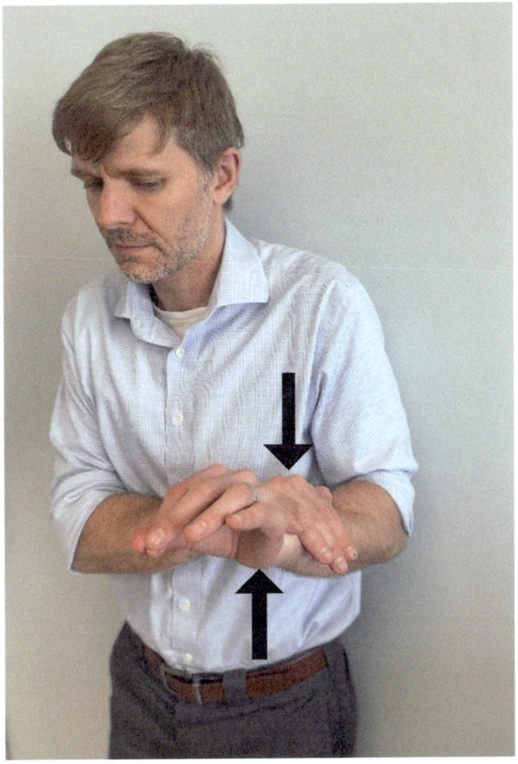

☐ **Active Donor + Passive Recipient Movement**: **Complete one or both of the below exercises 10 repetitions, 2–3 times per day.**

1. Use your opposite hand to bend the index and thumb together while you bend your elbow into a flexed position. The forearm should be palm down (pronated). Return to the start position, and repeat.

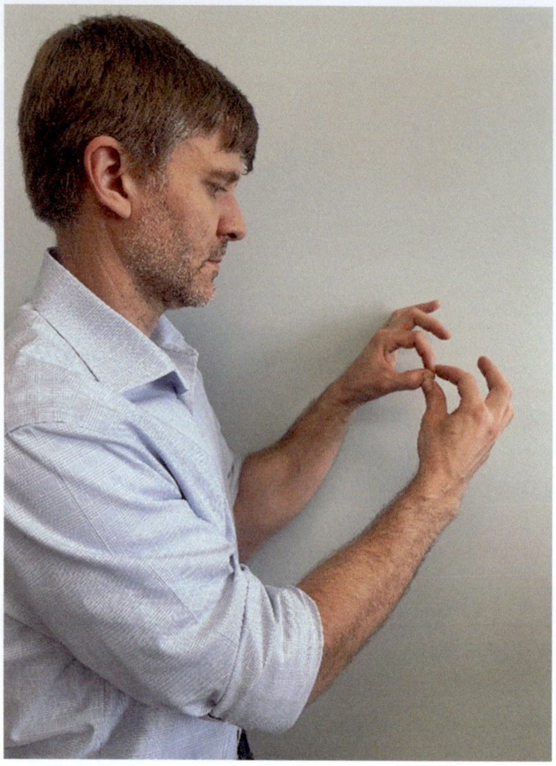

Phase 2 Brachialis-to-AIN Nerve Transfer Exercises

☐ **Active or Resisted Donor + Active-Assisted Recipient Movement**:

Complete the below exercises 1–10 repetitions, 2–3 times per day.

1. Bend your elbow with the forearm in a palm-down position while trying to independently bend the tip of the **thumb**. Once you cannot bend it further, use your opposite hand to assist the **thumb** into a fully bent position.

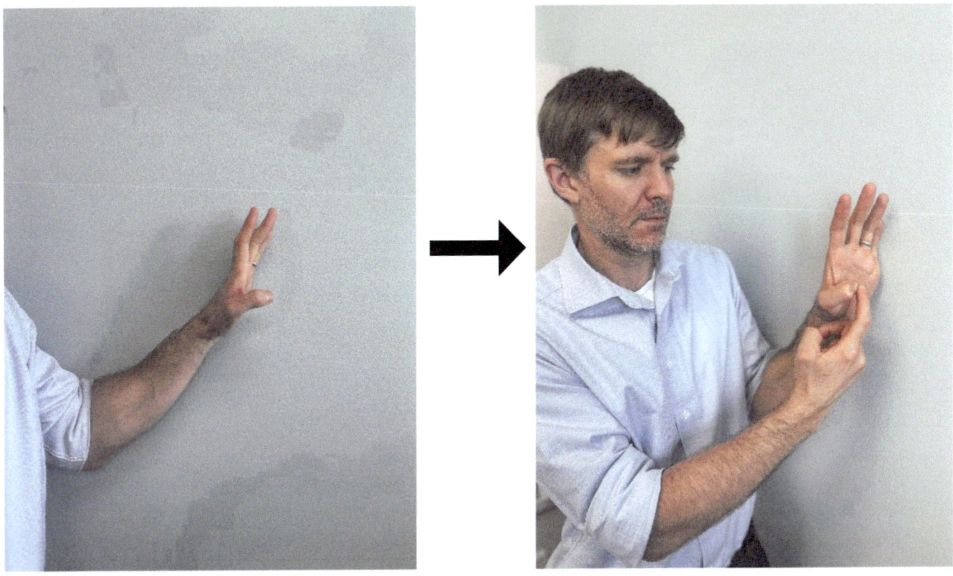

2. Bend your elbow with the forearm in a palm-down position while trying to independently bend the **index finger** into the palm. Once you cannot bend it further, use your opposite hand to assist the **index finger** into a fully bent position.

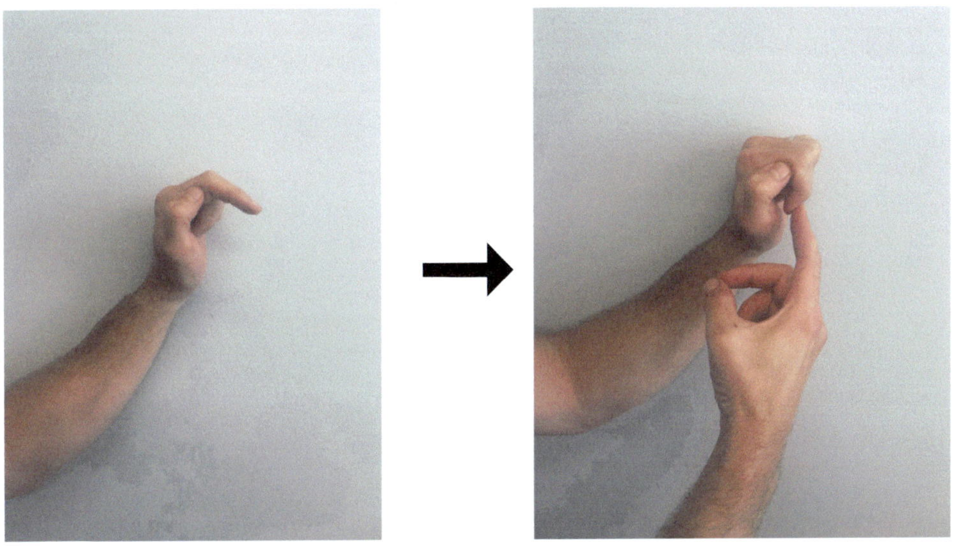

3. **"Place-and-Hold" Exercise**

Use your opposite hand to manually stretch the thumb into a bent position while bending your elbow. Let go with the opposite hand, and try to maintain this bent position of the thumb for a count of 5 seconds.

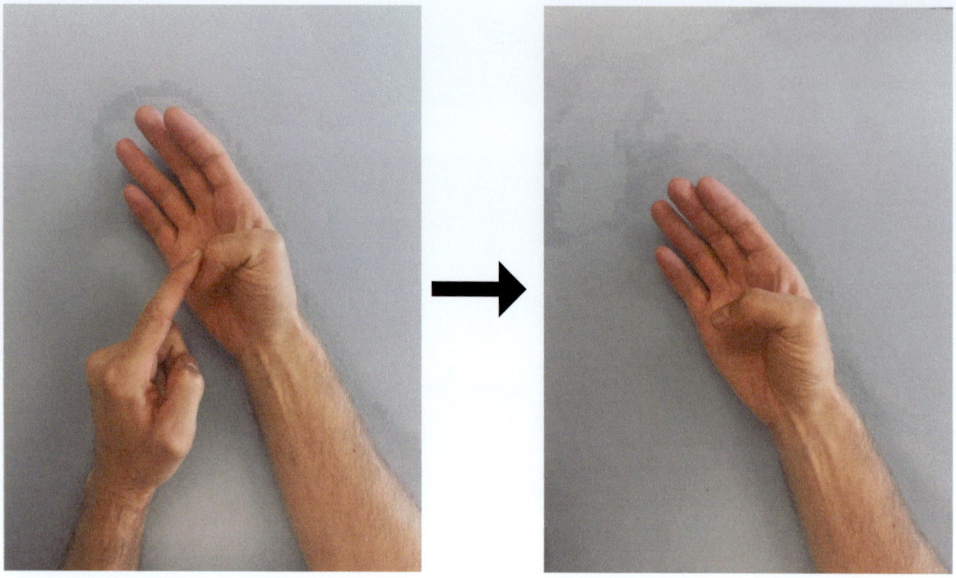

Do the same exercise for the index finger. Use your opposite hand to manually stretch the index finger into the palm while bending the elbow. Let go with the opposite hand, and try to maintain this bent position for a count of 5 seconds.

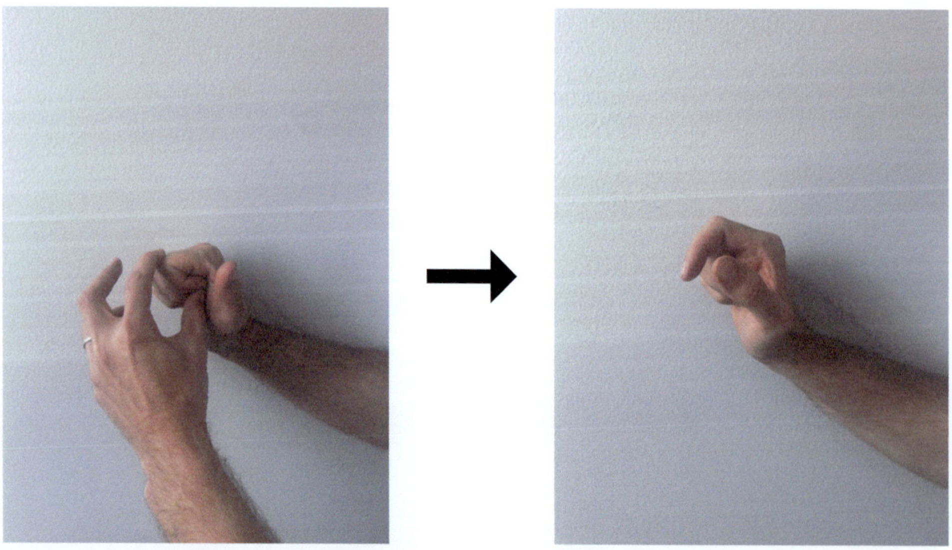

□ **Active Donor + Active Recipient Movement**:

Complete the below exercises 1–10 repetitions, 2–3 times per day.

With your arm beginning down by your side, bend your elbow with the forearm in a palm-down (pronated) position. Simultaneously try to pinch the thumb and index finger together, making an "O" shape. Try this while holding a light object between the fingers.

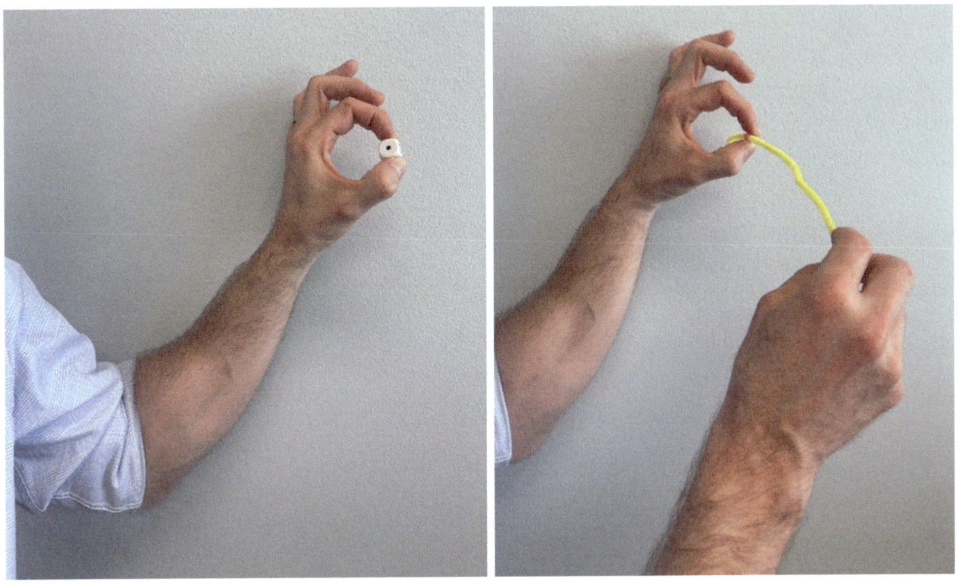

Phase 3 Brachialis-to-AIN Nerve Transfer Exercises

☐ **Resisted Donor + Resisted Recipient Movements**:

Complete the below exercises <u>1–10</u> repetitions, <u>2–3</u> times per day.

Only complete the exercises approved by your therapist.

1. Putty: With the elbow in a bent position and the palm facing away from you, pinch therapy putty between the thumb and index finger. Try to maintain an "O" shape while pinching the putty.

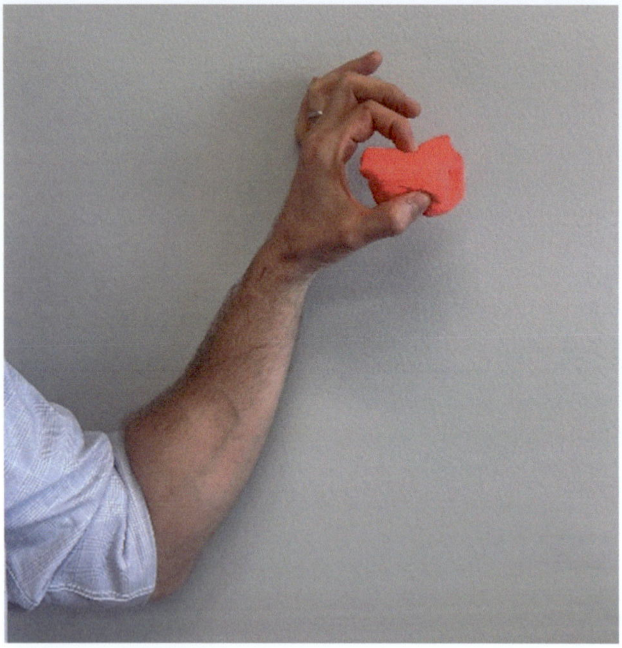

2. Theraband with gripper: Attach a piece of resistance band to a gripper device, such as a Hand Helper™. Secure the opposite end of the band to a doorknob. Squeeze the gripper while simultaneously pulling the elbow into flexion.

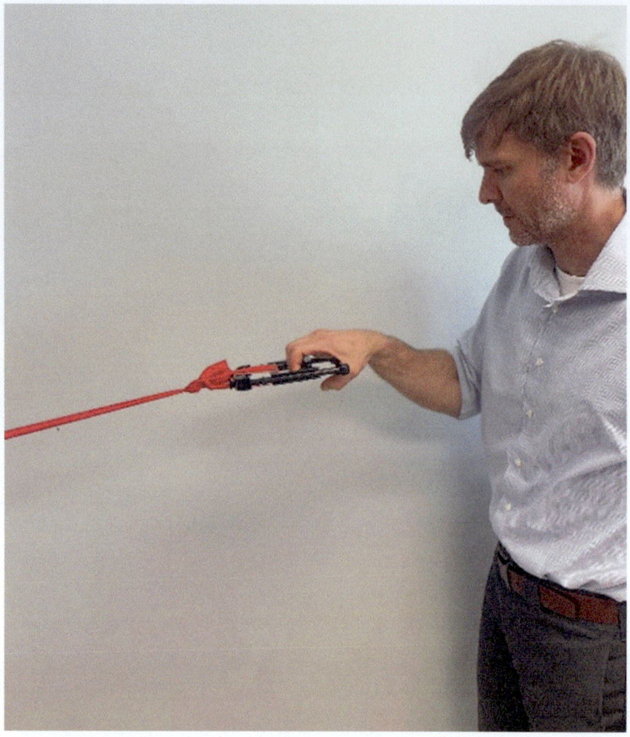

3. Clips: Pinch a chip-clip or clothespin, maintaining an "O" shape between the thumb and index finger.

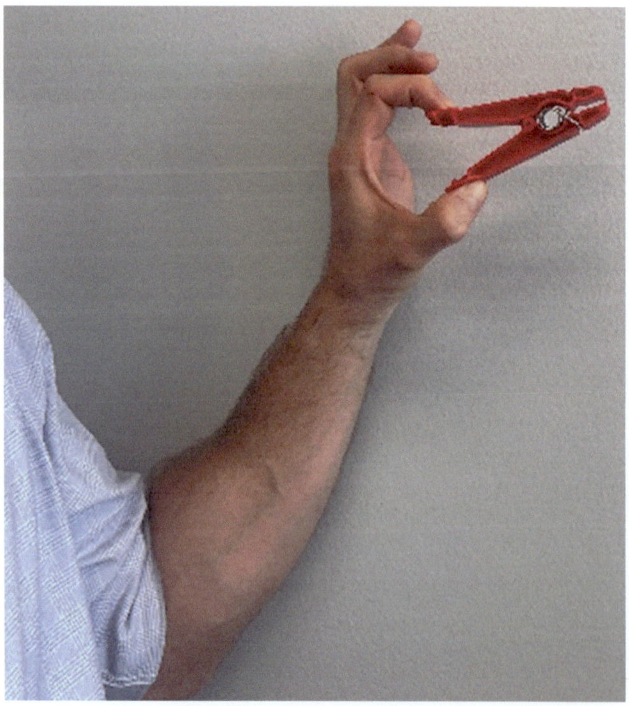

☐ **Isometric Recipient Movement**:

Practice an activity that requires sustained pinching of the thumb and index finger, such as writing, needlework, or stabilizing a nail while using a hammer.

Complete 3–5 min, 2–3 times per day.

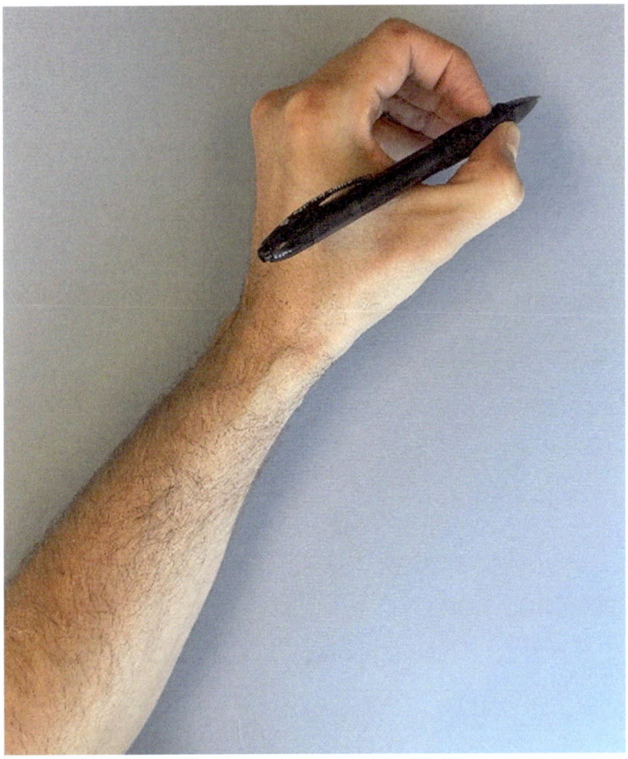

☐ **Resisted Recipient Movement**:

Complete the below exercises 5–10 repetitions, 2–3 times per day.

1. Putty: Pinch therapy putty between the thumb and index finger with the elbow in a straight position. Try to maintain an "O" shape while pinching the putty.
2. Functional activity: Work on reaching away from your body while using the hand to squeeze, pinch, or twist an object. Consider reaching to unscrew a lightbulb or plug in a power cord.

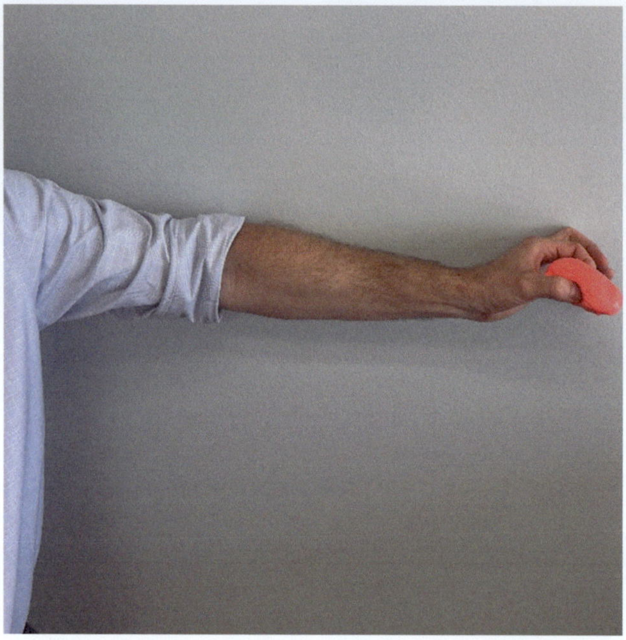

References

1. Kim DH, Murovic JA, Tiel RL, Kline DG. Infraclavicular brachial plexus stretch injury. Neurosurg Focus. 2004;16(5):1–6.
2. Warade AC, Jha AK, Pattankar S, Desai K. Radiation-induced brachial plexus neuropathy: a review. Neurol India. 2019;67(7):47.
3. Rodner CM, Tinsley BA, O'Malley MP. Pronator syndrome and anterior interosseous nerve syndrome. J Am Acad Orthop Surg. 2013;21(5):268–75.
4. Moore AM. Nerve transfers to restore upper extremity function: a paradigm shift. Front Neurol. 2014;5(40):1–2.
5. Gu Y, Wang H, Zhang L, Zhang G, Zhao X, Chen L. Transfer of brachialis branch of the musculocutaneous nerve for finger flexion: anatomic study and case report. Microsurgery. 2004;24(5):358–62.
6. Brown JM, Mackinnon SE. Nerve transfers in the forearm and hand. Hand Clin. 2008;24:319–40.
7. Hawasli AH, Chang J, Reynolds MR, Ray WZ. Transfer of the brachialis to the anterior interosseous nerve as a treatment strategy for cervical spinal cord injury. Global Spine J. 2015;5:110–7.
8. Ray WZ, Yarbrough CK, Yee A, Mackinnon SE. Clinical outcomes following brachialis to anterior interosseous nerve transfers. J Neurosurg. 2012;117(3):604–9.
9. Mackinnon SE, Yee A, Ray WZ. Nerve transfers for the restoration of hand function after spinal cord injury: case report. J Neurosurg. 2012;117(1):176–85.
10. Bertelli JA, Ghizoni MF. Nerve transfers for restoration of finger flexion in patients with tetraplegia. J Neurosurg Spine. 2017;26:55–61.
11. Bertelli JA, Ghizoni MF. Nerve transfers for restoration of finger flexion in patients with tetraplegia. J Neurosurg. 2017;26(1):55–61.
12. Kahn L, Moore A. Donor activation focused rehabilitation approach: maximizing outcomes after nerve transfers. Hand Clin. 2016;32(2):263–77.
13. Novak CB. Rehabilitation following motor nerve transfers. Hand Clin. 2008;24(4):417–23.
14. Kahn LC, Stonner MM, Miller VA. Chapter 21: Tendon and nerve transfers. In: Jacobs MLA, Austin NM, editors. Orthotic intervention for the hand and upper extremity, splinting principles and process. 3rd ed. Wolters Kluwer; 2022. p. 477–91.
15. Avers D, Brown M. Muscle testing: techniques of manual examination and performance testing. 10th ed. Saunders; 2018.

Abductor Digiti Minimi (ADM) Branch of the Ulnar Nerve to the Thenar Branch of the Median Nerve Transfer

Macyn M. Stonner

Background

The thenar or recurrent branch of the median nerve innervates the abductor pollicis brevis (APB), opponens pollicis (OP), and superficial head of the flexor pollicis brevis (FPB). Axonal injury to the median nerve may result in the loss of thumb opposition and functional pinch. Patients often develop first web space contractures, weakness, and poor thumb mechanics due to the dominant adductor pollicis unopposed by weak or absent thenar muscles. Unfortunately, native recovery of thumb opposition is uncommon following proximal median nerve injuries due to distance to the end target [1, 2]. Tendon transfers using the extensor indicis proprius (EIP) or extensor digiti minimi (EDM) have historically been used to restore palmar abduction in high median nerve injuries [3]. Palmaris longus (PL) and flexor digitorum superficialis (FDS) are frequently used as donors in low median nerve injuries. However, tendon transfers are often complicated by prolonged immobilization, joint stiffness, donor-site morbidity, transfer failure, and pinch weakness [4, 5]. Tendon transfers are unable to restore rotation of the first metacarpal that contributes to true opposition [6]. Alternatively, nerve transfers have the potential to restore multidirectional thenar function. They have therefore gained considerable recognition in recent years [7].

Outcomes

In 2018, Bertelli first described the transfer of the abductor digiti minimi (ADM) branch of the ulnar nerve to the thenar branch of the median nerve [8]. This pioneer study of five patients showed that all patients obtained a minimum 4/5 thenar manual muscle testing (MMT) grade and 75% of pinch strength recovery [8]. Power and colleagues additionally obtained excellent results from ADM to thenar nerve transfer following median nerve sarcoma resection, demonstrating 4+/5 strength and return to functional activities, including writing and crafting within 15 months [9]. Because this nerve transfer is a relatively new procedure, large-population outcome data is not yet available.

M. M. Stonner (✉)
Milliken Hand Rehabilitation Center, WashU Medicine, St. Louis, MO, USA
e-mail: macyn.stonner@wustl.edu

L. C. Kahn et al. (eds.), *Rehabilitation for Nerve Transfers of the Upper Extremity*,
https://doi.org/10.1007/978-3-031-92008-0_24

Surgical Graphic

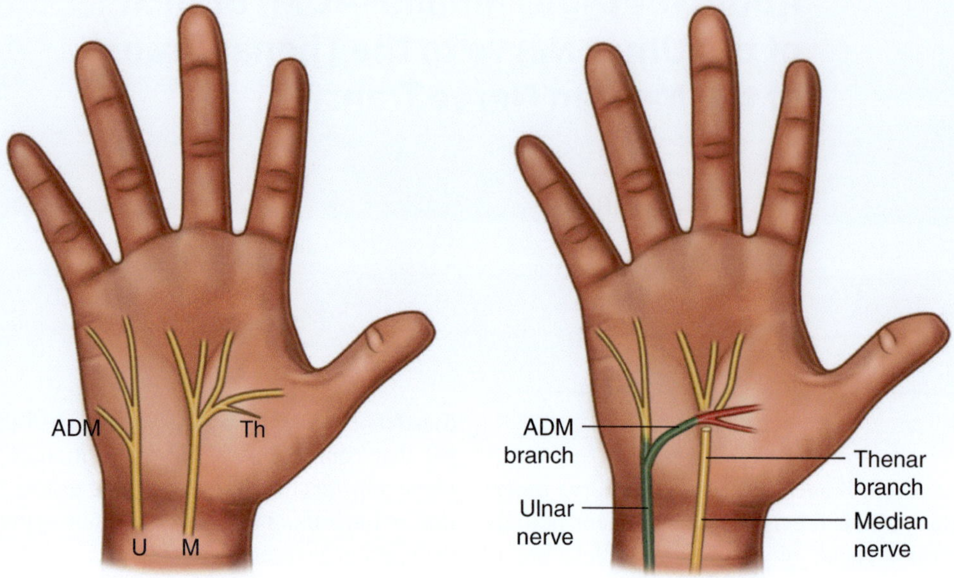

Microsurgical technique of Abductor Digiti Minimi (Adm) Branch of the Ulnar Nerve to the Thenar Branch of the Median Nerve Transfer

A curvilinear incision is made at the base of the palm, centered just radial to the hook of the hamate. The superficial palmar fascia is divided, and the transverse carpal ligament is released along its ulnar aspect. The median nerve is identified within the carpal tunnel and is inspected to identify the recurrent motor branch, which may have an extraligamentous, subligamentous, or transligamentous origin. The nerve branch is then visualized to enter the thenar musculature. A handheld nerve stimulator is used to confirm the absence of thenar function when stimulating the recurrent motor branch, ensuring that the anesthesia team is not using muscle paralytics. This stimulation must be performed within 30 min of the tourniquet being inflated, if one is being used. The ulnar neurovascular bundle is then identified. Release of zones 1, 2, and 3 of Guyon's canal is typically performed. Near the bifurcation of the ulnar motor branch from the ulnar nerve proper, the motor branches to the ADM are identified. A handheld nerve stimulator is used to confirm isolated ADM function (and no other ulnar intrinsic function) when stimulating the donor nerve. This stimulation must be performed within 30 min of the tourniquet being inflated, if one is being used. The donor nerve is dissected as distally as possible, divided, and transposed to meet the median nerve. The recipient recurrent motor branch is neurolyzed as proximally as possible from the median nerve proper and divided. Coaptation of the ADM branch of the ulnar nerve to the recurrent motor branch of the median nerve is performed using microsurgical technique.

Phases of Rehabilitation

Phase 1

Pre-op to 1/5 MMT in the Recipient Muscle

Both the surgeon and therapist should provide thorough yet simplified education about the anatomy involved in the nerve transfer and therapy/timeline expectations. Patients should be educated on thumb mechanics as patients with median nerve insufficiency often pinch using an inefficient, adducted posture due to lack of palmar abduction. After surgery, the thumb is positioned in palmar abduction in the postoperative dressing, which is removed after 1–2 weeks. Patients may be referred to an initial therapy visit at this time, often in conjunction with their appointment with the surgeon. A custom hand-based thumb spica orthosis is fabricated with the thumb CMC joint in full palmar abduction and the IP joint free (Image 1). Some prefer a forearm-based thumb spica orthosis to protect the carpal tunnel. Two weeks after surgery, the orthosis does not need to be worn full time; rather, it can be used for comfort and/or function. The orthosis is helpful to prevent web space (adductor) tightness as the patient awaits thenar return. It also reinforces the new, proper functional position that the thumb should maintain for effective pinch and prehension.

Between 10 days and 3 weeks (pending wound healing and surgeon preference), sutures are removed. Scar management may begin once the wound is fully healed.

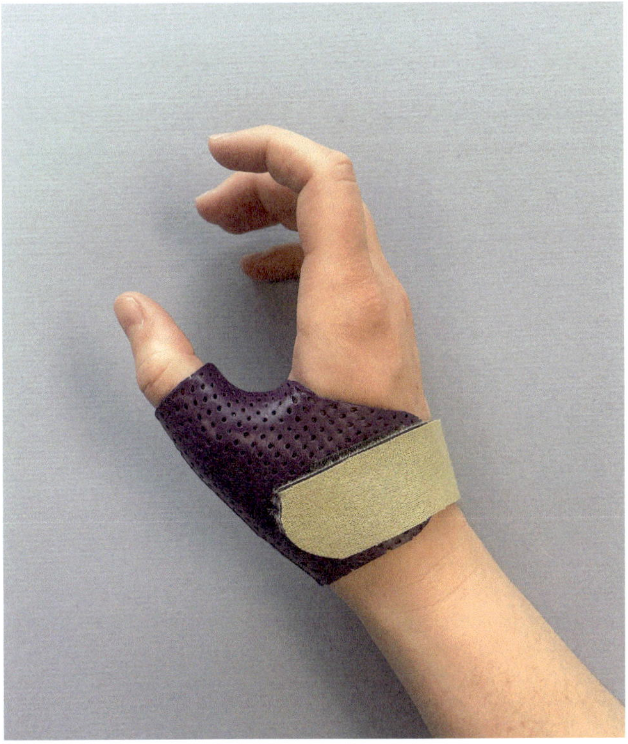

Image 1 At 2–3 weeks post-op, a custom hand-based orthosis that positions the thumb in opposition may be helpful to promote functional grasp/pinch and prevent web space tightness as the patient awaits thenar return

Instrument-assisted soft tissue mobilization (IASTM) is not recommended after nerve surgery. The therapist may provide a general timeline about the anticipated timeframe for functional return of thumb opposition, which has been published to be approximately 9–13 months [8]. At the completion of the first therapy visit, the patient should be able to identify the action of the donor (small-finger abduction) and demonstrate an understanding that performing this movement amplifies neural messages to the thenar muscles [10, 11].

Exercises

- ROM of Uninvolved Joints
  Patients are instructed to perform active range of motion (AROM) of uninvolved joints immediately following the postoperative rest period. Exercises include flexion and extension of the wrist and digits. If the patient has web space tightness, passive palmar abduction should be initiated.
- Donor Activation
  As early as 2 weeks from surgery, patients should be instructed in "flooding the donor" exercises. Donor activation is performed with active small-finger abduction recommended at a frequency of ten repetitions every hour. Instruction in four-finger abduction is a simple way to achieve this.

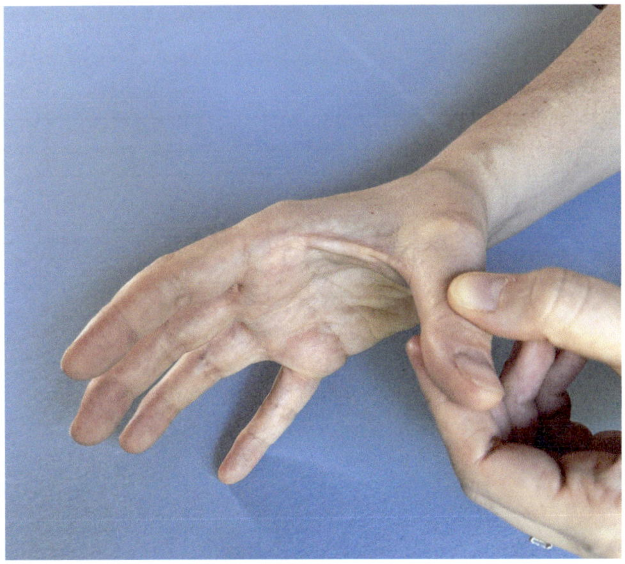

Image 2 Active donor with passive recipient muscle exercise is performed with the hand resting on the ulnar side. The patient is instructed to abduct the small finger into the table while assisting the thumb into abduction and opposition

- Combined Donor with Passive Recipient Exercise
  At follow-up therapy visits, the patient is instructed in combined donor-recipient exercises to strengthen the new motor pathway. This would include active small-finger abduction with passive or "assisted" thumb palmar abduction, performed at a high frequency (10–20 repetitions, 6–8 times per day). With the hand resting on the ulnar side, the patient is instructed to abduct the small finger into a table while assisting the thumb into abduction and opposition (Image 2).

Clinical Pearl

During this phase, a hand-based thumb opposition orthosis is beneficial to reduce the substitution pattern of the adductor and to retrain the thumb in the normal position for functional activities. With this on, the patient is instructed in functional activities involving pinch with active small-finger abduction.

Assessment of Recovery

Thenar motor function is reassessed after a few months either in the therapy or in the surgery clinic. Reinnervation is assessed as the patient touches the small finger and thumb together while attempting to bring the thumb away from the palm. Resistance to small-finger abduction may improve a response in the recipient as the examiner simultaneously palpates the thenar region to evaluate for a muscle contraction (Image 3). In low median nerve injuries, a common substitu-

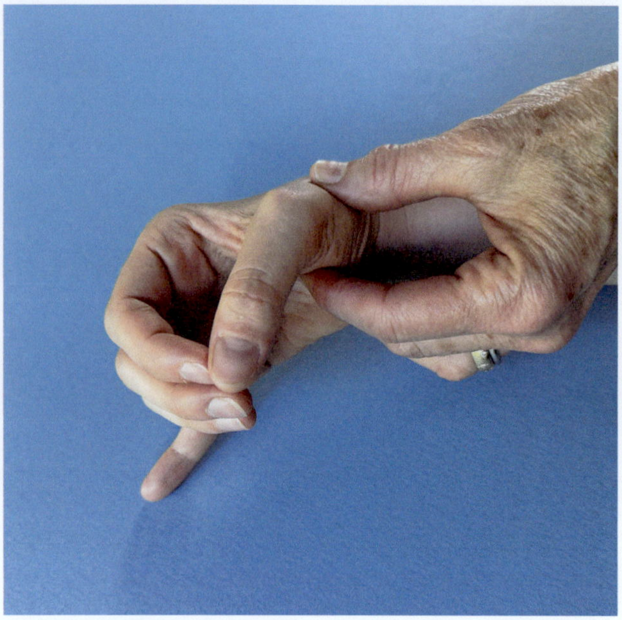

Image 3 Assessment of recovery is performed by applying resistance to small-finger abduction as the examiner simultaneously palpates the thenar region for any muscle contraction

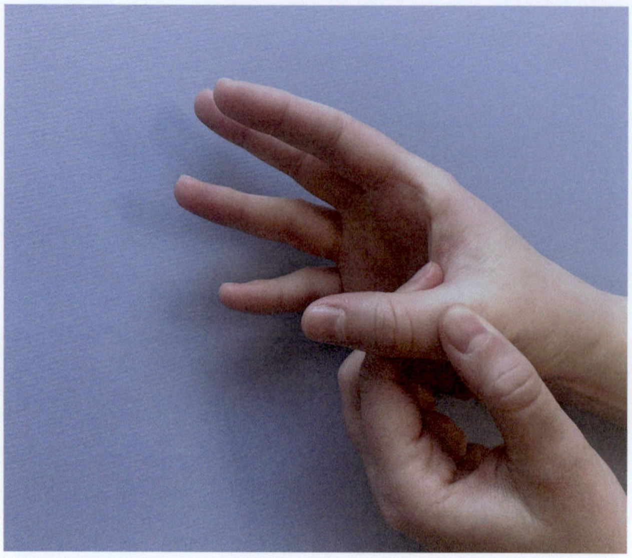

Image 4 The patient is instructed to attempt to touch the thumb and small finger together while assisting the CMC joint into end-range palmar abduction

tion pattern for thumb opposition is thumb flexion with the flexor pollicis longus (FPL) muscle. When assessing recovery of thenar function, the examiner should observe the quality of the movement and palpate the radial aspect of the thenar muscles. When the FPL is dominant, the thumb tip will oppose the radial aspect of the digit, whereas with true opposition, the thumb tip will oppose the digit tip and the fingernails will meet [12].

Therapy Frequency

The ADM-to-thenar nerve transfer is a very intuitive, synergistic transfer. Frequent therapy is often not necessary. Over the course of recovery, an average total number of therapy visits of three to six is reasonable. Phase 1 of rehabilitation could be completed in one therapy visit, addressing education, orthotic needs, donor-recipient exercises, and ROM as needed. Patients may be seen more frequently if they have a webspace contracture, high pain or nerve sensitivity, excessive swelling, and/or stiffness in uninvolved joints. Additional therapy is warranted if multiple nerve transfers were performed at the same time.

Phase 2

2−/5 to 3/5 MMT in the Recipient Muscle

Patients may progress to phase 2 of rehabilitation once they show any active palmar abduction. Exercises are typically performed in a gravity-minimized plane for wrist, elbow, and shoulder conditions. However, the role of anti-gravity versus gravity-minimized movement is not a crucial factor with digital movement. At this point in recovery, the patient should be reliable with his or her home exercise program and demonstrate a good understanding of the donor-recipient muscle relationship. The hand-based thumb spica orthosis should be worn intermittently to maintain proper positioning of the CMC joint, reduce fatigue in the recovering thenar muscles, and assist with functional tasks requiring pinch.

Exercises

- Active Donor with Active-Assisted Recipient
  Abductor Pollicis Brevis MMT = 2−/5 to 2/5
  Phase 2 exercises advance from passive to active-assisted thenar movement while simultaneously contracting the ADM. The patient should frequently attempt to touch the thumb and small finger together while attempting independent palmar abduction and then passively assisting the CMC joint into full-range palmar abduction or opposition (Image 4).
- "Place and Hold" Exercise
  Abductor Pollicis Brevis MMT = 2+/5
  At this point in recovery, a "place and hold" exercise may begin. The patient passively places the thumb in full palmar abduction, releases the support from the contralateral hand, and then attempts to hold this position for 5 seconds (with small-finger abduction).
- Active Donor with Active Recipient
  Abductor Pollicis Brevis MMT = 3−/5 to 3/5
  As the thenar muscles increase in strength and can abduct through mid to full range, exercise includes simple active opposition to the small fingertip. This intuitively contracts the donor ADM with the recipient APB/opponens (Image 5).

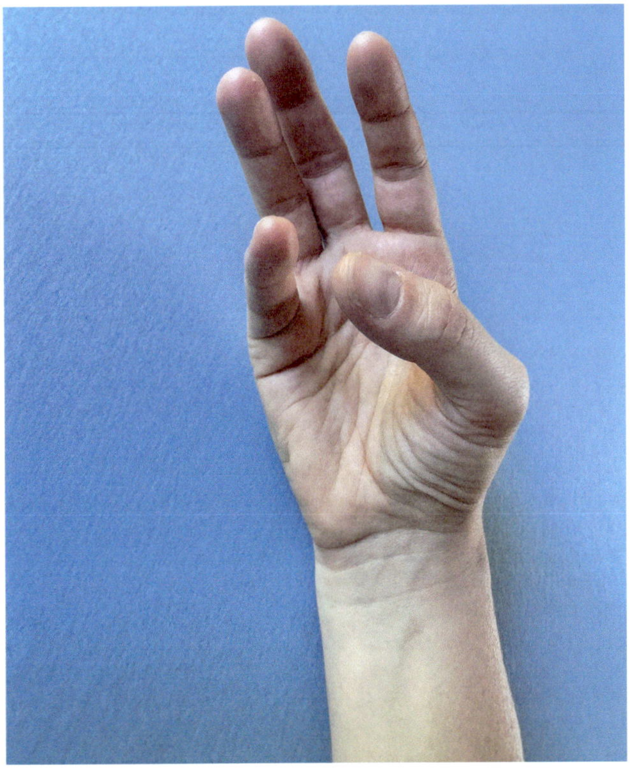

Image 5 Active donor with active recipient muscle exercise is performed with simple active thumb opposition to the small fingertip

- Functional Activity
  Patients are encouraged to activate their nerve transfer for functional activities requiring light pinch. Examples may include threading beads, buttoning a shirt, and/or picking up coins (Image 6). Patients should make their best attempt to avoid collapsing their CMC into adduction or flexion during attempted pinch.
- Therapy Frequency
  Patients may only need to attend formal therapy once or twice in phase 2. High emphasis is placed on short, frequent, independent exercises at home.

Phase 3

3+/5 MMT in the Recipient Muscle

Late-phase therapy begins once the thumb can palmarly abduct through full range against some resistance. Phase 3 is characterized by resistive exercise, which should not be initiated before the APB/opponens demonstrate 3/5 MMT strength. This would likely result in the CMC joint collapsing into adduction during pinch (Image 7), instead of maintaining a stable position in palmar abduction. To prevent fatigue, high repetition/low resistance should remain an important exercise parameter during this time.

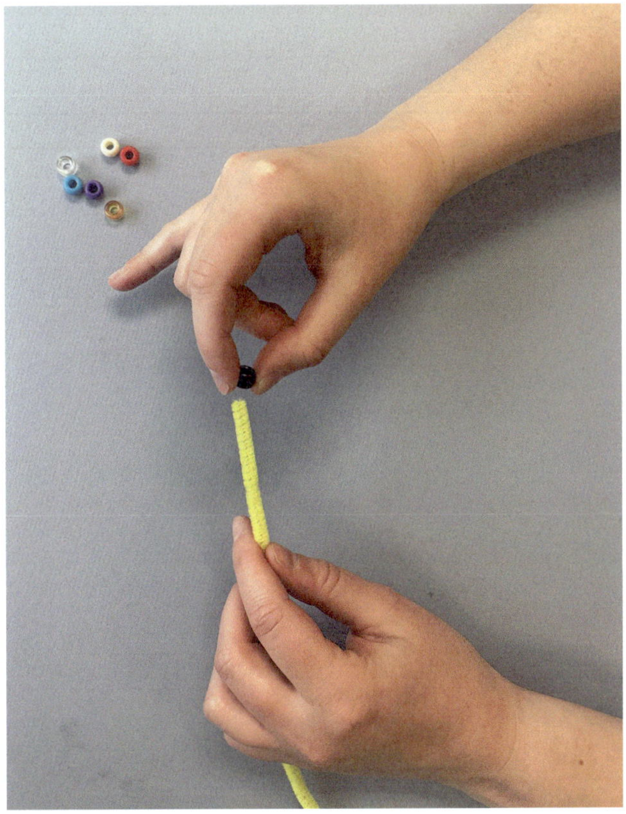

Image 6 Patients are encouraged to activate their nerve transfer with functional activities that require light pinch between the thumb and alternating fingers such as threading beads on a pipe cleaner

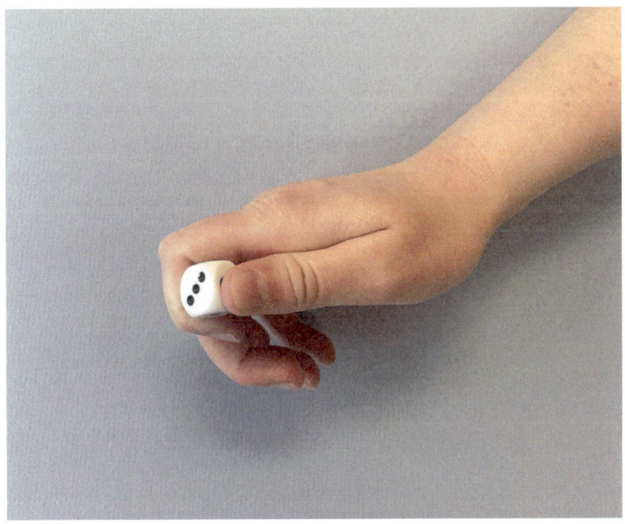

Image 7 Working on resisted pinch before a 3+/5 MMT grade is achieved in the thenars may result in the CMC joint collapsing into adduction during pinch as shown here

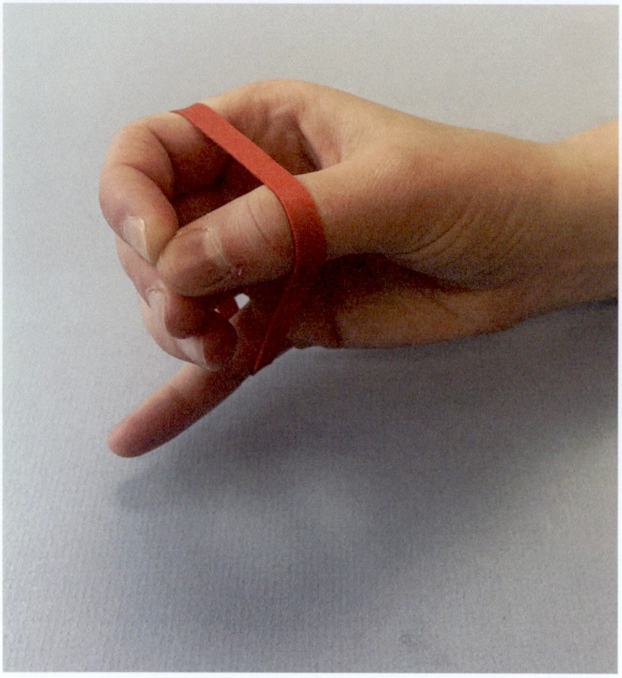

Image 8 Resistance may be introduced with simultaneous contraction of the ADM and thenars by wrapping a rubber band around the thumb and small finger while making an "O" shape

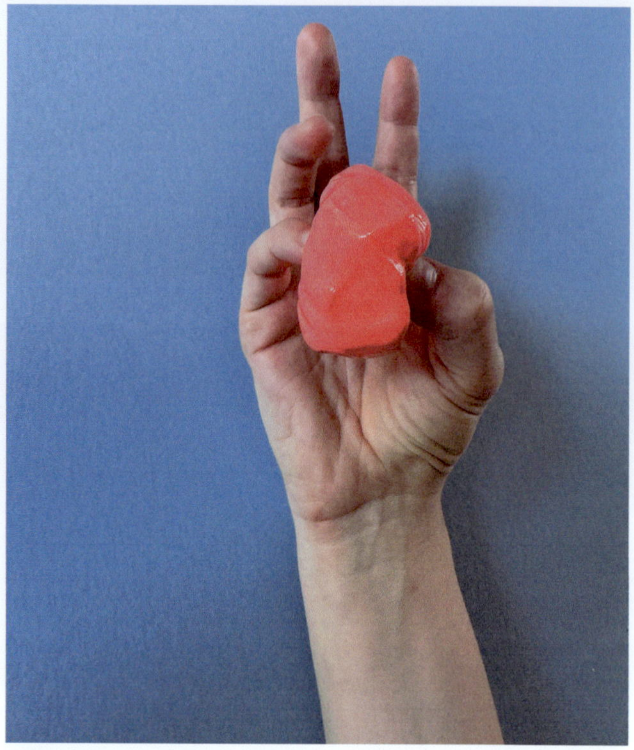

Image 10 Ultimately, the patient is encouraged to strengthen the hand with functional pinching activities involving the thumb and small finger, such as with therapy putty

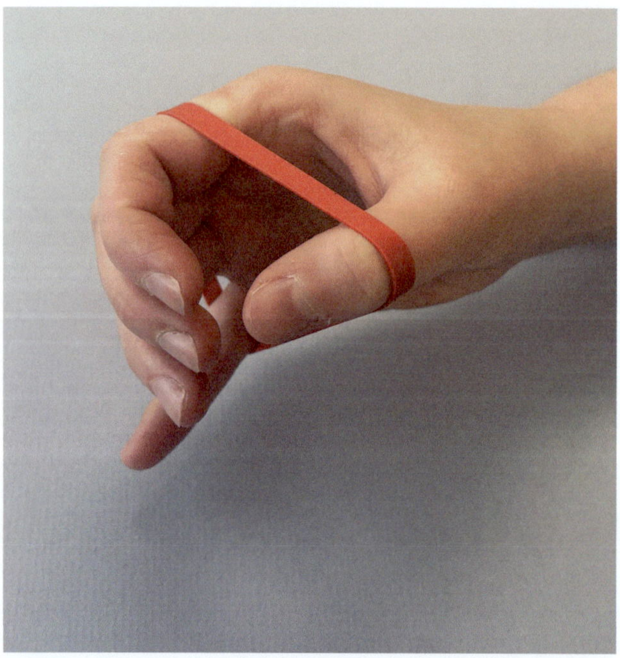

Image 9 The next level of resistance is to attempt a "C" shape with both small finger and thumb abducting against the force of a rubber band

Exercises

- Resistive Recipient Activity with Donor Contraction
  Resistive palmar abduction begins with simultaneous contraction of the ADM. This may involve wrapping a rubber band around the thumb and small finger while first making an "O" shape (Image 8). The patient is then instructed to make a "C" shape, which activates both CMC palmar abduction and small-finger abduction (Image 9). Patients may also work on pinching items between the thumb and small finger, such as putty or clips (Image 10). Engaging the ADM will augment thenar strength, which may be functionally useful when additional pinch strength is needed.
- Resistive Recipient Activity Without Donor Contraction
  Once patients demonstrate reliable activation of their transfer using simultaneous small-finger abduction, they may learn to separate the two functions. Patients may begin to work on resistive tasks with the thumb and index finger (rather than the small finger), such as putting on earrings, opening ziplock bags, or stabilizing a nail while hammering.
- Therapy Frequency
  Patients may only need to attend formal therapy once or twice in phase 3. High emphasis is placed on frequent, independent exercises at home.

ADM-to-Thenar Nerve Transfer

Nerve transfer overview					
Donor nerve	Donor action	Recipient nerve	Recipient action	Indications for functional restoration	Approximate months to functional movement
Deep branch of the ulnar nerve to the ADM	Small-finger abduction	Thenar branch of the median nerve	Thumb palmar abduction and opposition	Pinch strength and coordination	9–13 months [8]

Information below is suggested guidelines. Precautions may vary according to surgeon preferences and patient factors

	Preoperative therapy	Early phase	Middle phase	Late phase
Criteria	Before surgery	0/5 to −1/5 MMT	2−/5 to 3/5 MMT	>3/5 MMT
Purpose of phase	Educate and establish baseline function	Understand donor-recipient relationship Activate donor [10]: small-finger abduction	Activate nerve transfer for functional activities requiring light pinch	Isolate recipient through resistance Separate thumb opposition from donor activation
Precautions	N/A	No thumb/wrist ROM for the first 2 weeks Thumb should be positioned in palmar abduction for at least the first 2 weeks with a neutral wrist	Avoid collapsing the CMC into adduction or excessive MCP/IP flexion during attempted pinch	Resistive exercise should not be performed before the APB has a 3/5 MMT strength Avoid CMC joint collapsing into adduction or excessive MCP/IP flexion during pinch
Frequency of visits (considerations)	1 visit; more if PROM limitations are present	1–2 visits total	1–2 visits total	1–2 visits total
Orthosis considerations	Custom hand-based thumb spica orthosis with the CMC joint in full palmar abduction. The orthosis does not have to be worn full time. It may be worn for comfort and function and to prevent web space contracture	Custom forearm-based thumb spica orthosis (or post-op dressing) is fabricated with the CMC joint in full palmar abduction. It is worn full time for 2 weeks. It may then be replaced with a hand-based orthosis and worn for comfort and function and to prevent web space tightness This will reinforce the proper thumb position for effective pinch and prehension	Hand-based thumb spica orthosis is worn intermittently to maintain proper positioning of the CMC joint and assist with functional tasks requiring pinch	N/A
Interventions		**Donor activation**: Small finger abduction (isometric, active, and resisted) 10× every hour **Donor-recipient pairing**: Active small-finger abduction with passive thumb palmar abduction 10–20 reps, 6–8×/day	**Active/resisted donor with active assist recipient**: Passive progresses to active-assisted thumb palmar abduction (with active and/or resisted small-finger abduction) **Place and hold**: Place thumb in palmar abduction. Remove the support, and maintain this position (with simultaneous small-finger abduction)	**Resisted donor and recipient**: Resisted small-finger abduction while trying to oppose the thumb toward the small finger Can isometrically hold a small object between the thumb and small finger **Resisted recipient without donor contraction**: Thumb to index finger tip pinching into resistance (putty, clip, functional items) without involvement of the small finger
Additional intervention considerations			This transfer is very intuitive and synergistic. Therapy emphasizes high repetition for exercises at home Frequent formal therapy is not necessary in most cases (unless multiple nerve transfers were performed at the same time)	Therapist facilitation of movement is encouraged due to prolonged time of disuse (may still need to activate donor for stronger contraction but continue to work on selective activation) Focus on high repetitions, low resistance

ADM-to-Thenar Nerve Transfer

Goal of Surgery: To restore the ability to perform tip-to-tip pinch

Recipient Movements = Touch tip of thumb to tip of small finger (thumb opposition)

= Move thumb away from palm (thumb palmar abduction)

Recipient Muscles: Opponens pollicis (OP) and abductor pollicis brevis (APB)

Recipient Nerve: Median nerve

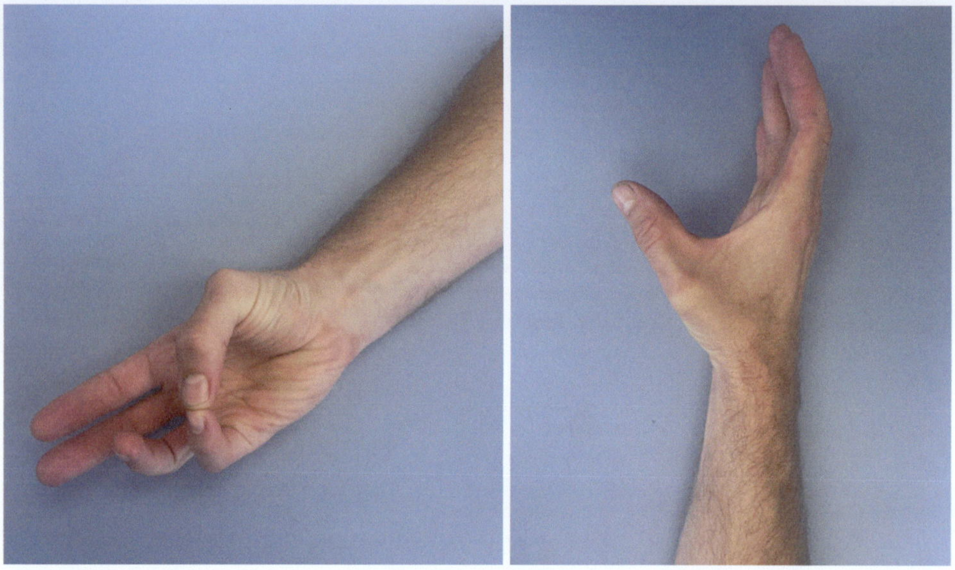

Donor Movement = Move small finger out to side (small finger abduction)

Donor Muscle: Abductor digiti minimi (ADM)
Donor Nerve: Ulnar nerve

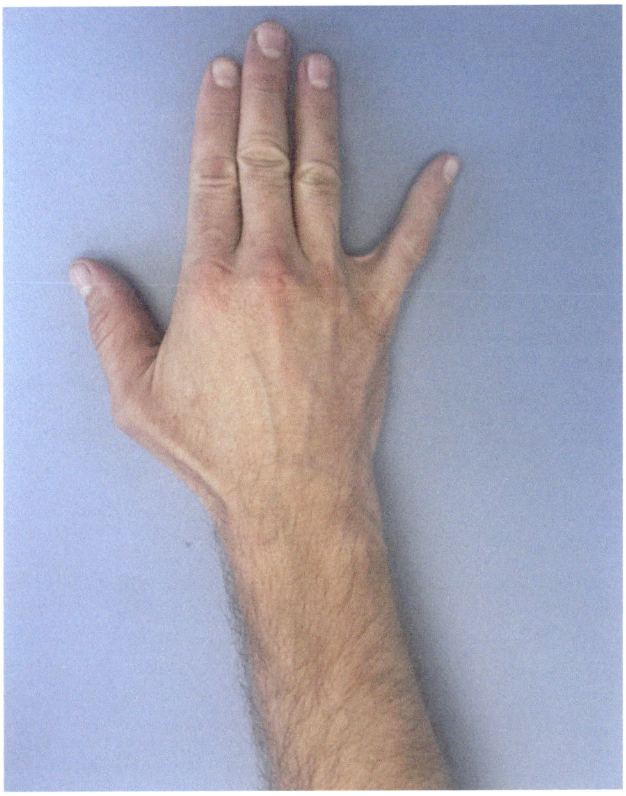

Phase 1 ADM-to-Thenar Nerve Transfer Exercises

☐ **Active Donor Movement**:

- Begin with your palm resting on a table. Move your small finger out the side. Return to the start position, and repeat.

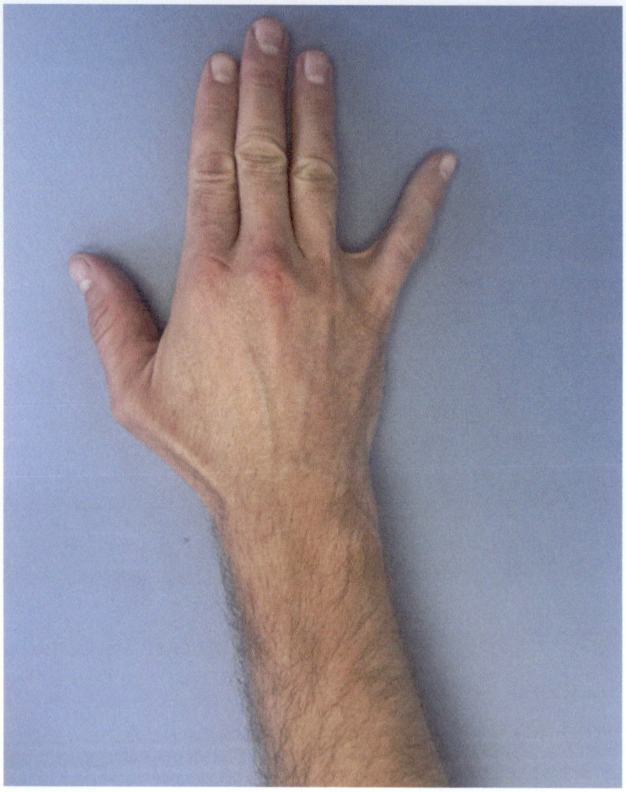

Complete 10 repetitions, every waking hour

☐ **Isometric Donor + Passive Recipient Movement**:

- Begin with the small finger side of the hand resting on a table, your leg, or another surface. Gently press the small finger down into the surface. At the same time, use your other hand to move your thumb away from the palm.

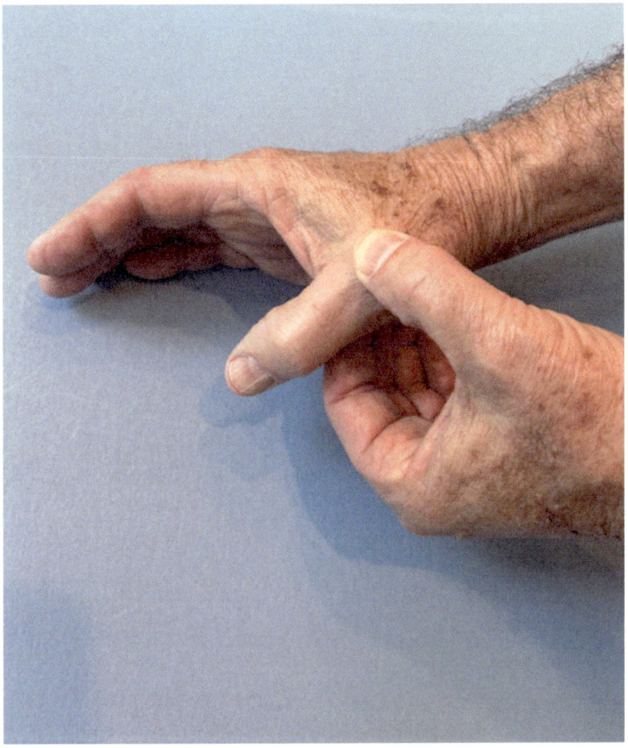

Complete 10–20 repetitions, 6–8 times per day.

Phase 2 ADM-to-Thenar Nerve Transfer Exercises

☐ **Active Donor + Active-Assisted Recipient Movement**:

- First spread your fingers and move the thumb toward the small finger. Use your opposite hand to help the thumb move away from your palm. Try to hold the base of the thumb to rotate it further so you can better reach the tip of your small finger.

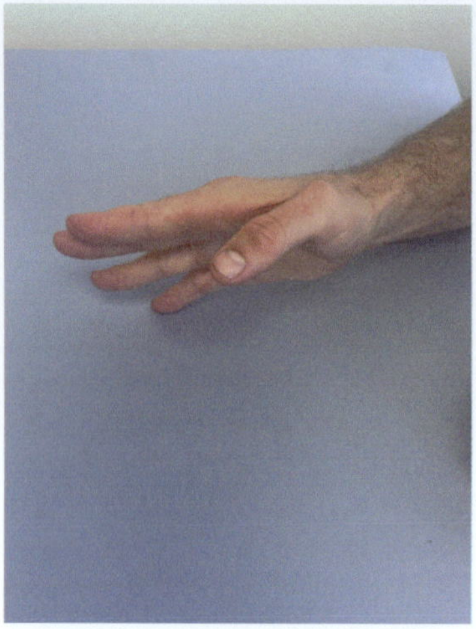

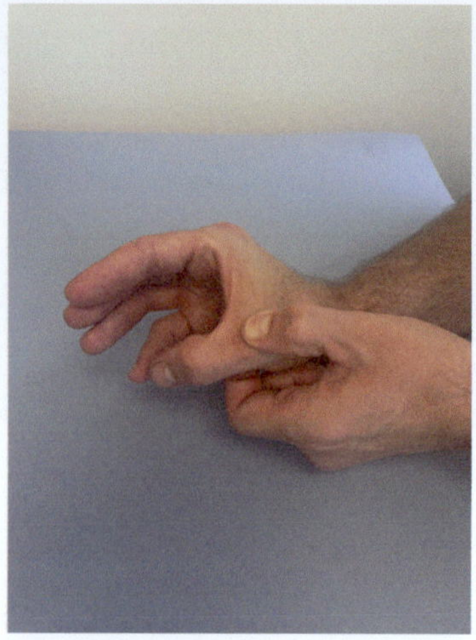

Complete the below exercises 10 repetitions, 3 times per day.

☐ **Isometric Donor + "Place-and-Hold" Recipient Movement**:

- Begin with the small finger side of the hand resting on a table. Using your other hand, bring your thumb away from the palm. Press your small finger into the table. SLOWLY let go of your thumb as you try to keep it away from the palm without the help of your other hand. Hold for 3–5 seconds.

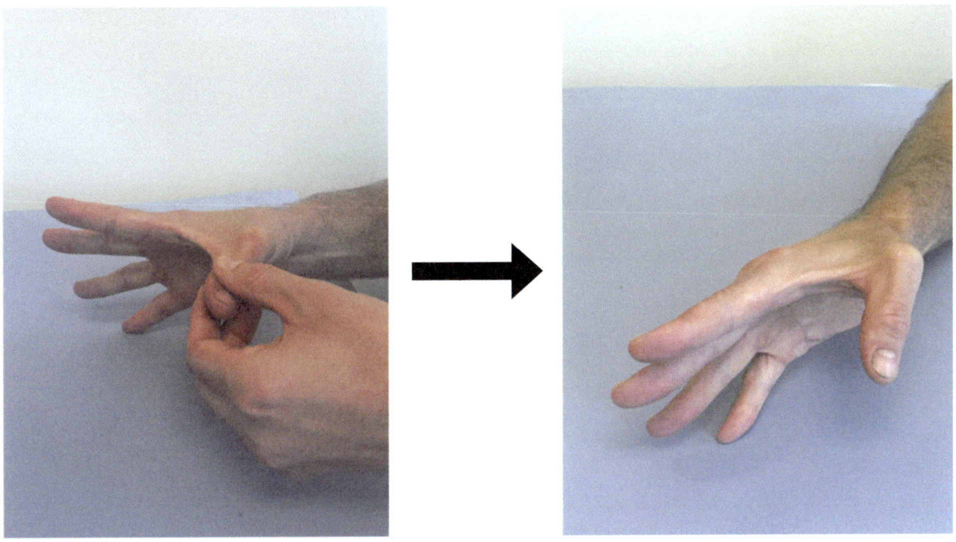

Complete 10 repetitions, 3 times per day.

☐ **Active Donor + Active Recipient Movement**:

- Begin with your forearm supported on a table and hand facing the ceiling. Touch the tip of your thumb to the tip of your small finger, attempting to touch the fingernails together. Return to the start position, and repeat.

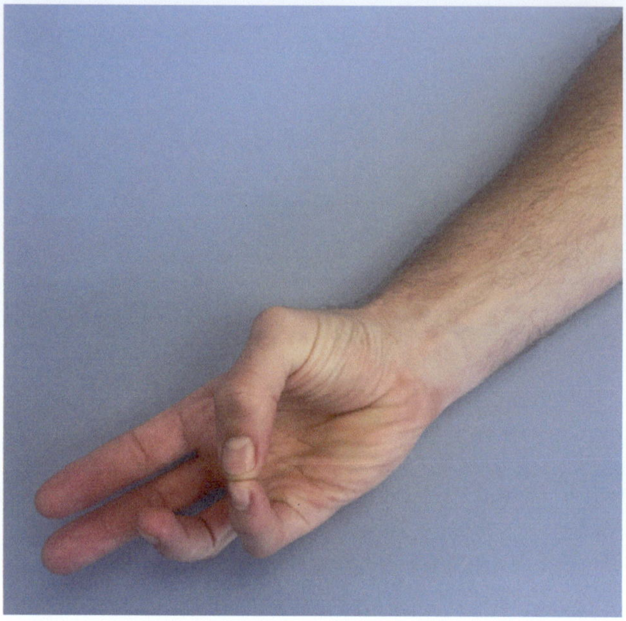

Complete 5–10 repetitions, 3 times per day

Phase 3 ADM-to-Thenar Nerve Transfer Exercises

□ **Resisted Donor + Resisted Recipient Movement**: **Complete one of the below exercises <u>3–10</u> repetitions, <u>2</u> times per day.**

1. Wrap a rubber band around your hand so it is positioned at the base of your thumb and small finger. While pushing the **small finger away from the hand**, make an "O" shape with the tip of your **thumb** and **index** finger. Then, make a "C" shape with your hand. Return to the start position, and repeat.

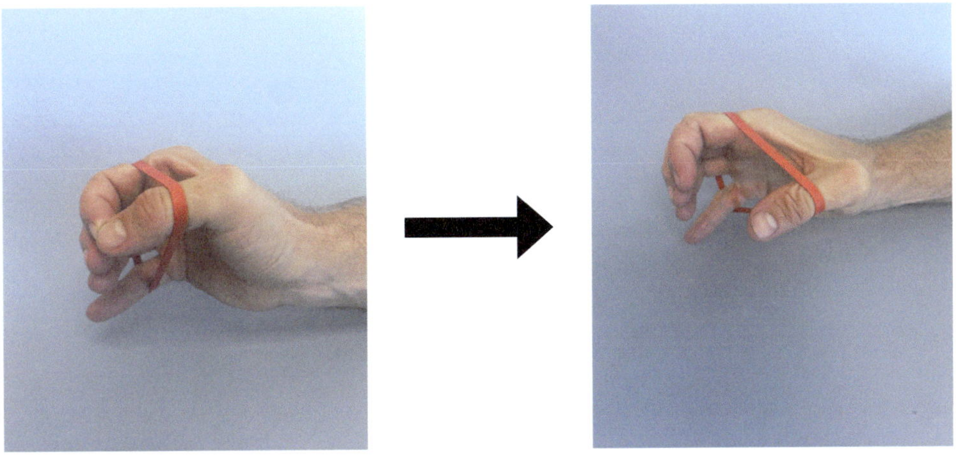

2. Pinch therapy putty between the tip of your **thumb** and the tip of your **small** finger.

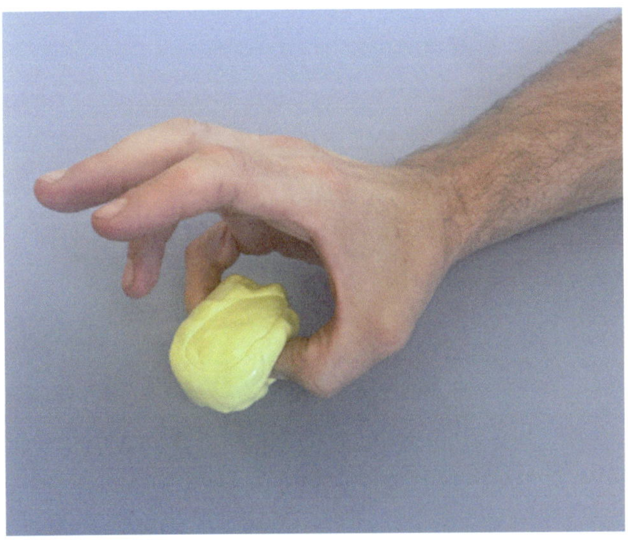

☐ **Resisted Recipient Movement**:

- Pinch therapy putty between the tip of your **thumb** and the tip of your **index** finger while maintaining an "O" shape.

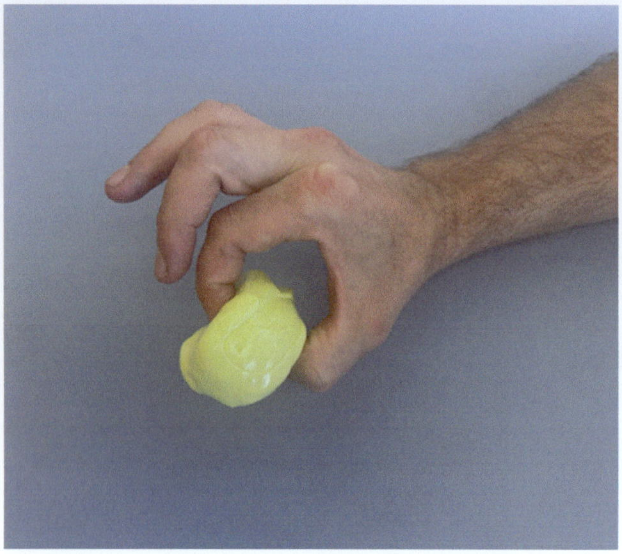

Complete 3–10 repetitions, 2 times per day.

References

1. Boswick JA, Stromberg WB. Isolated injury to the median nerve above the elbow: a review of thirteen cases. J Bone Joint Surg. 1967;49(4):653–8.
2. Hundepool CA, Ultee J, Nijhuis TH, et al. Prognostic factors for outcome after median, ulnar, and combined median–ulnar nerve injuries: a prospective study. J Plast Reconstr Aesthet Surg. 2015;68(1):1–8.
3. Ratner JA, Peljovich A, Kozin SH. Update on tendon transfers for peripheral nerve injuries. J Hand Surg Am. 2010;35(8):1371–81.
4. Abou-Al-Shaar H, Dorius GT, Morton DA, Mahan MA. Distal nerve transfer for thenar palsy: a cadaveric study. Clin Anat. 2020;33(3):414–8.
5. Coulshed N, Xu J, Graham D, Sivakumar B. Opponensplasty for nerve palsy: a systematic review. Hand. 2023;19:1037–43. https://doi.org/10.1177/15589447231174481.
6. Jones NF, Machado GR. Tendon transfers for radial, median, and ulnar nerve injuries: current surgical techniques. Clin Plast Surg. 2011;38(4):621–642e.
7. Soldado F, Bertelli JA, Ghizoni MF. High median nerve injury: motor and sensory nerve transfers to restore function. Hand Clin. 2016;32(2):209–17.
8. Bertelli JA, Soldado F, Rodrígues-Baeza A, Ghizoni MF. Transfer of the motor branch of the abductor digiti quinti for thenar muscle reinnervation in high median nerve injuries. J Hand Surg Am. 2018;43(1):8–15.
9. Power HA, Fox IK, Kahn LC, Mackinnon SE. Restoration of sensation and thumb opposition using nerve transfers following resection of a synovial sarcoma of the median nerve. J Hand Surg Am. 2019;1(3):185–9.
10. Kahn L, Moore A. Donor activation focused rehabilitation approach: maximizing outcomes after nerve transfers. Hand Clin. 2016;32(2):263–77.
11. Novak CB. Rehabilitation following motor nerve transfers. Hand Clin. 2008;24(4):417–23.
12. Bourrel P. Two objective "archivable" tests for voluntary muscle testing in ulnar and median nerve paralysis. Indian J Lepr. 1997;69(1):13–23.

Anterior Interosseous Nerve (AIN) Branch of the Pronator Quadratus to the Ulnar Motor Nerve Transfer

Lorna C. Kahn

Background

The deep motor branch of the ulnar nerve provides innervation to the palmar and dorsal interossei, lumbricals to the ring and small fingers, hypothenars, and adductor pollicis muscles. Proximal compression or injury to the ulnar nerve may result in loss of pinch and grip strength and loss of dexterity. In cases where the extrinsic muscles are intact (ring and small-finger FDP) but intrinsic ones are weak or absent, there will likely be some degree of ulnar digital clawing. Primary repair of ulnar nerve injuries occurring in the forearm or proximal arm can take many months to recover to the hand due to distance and slow pace of axonal growth [1, 2]. This can lead to permanent denervation of the ulnar intrinsic muscles and ulnar nerve palsy. Distal nerve transfers move the timeline of motor recovery closer to the motor end plate and can "rescue" the intrinsic muscles by providing alternate innervation sooner than a recovering native nerve repair [3, 4].

Surgical Technique

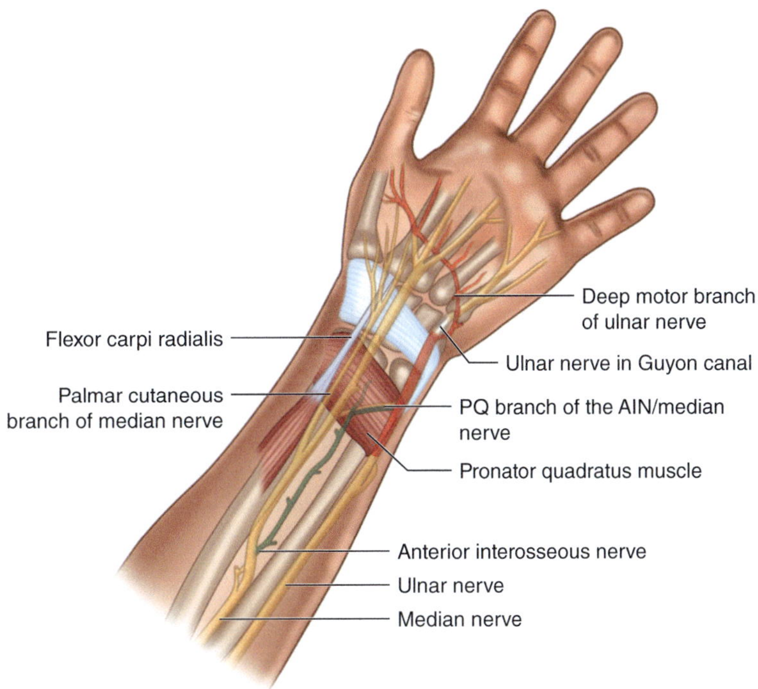

L. C. Kahn (✉)
Milliken Hand Rehabilitation Center, WashU Medicine, St. Louis, MO, USA
e-mail: Kahn.lorna.c@wustl.edu

L. C. Kahn et al. (eds.), *Rehabilitation for Nerve Transfers of the Upper Extremity*,
https://doi.org/10.1007/978-3-031-92008-0_25

A curvilinear incision is made at the base of the palm, centered over the hook of the hamate, continued proximally with a zigzag at the wrist crease, and carried proximally along the flexor carpi ulnaris tendon. The ulnar neurovascular bundle is identified, and Guyon canal release is performed, including a thorough decompression of the deep motor branch of the ulnar nerve from the overlying hypothenar fascia. Intraoperative stimulation is used to confirm whether the ulnar motor branch is functioning. It is important to stimulate the ulnar motor branch within 30 min of the tourniquet being inflated (if one is being used) and to ensure that the anesthesia team is not using any muscle paralytics. The ulnar motor branch is then neurolyzed from the ulnar nerve proper in a retrograde (distal to proximal) manner. Given the reliable topography of the ulnar nerve in the distal forearm, many surgeons choose to perform a "skip" neurolysis to minimize surgical trauma to the ulnar nerve. Typically, neurolysis is performed to the level at which the dorsal cutaneous branch of the ulnar nerve is branching from the ulnar nerve proper. The flexor tendons are then retracted, and the pronator quadratus muscle is identified. The anterior interosseous nerve is identified proximal to the pronator quadratus muscle belly. A handheld nerve stimulator can be used to ensure functioning of the AIN. The pronator quadratus muscle belly is then divided to expose the AIN. The AIN is divided distally after it begins to arborize and is transposed to meet the ulnar nerve. Coaptation of the AIN to the ulnar motor branch is performed using microsurgical technique, either in an end-to-end or reverse end-to-side manner based on the clinical scenario and surgeon preference.

Outcomes

Outcome measures for this nerve transfer should be evaluated carefully. Following a proximal traumatic (Sunderland grades IV–V) injury to the ulnar nerve, an end-to-end nerve transfer (ETE) is typically performed because there is little to no chance of the native nerve recovering from the site of injury all the way into the hand. Any recovery of intrinsic function, therefore, would be due to the nerve transfer. Contrast this with patients who undergo a supercharged (reverse) end-to-side transfer (SETS) in the case of severe compression at the elbow or wrist level. In such cases, a "window" is created in the epineurium of the recipient ulnar nerve, and the AIN branch to the pronator quadratus is coapted here [3]. This procedure preserves an opportunity for the native nerve to recover and restore function. The timing of the recovery would then guide any interpretation of the source of the recovery (native ulnar nerve or AIN input from the nerve transfer).

In a 2021 review of 16 patients with traumatic proximal ulnar nerve injuries that underwent primarily ETE nerve transfers to restore ulnar intrinsic function, George et al. reported "good motor recovery" in 81.3% of patients. Five patients recovered an MMT grade of 4/5 in their ulnar intrinsic muscles, and 13 of the 16 achieved at least a 3/5 MMT grade [5]. Similarly, a systematic review by Thakkar reported that 85% of patients achieved an MMT intrinsic grade of 3/5 or better following this ETE nerve transfer [2].

Thakkar's systematic review also addressed outcomes for ETS and SETS AIN-to-ulnar nerve transfers. In the SETS group, 145/156 patients (93%) achieved an MMT grade greater than 1/5. From seven studies reviewed, 75% of patients undergoing the SETS procedure achieved at least a 3/5 MMT grade in the first dorsal interosseous muscle [2]. No recovery was noted in 11 individuals. Outcomes were better in both procedures when the surgical intervention was performed prior to a year from the onset of symptoms [6].

Phases of Rehabilitation

Phase 1

Pre-op to 1/5 MMT in the Recipient Muscle

Preoperative

The following measures are taken at the first visit: assessment of hand girth (at the distal palmar crease), baseline donor and recipient muscle strength, joint ROM, and grip and lateral pinch strength. Additionally, a list of functional deficits is recorded. Active joint measures will include active MCP and IP joint extension of the ring and small digits to assess the degree of claw deformity that may be present. Lumbrical function is assessed by demonstrating and measuring the individual's ability to position the ring and small digits in the intrinsic plus position (MP flexion and IP extension). The distance of digital spread [7] (Image 1) from the center of the index fingertip to the small fingertip may also be included. These measures will form the baseline for comparison with monthly visit measurements.

If preoperative joint contractures are present, hand therapy treatment is initiated to address this with ROM exercises and orthoses, as needed. An anti-claw orthosis is recommended, if clawing is present, to facilitate active PIP extension (Image 2). A dynamic PIP extension orthosis, such as an LMB™ (Image 3), may also be used to improve passive PIP extension if needed. Donor and recipient muscle function and nerve transfer concepts may be introduced at this time. Donor activation in the form of active forearm pronation exercises is demonstrated to strengthen the new neural pathway created by the nerve transfer [8].

Postoperative

Once postoperative dressings are removed, patients are fit with a prefabricated neutral wrist orthosis. Orthosis use is encouraged for 3 weeks to protect the nerve coaptation, min-

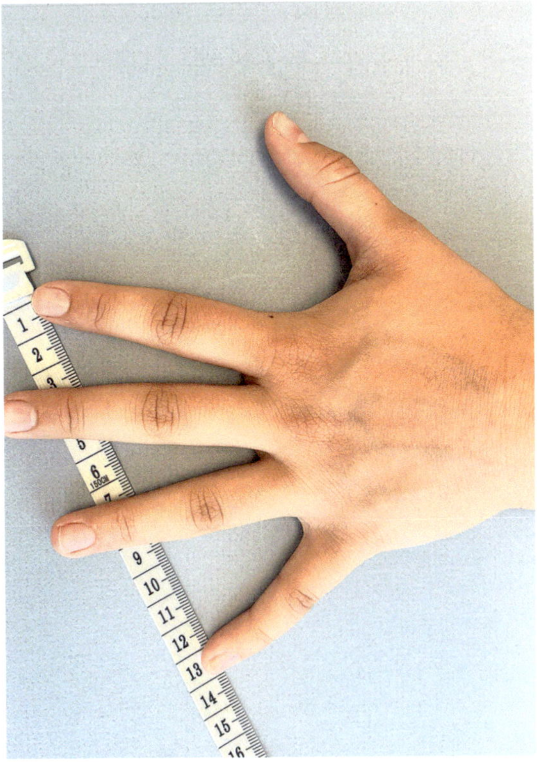

Image 1 Measuring the distance of digital spread from the center of the index fingertip to the small fingertip provides one form of baseline function for comparison with monthly visit measurements

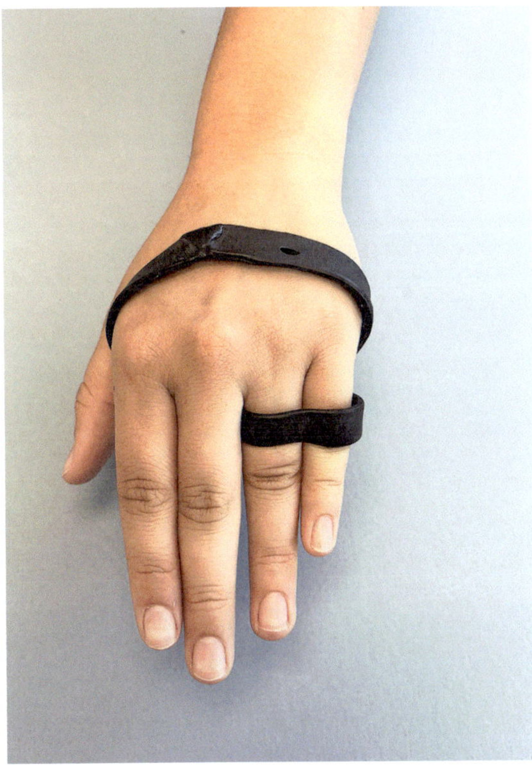

Image 2 An anti-claw orthosis is recommended if clawing is present, to facilitate active PIP extension and prevent PIP joint contracture

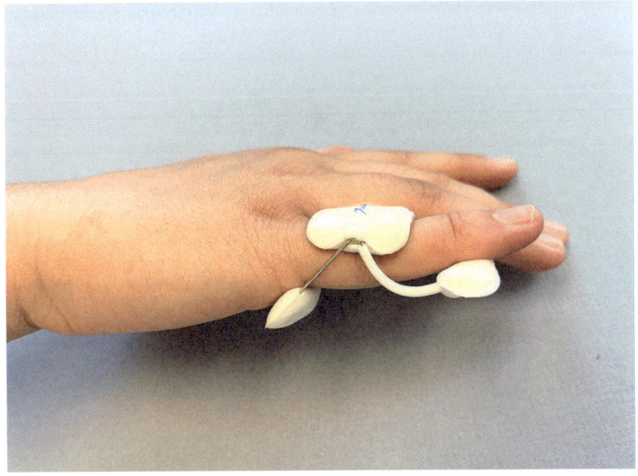

Image 3 A prefabricated PIP dynamic extension orthosis such as the LMB™ shown here is recommended for patients who present with PIP joint contracture to improve PROM. Recommended frequency of use is 4–6×/day for 10–30 min

imize edema, and discourage functional use of the hand but not completely limit finger ROM. Once sutures have been removed, scar management is addressed. Given the location of the incision in the volar distal third of the forearm, there is a potential for scar adherence to the flexor tendons. Tendon gliding exercises and scar massage in this area are encouraged. IASTM devices are not recommended near a nerve repair or transfer. If hand or wrist edema is present, standard edema management techniques are employed with compression, retrograde massage, and education about proper positioning and elevation.

Patient education is initiated with a review of the anatomy of the involved structures. The donor and recipient muscle groups are named, and written descriptions are issued for reference.

Exercises

- Donor Activation

  Donor activation exercises begin with active forearm rotation. Hourly performance of ten repetitions of active pronation is recommended. Early-phase donor activation exercises are completed with low resistance, high repetitions, and high frequency to maximize neural signals to the donor muscle [9, 10]. During subsequent visits, isometrics and resistance exercises with weight or a dowel can be added to augment donor activity.
- Combined Donor with Passive Recipient Exercise

  These exercises are relatively simple because they are performed with the palm on a table, which inherently requires forearm pronation and thus some degree of donor activation. Interossei exercises involve passively moving each finger into abduction and adduction with the opposite hand. A coin or small tab of Velcro is recommended

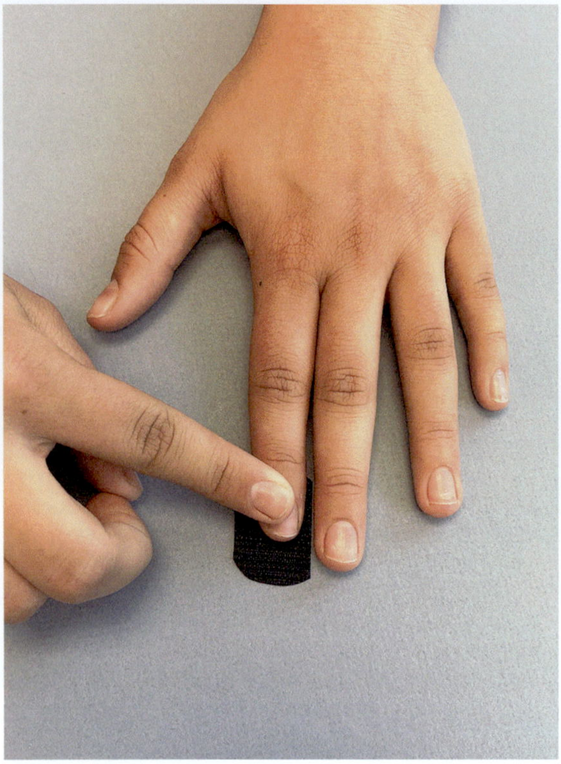

Image 4 Combined donor with passive recipient exercise is demonstrated with the forearm in pronation as the individual assists the finger into abduction

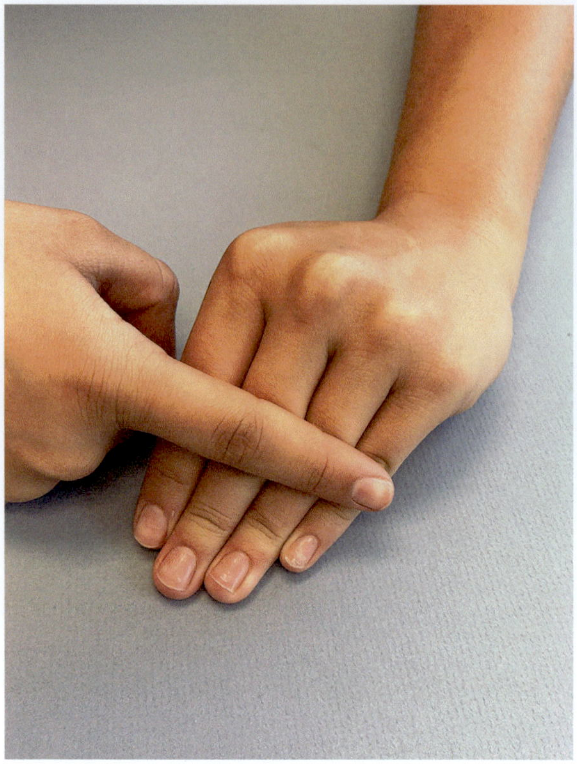

Image 5 Passive lumbrical exercises are performed in pronation with passive assistance to the ring and small fingers into IP extension and MCP flexion

to reduce friction under the fingertip (Image 4). Lumbrical exercises are performed in pronation as well; the ring and small fingers are passively assisted into IP extension and MCP flexion (Image 5).

These exercises are challenging and frustrating in the early period when there is no active participation of the ulnar intrinsic muscles. Circumferential extension tube splints are recommended for those who demonstrate a strong claw deformity (Image 6). These can be fabricated easily with scraps of thermoplastic material. By maintaining the IP joints in extension, the patient can more easily and successfully focus on digital abduction/adduction, MCP flexion, and IP extension. This aids in training the hand to avoid the strong substitution patterns created by the extrinsic flexor (FDS, FDP) and extensor muscles (EDC, EIP, EDM).

Assessment of Recovery

Reinnervation of the muscle is assessed by resisting forearm pronation (isometrically against a table) while attempting to activate one of the intrinsic muscles as it is observed and palpated by the therapist. Given that the ulnar nerve route begins in the hypothenar muscles before growing across the palm toward the first dorsal interossei [11], it makes sense to check for muscles on the ulnar side of the hand first in the early phases. Keep in mind that although the estimated timeline for

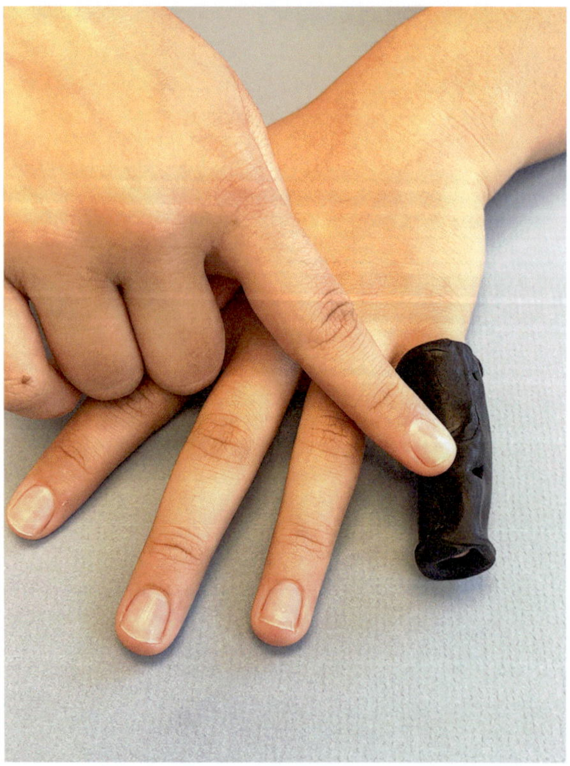

Image 6 Extension tube splints are helpful for individuals with a strong claw deformity to aid with isolation of the intrinsic muscle exercises

this nerve transfer recovery is 9–18 months [12], if the nerve transfer is performed in an end-to-side fashion, there is a possibility that the native nerve will recover sooner. If a response or change in motor function is seen in the first month, it is likely due to improved blood flow to the nerve from the decompression at Guyon's canal [13]. If there is improvement between 3 and 6 months, it is likely due to recovery of myelin sheath which restores conductivity in the nerve in this time frame [14]. After 6 months, improvement in intrinsic motor function is likely due to the nerve transfer.

To test this hypothesis, the therapist may look for donor dominance [15]. The patient's ability to maintain an intrinsic plus position should be compared in both pronation and supination. Have the patient perform the movement in supination and then in pronation (with resistance to pronation), and compare the finger positions (Image 7). If there is greater control of MP flexion and IP extension with pronation, then the nerve transfer is likely innervating these muscles (Image 8).

Therapy Frequency

In phase 1, patients may require hand therapy once a week until the wound is healed, excessive joint restriction is resolved, and the patient demonstrates an understanding of all exercises. Patients should be able to verbalize an understanding of the timeline for recovery. Once these goals are achieved, monthly visits may commence.

Phase 2

From 2−/5 to 3/5 MMT in the Recipient Muscles

Precautions

Avoid prolonged or high-intensity exercises that involve the recipient muscles. Intense exercise leading to recipient muscle fatigue may impair the regeneration of axons, inhibiting reinnervation of recipient musculature [10, 15, 16].

Orthosis

Daytime use of the anti-claw orthosis is recommended until the claw deformity is resolved.

Exercises

Once a response is visualized in the intrinsic muscles, phase 2 of therapy may begin. A response in this context is considered to be an intrinsic joint motion beyond a twitch.

- Combined Active Donor with Active-Assisted Recipient Ulnar Intrinsic MMT = 2−/5 to 2/5
  With the patient seated at a table, a piece of foam or therapy-putty is placed under the thenar muscles. This provides the patient with a tactile cue to press down, thus activating the donor muscle with forearm pronation. Instruction is given to simultaneously attempt active

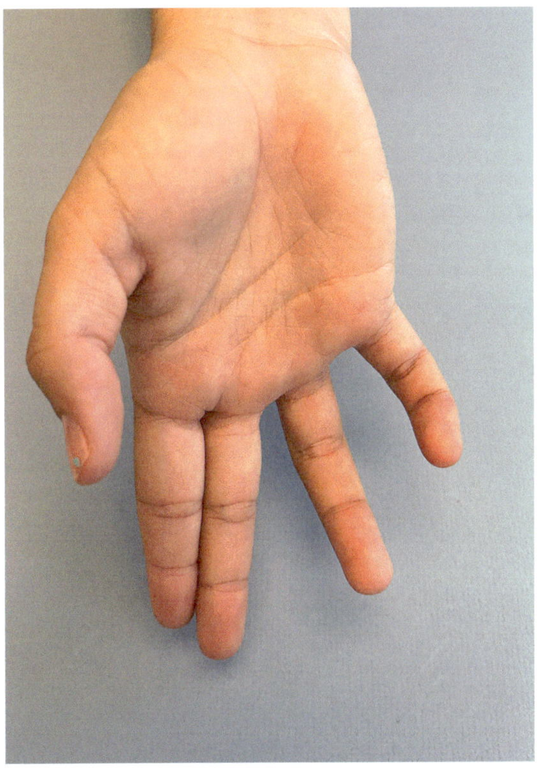

Image 7 Assess for recovery in supination and pronation. If there is equal or greater reduction in claw deformity, the recovery is possibly not related to the nerve transfer but more likely to the decompression at Guyon's canal

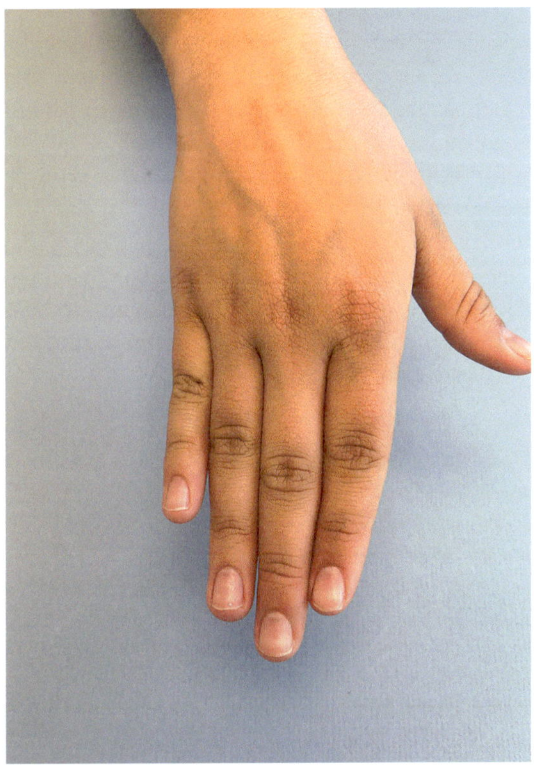

Image 8 If the individual demonstrates greater control of IP extension (reduction in claw) in pronation, at 6 months or more post-op, the response is more likely related to the AIN-to-ulnar nerve transfer

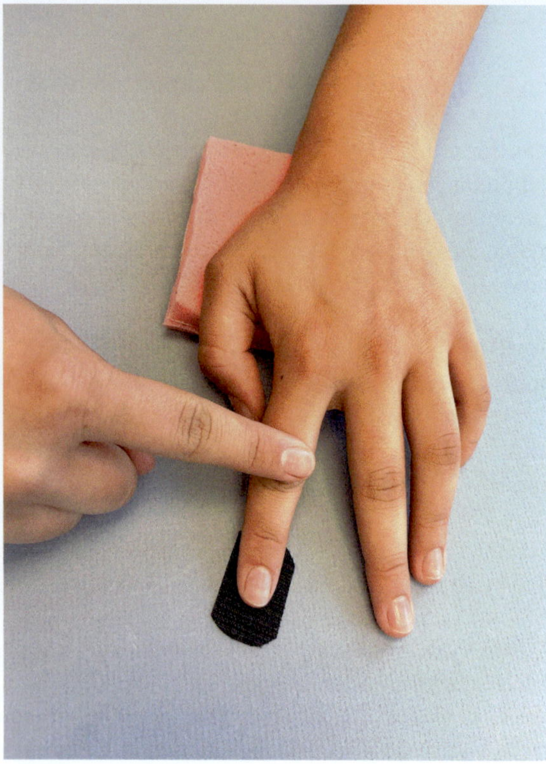

Image 9 Active donor with active-assisted recipient exercises are performed in pronation with assistance to each finger into abduction/adduction. A coin or Velcro tab beneath the fingertip will allow it to slide more easily, making it easier for the weak recipient interossei muscle to move the finger

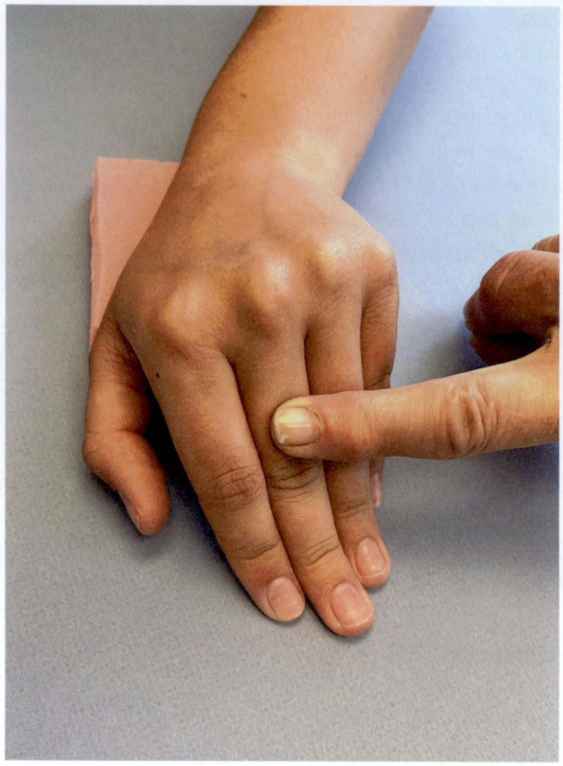

Image 10 Active donor with active-assisted lumbrical exercise is demonstrated here with the forearm in pronation

finger abduction with the IP joints in extension (dorsal interossei) and to assist the finger to complete available abduction range (Image 9). The same is performed for finger adduction (palmar interossei) and "table-top" position for MP flexion and IP extension (lumbricals) (Image 10). Strategies that improve ease of effort for the recipient muscles are incorporated, such as placing a coin or Velcro™ tab under the finger pad to reduce friction [10]. IP joint extension tubes (Image 11) continue to be useful as the patient begins to regain some intrinsic control while trying to overcome extrinsic input.

Clinical Pearl
Place a 1–2 inch dowel directly beneath the volar MCP joints, which will support the hand in slight MCP flexion. This helps reduce the extrinsic substitution when performing assisted intrinsic exercises.

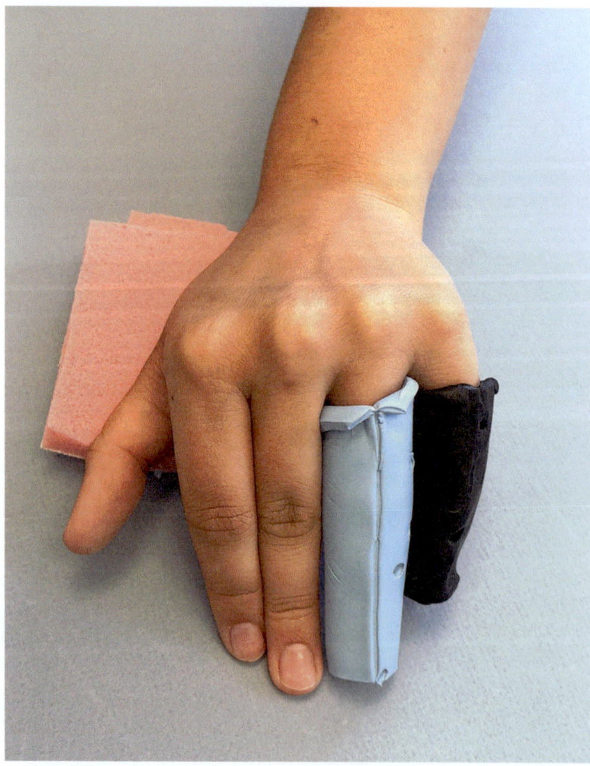

Image 11 Extension tube splints are useful to control clawing during exercise in phase 2

- "Place and Hold"
  Ulnar Intrinsic MMT = 2+/5
  Patients may progress from purely passive motion to a "place and hold" once there is some active joint move-

ment in the recipient intrinsic muscles. While isometrically resisting pronation into the table, the opposite hand passively places a finger into abduction. The patient is cued to maintain that position for a count of 3 seconds. Approximately six to ten repetitions are recommended or until fatigue is noted and/or the extrinsic muscles overpower the movement. While still demanding a strong contraction of the donor PQ, this exercise is repeated for each ulnar intrinsic muscle (outlined below) in isolation.
Thumb adduction (adductor pollicis)
Index-finger abduction (first dorsal interossei)
Index-finger adduction (first palmar interossei)
Middle-finger abduction (second and third dorsal interossei)
Ring-finger adduction (second palmar interossei)
Ring-finger abduction (fourth dorsal interossei)
Small-finger adduction (third palmar interossei)
Small-finger abduction (abductor digiti minimi)
Ring- and small-finger MP flexion and IP extension (third and fourth lumbricals)

- Active Donor with Active Recipient
  Ulnar Intrinsic MMT = 3−/5 to 3/5
  Beginning in supination while seated at a table, the patient pronates the forearm and simultaneously performs digital abduction (dorsal interossei, abductor digiti minimi), with care to avoid MP hyperextension and/or IP flexion. The same is performed for digital adduction (palmar interossei), MP flexion with IP extension "table top" (lumbricals), and thumb adduction (adductor pollicis) with care to avoid compensatory thumb IP flexion from the extrinsic flexor pollicis longus (FPL).
- Functional Activity
  Functional activities are advanced during phase 2 to maximize grip strength and hand use. Activities may include playing card draw/count (Image 12), "pinch and place" (alternating opposition) of light objects such as cotton balls, and use of small pegboards (Image 13). Patients are encouraged to hold light objects, like cotton balls or pencils, between their thumb and index finger to promote strength of the adductor pollicis and first dorsal interossei. Frequency should be a limited number of repetitions throughout the day to minimize fatigue.
  Donor activation continues throughout phase 2 to maximize the input to the weak ulnar intrinsic muscles. Resistive pronation exercises are encouraged along with exercises that combine resisted pronation with grasp, such as using a FlexBar® (Image 14).

Assessment of Recovery

Reinnervation of the recipient muscles is assessed by resisting forearm pronation while attempting to activate one of the intrinsic muscles as it is palpated by the examiner. The easiest intrinsic muscles to palpate are the hypothenars and first dorsal interossei. Manually blocking the dorsal hand throughout the assessment will limit substitution with metacarpal movement.

Therapy Frequency

Once active movement is observed in the intrinsic muscles, the frequency of therapy may be increased to every week or every other week, depending on the needs of the patient. Once the patient demonstrates an understanding of their motor reeducation program and their home exercise program, therapy visits may be reduced to once per month.

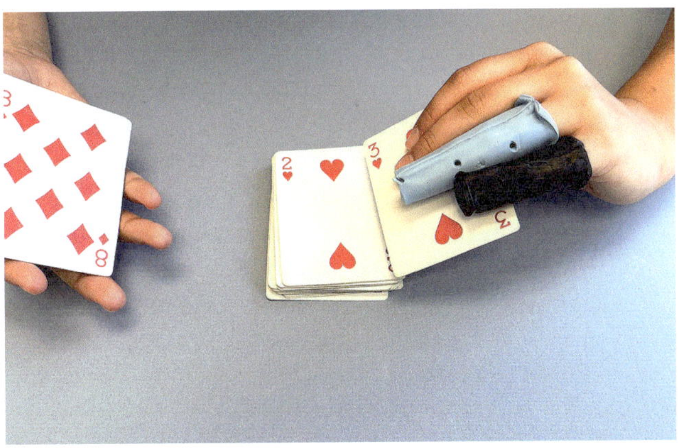

Image 12 Drawing or counting playing cards from a deck is an example of activities used in phase 2 to encourage lumbrical function

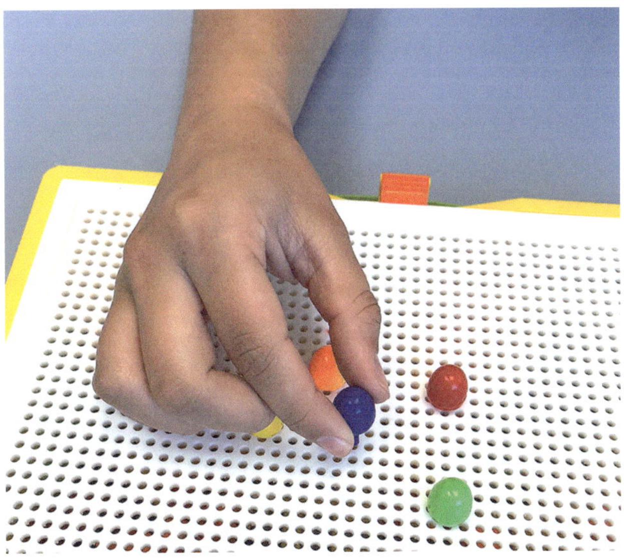

Image 13 Pegboards are used as a functional activity that encourages pinch in forearm pronation

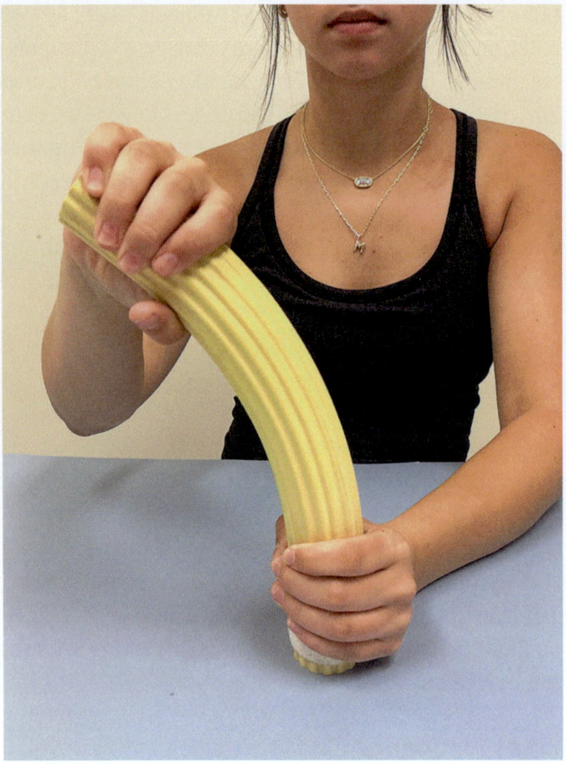

Image 14 A Flexbar™ is used for resisted pronation exercises. This image demonstrates an exercise that combines resisted pronation with grasp

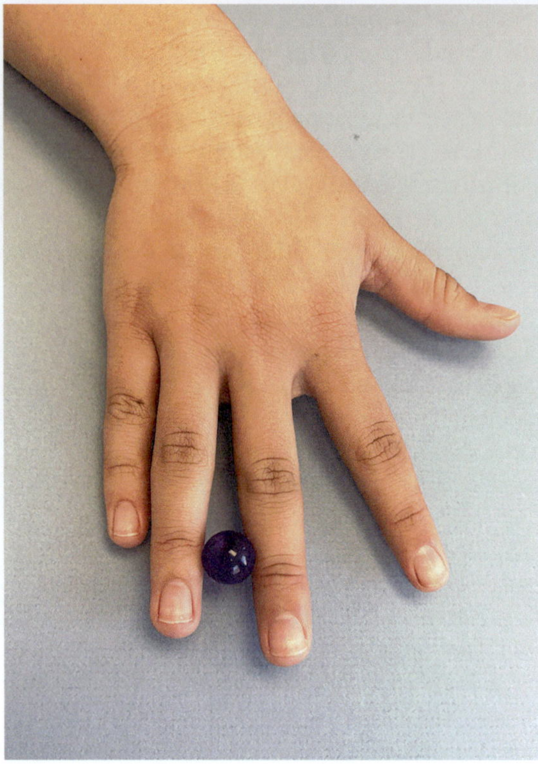

Image 15 One example of a resisted recipient activity with donor contraction is holding small objects between the fingers with the forearm pronated. Progressively making the object smaller will increase the challenge of this activity

Phase 3

3+/5 MMT in the Recipient Muscle(s)

Resistive activity may begin once the patient can move through the full active ROM and hold the ulnar digits in extension (without clawing) and in the intrinsic plus position.

Precautions

Continue to monitor and limit fatigue as resistive exercises are added.

Orthosis

The anti-claw orthosis is weaned gradually as endurance is achieved and clawing resolves.

Exercises

- Resistive Recipient Activity with Donor Contraction
  Retrieval of small objects between digits will promote palmar interossei (adduction) strength, but care must be taken to avoid MP hyperextension and IP joint flexion (Image 15). This activity can be advanced with heavier items, such as therapy-putty (Image 16).
  Exercises and activities that challenge the lumbricals are encouraged. One example is "table-top pulls." With the hand in intrinsic plus position, the fingers pull through therapy-putty while maintaining IP joint extension (Image 17).
  Resistive pinch activities include therapy-putty pulls. Both hands hold opposite ends of the putty, pinching to hold it in place while pulling apart. If the thumb defaults to the substitution pattern of excessive IP flexion due to FPL dominance, an IP flexion block orthosis such as an Oval8TM may be used to better isolate the adductor pollicis muscle [17] (Image 18).
- Resistive Recipient Activity Without Donor Contraction
  There will be instances in which ulnar intrinsic strength is needed when the forearm is not pronated. During phase 3, the patient may start trying to de-emphasize the assistive component of the donor PQ with exercises performed in forearm supination. Resisted finger abduction using a rubber band around the hand in a supinated position is one example of this (Image 19). Pinch and lumbrical strengthening may similarly be performed in supination or forearm neutral. Holding flat objects such as a book with the hand in intrinsic plus position requires resisted lumbrical activity and would naturally be done with the forearm supinated.

Assessment of Recovery

MMT strength of all the ulnar intrinsic muscles with and without donor activation should continue to be assessed. The greatest strength will likely be noted during co-contraction

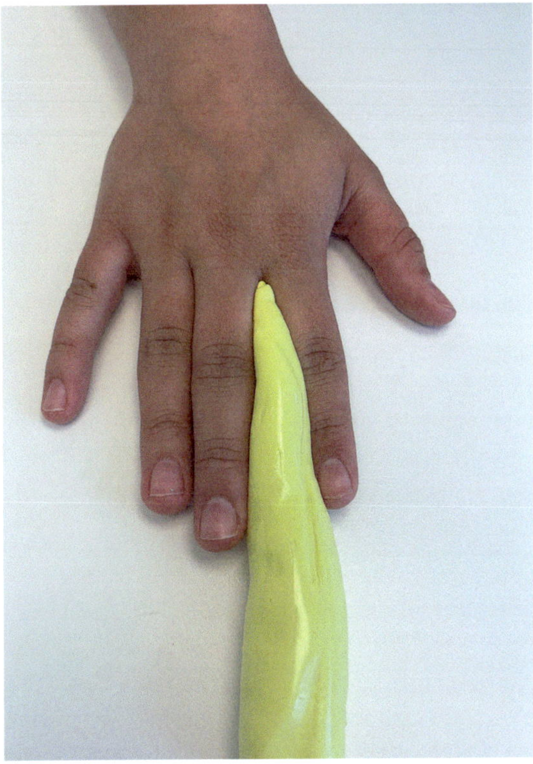

Image 16 Therapy putty is used to advance resistance in phase 3 for finger adduction

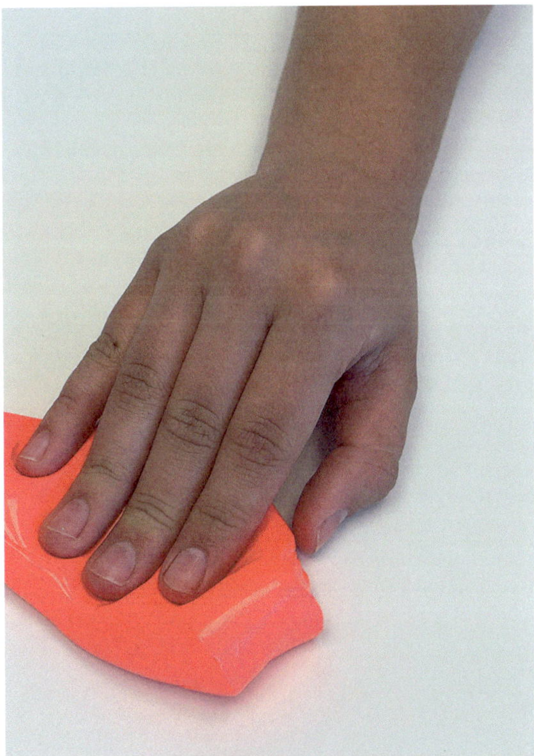

Image 17 Resisted lumbrical exercise includes "tabletop pulls" into therapy putty while maintaining IP joint extension

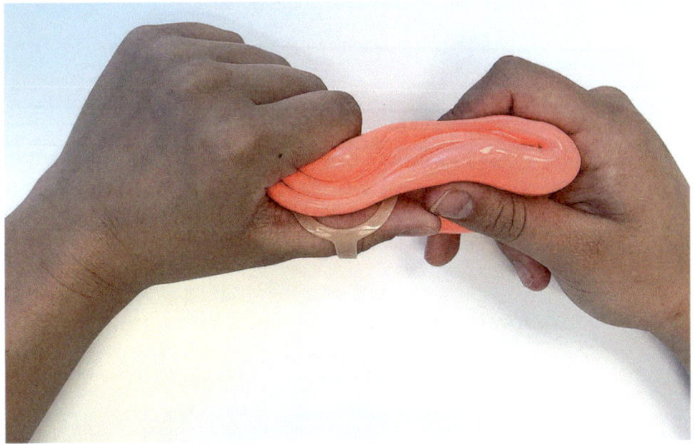

Image 18 An IP flexion block orthosis such as an Oval-8® splint is used to isolate the adductor pollicis muscle by limiting excessive thumb IP flexion due to FPL dominance during pinch activities

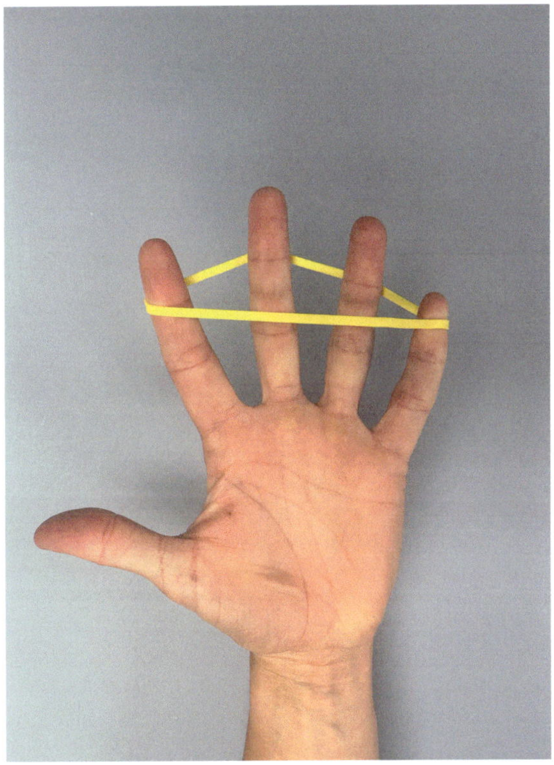

Image 19 To strengthen the intrinsic muscles in phase 3, a rubber band is used to resist finger abduction while the forearm is supinated

of donor and recipient muscle activation for 1–2+ years post-surgery.

Frequency

Frequency of therapy may continue once or twice per month in phase 3 until functional goals are mostly met or until the patient has plateaued.

AIN-to-Ulnar motor nerve transfer

Nerve transfer overview					
Donor nerve	Donor action	Recipient nerve	Recipient action	Indications for functional restoration	Approximate months to functional movement
AIN branch of the median nerve (to pronator quadratus)	Forearm pronation	Deep motor branch of the ulnar nerve	Finger abduction, adduction, RF/SF MCP flexion with IP extension, thumb adduction	Ulnar digital clawing, loss of pinch and grip strength, and loss of dexterity	9–18 months [12]

Information below is suggested guidelines. Precautions may vary according to surgeon preferences and patient factors

	Preoperative therapy	Early phase	Middle phase	Late phase
Criteria	Before surgery	0/5 to 1/5 MMT	2−/5 to 3/5 MMT	>3/5 MMT
Purpose of phase	Educate and establish baseline function	Understand donor and recipient relationship	Consistently activate recipient	Isolate recipient through resistance and separate from donor activation
Precautions	Prevent flexion contractures of IP joints to ring/small fingers	Limit wrist motion for 2–3 weeks	Respect fatigue and prevent dominance of extrinsics (EDQ/EDC/FDP)	None
Frequency of visits (considerations)	1–2 pre-op visits May increase if PROM limitations exist	1×/week until PROM is full and patient is independent with donor activation; then 1× monthly	1× per week to 1× per month based on patient needs and accurate, consistent demonstration of exercise program	1× every 1–2 weeks based on progress toward patient-specific goals
Orthosis considerations	PIP extension orthosis if joint contractures present Anti-claw orthosis to improve active PIP extension and limit extrinsic dominance	Volar wrist orthosis for 3 weeks to protect coaptation of the nerves	Continue with anti-claw orthosis until clawing is resolved Reverse Oval-8 orthosis to block the FPL while retraining the adductor pollicis	Wean from anti-claw orthosis
Interventions	Isolated passive PIP extension if contractures are present	**Donor activation**: Forearm pronation **Donor-recipient pairing**: Active pronation with passive finger abduction, adduction, and RF/SF MCP flexion with IP extension	**Active/resisted donor with active assist recipient**: Isometric pronation into a table with active assisted finger abduction/adduction and RF/SF MCP flexion with IP extension. Use "tube" orthoses to isolate intrinsics and maintain PIP extension **Place and hold**: Passively place individual fingers in abduction and adduction, then remove support, and maintain this position. The same is done with "table top" (RF/SF MP flexion and IP extension)	**Resisted donor and recipient**: While pronated, perform resisted pinch, finger abduction, adduction, and MCP flexion with IP extension Include therapy putty or small object retrieval **Resisted recipient**: While supinated, resisted pinch, finger abduction, adduction, and MCP flexion with IP extension. Introduce therapy putty or small objects for functional activities
Additional interventions		Scar management, desensitization for scar or nerve irritation	Visual motor feedback Mirror therapy Implement functional activities requiring lumbrical grasp	

During all phases, it is essential to continue cortical reorganization and psychological and psychosocial interventions and progress to incorporate donor/recipient with ADLs

AIN-to-Ulnar Motor Nerve Transfer

Goal of Surgery: Restore finger dexterity and hand strength

Recipient Movements = Spread fingers apart (finger abduction)

Bring fingers together (finger and thumb adduction)

Bend base joints and straighten end joints (intrinsic plus)

Recipient Muscles: Palmar and dorsal interossei, adductor pollicis, ring/small-finger lumbricals

Recipient Nerve: Ulnar nerve

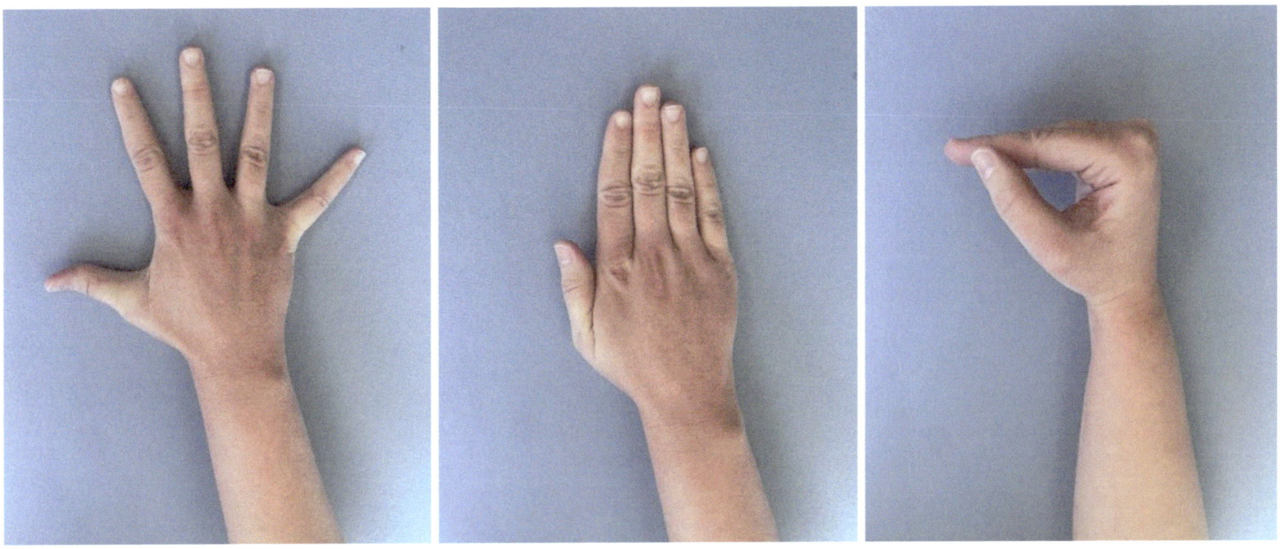

Donor Movement = Turn palm down (forearm pronation)

Donor Muscle: Pronator quadratus (PQ)

Donor Nerve: Anterior interosseous nerve (AIN)

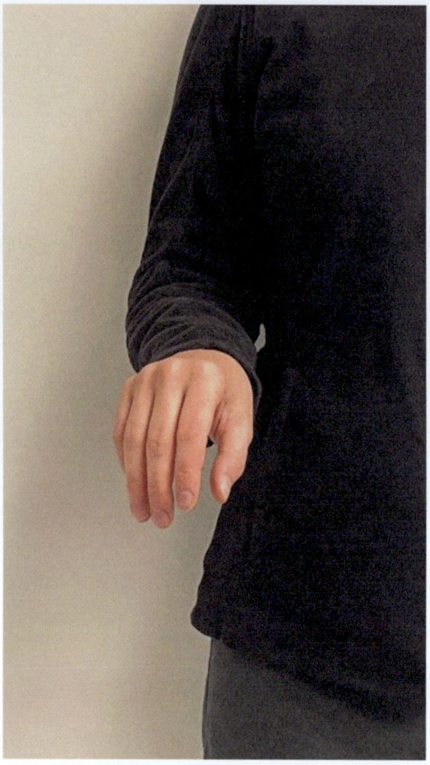

Phase 1 AIN-to-Ulnar Nerve Transfer Exercises

☐ **Active or Resisted Donor Movement**:

- Start with your elbow bent by your side and your forearm palm up. Turn your palm down. Return to the start position, and repeat.
  - You may use your other hand or a weight to provide resistance when performing this exercise if recommended by your therapist.

Complete 10 repetitions, every waking hour.

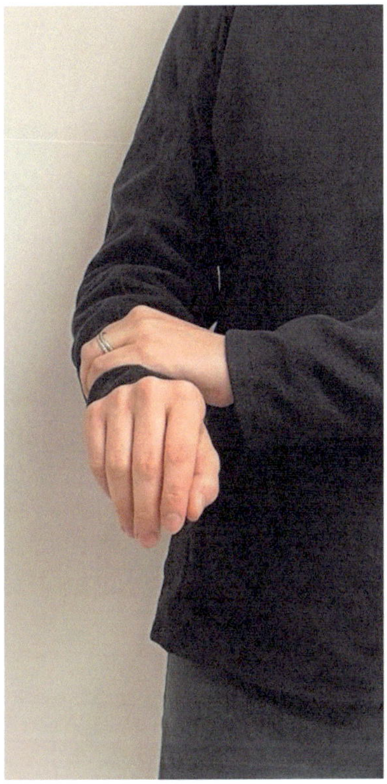

☐ **Active Donor + Passive Recipient Movement**: **Complete each of the below exercises <u>10</u> repetitions, <u>3</u> times per day.**

and small fingers for the following exercises, if needed, to prevent finger bending during the exercise.

1. Begin with your forearm resting on a table with palm facing down. You may wear finger tube splints on the ring and small fingers for the following exercises, if needed, to prevent finger bending during the exercise.

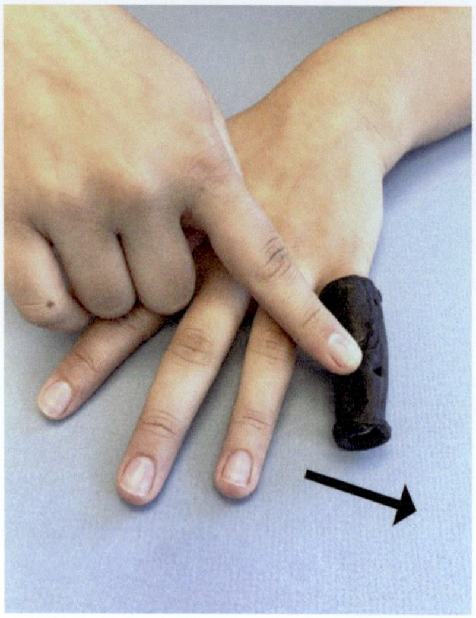

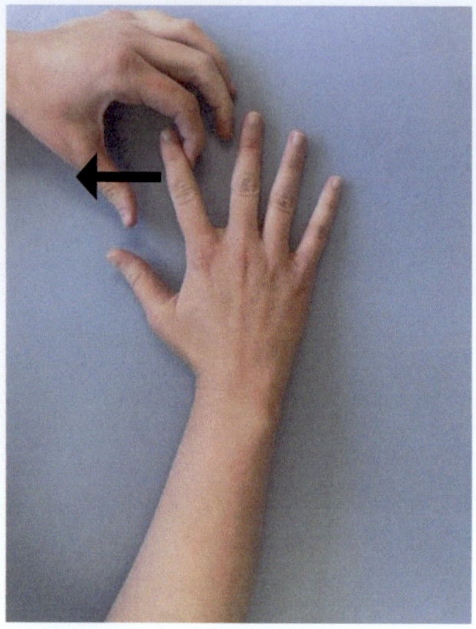

Use your other hand to move each finger side to side, focusing on one finger at a time. To reduce friction between your hand and the table, place a coin or Velcro tab beneath the pad of your finger. This will make it easier to slide.

2. Use your other hand to bend your big knuckles and straighten the end joints of your fingers. This creates a "tabletop" position with your hand.

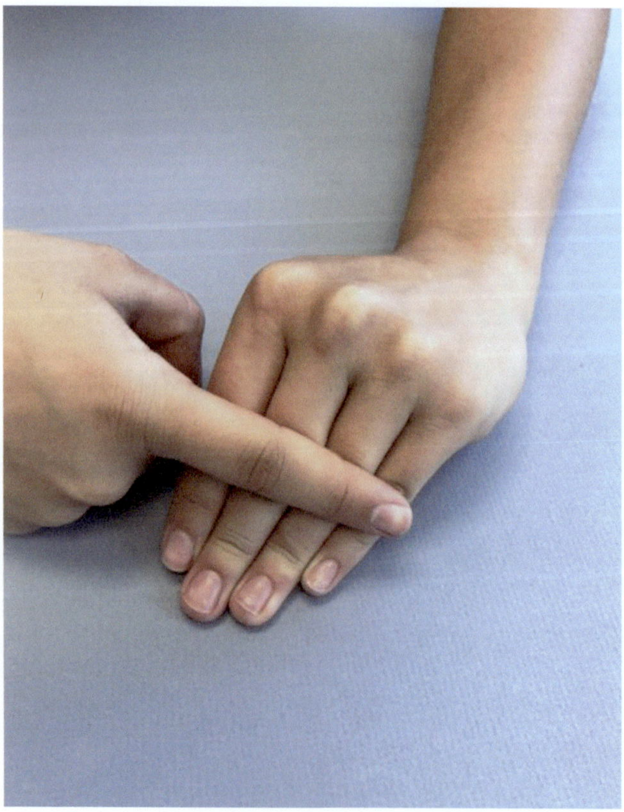

Phase 2 AIN-to-Ulnar Nerve Transfer Exercises

□ **Resisted Donor + Active-Assisted Recipient Movement**:

Complete the below exercises <u>10</u> repetitions, <u>3</u> times per day.

For the below exercises, begin with your forearm resting palm down on a table. Therapy putty or resistive foam is placed between the base of your thumb and the table. You may wear finger tube splints on the ring and small fingers for the following exercises to prevent finger bending.

1. Press the thumb side of your hand into therapy putty or resistive foam. One at a time, attempt to slide each finger out to the side. Then, use your other hand to complete the movement sliding as far as it will comfortably go. To reduce friction between your hand and the table, place a coin or Velcro® tab beneath the pad of your finger.

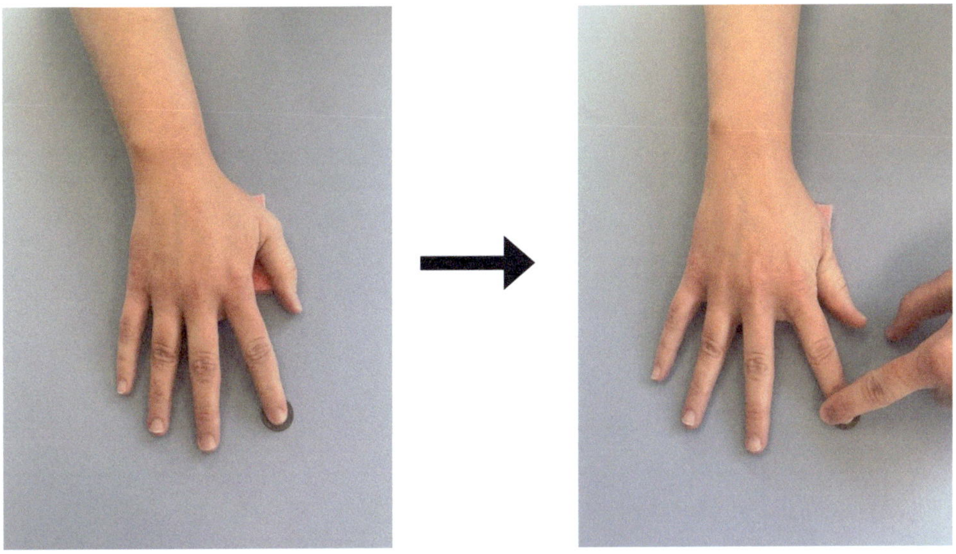

2. Press the thumb side of your hand into therapy putty or resistive foam. At the same time, attempt to slide your finger as close to the next finger as you can. Use your other hand to complete the movement, bringing your finger together. To reduce friction between your hand and the table, place a coin or Velcro® tab beneath the pad of your finger and the table.

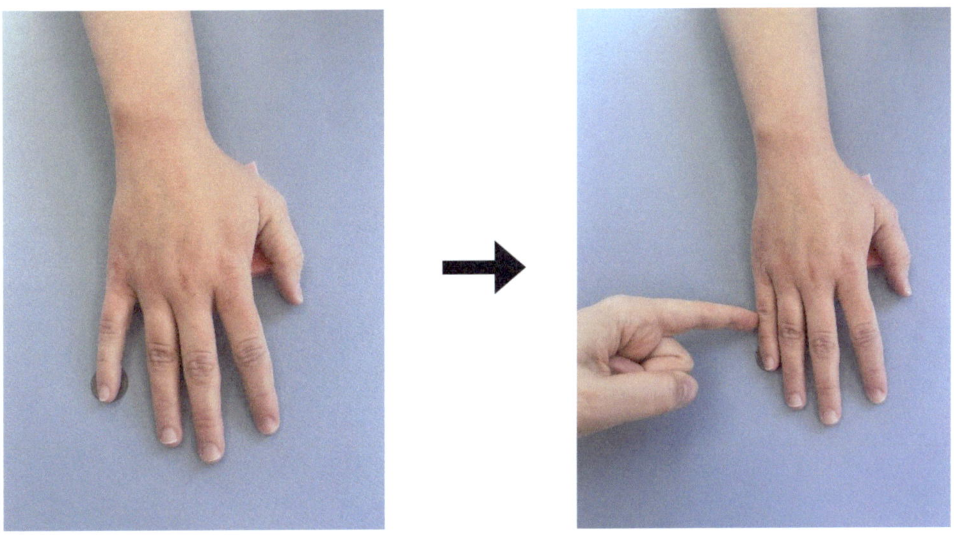

3. Press the thumb side of your hand into therapy putty or resistive foam. At the same time, attempt to bend the big knuckles and straighten the end joints of all the fingers making the "tabletop" position.

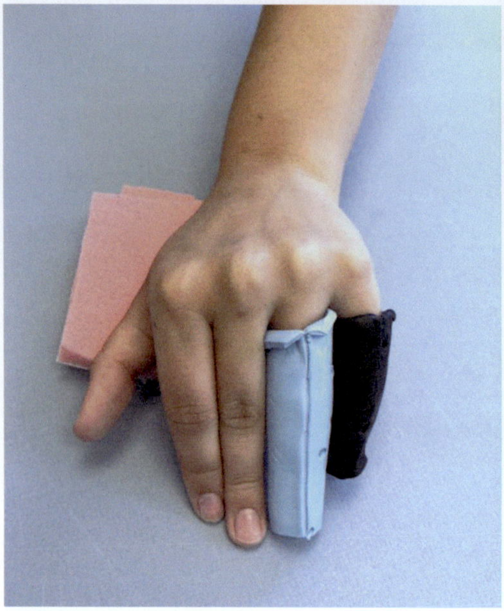
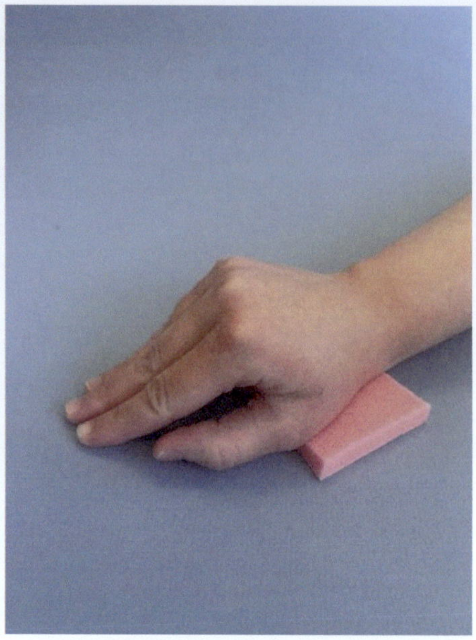

☐ **Isometric Donor + "Place-and-Hold" Recipient Movement**:

Complete the below exercises 6–10 repetitions, 2–3 times per day.

Hold for 3 seconds.

For the below exercises, begin with your forearm resting palm down on a table. Press the thumb side of your hand into the table to create resistance. At the same time, complete the following finger and thumb movements:

1. Use your other hand to place your **index finger out to the side**. As you let go with your other hand, try to maintain your index finger position out to the side.
2. Use your other hand to place your **index finger next to the middle finger**. As you let go with your other hand, try to maintain your index finger position next to the middle finger.
3. Use your other hand to place your **thumb next to the hand and index finger**. As you let go with your other hand, try to maintain your thumb position next to the hand and index finger.
4. Use your other hand to place your **middle finger toward the index finger**. As you let go with your other hand, try to maintain your middle finger position next to the index finger.
5. Use your other hand to place your **middle finger toward the ring finger**. As you let go with your other hand, try to maintain your middle finger position toward the ring finger.
6. Use your other hand to place your **ring finger toward the middle finger**. As you let go with your other hand, try to maintain your ring finger position toward the middle finger.
7. Use your other hand to place your **ring finger toward the small finger**. As you let go with your other hand, try to maintain your ring finger position toward the small finger.
8. Use your other hand to place your **small finger toward the ring finger**. As you let go with your other hand, try to maintain your small finger position toward the ring finger.
9. Use your other hand to place your **small finger away from the ring finger**. As you let go with your other hand, try to maintain your small finger position away from the ring finger.
10. Use your other hand to bend the big knuckles and straighten the end joints of your ring and small fingers. As you let go with your other hand, try to maintain your ring and small finger position in "**tabletop**" position.

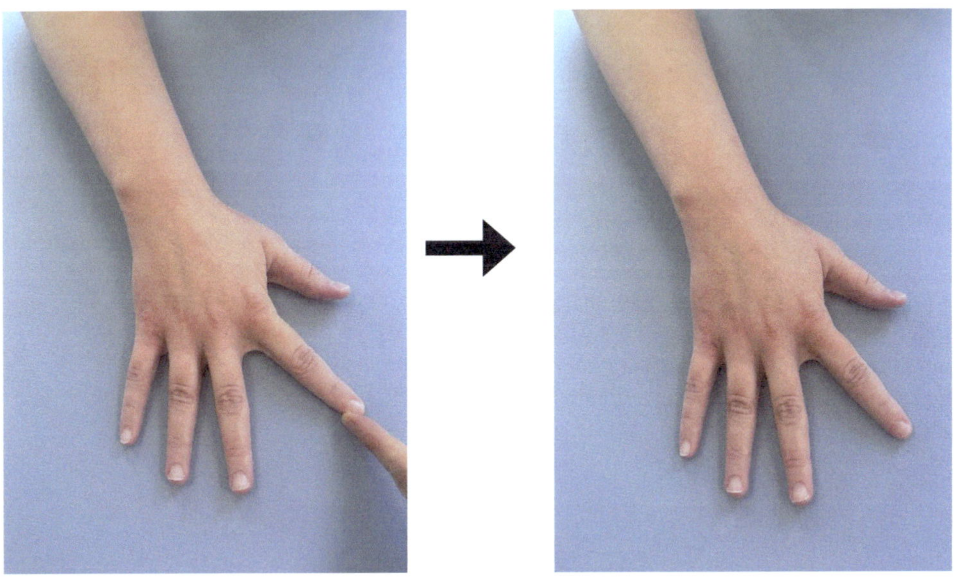

☐ **Active Donor + Active Recipient Movement**:

Complete the below exercises <u>5–10</u> repetitions, <u>3</u> times per day.

For the below exercises, begin seated at a table with your forearm turned palm up.

1. Turn your palm down, and at the same time, spread your fingers apart. Try to avoid lowering or lifting your fingers as you spread your fingers apart, and instead keep your finger movements parallel to the tabletop. Return to the starting position, and repeat.

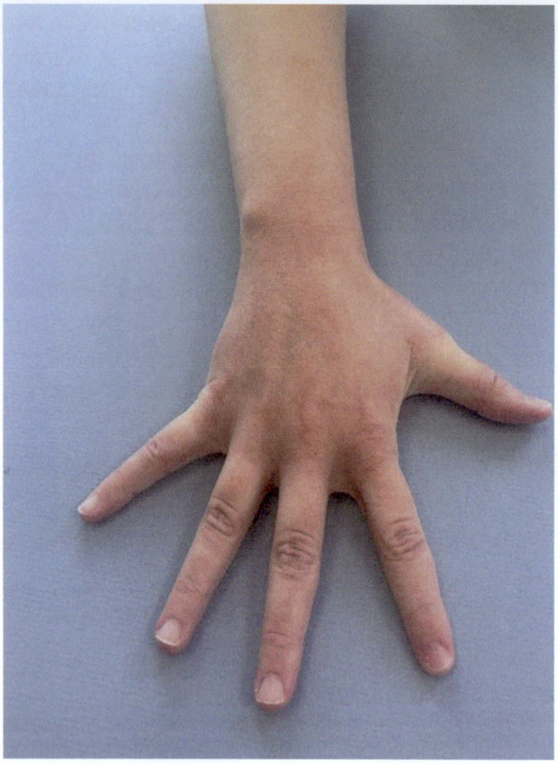

2. Turn your palm down, and at the same time, bring your fingers together. Avoid lowering or lifting your fingers as you bring your fingers together, and instead keep your finger movements parallel to the tabletop. Return to the starting position, and repeat.

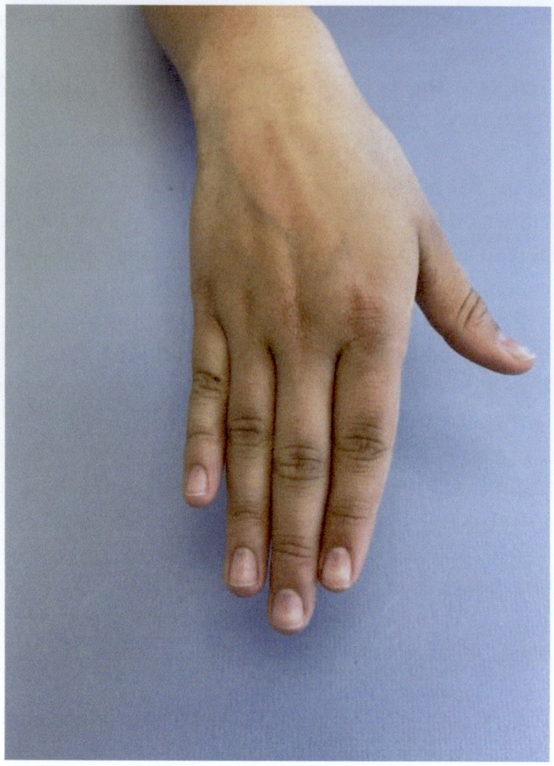

3. Turn your palm down, and at the same time, bend the big (base) knuckles and straighten the end joints into a "table-top" position. Return to the start position, and repeat.

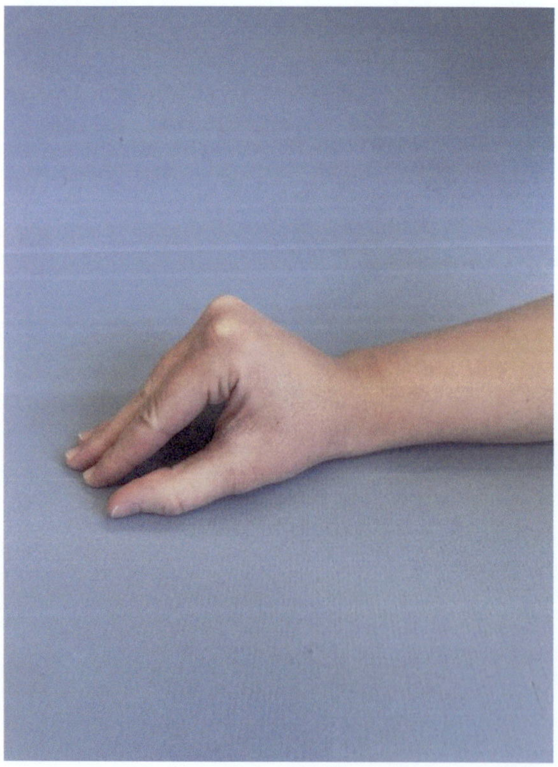

4. Turn your palm down, and at the same time, move your thumb toward the hand/index finger. Try to avoid bending at the tip of the thumb during this exercise. (Your therapist may provide you with a splint to prevent this.) Return to the start position, and repeat.

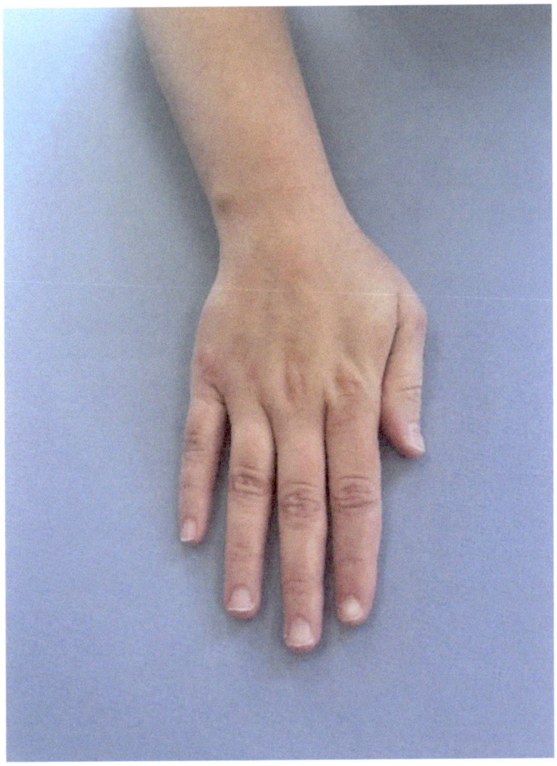

Phase 3 AIN-to-Ulnar Nerve Transfer Exercises

□ **Resisted Donor + Recipient Movement**:

Complete the below exercises 3–10 repetitions, 2 times per day.

1. Turn palm down, and bring fingers together to pick up small objects off a tabletop. Retrieve the object between index and middle fingers, between middle and ring fingers, and between ring and small fingers. Try to avoid lifting or lowering your fingers during this exercise, and instead keep your finger movements parallel to the tabletop.
   - You may use therapy putty to complete this exercise when recommended by your therapist.

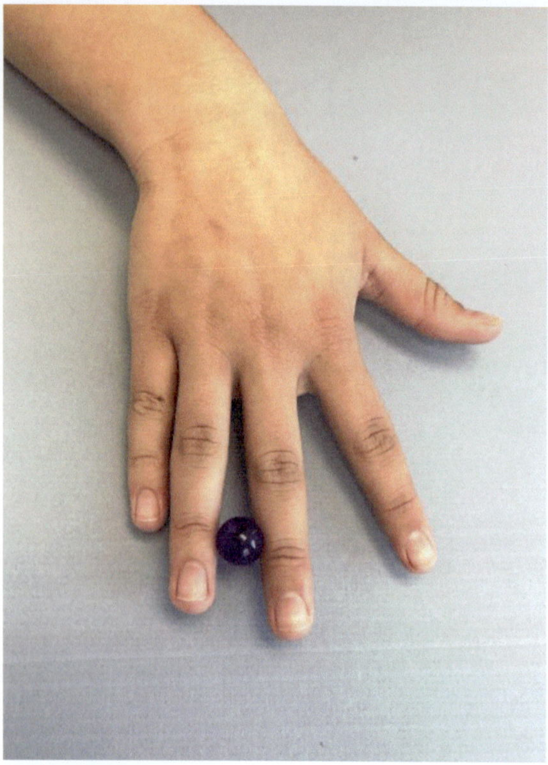

2. "Tabletop pulls": Begin palm down on a table with the hand flat and fingers resting on therapy putty. Bend big knuckles to pull your straight fingers gently toward you against the resistance of the putty. Keep the end joints of your fingers straight during this exercise. Return to the start position, and repeat.

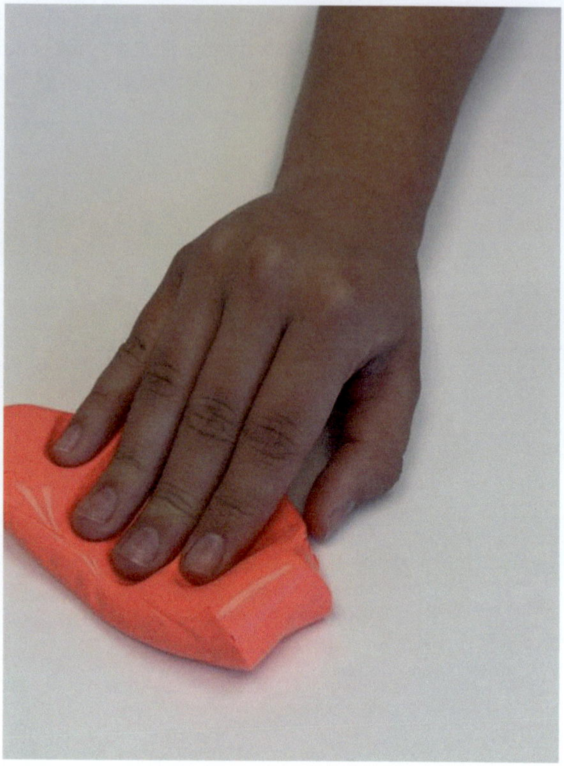

3. Position yourself with palms down as you pinch and pull therapy putty between the thumb and index finger of both hands.
   - You may wear an Oval-8® splint to keep the tip of the thumb straight to complete this exercise when recommended by your therapist.

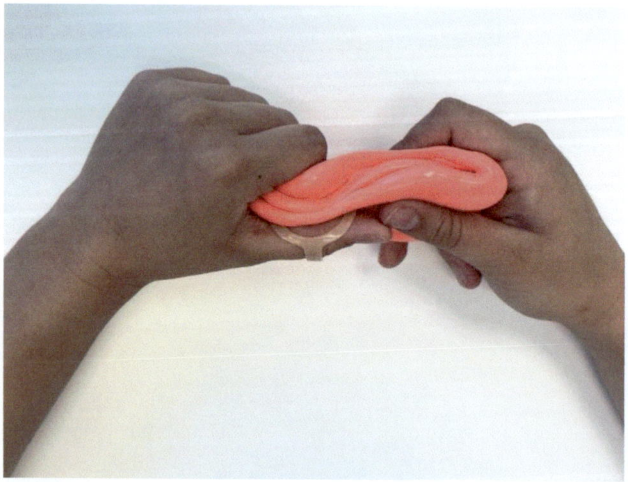

☐ **Resisted Recipient Movement**:

Complete the below exercises 5–10 repetitions, 2 times per day.

1. In a palm-up position, place a rubber band around your fingers. Spread your fingers apart against the resistance of the rubber band.

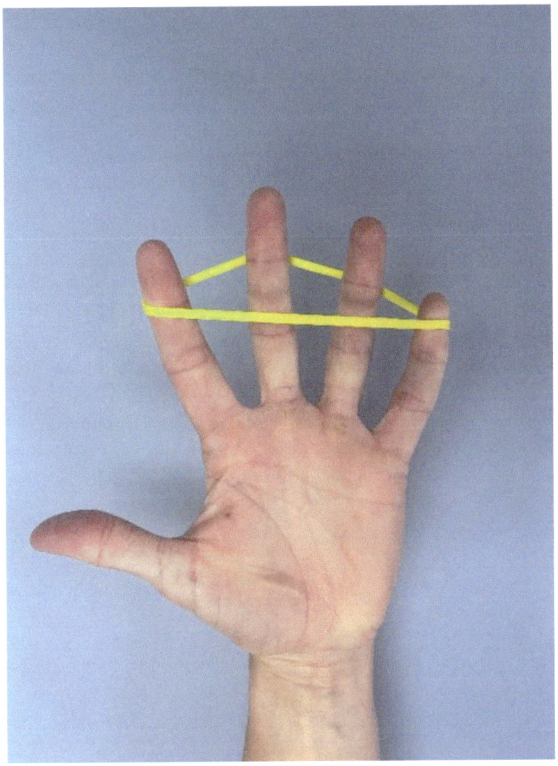

2. Position yourself with the palms of both hands facing each other as you pinch and pull resistive putty between the thumb and index finger of both hands. Avoid bending the tips of the thumbs.

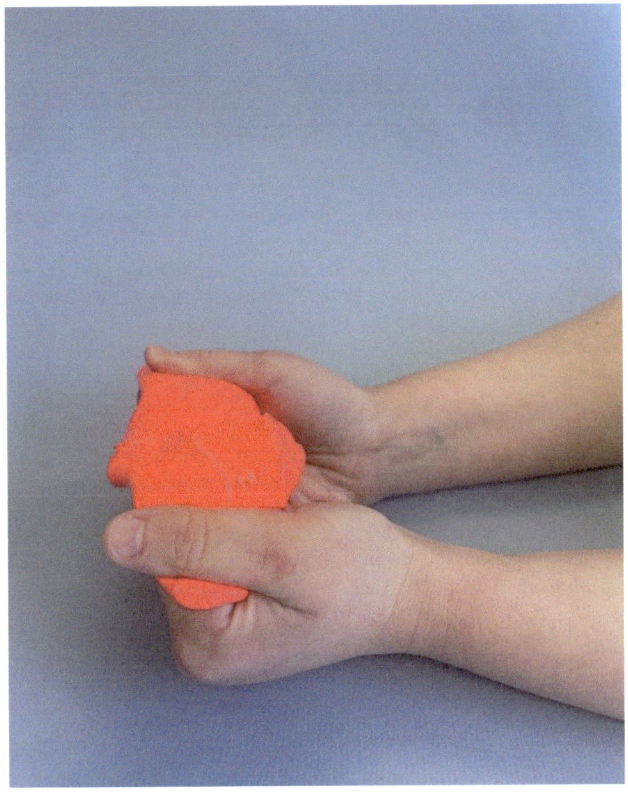

3. Position yourself with the palm up or thumb facing the ceiling. Press straight fingers into putty only bending at the big (base) knuckles.

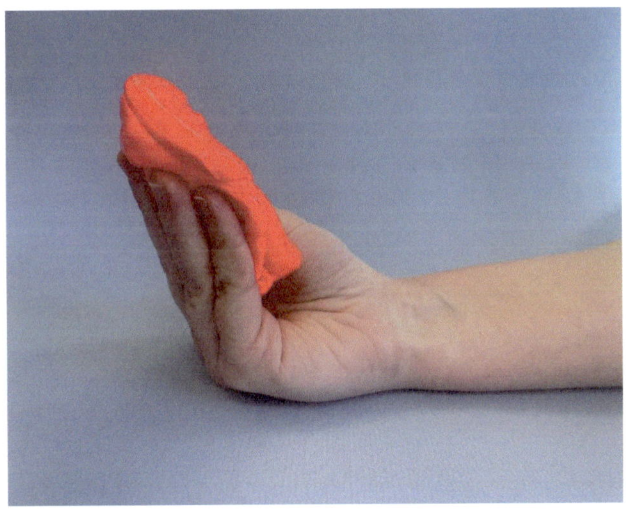

References

1. Koriem E, El-Mahy MM, Atiyya AN, Diab RA. Comparison between supercharged ulnar nerve repair by anterior interosseous nerve transfer and isolated ulnar nerve repair in proximal ulnar nerve injuries. J Hand Surg Am. 2020;45(2):104–10.
2. Thakkar M, Rose A, King W, Engelman K, Bednarz B. Anterior interosseous nerve to ulnar nerve transfer: a systematic review. JPRAS Open. 2022;32:195–210.
3. Barbour J, Yee A, Kahn LC, Mackinnon SE. Supercharged end-to-side anterior interosseous to ulnar motor nerve transfer for intrinsic musculature reinnervation. J Hand Surg Am. 2012;37(10):2150–9.
4. Chen SH, Mao SH, Lan CY, et al. End-to-side anterior interosseous nerve transfer: a valuable alternative for traumatic high ulnar nerve palsy. Ann Plast Surg. 2021;86(2S):S102–7.
5. George SC, Burahee AS, Sanders AD, Power DM. Outcomes of anterior interosseous nerve transfer to restore intrinsic muscle function after high ulnar nerve injury. J Plast Reconstr Aesthet Surg. 2022;75(2):703.
6. McLeod GJ, Peters BR, Quaife T, Clark TA, Giuffre JL. Anterior interosseous-to-ulnar motor nerve transfers: a single center's experience in restoring intrinsic hand function. Hand. 2022;4(17):604–19.
7. Knight S, Miller TA, McIntyre A, Larocerie-Salgado J, Ross DC. The hand diagram: a novel outcome measure following supercharged end-to-side anterior interosseous nerve to ulnar nerve transfer in severe compressive ulnar neuropathy. J Hand Ther. 2023;37:348.
8. Kahn LC, Evans AG, Hill EJ, Fox IK. Donor activation focused rehabilitation approach to hand closing nerve transfer surgery in individuals with cervical level spinal cord injury. Spinal Cord Ser Cases. 2022;8(1):1–9.
9. Davidge KM, Yee A, Kahn LC, Mackinnon SE. Median to radial nerve transfers for restoration of wrist, finger, and thumb extension. J Hand Surg Am. 2013;38(9):1812–27.
10. Kahn L, Moore A. Donor activation focused rehabilitation approach: maximizing outcomes after nerve transfers. Hand Clin. 2016;32(2):263–77.
11. Wolfe SW, Pederson WC, Kozin SH, Cohen MS. Green's operative hand surgery. Elsevier Health Sciences; 2021.
12. Hill JL, Turner LC, Jones RD, et al. The stages of rehabilitation following motor nerve transfer surgery. J Musculoskelet Surg Res. 2019;3:60.
13. Novak CB, Mackinnon SE. Distal anterior interosseous nerve transfer to the deep motor branch of the ulnar nerve for reconstruction of high ulnar nerve injuries. J Reconstr Microsurg. 2002;18(6):459–64.
14. Mackinnon SE. Nerve Surgery. Thieme; 2015.
15. Kahn LC, Stonner MM, Dy CJ. Key concepts for nerve transfer rehabilitation after surgical reconstruction for brachial plexus and peripheral nerve injuries. J Hand Surg Am. 2023;49:160.
16. Tam SL, Archibald V, Tyreman N, Gordon T. Tetrodotoxin prevents motor unit enlargement after partial denervation in rat hindlimb muscles. J Physiol. 2002;543(2):655–63.
17. Kahn LC, Stonner MM, Miller VA. Chapter 21: tendon and nerve transfers. In: Jacobs MLA, Austin NM, editors. Orthotic intervention for the hand and upper extremity, splinting principles and process. 3rd ed. Wolters Kluwer; 2022. p. 477–91.

Opponens Pollicis Branch of the Median Nerve to First Dorsal Interossei Branch of the Deep Ulnar Motor Nerve

Jamie Findeiss

Background

Isolated ulnar nerve lesions most commonly occur with compression at the cubital tunnel and/or Guyon's canal [1]. Ulnar nerve pathology can also present from laceration or traction injuries. Ulnar nerve lesions are separated into high (above elbow) and low (below elbow) nerve injuries [2, 3]. Ulnar intrinsic muscle weakness and atrophy may be present in both high and low ulnar nerve injuries. The first dorsal interossei (FDI) and adductor pollicis (AP) muscles are innervated by the furthest distal branch of the deep ulnar motor nerve, making reinnervation difficult to achieve from decompression or primary repair alone [4].

Ulnar nerve injuries have significant functional implications due to loss of intrinsic function, sensation, grip strength, and dexterity [3]. Additionally, lateral pinch is weak or absent because the primary muscles of lateral pinch, adductor pollicis (AP), and first dorsal interossei (FDI) are innervated by the deep ulnar motor branches [5]. These two muscles work synergistically to facilitate a strong, stable pinch between the thumb and index finger, providing as much as 75% of lateral or key pinch [2]. Loss of pinch strength is shown to impede functional use of the entire hand by 50–60% [3].

Whether compressive or neurotmetic, high ulnar nerve injuries are complex and have a tremendous impact on pain, psychosocial health, and employment [6, 7]. Direct repair, grafting, and transposition rarely result in native motor recovery of the AP and FDI due to excessive reinnervation distance. Adductorplasty tendon transfers (including ECRL to AP *or* APL to FDI) have historically been the accepted reconstructive approach to restore pinch function, yet they often produce unreliable and inferior outcomes, such as loss of abduction strength or transfer failure [4, 8]. Nerve transfers are a reliable surgical option to restore pinch function using a branch of the median nerve to the opponens pollicis muscle and coapting it to the deep ulnar motor nerve branch to the FDI.

Outcomes

This nerve transfer was first described by Bertelli in 2019 and included a sample of three patients who underwent OP-to-FDI nerve transfer following sharp neurotmetic injuries in the forearm [9]. All three patients had improved measures for all outcome variables, which included grip strength, key pinch strength, and FDI thickness (via a digital fat caliper). All patient complaints of hand weakness were resolved following surgery, and the authors attribute this to FDI and ADP reinnervation.

Bertelli later reported on this transfer in 2023, again showing promising findings. The 16 patients in this study demonstrated an average grasp and key pinch strength of 57% and 71%, respectively, compared to the contralateral hand [10]. Additionally, average FDI thickness was 11 mm prior to surgery and 18 mm after surgery, which was 86% of the contralateral side. Following nerve transfer, all patients had preserved thenar function and no pain. He also noted that patients achieved better outcomes if surgery was performed fewer than 6 months from the original injury [9].

J. Findeiss (✉)
Athletico Physical Therapy, St. Louis, MO, USA

L. C. Kahn et al. (eds.), *Rehabilitation for Nerve Transfers of the Upper Extremity*,
https://doi.org/10.1007/978-3-031-92008-0_26

Surgical Description

A curvilinear incision is made at the base of the palm, with the distal extent near the level of the distal palmar crease for the middle finger. The superficial palmar fascia is divided, and the transverse carpal ligament is divided. The recurrent motor branch of the median nerve is identified and dissected distally. Branching of the recurrent motor branch into individual branches to the abductor pollicis brevis and opponens pollicis is visualized. A handheld nerve stimulator is used to confirm robust response in both branches. It is important to stimulate these branches within 30 min of the tourniquet being inflated (if one is being used) and to ensure that the anesthesia team is not using any muscle paralytics. The surgeon then works along the radial side of the middle finger flexor tendons, identifying the lumbrical muscles and deep palmar arch. The adductor pollicis muscle is identified, and the terminal portion of the ulnar motor branch is visualized within the hiatus between the two heads of the adductor pollicis muscle. A handheld nerve stimulator is used to confirm absent response in the terminal portion of the ulnar nerve. It is important to stimulate these branches within 30 min of the tourniquet being inflated (if one is being used) and to ensure that the anesthesia team is not using any muscle paralytics. The ulnar nerve is then dissected as proximally as possible and divided. The opponens branch is neurolyzed from the recurrent motor branch and divided proximally. Coaptation of the opponens branch of the median nerve to the terminal portion of the ulnar motor nerve is performed using microsurgical technique.

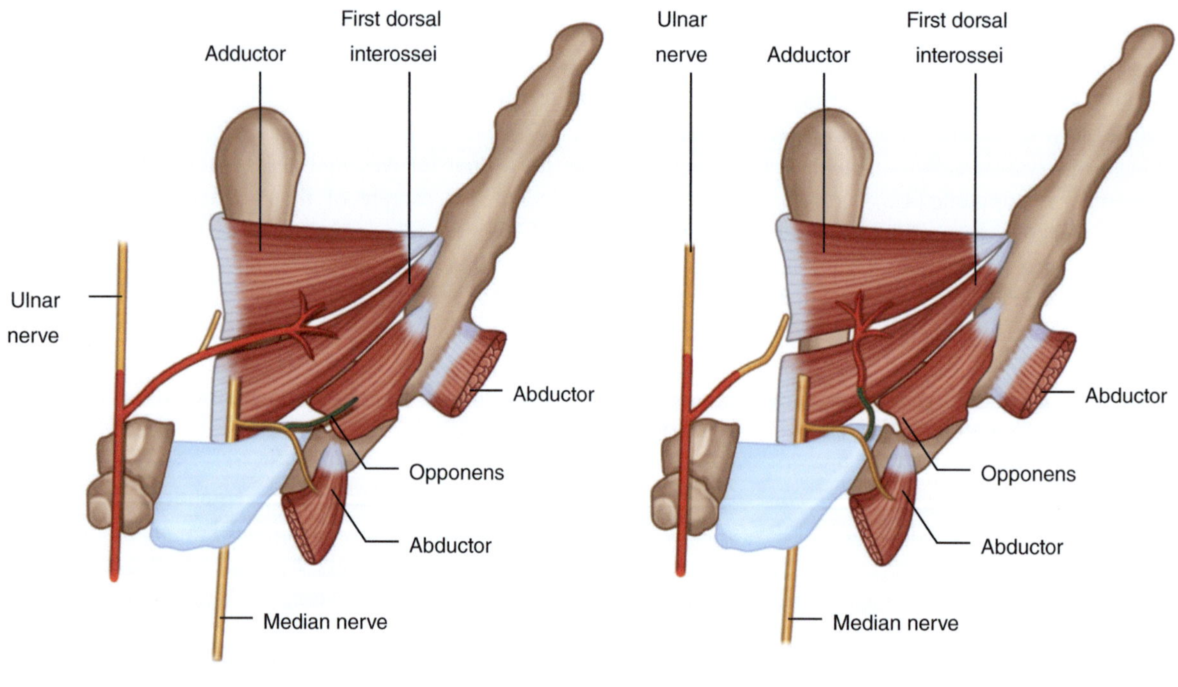

Before the nerve transfer **After the nerve transfer**

Phases of Rehabilitation

Phase 1

Preoperative to 1/5 MMT in Recipient Muscle

Preoperatively, it is important to educate the patient of the anatomy, therapy goals, and timeline for functional use. This particular nerve transfer is most commonly done in combination with other distal nerve transfers, along with decompression and neurolysis. It is beneficial to provide the patient with simplistic yet thorough education about the surgery and the donor-recipient relationship.

Postoperatively, patients are immobilized in a soft postoperative dressing that limits wrist, thumb, and index finger use for about 2 weeks. In this immediate postoperative stage, therapy may be minimal (two to three sessions as needed). Therapy focuses on education, passive range of motion of the hand (if limited), and edema/wound management. A protective orthosis is not required for this stage unless otherwise specified by the physician. Exercise instruction will focus on donor activation, followed by combining donor and recipient activity. This form of early donor-recipient pairing assists with neuro reeducation of the new motor pathway to augment long-term functional pinch [11].

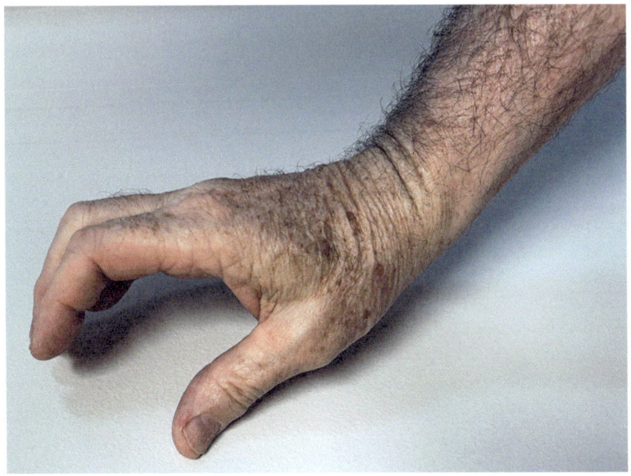

Image 1 Donor activation for the opponens pollicis muscle is performed with the palm facing down on a table. The patient is instructed to press the radial aspect of the thumb into a table

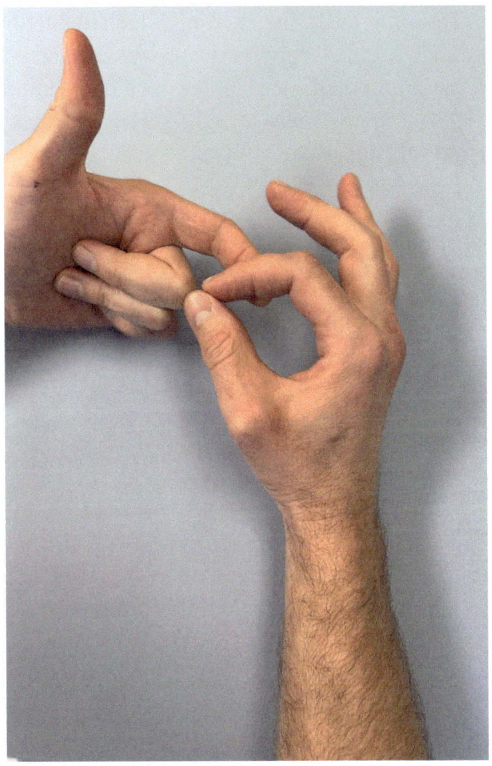

Image 2 Active donor/passive recipient exercise is performed with active abduction of the thumb while passively abducting the index finger to meet it for tip-to-tip pinch

Exercises

- Range of Motion

  Therapy should address any ROM limitations of the hand in the early postoperative period. If the index finger MCP joint is stiff in an adducted, ulnar-deviated position due to chronic abductor weakness, passive index MCP joint abduction is recommended.
- Donor Activation

  The patient should be performing active thumb opposition every 1–2 hours (20 repetitions) in order to "flood the donor." Isometric opposition is another good option to recruit the donor. This is easily performed with the palm facing down on a table. The patient is instructed to press the radial aspect of the thumb into the table (Image 1). The therapist should discourage excess flexor pollicis longus (FPL) or abductor pollicis longus (APL) substitution during donor activation.
- Active Donor with Passive Recipient Exercise`

  Once the patient is proficient with donor activation and demonstrates an understanding of its rationale, he or she should begin pairing the donor (opponens) with passive movement of the recipient (index-finger abduction). This can be as simple as trying to touch the thumb and index fingertip together. The therapist should encourage the patient to make good "pad-to-pad contact" with the thumb and index, which will have to be accomplished through passive assistance to index-finger abduction (Image 2).

When the patient lacks first dorsal interossei function, pinching may result in the index finger simply flexing toward the palm using the flexor digitorum profundus (FDP).

> **Clinical Pearl**
> An easy form of donor AROM with recipient PROM involves the use of a custom orthosis that places the index MCP joint in abduction. With the index finger in passive abduction, the patient is instructed to work on active or isometric thumb opposition (Image 3).

Assessment of Recovery

Reinnervation of the FDI should be monitored monthly in therapy sessions. To evaluate for FDI muscle return, the therapist asks the patient to make an "O" shape between the thumb and index fingers. This intuitively recruits the donor opponens pollicis, which isometrically contracts against pressure from the index finger, from which abduction force is generated. Manual support is provided as the patient pinches the thumb and index finger together. The therapist should palpate the first web space for signs of muscle contraction in FDI (Image 4).

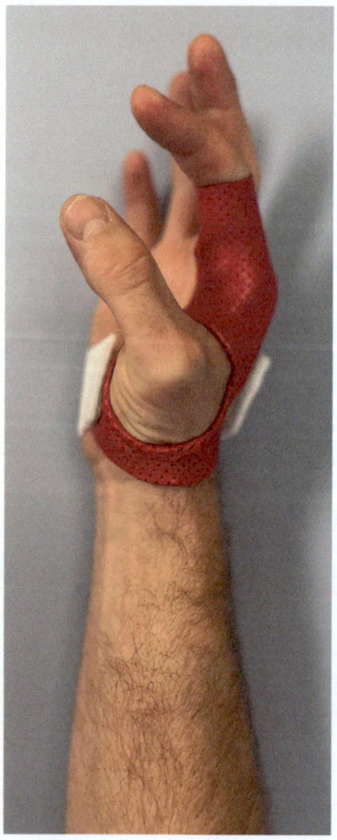

Image 3 A custom orthosis that places the index MCP joint in abduction is an easy way to position the index finger passively while the patient is encouraged to use the thumb actively for donor activation activities

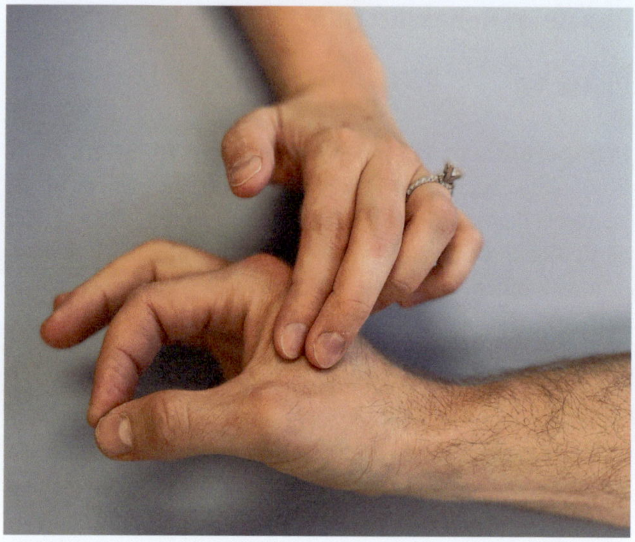

Image 4 To assess for reinnervation of the FDI, have the patient pinch the thumb and index finger together in an "O" shape while the therapist palpates the first web space for signs of muscle contraction

Therapy Frequency

Frequency of therapy visits depends on many factors. If the opponens-to-FDI nerve transfer was performed in isolation, most patients do well with a few sessions (two to three) in phase 1. When there are multiple nerve transfers performed simultaneously, therapy once a week is beneficial to ensure understanding of and compliance with a thorough home exercise program (HEP). If passive ROM is full, pain is negligible, and the patient has a good understanding of the donor-recipient relationship, therapy once per month is adequate. Due to the protracted length of motor recovery, consideration of insurance limitations is advised.

Phase 2

2−/5 to 3/5 MMT in Recipient Muscle

Phase 2 begins once the patient demonstrates a trace of active index-finger abduction. This stage of rehabilitation focuses on active and active-assisted motion (AROM/AAROM) of the recovering recipient (FDI) while still demanding a strong contraction of the donor. Exercises in phase 2 are routinely performed in a gravity-minimized plane for recipient muscles of the wrist, elbow, and shoulders. However, the role of antigravity versus gravity-minimized planes is not an important factor with digital movement. Due to the small range of index-finger abduction, the timing of MMT grade-based variations in exercises throughout this phase is less important.

Exercises

- Active Donor with Active-Assisted Recipient
  FDI MMT = 2−/5 to 2/5

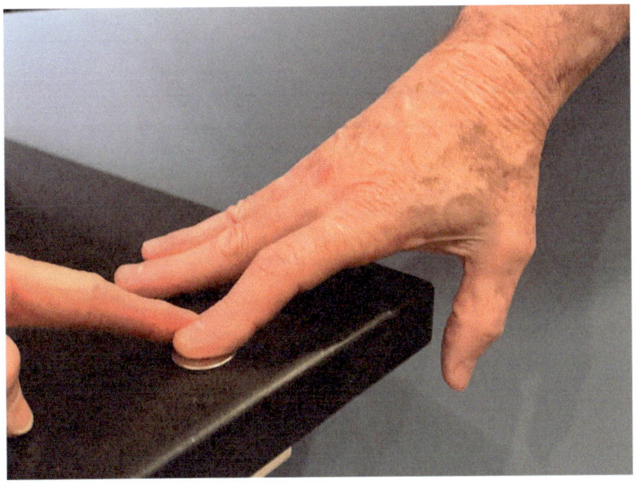

Image 5 Active donor with active-assisted recipient muscle exercise is performed with the thumb resting off the table. A coin is placed under the index finger to reduce friction and facilitate abduction. The patient is instructed to abduct the thumb in the direction of opposition while attempting to abduct the index finger across the table with assistance from contralateral hand

The patient is seated at a table with the forearm pronated, with the fingers resting on the table and the thumb positioned off the table. A coin or Velcro tab is placed under the index finger to reduce surface friction and facilitate abduction. The patient first moves the thumb in the direction of opposition (into the table) while trying to abduct the index finger across the table (Image 5). The contralateral hand then *assists* the index finger into further abduction range.

- "Place and Hold"
  FDI MMT = 2+/5
  The patient's contralateral hand places the index finger in full abduction while thumb opposition is performed, and the patient is instructed to maintain index finger abduction when the contralateral hand is removed.
- Active Donor with Active Recipient
  FDI MMT = 3−/5
  The patient is asked to make a "C" shape between the thumb and index finger. This intuitively contracts the donor into thumb opposition and the index finger into abduction (Image 6). The extensor indicis proprius (EIP) often compensates for abduction in the setting of FDI weakness, so the therapist should cue the patient to truly abduct (rather than extend) the index finger. Analogies may be helpful, such as telling the patient to pretend like they are unsticking glue between the index and middle fingers.
- Functional Activity
  Functional activities are encouraged once the patient reaches an MMT score of 3−/5. Because pinch requires thumb opposition and index-finger abduction, this nerve transfer is very intuitive. Patients should work on very light pinch activities, such as threading a needle, using tweezers, and/or picking up large beads or coins. In therapy, patients can grasp cones or cups to activate the transfer. The patient places the hand around a cone (which facilitates thumb opposition) and actively slides the index finger into abduction along the side of the cone (Image 7).

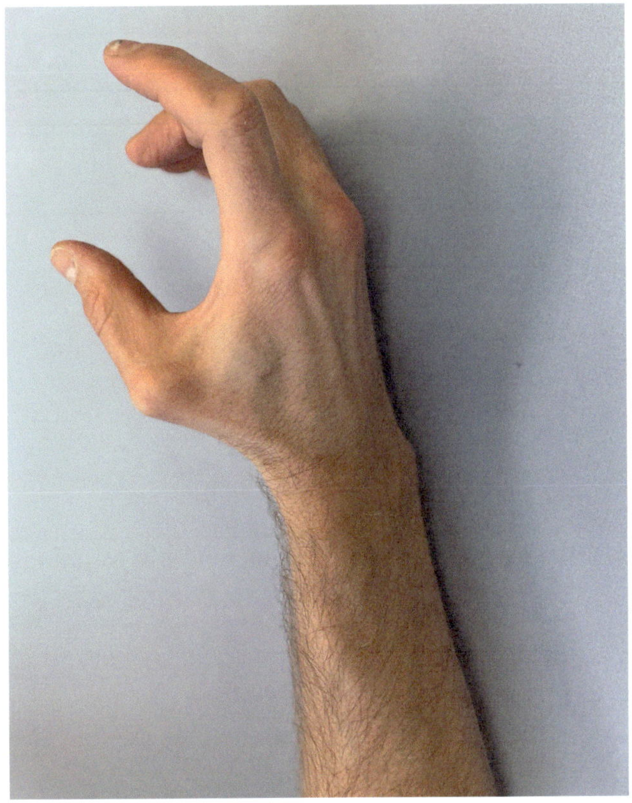

Image 6 Active donor with active recipient muscle exercise is performed by instructing the patient to form a "C" shape with the thumb and index finger

Assessment of Recovery

Reinnervation of the FDI should be monitored monthly in therapy sessions. To evaluate for muscle return, the therapist asks the patient to pinch between the thumb and index finger. This intuitively recruits the donor opponens pollicis, which isometrically contracts against pressure from the index finger as abduction force is generated. As the patient pinches the fingers together, the therapist palpates the FDI for muscle contraction. Monthly measures of degrees of index-finger abduction are helpful to monitor subtle advancement of recovery of FDI function and can be motivating for the patient.

Therapy Frequency

As stated previously, this nerve transfer is very intuitive. If this surgery was performed in isolation, patients may require only a handful of therapy sessions (once per month). A strong emphasis is placed on independent home exercises. If multiple procedures were performed at once, more frequent therapy sessions may be needed.

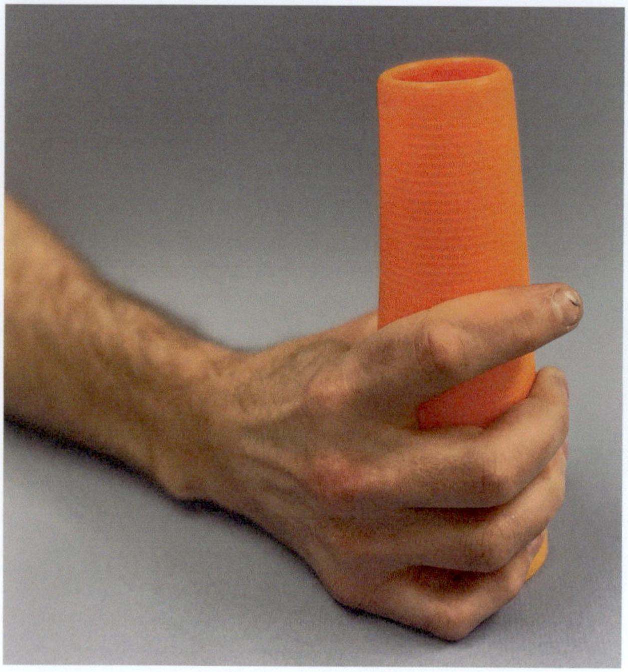

Image 7 Functional activities such as grasping a cone facilitate thumb opposition and actively position the index finger into abduction along the side of the cone

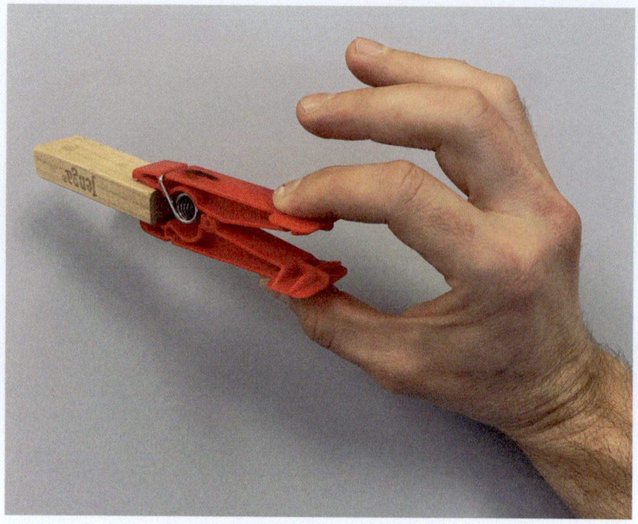

Image 8 Pinching clips may be used as a form of resisted recipient exercise that includes donor activation

Phase 3

3+/5 MMT in Recipient Muscle

Once the patient demonstrates full index-finger abduction against slight resistance, exercises are progressed to include resistance and functional strengthening. This stage of rehabilitation focuses on lateral pinch strengthening for application to ADL/IADL tasks.

Exercises

- Resistive Recipient Activity with Donor Contraction
  The patient practices lateral pinch using a clothespin to pick up small items. Thumb opposition is cued while pinching against the index finger (Image 8). The patient could also place a rubber band around the hand (specifically the thumb proximal phalanx and the index proximal phalanx). Starting in an "O" position, the patient is instructed to spread the index away from the middle finger while pushing the thumb into palmar abduction (Image 9). Therapy putty may be used for resistance with lateral pinch between the thumb and index finger while ensuring that the index finger abducts away from the middle finger.
- Resistive Recipient Activity Without Donor Contraction
  Because functional pinch involves thenar muscle action, it is not necessary to train the patient to eliminate the assistive action of the donor opponens during exercise. However, if independent FDI strength is desired, a rubber band may be looped around the proximal phalanges of all four fingers, and the patient is instructed to work on finger abduction. Fatigue should be monitored to prevent compensatory pinch patterns. Kinesiotaping the index finger into some abduction can be helpful during resistive or repetitive activities that might cause fatigue (Image 10).

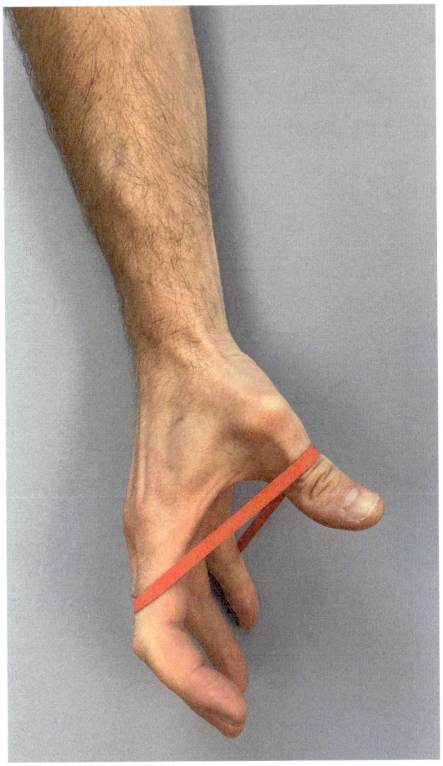

Image 9 A rubber band is used to provide resistance to the recipient, FDI, and the donor, OP. Starting in the "O" position, the patient is instructed to spread the index away from the middle finger while pushing the thumb into palmar abduction

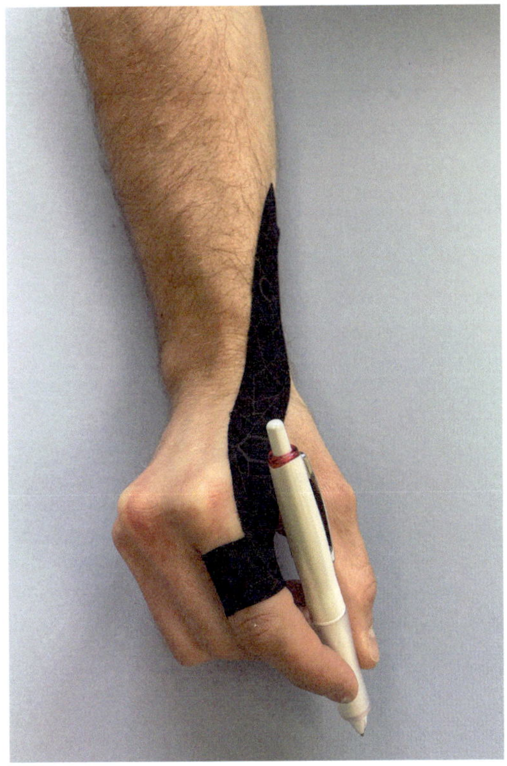

Image 10 Kinesiotape™ or other sports tape may be used to support the FDI as the individual advances to more resistive or repetitive activities

Opponens to First Dorsal Interosseous (FDI) nerve transfer

Nerve transfer overview					
Donor nerve	Donor action	Recipient nerve	Recipient action	Indications for functional restoration	Approximate months to functional movement
Deep branch of the median nerve to the opponens pollicis	Thumb opposition	Deep motor branch of the ulnar nerve to the first dorsal interossei	Index finger abduction	Pinch strength	12 [9, 10]

Information below is suggested guidelines. Precautions may vary according to surgeon preferences and patient factors

	Preoperative therapy	Early phase	Middle phase	Late phase
Criteria	Before surgery	0/5 to −1/5 MMT	2−/5 to 3/5 MMT	>3/5 MMT
Purpose of phase	Educate and establish baseline function	Understand donor-recipient relationship Activate donor: small-finger abduction	Activate nerve transfer for functional activities requiring light pinch	Isolate recipient through resistance Separate from donor activation
Precautions	NA	No resistance training	Minimize fatigue and force placed on the weak FDI	Resistive exercise should not be performed before the FDI demonstrates 3/5 MMT Avoid fatigue with resistance training
Frequency of visits (considerations)	NA	1×/week until PROM is restored, and patient is independent with HEP Decrease to 1×/month based on progress	1×/month to advance HEP	1×/month
Orthosis considerations	NA	Post-op dressing with wrist immobilization for 2 weeks	NA	No orthosis required, but kinesiotaping or a hand-based index finger abduction orthosis can be helpful during highly resistive or repetitive tasks
Interventions	NA	**Donor activation**: Thumb opposition and palmar abduction 10× every hour **Donor-recipient pairing**: Active thumb opposition with passive index finger abduction 10–20 reps, 6–8×/day	**Active/resisted donor with active assist recipient**: Active-assisted index finger abduction (with active and/or resisted thumb opposition) **Place and hold**: Manually place index finger in abduction. Remove the support, and maintain this position (with simultaneous thumb opposition) Continue **donor activation**	**Resisted donor and recipient**: Resisted thumb opposition with resisted index finger abduction Resisted pinch activities **Resisted recipient without donor contraction**: Index finger abduction strengthening without assistance of thumb; rubber band around digits 2–5 with resistive abduction
Additional intervention considerations	NA		If this transfer was performed in isolation with no other nerve or tendon transfers, frequent formal therapy is not necessary for many cases	Focus on high repetitions, low resistance

During all phases, it is essential to continue cortical reorganization and psychological and psychosocial interventions and progress to incorporate donor/recipient with ADLs

Opponens-to-First Dorsal Interossei Nerve Transfer

Goal of Surgery: Restore pinch strength
Recipient Movement = Index finger abduction
Recipient Muscle: First dorsal interosseous
Recipient Nerve: Deep motor branch of the ulnar nerve

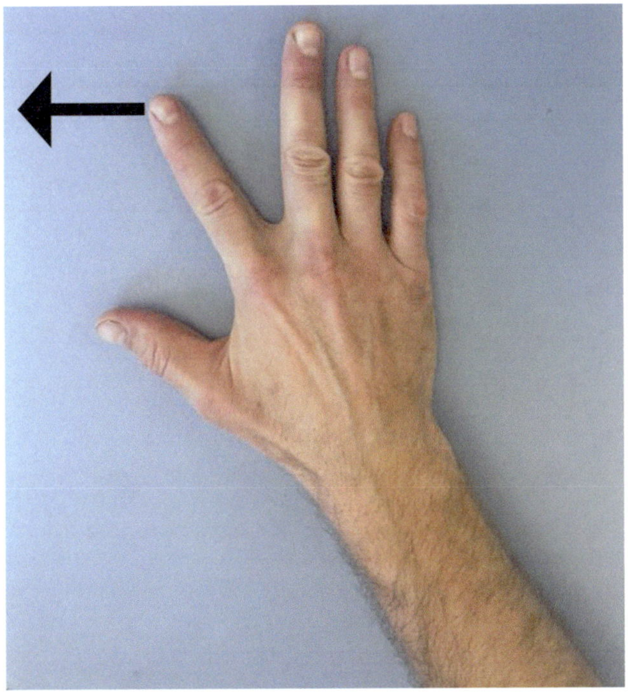

Spread your index finger away from the middle finger

Donor Movement = Thumb opposition
Donor Muscle: Opponens pollicis
Donor Nerve: Recurrent branch of the median nerve

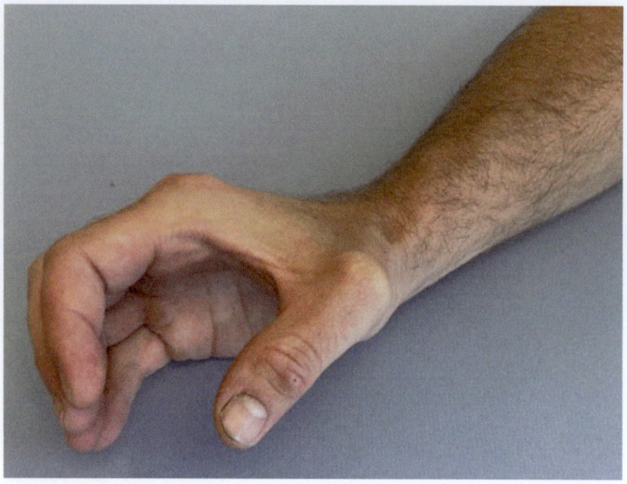

Move your thumb away from the palm

Phase 1 Opponens-to-FDI Nerve Transfer Exercises

☐ **Active or Resisted Donor Movement**:

- Touch your thumb to the tip of the index finger, trying to make an "O" shape. Next, touch your thumb to the tip of the middle finger, ring finger, and then pinky finger.

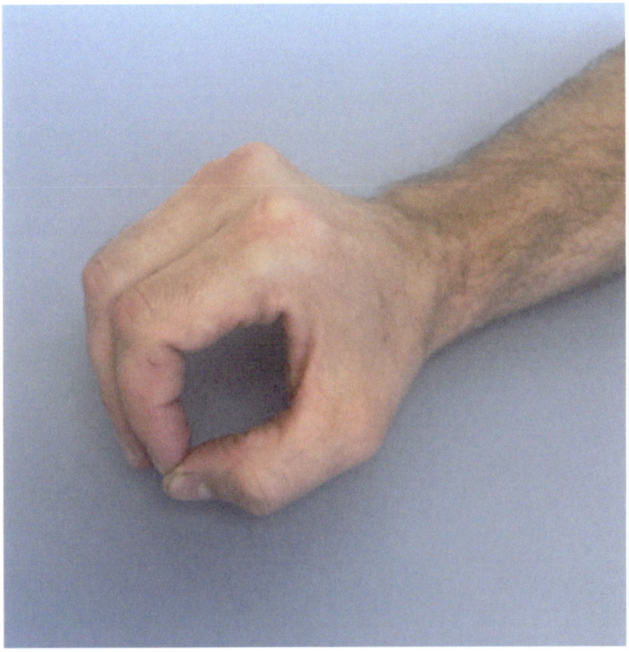

Complete 10 repetitions, every waking hour

- Once advised by your therapist, you may perform resisted thumb opposition. Bring your hand up from the table, and press your thumb into the table, away from the palm.

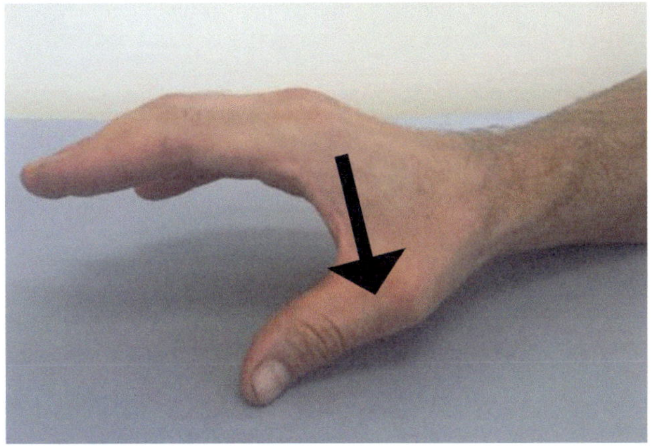

Complete 5 – 1 0 repetitions, hold for 5 seconds, 5 – 6 times per day

☐ **Active Donor + Passive Recipient Exercise**

- Touch your thumb to the tip of the index finger. Use your opposite hand to spread the index finger away from the middle finger, trying to make "pad-to-pad" contact with the thumb.

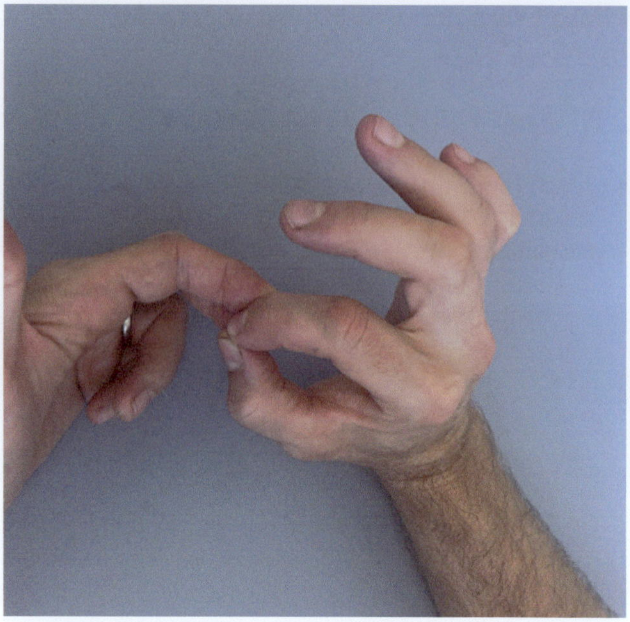

Complete 5 – 1 0 repetitions, hold for 5 seconds, 5 – 6 times per day

Phase 2 Opponens-to-FDI Nerve Transfer Exercises

☐ **Active Donor + Active-Assisted Recipient**:

- Begin seated at a table with the tip of your index finger touching the table edge. The thumb is off the table and facing the floor. Actively push your thumb down toward the floor while sliding the index finger away from the hand. Once the index finger cannot move on its own anymore, assist it further with your opposite hand. You can place a coin or Velcro tab under the finger pad to make the movement easier.

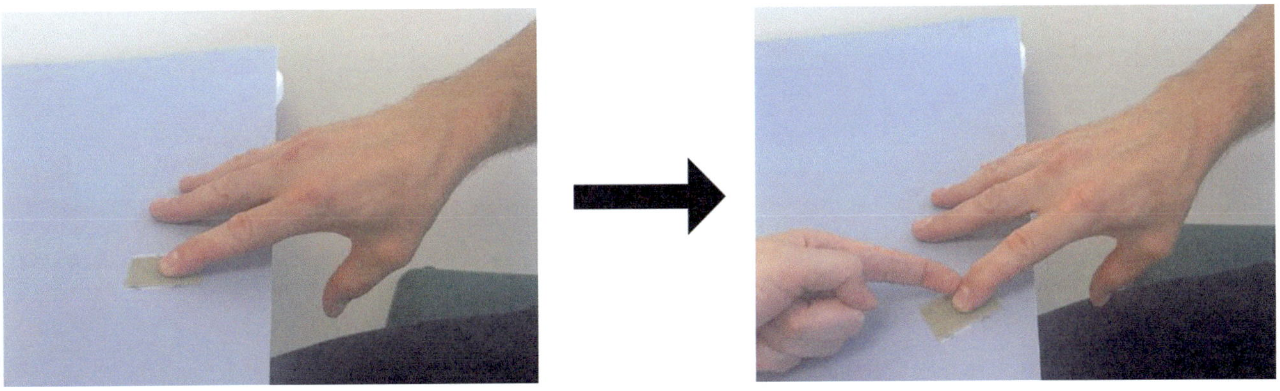

Complete 5 – 10 repetitions, hold for 5 seconds, 5 – 6 times per day

☐ **Place and Hold**

- Make an "O" shape between your thumb and index finger. Use your opposite hand to pull the index finger closer toward the thumb. Let go of the index finger, and try to keep it positioned away from the middle finger and toward the thumb.

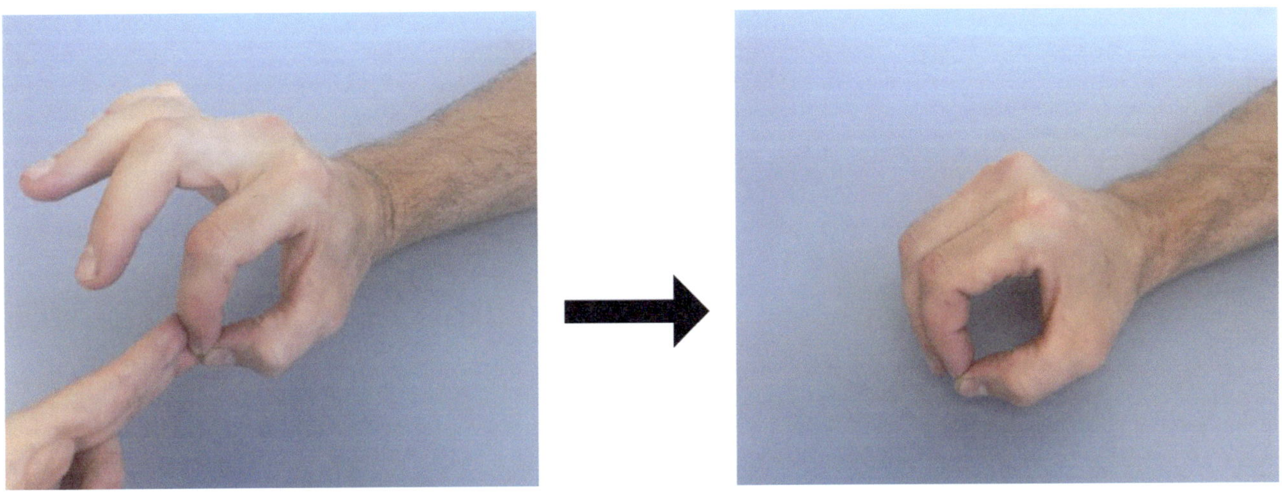

Complete 5 – 10 repetitions, hold for 5 seconds, 5 – 6 times per day

☐ **Active Donor + Active Recipient**

- Make a "C" shape between your thumb and index finger. Pretend like there is glue between your index and middle fingertips, and you are trying to unstick them.

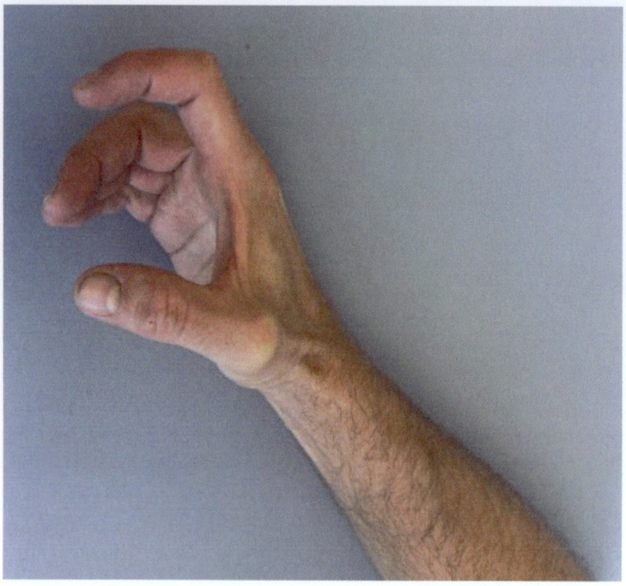

Complete <u>10</u> repetitions, <u>3</u> times per day

You may also begin pinching lightweight objects, such as coins or tweezers. Try to make pad-to-pad contact with the thumb and index finger.

Phase 3 Opponens-to-FDI Nerve Transfer

☐ **Resisted Recipient Activity with Donor Contraction**:

- Use your thumb and index finger to pinch a clip and pick up small objects. Try to maintain a "C" shape while pinching.

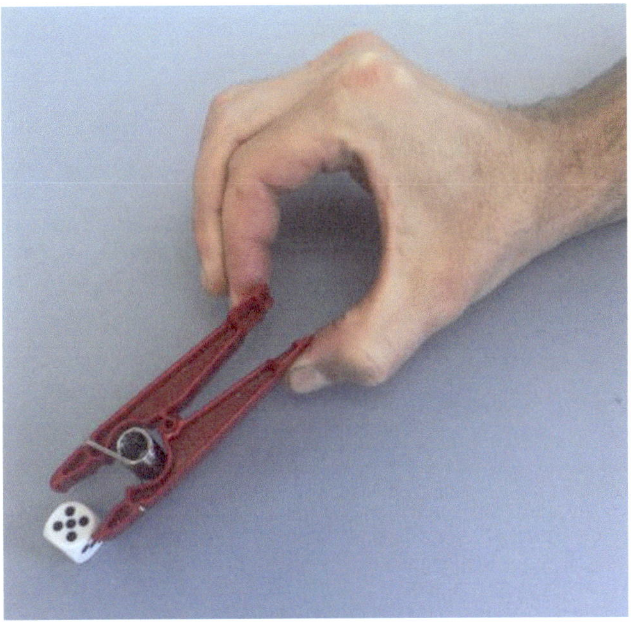

- You may also use therapy putty to pinch using your thumb and index finger.

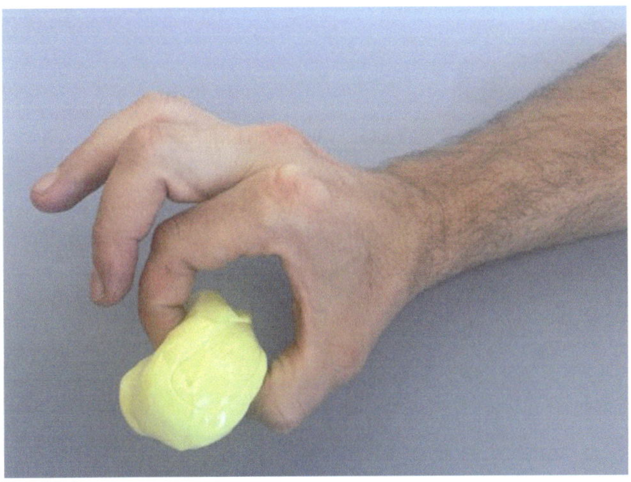

Complete 10 repetitions, 3 times per day

- Your therapist may consider applying kinesiotape to support your index finger in an abducted position (away from the middle finger and toward the thumb) while you pinch objects.

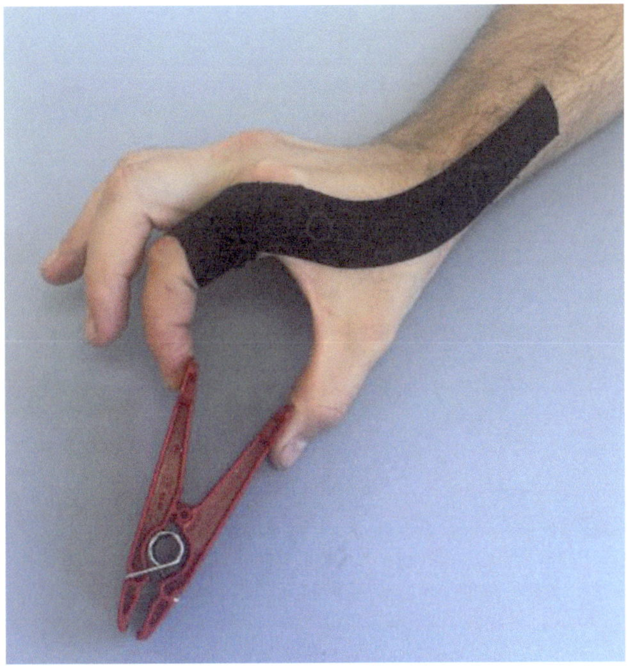

☐ **Resisted Recipient Without Donor Contraction**:

- Loop a rubber band around the base of your fingers, not including your thumb. Keep your hand completely flat on a table, and spread your fingers apart.

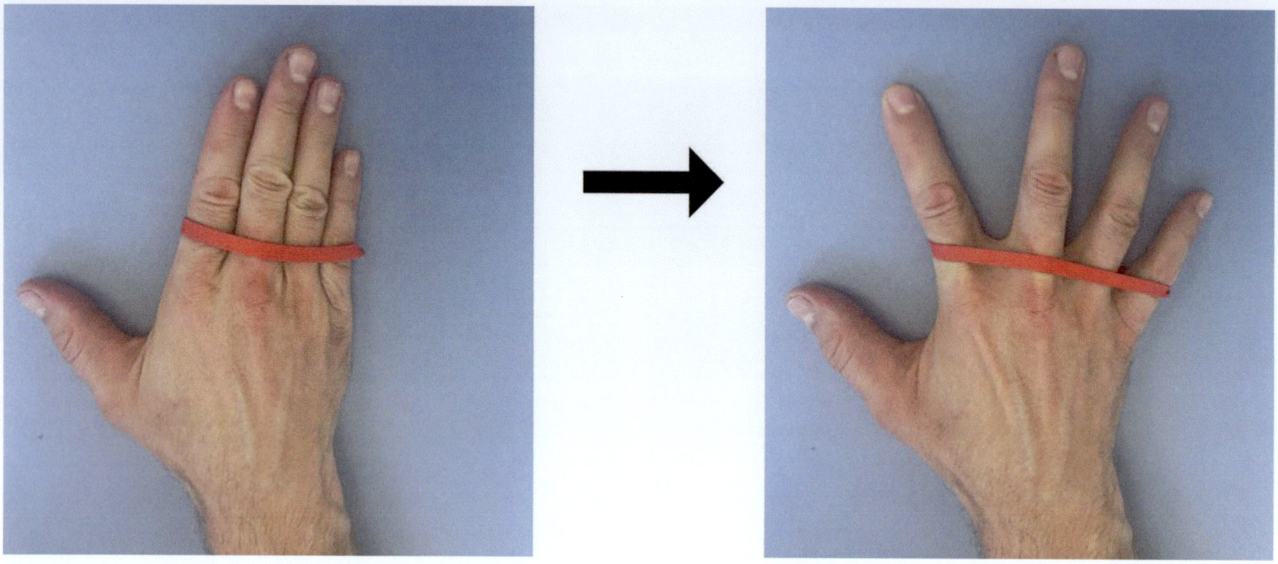

Hold for 3 s, complete 10 repetitions, 3 times per day.

References

1. Lan CY, Tien H, Lin Y, Hsu CC, Lin C, Chen SH. Prognosis of traumatic ulnar nerve injuries: a systematic review. Ann Plast Surg. 2019;82(1S):S45–52.
2. Puzovic V, Samardzic M, Jovanovic M, Zivkovic B, Savic A, Rasulic L. Etiology and mechanisms of ulnar and median forearm nerve injuries. Vojnosanit Pregl. 2015;72(11):961.
3. Bertelli JA. Prior to repair functional deficits in above- and below-elbow ulnar nerve injury. J Hand Surg. 2020;45(6):552.e1–552.e10.
4. Gaul JS Jr. Intrinsic motor recovery—a long-term study of ulnar nerve repair. J Hand Surg Am. 1982;75(5):502–8.
5. Kozin SH, Porter S, Clark P, Thoder J. The contribution of the intrinsic muscles to grip and pinch strength. J Hand Surg Am. 1999;24(1):64–72.
6. Heinzel JC, Dadun LF, Prahm C, et al. Beyond the knife—reviewing the interplay of psychosocial factors and peripheral nerve lesion. J Pers Med. 2021;11(11):1200.
7. Stonner MM, Mackinnon SE, Kaskutas V. Predictors of disability and quality of life with an upper-extremity peripheral nerve disorder. Am J Occup Ther. 2017;71(1):7101190050p1–8. https://doi.org/10.5014/ajot.2017.022988.
8. Fischer T, Nagy L, Buechler U. Restoration of pinch grip in ulnar nerve paralysis: extensor carpi radialis longus to adductor pollicis and abductor pollicis longus to first dorsal interosseus tendon transfers. J Hand Surg. 2003;28(1):28–32.
9. Bertelli J, A., Soldado F, Rodrígues-Baeza A, Ghizoni MF. Transferring the motor branch of the opponens pollicis to the terminal division of the deep branch of the ulnar nerve for pinch reconstruction. J Hand Surg. 2019;44(1):9–18.
10. Bertelli JA. Reconstructing pinch strength after ulnar nerve injury by transferring the opponens pollicis motor branch. Plast Reconstr Surg. 2023;154:10–1097.
11. Kahn L, Moore A. Donor activation focused rehabilitation approach: maximizing outcomes after nerve transfers. Hand Clin. 2016;32(2):263–77.

Index

L. C. Kahn et al. (eds.), *Rehabilitation for Nerve Transfers of the Upper Extremity*, https://doi.org/10.1007/978-3-031-92008-0

L

M

N

O

P

MIX
Papier aus verantwortungsvollen Quellen
Paper from responsible sources
FSC® C105338

If you have any concerns about our products,
you can contact us on
ProductSafety@springernature.com

In case Publisher is established outside the EU,
the EU authorized representative is:
Springer Nature Customer Service Center GmbH
Europaplatz 3, 69115 Heidelberg, Germany

Printed by Libri Plureos GmbH
in Hamburg, Germany